Issues in Nutrition for the 1980s
An Ecological Perspective

Alice L. Tobias, Ed.D., R.D.
Medical and Health Research Association
of New York City, Inc.

Patricia J. Thompson, M.S., M.Ed.
Herbert H. Lehman College of The City University of New York

Wadsworth Health Sciences Division
Monterey, California

Dedication

To our parents, Beatrice and Herbert Tobias and Elizabeth and Henry Peters,
for their unselfish love, unfailing support, and cheerful encouragement

Issues in Nutrition for the 1980s was prepared for publication by the following people:
copy editor, Ellie Connolly; interior designer, Elizabeth Rotchford; cover designer, Trisha
Hanlon; cover photographer, Grant Heilman.

Wadsworth Health Sciences Division
A Division of Wadsworth, Inc.

Library of Congress Cataloging in Publication Data
Main entry under title:
Issues in nutrition for the 1980s.

    Bibliography: p.
    Includes index.
    1. Nutrition. 2. Food. 3. Food supply. 4. Diet.
I. Tobias, Alice L., 1940–   II. Thompson,
Patricia J. [DNLM: 1. Nutrition. QU145 B311]
TX354.I84   641.1   80–15864
ISBN 0-87872-239-4

Printed in the United States of America
1   2   3   4   5   6   7   8   9 — 84   83   82   81   80

Contents

Part IV   Consumer Perspective on Food   215

Part V   Alternatives for the Future   349

Appendix Tables   485

Glossary   499

Bibliography   525

Index   534

Preface

On the threshold of the 1980s with the world's population exceeding 4.5 billion people, critical issues related to food, nutrition, and health have assumed a magnitude never before experienced by humankind. Many taken-for-granted assumptions about human populations and the food supply are undergoing reexamination and reevaluation. The general public has become increasingly alert to the linkages among energy, the environment, food, nutrition, and health. The media focus attention on the consequences of human intervention in natural systems and the subsequent effects on food and water supplies—for example, recent news stories such as the following:

— Canadian researchers link artificial food dyes with behavioral problems in children;
— Funds are allocated to develop a variety of alfalfa that would put enough nitrogen into the ground to eliminate the need for costly chemical fertilizers whose manufacture requires huge energy expenditures;
— Sale of at least 70,000 head of cattle is curbed due to use of DES;
— A major food company reassures the public that a spill of antimony trioxide onto stockpiled bags of green coffee beans caused no product damage;
— A LANDSAT spacecraft orbits the earth watching the development of planted crops everywhere;
— China's ecology is upset by a food drive that cut down forests to reclaim land for agriculture and a regional drop in annual rainfall that resulted in soil erosion and crop failure.

These and like stories reveal the complex agricultural, political, and economic problems confronting food and nutrition scientists today.

Issues in Nutrition for the 1980s places nutrition study within a conceptual framework that allows professionals and lay readers alike to identify the linkages that exist among seemingly disparate phenomena. This book views nutrition from an ecological perspective.

In the 1780s the great French scientist Antoine Lavoisier recognized the chemical basis of life. He termed life a "fonction chemique" or chemical process. A basic discovery of nutrition science has been the knowledge that the chemical breakdown of food in the body supplies the energy necessary to sustain life. Early scientists analyzed the chemical composition of food to ascertain its caloric or energy value. We now know that all energy derives from solar energy; solar energy drives and sustains the cycling of the earth's chemical elements: Carbon, oxygen, hydrogen, nitrogen, sulfur, and phosphorus are among the most important of these elements for human nutrition. The fragile web of life, the biosphere on which humankind depends for life, operates within finite limits. Chemical elements are fixed-sum resources. Therefore, the continued availability of chemical elements in nutrients depends on the elements' continuous cycling from their original reservoirs of air, earth, and water through food chains and food webs and back again.

In the 1980s the fact that nutrition goes beyond chemistry and biology is accepted. Foodstuffs come from living things, and all living things are interconnected, interrelated, and interdependent. Energy from the sun flows through our ecosystem in a series of steps from one organism to another. Survival of the human species depends on an awareness of how food and nutrition are related to these steps termed *trophic levels*. All life is related through energy flow and biogeochemical cycles. Nutrition can be viewed from this encompassing perspective.

The concept of ecology provides a means of viewing the interrelationships among organisms and their environments in their totality. A holistic pattern in which a multiplicity of causes and effects occur simultaneously begins to emerge. Parts and processes comprise aggregates called *systems*. This book reflects the ecological systems perspective on nutrition. This approach provides a comprehensive yet simplifying conceptual framework for viewing the many determinants that affect food, nutrition, and people in today's rapidly changing world. In studying food from an ecological perspective, it is useful to look at the variables that must be considered in providing the world's people with a diet adequate to promote both physical and mental health. These variables may be examined from a variety of disciplinary vantage points, including physical and life sciences, social and behavioral sciences, and arts and humanities.

The physical and life sciences (chemistry, physics, geology, and biology) provide basic concepts and information concerning the ways in which food meets the survival needs of humankind. The social and behavioral sciences (anthropology, sociology, psychology, economics, geography, and political science) provide knowledge concerning the security, ego, and affiliation needs met through food-related behaviors. Such behaviors may be observed at the personal, family, community, national, and global levels. Social scientists study the geopolitical factors that influence the production, distribution, and consumption of foodstuffs throughout the world. The arts and the humanities (history, literature, poetry, philosophy, and the sense-satisfying arts of food preparation and service) increase our appreciation of the ways in which food and nutrition uplift our spirits and contribute to meeting our higher needs for self-actualization and altruism. They extend our understanding of food from the quantitative measures related to meeting nutritional requirements to the qualitative issues concerning the ethics and aesthetics of food, nutrition, and ecology. Thus they raise our consciousness concerning the quality of life enjoyed by human beings the world over.

Although the ecological approach has been touched on by many nutrition educators and writers, it has not previously provided the focus for a basic introductory text in food and nutrition. There has long been a need for such a text that introduces the basic concepts, principles, and issues of nutrition science not only to majors but also to nonmajors who may take only one course in the subject.

The selections in this book, although they come from a variety of popular and professional sources, together should not be viewed as a "book of readings" in the conventional sense. They may be read individually for their topical interest, but they also are unified by virtue of their thematic relevance to the book's conceptual framework. Through their sequential and systematic arrangement, the selections present the basic principles of nutrition science within a comprehensive ecological perspective. Each selection is preceded by an Editors' Introduction, or concept frame, that focuses the reader's attention on the major ideas of the selection. The concept frames clarify principles and also supply the information necessary to view the material in ecological perspective. Thus the introductions provide bridging rather than interstitial material.

The text also offers suggestions through recipes and menu plans for practicing ecologically sound eating habits. The "Survival Seven" model for ecological eating is introduced and offered as a self-check chart that, combined with the model, will help the reader to make ecologically informed food choices. The model provides a basis for selecting low-fat, low-sugar diets with an adequate, but not extensive, protein intake and thus offers both the theory and praxis essential for eating lower on the food chain.

The authors' aim is to promote the concept of nutritional literacy. By this we mean the basic body of knowledge that must be shared by professionals and the general public. The nutritionally literate person can (1) understand the role of essential nutrients in the diet, (2) identify affordable sources of essential nutrients, (3) appreciate the contributions of varied cultural food patterns to a nutritionally adequate diet, (4) select a varied and sound diet that is both pleasing and nutritionally adequate, (5) evaluate nutritional claims in the media and on food products, (6) recognize that sound nutrition knowledge is based on empirical evidence and not just so-called "common sense," (7) refer to respected sources and authorities in the field for accurate, up-to-date information, (8) respond intelligently to relevant new information, (9) incorporate such information into appropriate conceptual categories, and (10) act on this knowledge. Thus, nutritional literacy promotes positive aspects of total well-being and not just the absence of nutritional deficiency.

We wish to thank our many friends and colleagues who gave their enthusiasm, support, and assistance throughout the development of this text. Although we accept full responsibility for the final product, we would like to thank those who read working outlines and drafts of the work and made constructive suggestions. Among these helpful colleagues to whom our appreciation goes are Susan J. Crockett, M.S., R.D., North Dakota State; Sara Hunt, Ph.D., R.D., Georgia State University; Tom R. Watkins, University of Delaware, Dr. Beatrice Paolucci, Michigan State University, and Mrs. Anne Knudson, Herbert H. Lehman College.

Special thanks are due to Dr. G. Tyler Miller, Jr., St. Andrews Presbyterian College, and Dr. Orrea Pye and Dr. Joan Gussow, Teachers College, Columbia University, for stimulating our interest in the relationships between nutrition and ecology. Our gratitude is extended also to Mrs. Annette Cummings of Herbert H. Lehman College who assumed the role of peacemaker when the authors' views diverged and who remained a helpful, loyal, and principled friend to both throughout a difficult time.

Alice L. Tobias
Patricia J. Thompson

Introduction

Food—how do you respond to this simple word? With a sense of anticipation for a favorite snack? A plan to prepare a pleasurable meal to share with family or friends? A concern for health, fitness, and appearance related to your diet? Awareness of food's cost in your weekly budget? Desire to contribute money and surplus foods to alleviate the deprivation of those suffering from starvation in various parts of the world? If so, you are already involved in food at many levels. Your involvement may go further as circumstances change, your knowledge increases, and opportunities arise.

Interest in food can be seen from college cafeterias to corporate dining rooms, from candlelit off-campus hangouts to elegant gourmet restaurants and family dinner tables, from farmers' markets to supermarkets and health food stores. People ask: How can I keep fit and attractive? Will my new diet really work? Why is food so expensive? How safe is the food I eat? Can we maintain a healthful environment and still produce enough food? There are no simple answers to such questions. Much myth and food faddism exist to cloud sound judgment about what people should eat. As food scientist Magnus Pyke has observed, "People must eat what they need, but in real life they choose what they like. Health will be maintained only when they like what they need." This is not an easy thing to bring about.

Food and *nutrition* are not synonymous. Food provides the human body with chemical substances called *nutrients*. Nutrition is the scientific study of the substances required for the normal functioning and optimal health of the body. It deals both with the foodstuffs consumed by human beings and the body's use of their nutrients. It focuses on the relationships of the nutrients obtained in food to health. Intricate interrelationships among nutrients affect health. Excess of some nutrients can damage health. Thus nutrition study requires knowledge based on sound facts applied to highly personal and individualized situations. Nutrition is concerned with maintaining homeostasis—that is, a balanced internal biological environment. But nutrition cannot be separated from the many external environmental determinants of food production and distribution nor from the behavior associated with the selection, preparation, and consumption of food.

Interconnected, interrelated interdependent components make up systems. A systems approach allows us to examine these interlocking parts and processes and helps us to see how a change in one part of the system affects other parts of the system. Human ecology is the study of human beings' relationships to both their internal and external environments and the processes that link each environment to the other. The term *ecology* derives from the Greek root *oikōs* 'house' combined with the root *logy* and means "the study of" or "the science of" households. Today the term *ecology* embraces the notion of the earth's natural households or ecosystems. Ecosystems are made up of all the microorganisms, plants, animals, and people involved in the process of living together. In combination ecosystems make up life-support systems—including forest ecosystems, marine ecosystems, and desert ecosystems. Because the family is also a life-support system for its members, it, too, can be regarded as an ecosystem.

This text views the study of human diets from an ecological systems perspective and from a variety of disciplinary viewpoints. It examines the problem of providing people from various geographic, cultural, and socioeconomic backgrounds with the kinds and amounts of foods necessary to assure optimum physical and mental health. Each of its five parts presents a major facet of the food-ecology problem and opens with a broad overview setting forth the major concepts to be discussed. The selections in each part were drawn from a variety of popular and professional sources. The information in each selection contributes to an understanding of food and nutrition in ecological perspective. The selections are not offered as topical readings in the conventional sense. Rather, they are organized to be synergistic so that in combination they add more to our understanding than they would individually or even than they may have done in their original context. Each selection is preceded by an Editors' Introduction, or concept frame, that bridges the selections, reinforces basic concepts, and adds information necessary for a more complete understanding of the content in an ecological perspective. Because the text emphasizes conceptual relationships, this framework is flexible enough to permit introduction of new knowledge as new ideas are disseminated and innovations introduced to the world's ecosystems on a day-to-day basis.

Part I examines food and nutrition in the broadest possible ecological perspective. It introduces the basics of nutrition science.

Part II explains the relationship between human populations and their food supply. It deals not only with problems associated with food shortages and lack of nutrients but also with the other ecological extreme—overnutrition and the health risks associated with what is now called the "affluent diet."

Part III examines the ways in which our food supply has been affected by technological change and the dangers inherent in relying too heavily on short-range technological solutions with the risk of long-range ecological damage.

Part IV deals with the complex sociocultural and economic factors that affect consumer food choices. The family itself is viewed as an ecosystem that influences the nutritional status of its members. This part includes suggestions for improving both individual and family menu planning.

Part V emphasizes the fact that ecological eating can also be healthful and economical for the average North American. It illustrates with selected recipes ways to eat less animal and more vegetable protein. It, too, emphasizes the unity of nature's systems that depend on energy flows and biogeochemical cycles to maintain their balance. It presents possible unconventional alternatives that may prove significant food sources for the future.

In one sense the nutrition-ecology argument is simple. Survival of the human species rests on this imperative: Sufficient energy, protein, and other nutrients as well as other vital necessities must be available for the perpetuation of the species. The intricate interdependencies, however, are not always obvious and have not previously been systematically developed as the basis for an introductory nutrition textbook. This book is intended to define and elucidate the dimensions of the food problem for the 1980s, and in so doing the authors hope to suggest alternatives that will help in promoting health and well-being through the adoption of food practices that maintain the health of both individuals and their families and the environment on which they depend for food.

Part I

The Man-Food Continuum

Ecology is the study of the interaction between living organisms and their environments. The physical environment includes living components (plants and animals) and nonliving components (air, water, soil, and various chemicals) together with such dynamic factors as solar energy, heat, and wind that operate upon them.

Ecology is studied in systems terms. A system is anything that is made up of interdependent parts that function as a whole. Parts of any system are uniquely related. No part of the system can be affected without all other parts being less, equally, or more affected. The system remains functional only so long as it remains dynamic and each part is perpetuated. The parts of a system are related through *inputs*, which enter the system, *throughputs*, which are processes that act upon inputs, and *outputs*, which are processed inputs that leave the system. All systems maintain themselves through *feedback*. Feedback is the unique ability of a system to allow output to reenter the system as input. Feedback helps to regulate and maintain the system.

Systems may be closed or open. In a closed system there are no inputs from outside and no outputs to the outside. An open system has the unique capacity to maintain itself despite inputs from and outputs to one or more systems outside itself. All living things—including human beings—are open systems.

The human body can be viewed as an open system. The nutrients in food are inputs to that system. Food, in the throughput phase, is acted on by physiological processes such as digestion, absorption, assimilation, circulation, and the utilization of nutrients at the cellular level. The by-products of these processes—waste materials such as carbon dioxide, water, urea, uric acid, and other nitrogenous wastes—pass out of the cell into the circulatory system where they are disposed of by either the respiratory or excretory system and become outputs. From the breakdown (metabolism) of the nutrients the body derives energy for work and other substances essential to health, maintenance, repair, and growth of the body throughout life. The body experiences feedback through such mechanisms as hunger, thirst, and satiety.

In ecology, the unit of study is the *ecosystem*—that is, the plants and animals occupying a particular environment or *habitat.* Together these constitute a *life-support system.* Human ecology emphasizes humankind's relationship with other organisms and the natural as well as the man-made environment. Human exploitation of the natural environment, the creation of man-made systems such as transportation and irrigation, and the introduction of chemicals through fertilization and pest control have interfered with natural ecosystems. These interferences have resulted in serious ecological disruptions termed *ecocatastrophe.*

Essential to an understanding of the man-food continuum is the idea that human beings are a part of nature and in fact cannot exist apart from nature. In the readings that follow, we will examine the factors that have affected our *global ecosystem*—the totality of all the ecosystems supported on our planet. We will learn why food production and consumption are among the most important aspects of this life-support system and discover the effect of the man-food continuum on human survival.

Selection 1 The Ecosphere: Our Life-Support System

G. Tyler Miller

Editors' Introduction

The two basic components of the entire universe are matter and energy. Matter is anything that has mass (i.e., has weight when subjected to gravitational forces and occupies space). The various forms of matter make up the living (biotic) and nonliving (abiotic) components of the environment. When a change in matter occurs, energy becomes available for work. Energy takes many forms, such as nuclear energy, chemical energy, electrical energy, and radiant energy. When organisms interact with other organisms and with the environment, changes take place in the different forms of energy.

Source: Adapted from *Living in the Environment: Concepts, Problems, and Alternatives,* by G. Tyler Miller, Jr. © 1975 by Wadsworth Publishing Company, Inc., Belmont, California 94002. Reprinted by permission of the publisher. Figures and complete notes and references appearing in this article are not included here; for further information consult the original version.

Energy processes are controlled by two very general physical laws that are called the *laws of thermodynamics*. Unlike man-made laws, the laws of nature cannot be repealed. The laws of thermodynamics describe the relationship between the different forms of energy. Simply stated, the first law says that energy can neither be created nor destroyed. In effect, you cannot get something for nothing. Indeed, "there is no free lunch." The second law states that whenever energy is transferred from one form to another, some usable energy is dispersed.

The ultimate source of energy is radiant energy from the sun, which is called *solar energy*. We identify solar energy in the form of sunlight. The first and second laws of thermodynamics explain the one-way flow of solar energy through the global ecosystem. The sun's energy is not destroyed as it flows through the earth's ecosystem. It is, instead, degraded from a more concentrated form of energy that is capable of driving reactions and doing work into the most diffuse kind of energy—heat. The first law states that the total amount of energy in the universe remains constant. The second law states that concentrated, usable energy must continually diminish.

Green plants that contain a substance called *chlorophyll* convert solar energy into chemical energy in the form of glucose. All food energy is chemical energy. When food enters an organism's system, energy conversions take place. There are ongoing exchanges taking place between the organism's system (internal environment) and the external environment of the global ecosystem *(ecosphere)*. These exchanges make life as we know it possible. Lower life forms break down once-living matter and return vital materials into the ecosphere. All life forms are linked through such exchanges. In the following excerpt G. Tyler Miller explains some of these fundamental processes.

What keeps all species alive on this tiny planet hurtling through space at 66,000 miles per hour? All life exists only in a thin film of air, water, and soil having an approximate thickness of only nine miles. This spherical shell of life is known as the *ecosphere*, or *biosphere*. The ecosphere concept includes every relationship that binds together all living things.

The earth can be divided into three major spherical layers—the *atmosphere* (air), the *hydrosphere* (water), and the *lithosphere* (soil). Our life-support system, the ecosphere, is a thin spherical shell within this system. It consists of three major layers: . . . (1) above us a thin layer of usable atmosphere no more than seven miles (about twelve kilometers) high; (2) around us a limited supply of water in rivers, glaciers, lakes, oceans, and underground deposits; and (3) below us a thin crust of soil, minerals, and rocks extending only a few thousand feet into the earth's interior. This incredibly intricate film of life contains all of the water, minerals, oxygen, nitrogen, carbon, phosphorus, and other chemical building blocks. Because we live in a closed system these vital chemicals must be recycled again and again for life to continue. If we liken the earth to an apple, then all life and all of the supplies necessary for maintaining life are found within the skin of the apple. Everything in this skin is interconnected and interdependent: the air helps purify the water; the water keeps plants and animals alive; and the plants keep animals alive and help renew the air. It is a remarkably effective and enduring system—and endure it must.

Solar Energy: The Source for All Life

A Nuclear Fusion Reactor

The source of the radiant energy that sustains all life on earth is the sun. The sun warms the earth and provides energy for photo-synthesis in plants, which in turn provides the food or carbon compounds that sustain all life.

The sun is a medium-sized star composed mostly of hydrogen. At its center, the sun is so hot that a pinhead of heat at this temperature could kill a man 100 miles (166 kilometers) away. Under such temperatures (and pressures) light hydrogen nuclei can be "fused" together to form heavier helium nuclei. In this process, called *nuclear fusion,* some of the mass of the nuclei is converted to energy. . . .

The sun is really a gigantic thermonuclear reactor some 93,000,000 miles (155,000,000 kilometers) away that liberates about 100,000,000,000,000,000,000,000,000 (or 10^{26}) calories* of energy per second. If we could completely harness this energy, each person on earth each second would have for his own personal use over 70,000 times the annual power consumption of the United States. The sun uses up about

* The calorie is a standard unit for heat. It is equivalent to the amount of heat needed to raise the temperature of 1 gram of water from 14.5° to 15.5°C. The calories stated for food values are actually kilocalories, often represented by using a capital C:

1 kilocalorie (kcal) = 1 Calorie = 1,000 calories

A piece of pie listed as 200 Calories is actually 200 kcal or 200,000 calories. The internationally approved unit for energy is the joule (pronounced *jool*). Calories can be easily converted to joules and vice versa:

1 calorie = 4,184 joules
1 kilojoule = 1,000 joules

4.2 million tons (4.1 billion kilograms) of its mass every second in producing this enormous amount of energy. . . .

   The solar electromagnetic spectrum. This radiant energy from the sun is traveling at a speed of 300,000 kilometers per second (186,000 miles per second) in the form of *electromagnetic waves* with a whole range of energies. At this speed the light striking your eyes made the 93-million-mile (155-million-kilometer) trip from sun to earth in about eight minutes. What we observe as sunlight and refer to as visible light is only a tiny portion of the continuous spectrum of energies given off by the sun and known as the *electromagnetic spectrum*. . . . These various forms of electromagnetic radiation differ from one another in energy and in *wavelength*, the distance between the crest of one wave and the next. The higher energy, shorter wavelength rays—gamma rays, X-rays, and most ultraviolet rays—are harmful to life. Fortunately, various chemical molecules in our present atmosphere absorb these rays and thus prevent them from reaching the surface of the earth. Without this atmospheric screening process, essentially all present forms of plant and animal life on this planet would be destroyed.
   The only portion of the solar energy spectrum used to support life is a narrow band in the visible spectrum. And this energy can be captured and used only by plants containing chlorophyll or chlorophyll-like substances. Even so, plants use 100 times more energy than that used by all man-made machines and make more efficient use of their share of the energy than any man-made machine does.

Global Energy Flow

   The first law of thermodynamics (the law of conservation of energy) requires that eventually the earth must lose energy to space at the same rate that it receives radiant energy from the sun. But although energy in must equal energy out the useful short wavelength incoming solar energy is degraded to almost useless heat energy with a longer wavelength in accordance with the second law. The earth and its atmosphere can then be viewed as a giant thermodynamic engine driven by sunlight. . . . let us look at how solar energy is used by living organisms after it enters the ecosphere.

What Is an Ecosystem?

Levels of Organization

   Looking at earth from space we see a predominately blue sphere with an irregular pattern of green, red, and white patches on its surface. As we zoom closer these colorful patches are resolved into deserts, forests, grasslands, mountains, seas, lakes, oceans, farmlands, and cities. Each subsection is different, having its own characteristic set of organisms and climatic conditions. Yet, as we shall see, all of these subsystems are interrelated. As we move in closer, we can pick out a wide variety of living organisms. Continuing the magnification process would reveal that plants and animals are made up of cells, which in turn are made up of molecules, atoms, and subatomic particles. One theme running through the universe is that matter is organized in identifiable patterns that vary in complexity from subatomic particles to galaxies. The idea that matter can be classified according to various *levels of organization* is especially useful in helping us identify and understand the function of various components of the ecosphere. . . .

Ecology and Ecosystems

Ecology, a term coined by Ernest Haeckel in 1869, is derived from two Greek words, *oikos,* meaning house or place to live, and *logos,* meaning study of. Literally then, ecology is a study of organisms in their homes. It is usually defined as the scientific study of the relationships of living organisms with each other and with their environment. One of our most prominent ecologists, Eugene P. Odum, defines it as a study of the structure and function of nature. It considers how organisms and groups of organisms are structured and how they interact with one another and with their environment. . . .

[T]he ecologist is concerned primarily with interactions between only five levels of organization of matter—organisms, populations, communities, ecosystems, and the ecosphere. A group of individual organisms (pine trees, sheep, geese) of the same kind is called a *population* (grove, herd, flock). In nature we find a number of populations of different organisms living together in a particular area. This group of plant and animal populations occupying and functioning in a given locality is called a *natural community.* Any organism, population, or community also has an environment. It consists of two major categories: the nonliving *(abiotic)* components such as solar energy, air, water, soil, heat, wind, and various essential chemicals and the living *(biotic)* components—plants and animals. If we consider the living and nonliving environment together with the population or community we have an *ecosystem* or ecological system, a term first introduced by A.G. Tansley in 1935.

Types of ecosystems. An ecosystem may be a planet, a forest, a pond, a fallen log, a garden, or a petri dish. It is any area with a boundary through which the input and output of energy and materials can be measured and related to some unifying environmental factor. The boundaries drawn around ecosystems are arbitrary and selected for convenience in studying them.

The large major aquatic ecosystems are lakes, ponds, rivers, springs, swamps, estuaries, coral reefs, seas, and oceans. On land the large major ecosystems—usually called *biomes*—are the forests, grasslands, savannas (combinations of grasslands with scattered trees or clumps of trees), chaparral (shrublands), tundra, and deserts. . . .

All of the various ecosystems on earth are connected to one another. Thus, if we group together all of the various ecosystems on the planet, we have the largest life unit, or planetary ecosystem, the *ecosphere*. The ecosphere can then be visualized as a vast graduation of diverse ecosystems all interconnected in a complex fabric of life. These connections help preserve the overall stability of an ecosystem. But disrupting or stressing an ecosystem in one place can have some complex, often unpredictable, and sometimes undesirable effect elsewhere. This ecological backlash effect has been eloquently stated by the English poet Francis Thompson: "Thou canst not stir a flower without troubling a star." The goal of ecology is to find out just how everything in the ecosphere is connected.

Ecosystem Structure

An ecosystem has two major components, nonliving and living. . . . The nonliving, or abiotic, component includes an outside energy source (usually the sun), various physical factors such as wind, and the chemicals necessary for life. The living, or biotic, portion consists of producers and consumers. Consumers are usually divided into macroconsumers (animals) and the microconsumers or decomposers (chiefly bacteria and fungi). . . .

Habitat and Niche

How would you get to know an organism in a biotic community? You would want to know where it lives and how it lives, what its occupation, function, and role in the community are, how it gets energy and necessary chemicals, and what its impact on the ecosystem is.

Ecologists call the specific place where an organism can be found its *habitat*. A habitat can be as large as an ocean or a desert or as small as a fallen log or the intestine of a termite.

An organism's profession, or total role in a biotic community, is known as its *ecological niche*. The organisms on which it feeds, the organisms that feed on it, whether it is a producer, macroconsumer, or microconsumer, the chemicals it extracts from the environment, the chemicals it returns to the environment, its energy requirements and outputs are all facts that help establish the organism's precise niche. The ecological niche then includes all of the chemical, physical, and biological factors that represent the position and function of an organism or population of organisms within the community structure.

Unrelated species in different parts of the world can occupy the same or similar ecological niches, and such species are known as *ecological equivalents.* . . . But no two species can occupy precisely the same niche in a particular community.* One will always be dominant and drive the other into local extinction through competition for food, shelter, and space.

Knowing about the niches of species in a given ecosystem can allow the ecologist to predict changes that might occur if some new factor is added — if heated water from a nuclear power plant or sewage is added to an aquatic ecosystem, for example, or if a new plant or animal species is introduced.

Ideally, no foreign species or new physical or chemical factor should be introduced into any area until a careful study of its niche indicates that its activities will not upset the existing ecosystem. In its new habitat, an organism may change its nesting or feeding habits. It may lack major predators or parasites and thus grow rapidly in population size so that it could become a pest. In practice, however, many organisms have been transported from continent to continent, some intentionally and some accidentally. Many of these have become pests or unwanted species, but a few are beneficial.

Man's ecological niche. What niche does man occupy? Most plants and animals are limited to specific habitats in the ecosphere because of their intolerance to a wide range of climatic and other environmental conditions. Some species such as flies, cockroaches, mice, and man are very adaptable and can live over much of the planet. Man's dominant position has resulted from his occupation of a new energy niche, never before occupied by any species. By learning how to use the stored solar energy of fossil fuels and more recently of atomic energy, we have ceased to depend directly on solar energy. We draw on solar energy stored millions of years ago as chemical energy in coal, oil, and natural gas.

With this energy subsidy man has been able to alter major portions of the earth's land surface. Now with man's large population and growing thirst for affluence, competition and conflict over limited energy and other resources have increased. In effect less than one-third of the world's people occupies a high energy niche, with the remaining two-

* The niches of two different populations in the same community can overlap somewhat, but not completely.

thirds in a lower energy niche. This is why the environmental crisis is basically an energy crisis. . . .

Selection 2 Ecosystem Function: What Happens in Them?

G. Tyler Miller

Editors' Introduction

Living things need energy to survive. Food is a source of energy. Green plants that convert inorganic (nonliving) substances into food for themselves are called *primary producers*. All other organisms are consumers. Animals depend on green plants to produce their food. Animals that consume only plants are called *herbivores*. They break down plants to obtain energy-rich substances that they can use. Animals that eat other animals are called *carnivores*. Humankind, like some other animal species, belongs to a special group called *omnivores*. Omnivores eat a mixed diet of plant and animal food. Each link in the chain by which food energy is transferred from one form of life to another is called a *trophic level*. Energy flows passing from one trophic level to the next (from the primary producers to other consumers) form *food chains*. Depending on the number of trophic levels food chains involve, they vary in their overall energy-use efficiency.

With each added link in the food chain, there is a decrease in the efficiency of energy transfer that is similar to the fee charged when transferring funds through a money order. The energy lost is the cost of the transfer. In terms of food energy we pay a very high cost with each transfer. Approximately 10 percent (from 5 to 30 percent) of the energy available to an organism at one trophic level can be captured by an organism on the next level. The energy costs are highest at the end of a food chain with many links. Interlocking food chains form *food webs*. An understanding of

Source: Adapted from *Living in the Environment: Concepts, Problems, and Alternatives* by G. Tyler Miller, Jr. © 1975 by Wasdworth Publishing Company, Inc., Belmont, California 94002. Reprinted by permission of the publisher. Figures and complete notes and references appearing in this article are not included here; for further information consult the original version.

these concepts, as presented by G. Tyler Miller, is basic to dealing with the ecological issues related to food.

For all practical purposes the total amount of matter on our planet is fixed. The earth is a closed system . . . with no matter entering or leaving. (The amounts of matter represented by incoming meteors and other materials from space and the spaceships and satellites we have launched are negligible.) So the chemicals necessary for life must be continuously cycled and recycled throughout the ecosphere. Vital chemicals such as carbon, oxygen, nitrogen, water, and phosphorus are recycled with the sun's energy being used to drive and sustain these *biogeochemical* cycles (*bio* for living; *geo* for water, rocks, and soil; and *chemical* for the processes involved). Note, however, that although some chemicals are cycled, energy is not; it flows in one direction through the ecosphere back into space. . . .

Thus, an ecosystem functions through the two important processes of *chemical cycling* and *energy flow.* These two processes connect the various structural parts of an ecosystem together so that life is maintained. . . . A study of ecosystem function involves an analysis of the rates and regulation of energy flow through the system and of chemical cycling within the system.

Two major processes in any ecosystem are

1. Chemical cycling
2. One-way flow of energy

. . .

Food Chains

Let us look more closely at what happens to energy as it flows through an ecosystem. Each link where energy is transferred from one organism to another is called a *trophic level,* and a particular sequence of transfers from one trophic level to another is a *food* or *energy chain.* . . .

It is convenient to distinguish between two major food chains in an ecosystem. The *grazing food chain* . . . is the familiar *plant → animal → animal* sequence. We think of this as the major food chain in a terrestrial ecosystem (such as a forest), but in most terrestrial systems more energy is transferred by the *detritus* or *decomposer food chain.* . . . In most aquatic ecosystems, however, the grazing food chain is dominant. In any ecosystem both chains are present and they are usually interconnected. . . . In addition, terrestrial and aquatic food chains can be mixed. . . .

Food Chains and the Second Law

One of the most important features of a food chain is that the transfer of energy from one trophic level to another is incomplete. In accordance with the second law of thermodynamics . . . as energy is transferred from one form to another some usable energy is lost. Most of it is degraded to heat energy that ends up in the environment. Typically, the energy actually available for use by the organism of the next trophic level is only 5 to 20 percent of the initial input.* In other words 80 to 95 percent of the energy is either stored, used for respiration, or lost as heat. All is ultimately transferred as heat to the environment. This loss of usable energy at each step in the food chain is frequently summarized in an *energy* or *food pyramid* diagram. . . . The size of each compartment is a relative measure of the usable energy available at each trophic level.

The same loss of useful energy can also be expressed as the number of organisms that can be supported per acre or other unit of area at each trophic level from a given input of solar energy. This representation becomes a *pyramid of numbers.* Both pyramids are ways of depicting the effects of the second law of thermodynamics.

Two important principles emerge from the food chain concept. First, the concept shows why all life begins with sunlight and green plants. All of our food can eventually be traced back to green plants, and the statement that "all flesh is grass" is a concise summary of the food chain concept. Second, we can see that the shorter the food chain, the more efficient it is. For example, in the typical Asian food chain *rice → man,* far less energy is wasted than in the typical Western food chains that are animal oriented such as *grain → steer → man.* Thus, the ultimate size of the human (or other population that can be supported) is related to the number of steps in the food chain. . . .

Food Webs

Although the concept of a simple food chain is very important and useful, such isolated linear food chains rarely exist in nature. Many animals feed on a number of different species, and generalists or omnivores such as man, bears, and rats can eat plants and animals at several different trophic levels. As a result, many different food chains crosslink and intertwine to form a complex system called a *food web.* . . .

* Actually the figures vary with different species. Typically, only 10 percent of the energy entering the plant population is available to herbivores as food. For warm-blooded carnivores the conversion efficiency is likely to be lower than 10 percent, while for cold-blooded predators it may be as high as 20 and in some cases 30 percent. Some sulfur bacteria have an energy transfer of only 2 percent. In any case, the efficiency of energy transfer is low and 10 percent is representative.

Selection 3 Nutrient Cycles

Clair L. Kucera

Editors' Introduction

A nutrient is a substance necessary for the normal growth, development, and reproduction of cells, tissues, organisms, and species. Plants get their nutrients from the soil. Animals obtain their nutrient supply from food. Nutrients in sufficient quantities are essential for health. Thirty to fifty nutrients have been identified. Among the most important are nitrogen (N), carbon (C), oxygen (O), hydrogen (H), phosphorus (P), and sulfur (S). Since we live in an ecosystem with fixed amounts of these elements, nutrients must continually be recycled through the life-support system of each species. This process occurs by means of *biogeochemical cycles* that involve biological organisms, their geological environment, and chemical transformations. Nutrients thus pass through one or more of these sectors of the environment: air, land, sea, and living systems. These movements of nutrients from the environment to the organism and back from the organism to the environment are called *nutrient cycles*. For life to continue, these vital elements must be recycled again and again. The force that drives these cycles is solar energy.

Green plants contain a substance called *chlorophyll*. Chlorophyll is essential for the production of carbohydrates by the process of photosynthesis. Through photosynthesis green plants convert CO_2 and H_2O to carbon, hydrogen, and oxygen compounds known as sugars. These energy-rich compounds and their derivatives are passed through the food chain from plants to herbivores and carnivores. At each step of the food chain, the organism derives energy from the carbon, hydrogen, and oxygen compounds by breaking them down through a process known as *cellular respiration*. Through this process carbon dioxide and water are recycled through the environment. Thus plant and animal life are involved in an ongoing exchange that makes life, as we know it, possible. In the following excerpt, Clair L. Kucera shows the importance of the phosphorus, nitrogen, and carbon-oxygen cycles. Each of these cycles is essential to the man-food continuum.

Source: Adapted from Kucera, Clair L.: *The Challenge of Ecology*, ed. 2, St. Louis, 1978, The C.V. Mosby Co. Reprinted by permission of the publisher and the author. Figures and tables appearing in this article have been omitted here; for further information consult the original version.

The elements essential to life are interwoven through a series of intersecting cycles. Carbon, hydrogen, oxygen, nitrogen, and sulfur move through living matter, entering and leaving their respective sinks (storage compartments) of air, water, and soil in the process. These five elements appear in various chemical forms, but all have in common a volatile or gaseous phase. Note that of the six elements that constitute 99 percent of living matter, only phosphorus is limited to soil and water by the nature of its cycling process. At one time or another in the cycle, carbon dioxide, sulfur dioxide, hydrogen sulfide, water vapor, molecular oxygen, and nitrogen are the transported agents. The other requirements of plant nutrition are restricted primarily to soil and water systems. Dust may on occasion carry nutrients aloft into the atmosphere for varying periods before they settle again on land or water surfaces. Oxygen and nitrogen are the main constituents of the atmosphere. . . . Carbon dioxide occurs as a minute percentage. . . . All other gases make up the balance. The concentration of water vapor alone may vary widely since it is affected by local climatic conditions on a day-to-day basis.

In the following pages [four] elements [are] discussed. . . .

Phosphorus

Phosphorus is the only plant nutrient utilized in relatively large quantities (a macronutrient) of which shortages in supply may well develop in the future. Although in the future other elements required for agriculture and industry may be extracted from seawater (as magnesium and sodium chloride, common table salt, are extracted now), it is unlikely that phosphorus can be obtained in this manner. Phosphorus is relatively scarce in the oceans. . . . Its average concentration is approximately one-half pound per million gallons, compared to about forty-five tons of sodium and more than eighty-five tons of chlorine. This comparison emphasizes some serious obstacles to man's modification of the landscape. On the one hand, phosphorus is essential to plant growth, and the supply may become limited. On the other hand, seawater has such high concentrations of nonessential salt (for plant growth) that it cannot be used for irrigation in arid regions where expanded crop systems are contemplated. . . .

The phosphorus cycle is relatively simple. . . . Unlike nitrogen, phosphorus has no atmospheric interface with land and water. When it is removed from the normal cyclic processes of the biosphere, the results are not easily overcome. Another factor to be considered in the conservation of phosphorus is the manner in which it is currently being used. In the United States about four-fifths of the phosphate extracted from deposits is used in fertilizers. Approximately 10 percent to 15 percent is used in the manufacture of detergents, and the remainder is used for other industrial purposes. These nonfood uses are an additional drain on phosphorus reserves and are also an important factor in the accelerating eutrophication in aquatic systems.

If phosphorus shortages develop, and no new deposits are discovered, will native ecosystems be able to maintain themselves as they have for millions of years without exhausting the supply of phosphorus? Some deficiencies certainly do exist in nature, but in general the answer lies in the characteristics intrinsic to native ecosystems. One is the "closed" nature of cycling in stable communities, which means that phosphorus and other mineral elements tend to remain within the system. They are not dispersed here as readily as they are in crop systems, which are more vulnerable to erosion and nutrient losses. Minerals gradually released through the decomposition of organic matter again become available to plants. The losses that do occur as a result of leaching are gradually made up by minerals released by weathering of the parent material. . . .

Nitrogen

Nitrogen is an inert, colorless, tasteless gas. Alone, it is incapable of supporting life, yet it is an essential component of all living organisms that is involved in the synthesis of proteins and the production of enzymes and nucleic acids. It is the main constituent of the earth's atmosphere, totaling almost four-fifths by volume. In a sense atmospheric nitrogen is a lifeless envelope on which a viable biosphere depends. Certain steps or transformations are necessary to convert nitrogen from an unavailable state to one that is usable by green plants. In nature these steps are accomplished principally through the process of nitrogen fixation that is carried out by several types of soil microorganisms. These are certain bacteria and the blue-green algae.

Among the bacteria are two important and well-known genera, Azotobacter and Clostridium. These are free-living organisms. The first occurs in aerated soils, and the second is an anaerobe found in environments devoid of oxygen. Other bacteria living in the soil are also able to fix certain quantities of atmospheric nitrogen in forms that can be used by green plants. An important group of nitrogen-fixing bacteria belong to the genus Rhizobium. In contrast to the free-living types, these bacteria live in a symbiotic association on the roots of legumes such as peas, beans, and clover. Bacterial cells can invade the fine roots of these plants, producing nodules in which nitrogen is fixed. Since plants of the legume family are found around the world, their importance in the nitrogen enrichment of a wide variety of soils is apparent. Symbiotic relationships in nitrogen fixation also occur in other plants . . . but leguminous species are the best known. Natural systems such as forests and grasslands rely to a great degree on the sustained activity of these nitrogen-fixing microorganisms in the soil. In addition to the bacteria, the blue-green algae can also fix nitrogen and are especially valuable in old fields, where soils have been worn out by poor farming practices. These organisms restore nitrogen to the soil from the atmosphere.

The nitrogen cycle includes two other significant processes, nitrification and denitrification, that involve soil microorganisms. In a sense these are two distinct and opposing processes, as nitrification increases the availability of nitrogen to plants and denitrification returns it to its original state as nitrogen gas (N_2) in the atmosphere. When plant and animal matter decay, the nitrogen locked up in complex molecules is progressively oxidized in a series of steps, each relying on a different group of soil microorganisms. Liberated ammonia is transformed by species of Nitrosomonas to nitrite salts (NO_2), which in turn are oxidized to the nitrate form (NO_3) by the genus Nitrobacter. The energy released through these oxidations can be used by the organisms in synthesizing organic energy from carbon dioxide and water. This sequence proceeds readily in well-aerated soils. Under waterlogged conditions in which the soil lacks oxygen, the process is reversed and denitrification occurs. Nitrates are converted to nitrites, releasing the oxygen required for the metabolism of organic compounds in the soil. . . .

Nitrogen in nitrate form is very soluble and readily leached from the soil. In cropping systems where heavy applications are required for high yields, these losses are considerable. . . .

In recent years nitrogen fixation by industrial methods has increased greatly, adding to the volume of transfer in the nitrogen cycle. If more nitrogen is being fixed by combined microbial and industrial activities than is being denitrified by microorganisms, accumulation obviously is occurring at particular points in the cycle. Two problems are implied. If the biosphere is indeed experiencing a gain in nitrogen, then enrichment, especially of aquatic systems, is a probable result. . . .

The second problem involves the nitrate contamination of underground water that is the source of some municipal water supplies. In the human body, nitrates are converted to nitrites, which in excess may lead to the development of deficiencies in oxygen metabolism, causing methemoglobinemia. This is the so-called blue baby condition that occurs in newborn infants. In some localities, including the San Joaquin Valley in California, nitrate poisoning is causing concern. Water in many of the valley's wells has been shown to exceed nitrate levels acceptable for human health.

The oxides of nitrogen emitted in automobile exhaust and by factories, electric power plants, and other consumers of fossil fuels are another source of pollution. The automobile contributes almost one-half of the total. Oxides of nitrogen enter the atmosphere and, in a series of complex reactions in the presence of visible light, produce photochemical oxidants, including ozone (O_3). When hydrocarbons are brought together with ozone and the nitrogen oxides, a "smog" condition develops. Nitric acid and sulfuric acid (in the presence of sulfur dioxide) are critical constituents of smog and cause human discomfort, widespread damage to crops and native vegetation, and the accelerated degeneration of rubber. Certain plant species are very sensitive to ozone. Concentrations as small as 0.05 ppm can reduce radish crop yields by one-half. Increasing amounts of nitrogen oxides are entering the atmosphere; more than 20 million tons were emitted in 1968 in the United States alone. . . .

The nitrogen cycle is dependent on several specialized groups of soil organisms. Without the benefit of their diversified activities, native ecosystems would soon experience a disruption of the nitrogen cycle. Shortages would develop where nitrogen fixers and nitrifiers were lacking, and surpluses would appear in the absence of denitrifiers. . . .

It has been shown that residual amounts of DDT remain in certain soils for 10 years or more. Even after 14 years, 50 percent of the original application may still remain. . . . Fortunately rates of application in the field are not generally detrimental to the bacteria involved in the nitrogen cycle, for the rate of disappearance maintains an equilibrium at a level within the range of tolerance of these organisms. Yet studies show that the activities of some organisms are sharply reduced when certain levels are reached. . . . Based on these data, bacteria were curtailed when DDT was present at levels above 0.01 percent by weight of dry soil. This value is equivalent to 200 pounds per acre, far in excess of most practices. However, some cotton-growing areas have averaged 100 pounds of DDT per acre over a 10-year period because of repeated applications during each growing season. The long-range effects of these sustained applications on nutrient cycles and on soil organisms in general are not yet fully determined.

Carbon [and Oxygen]

The entry of carbon into the cyclic process begins with atmospheric carbon dioxide that is reduced in photosynthesis involving hydrogen that is split from water molecules. This process initiates the dissemination of carbon-based energy through the food chains of the biosphere. . . . Carbon accounts for approximately 40 percent to 50 percent of the dry weight of all living matter.

The ratio of carbon to nitrogen (C:N) provides some interesting insights regarding trophic position and organic turnover. The C:N ratio for certain plant products may be as great as 100:1. The ratio is less in the conversion of plants to animal tissue. However, in the breakdown and humification of these materials by soil detritus animals and microorganisms, the C:N ratio always tends to become narrower because the nitrogen concentration increases, relative to total weight. The reason for this lies in the fact that at all trophic levels energy is being extracted from the system and dispersed as heat. Carbon dioxide is released to the external environment as a by-product [output] of metabolism.

When carbonaceous materials of plant origin such as oat straw or corn stalks are incorporated into the soil, the availability of nitrogen as a nutrient may be decreased for a time. This shortage occurs because the high carbon content of plant debris supplies the energy for an expanding population of microbes that release carbon dioxide in respiration but utilize nitrogen to make more cells. Until the bacteria themselves die and decompose, the nitrogen is tied up in their protoplasm and is not available for uptake by plants. . . . [Over several years of field weathering C:N ratios for plant material being decomposed change.] Although both elements are being lost, it is carbon, as a principal component of the total biomass, that is disappearing at the faster rate.

The carbon cycle is an intrinsic part of the world food picture. As greater demands are made for plant production, the interaction of carbon and the cycles of other elements such as phosphorus and nitrogen become sensitive areas of human concern. Sustained cycling processes determine the availability of nutrients throughout the biosphere. These cycling processes in turn are dependent on the turnover of plant and animal products that is accomplished by various populations of microorganisms and soil invertebrates such as earthworms and mites. Poisoning the soil environment adversely affects the ability of these key organisms to effect the turnover of carbon that leads to nutrient release. Dysfunction of the affected ecosystems may result.

Experimental evidence indicates that the decomposition processes associated with organic turnover and nutrient cycling can be modified through the application of soil chemicals. The results of one study conducted in the Soviet Union indicated that treated litter lost only one-sixth as much weight as untreated samples because the depleted populations of soil organisms were inadequate to achieve the natural breakdown of organic matter. . . . [The effects of pesticides on several groups of soil invertebrates have been studied.] Decreasing populations indicate that a majority of these organisms are seriously affected. In cases in which no direct adverse effect is registered (the effect of DDT and several other chemicals on earthworms is an example), adverse results may be manifested in secondary consumers such as birds. Since earthworms are immune to relatively high concentrations of these chemicals, they store and transfer the deleterious effects of DDT to consumers farther up in the food chain. In several soils of the cotton region where heavy applications of DDT are routine, the ratio of pesticide in the earthworm to pesticide in the soil is as high as 40:1. . . .

Selection 4 The Ecological Facts of Life

Barry Commoner

Editors' Introduction

Our global ecosystem is made up of interacting ecosystems. In it, many species of plant and animal life interact continuously with others and with the nonliving factors in the environment. Together they comprise a single whole—the global ecosystem. Natural systems are open systems because they depend on the external environment to provide inputs and to accept outputs. In an open system the amount of output produced is directly related to the amount of input received. Ecosystems and their subsystems are dynamic. Dynamic systems are always changing.

You are part of an ecosystem. Your body, too, is a system. It depends on input from the environment in the form of air, water, and food, and it depends on the environment to accept output resulting from processed air, water, and food in the form of carbon dioxide and body wastes. The amount of carbon dioxide exhaled and the amount of waste eliminated are directly related to the amount of food consumed and the amount of oxygen utilized in processing food in the body. For example, the energy available to your body for work and for growth or gain in body weight or size is directly related to the amount of food taken in.

Natural systems have a limited amount of matter. There is only a limited amount of oxygen, carbon, hydrogen, nitrogen, and other elements on the earth. These must be used over and over again. As natural systems evolved, they developed various cycles as strategies for dealing with the exchanges of matter and energy required to sustain life. Cycling is the step-by-step conversion of matter within a system until it is available for reuse in its original

Source: Adapted from Barry Commoner, "The Origin of the Ecosystem," prepared for 13th National Conference, U.S. National Commission for UNESCO, Washington, D.C., 1969. Reprinted by permission of the U.S. National Commission for UNESCO and the author.

form. Such conversions depend on the use of energy as it flows through the system.

In the following reading Barry Commoner describes the evolution and interrelationships of the physical, chemical, and biological cycles. He emphasizes that these circular, self-perpetuating processes form the grand scheme for the remarkable continuity of life.

The Origin of the Ecosystem

The global ecosystem in which we now live is the product of several billion years of evolutionary change in the composition of the planet's skin. Following a series of remarkable geochemical events, about two billion years ago there appeared a form of matter, composed of elements common on the earth's surface, but organized in a manner which set it sharply apart from its antecedents—life. Themselves the products of several billion years of slow geochemical processes, the first living things became, in turn, powerful agents of geochemical change.

To begin with, they depleted the earth's previously accumulated store of the organic products of geochemical evolution, for this was their food. Converting much of this food into carbon dioxide, the earth's early life forms sufficiently increased the carbon dioxide content of the planet's atmosphere to raise the average temperature—through the "greenhouse" effect—to tropical levels. Later there appeared the first photosynthetic organisms, which reconverted carbon dioxide into the organic substances that are essential to all living metabolism. The rapid proliferation of green plants in the tropical temperature of the early earth soon reduced the carbon dioxide concentration of the atmosphere, thereby lowering the earth's temperature and depositing a huge mass of organic carbon which became in time the store of fossil fuels. And with the photosynthetic cleavage of water, the earth for the first time acquired free oxygen in its atmosphere. By shielding the earth's surface from solar ultraviolet radiation (through the concurrent appearance of ozone), this event enabled life to emerge from the protection of an original underwater habitat. With free oxygen available new, more efficient forms of living metabolism became possible and the great evolutionary outburst of proliferating species of plants and animals began to populate the planet. Meanwhile terrestrial plants and microorganisms converted the earth's early rocks into soil and developed within it a remarkably complex ecosystem; a similar system developed in surface waters. Taken together, these ecosystems control the composition of the soil, of surface waters and the air, and consequently regulate the weather.

There is an important lesson here. In the form in which it first appeared, the earth's life system had an inherently fatal fault: The energy it required was derived from the destruction of a nonrenewable resource, the geochemical store of organic matter. The primeval life system became capable of continued existence only when, in the course of evolution, organisms appeared that converted carbon dioxide and inorganic salts to new organic matter—thus closing the loop and transforming what was a fatally linear process into a circular, self-perpetuating one. Here in its primitive form we see the grand scheme which has since been the basis of the remarkable continuity of life: the reciprocal interdependence of one life process on another.

In the course of further evolution the variety of living things proliferated; new interactions became possible, greatly enriching the network of events. Cycles were built on cycles, forming at last a vast and intricate web, replete with branches, interconnections, and alternate pathways; these are the bonds that link together the fate of all the numerous animals, plants, and microorganisms that inhabit the earth. This is the global ecosystem. It is a closed web of physical, chemical, and biological processes created by living things, maintained by living things, and through the marvelous reciprocities of biological and geochemical evolution, uniquely essential to the support of living things.

The Basic Properties of the Ecosystem

We know enough about some parts of this vast system to delineate the fundamental properties of the whole. These properties define the requirements of any activity—including human society—which is to function successfully within the ecosystem of the earth.

Because they are fundamentally circular processes and subject to numerous feedback effects, ecosystems exhibit nonlinear responses to changes in the intensity of any single factor. Consider, for example, the ecological processes which occur in surface waters, such as lakes and rivers. This is the cycle which links aquatic animals to their organic wastes; these wastes to the oxygen-requiring microorganisms that convert them into inorganic nitrate, phosphate, and carbon dioxide; the inorganic nutrients to the algae which photosynthetically reconvert them into organic substances (thereby also adding to the oxygen content of the water and so providing support for the animals and the organisms of decay); and algal organic matter to the chain of animals which feed on it, thus completing the cycle.

Since it is a cyclical system with closed feedback loops, the kinetic properties of this ecosystem are strikingly nonlinear. If the load of organic waste imposed on the system becomes too great, the demand of the bacteria of decay for oxygen may exceed the limited oxygen content of the water. When the oxygen content falls to zero, the bacteria die, the biological cycle breaks down, and organic debris accumulates. A similar nonlinearity is observed in the growth of algae. If the nutrient level of the water becomes so great as to stimulate the rapid growth of algae, the dense algal population cannot be long sustained because of the intrinsic limitations of photosynthetic efficiency. As the thickness of the algal layer in the water increases, the light required for photosynthesis that can reach the lower parts of the algal layer becomes sharply diminished, so that any strong overgrowth of algae very quickly dies back, again releasing organic debris. These are relatively simple examples of the ubiquitous propensity of ecosystems for strongly nonlinear responses, for dramatic overgrowths, and equally dramatic collapse.

Because the chemical events that occur in an ecosystem are driven by the metabolism of living things, they are subject to the special constraints of biological chemistry. One important characteristic is that the rate of chemical reactions in living cells, being determined by the catalytic action of enzymes, is subject to the considerable specificity of enzymes for their substrates. Another feature is a consequence of the long course of evolutionary selection which has been at work in living things. Living cells are capable of carrying out an enormous variety of particular chemical reactions. What is remarkable, however, is that the number of different biochemical substances which are actually synthesized in living cells is *very much smaller* than the number of substances which could, in theory, be formed—given the types of reactions which can occur. . . .

Thus, living systems have had a long opportunity to, so to speak, try out the enormous variety of biochemical reactions that *could* take place in the cell. In effect, the biochemical constituents now found in living cells represent the survivors of this evolutionary trial, presumably selected for their compatibility with the essential features of the overall system of cellular metabolism. This situation is analogous to the tendency of genes found in current organisms to be maximally advantageous—i.e., that nearly all mutations to alternative genes are lethal. Therefore in the same sense, we can expect that the entry into an ecosystem of an organic reagent not normally found in living systems is likely to have [damaging] effects on some living organisms.

The feedback characteristics of ecosystems result in amplification and intensification processes of considerable magnitude. The fact that in food chains small organisms are eaten by bigger ones and the latter by still bigger ones inevitably results in the concentration of certain environmental constituents in the bodies of the largest organisms at the top of the food chain. Smaller organisms always exhibit much higher metabolic rates than larger ones, so that the amount of their food which is oxidized relative to the amount incorporated into the body of the organism is thereby greater. Consequently, an animal at the top of the food chain depends on the consumption of an enormously greater mass of the bodies of organisms lower down in the food chain. Therefore, any nonmetabolized material present in the lower organisms of this chain will become concentrated in the body of the top one.

Because of the circularity of ecosystems and their complex branching patterns, the behavior of any given living member of the system is dependent on the behavior of many others. The specific relationships are varied: one organism may provide food for another; one organism may parasitize and kill another; two organisms may cooperate so closely in their livelihood as to become totally dependent on each other. As a result of such relationships, a change in the population of any one organism is likely to have powerful effects on other populations. Because of these numerous interconnections, a singular cause-and-effect relationship is rare. Instead a given intrusion on an ecosystem is likely to have effects which spread out in an ever-widening circle from its original source, affecting organisms and parts of the environment often very remote from the initial point of intrusion.

The stability of an ecosystem is achieved by a complex network of dynamic equilibriums, which permits alternative relationships to develop when any particular link in the network becomes inoperative. In a very simple form, this relationship is illustrated by a common farmyard practice. The farmer who wishes to maintain cats in order to control mice will provide for the cats an alternative source of food, in the form of a doorstep dish of milk. Otherwise, the cats might kill so many mice as to run out of food; they would then leave the farm in search of richer fields, if it were not for the milk on the doorstep. There is an increasing body of more sophisticated evidence to support the generalization that the stability of an ecosystem depends closely on its degree of complexity, on the fineness of the ecological web.

The cyclical processes of an ecosystem operate at an overall rate which is determined by the intricate coupling of the numerous separate events that constitute the whole. One result is that the ecosystem web has a kind of natural resonance frequency which may become evident in periodic fluctuation in a particular population of organisms—for example, seven-year locusts. Similarly, an ecosystem seems to be characterized by a specific "relaxation time"—that is, a rate at which it can successfully respond to an external intrusion by means of internal readjustment. Hence, we can expect the system to maintain its integrity only so long as external intrusions impinge on it at a rate which is compatible with the natural time constant of the cycle as a whole. Thus, an environmental change—for example, in temperature—which develops slowly may permit organisms to adapt or to evolve adaptive forms, and the system as a whole can persist. In contrast, a rapid, cataclysmic environmental change, such as that which trapped the arctic mastodons in fields of ice, can override the system's natural rate of adaptation and destroy it.

Human Intrusions on the Ecosystem

This brief summary gives us a working knowledge of the system that constitutes the environment—a system generated by the evolution of the vast variety of living things on the earth. But among these living things is man, an organism which has learned how to manipulate natural forces with intensities that go far beyond those attainable by any other living thing. For example, human beings expend in bodily energy roughly 1,000 kilowatt-hours per year. However, in a highly developed country such as the United States the actual expenditure of energy per capita is between 10,000 and 15,000 kilowatt-hours per year. This extension of the impact of human beings on the ecosphere is, of course, a consequence of technology. Prehistoric man withdrew from the atmosphere only the oxygen required for respiration but technological man consumes a far greater amount of oxygen to support fires, power plants, and chemical processes. The carbon dioxide produced by technological processes has measurably altered the carbon dioxide concentration of the atmosphere. Technology has had effects on the ecosystem which approach the magnitude of the natural processes themselves. Technology has also introduced into the environment substances wholly new to it such as synthetic pesticides, plastics, and man-made radioisotopes.

What we mean by environmental deterioration is the untoward effect of human activities, especially technology, on the quality of the environment and on the stability of the ecological processes which maintain it.

Selection 5 The ABCs of Nutrition

Medcom

Editors' Introduction

Although foods are eaten to satisfy a variety of psychological and social needs, their basic function is to provide the nutrients essential for life. The nutrients in food are needed to make the body function properly. They function in one or more of the following

Source: Medcom, Inc., "The ABCs of Nutrition," *Three Times a Day* (Englewood Cliffs, N.J.: Best Foods Corporation, 1970), pp. 12–13. Copyright, Medcom, 1970. Reprinted by permission of Medcom. Diagrams and illustrations appearing in this article have been omitted here; for further information consult the original version.

ways: as sources of energy (calories), as building materials, and as body regulators. The six classes of nutrients are: carbohydrates, proteins, fats, water, vitamins, and minerals.

Only three of these nutrient classifications (carbohydrates, proteins, and fats) yield energy for the body's use. When work must be done, energy is necessary. The body works when it carries on vital internal processes and when selected activities such as walking, running, dressing, or typing are undertaken. Proteins, some minerals, and water are present in body tissues. Therefore, these nutrients are required for building new tissues and for the repair of existing tissues. Vitamins, minerals, proteins, and water serve as body regulators and facilitate vital physical and chemical reactions within the body.

There are many complex interrelationships among the nutrients. In fact, they work together to perform vital functions. For example, while vitamins and minerals do not yield energy, they play an important role in utilizing carbohydrates, fats, and proteins as sources of energy. Vitamins, in their role as body regulators, make it possible for proteins and minerals to be used in the growth and repair of body tissues.

In addition to the nutrients, there are certain nonnutritive substances in food that are important for health but not essential for the maintenance of life. For example, fiber—the nonnutritive substance found in vegetables, fruits, and cereals—is important for facilitating elimination.

Carbohydrates, fats, and proteins occur abundantly in various foods. Vitamins and minerals are present in relatively small amounts in food. Fortunately, the body requires only minute amounts of these nutrients. Water, which we drink in its natural form, is also a major constituent of many beverages and foods. Carbohydrates, fats, and proteins can be used by the body more or less interchangeably to supply energy depending on the composition of the diet.

Proteins must be present in adequate amounts to perform the role of body builder. Fats and carbohydrates cannot be interchanged with proteins in fulfilling this function. Proteins are really protein chains. They are built up from twenty-two building blocks called *amino acids*. The process by which proteins are built up from amino acids is called *protein synthesis*. Therefore, the amino acids, rather than protein itself, are used in making and repairing tissues. The body's proteins are built up by linking one amino acid to another until a long chain of amino acids is assembled. All the different kinds of amino acids, the building blocks for a particular protein, must be available at the same time and in the correct proportion for protein synthesis to take place.

Of the twenty-two amino acids from which proteins are built, eight (nine in infants) cannot be synthesized by the body to any significant extent. Thus eight or nine essential amino acids must be supplied by the diet. Amino acids are not stored by the body. Those that are not utilized for protein synthesis are either utilized for energy or converted to fat, a potential source of energy.

No one food contains all the essential nutrients in the amounts required by the human body, but some foods are richer in certain nutrients than others. In order to obtain all the nutrients in the correct proportions to perform all the functions of the body, it is necessary to eat a varied diet. The following reading explains the functions of the nutrients in your body.

Water

. . . All the chemical reactions in your body that convert food to energy and body tissue require the presence of water. Man can live approximately two weeks without food, but not without water. About 60 percent of total body weight is water. It's divided more or less into special body compartments:

- *Cell water:* located inside the body cells;
- *Extracellular water:* located outside cells and actually bathes every body cell with a solution containing vital nutrients and oxygen;
- *Blood water:* the fluid portion of blood in which the red blood corpuscles, white blood corpuscles, and body nutrients such as fats, protein, and carbohydrates are suspended.

Just the right amount of water is kept in the body at all times — thanks to a rather remarkable brain computer called the Thirst Control Center. When the body is running low on water, you're thirsty. When there is too much water being ingested, the kidney receives a special hormonal message to start getting rid of the excess in the urine.

Elderly or ill people will sometimes develop abnormalities of thirst control; otherwise people go a lifetime without developing any problems of water metabolism.

Important terms for every budding nutritionist to know [include] *overhydration,* means too much body water, [and] *dehydration,* means too little body water.

Old health nostrums extolling "seven full glasses of water every day" are just that. Old. Nutritionists now know that healthy people need just follow the dictates of the Thirst Control Center. After that, nature takes over.

Minerals

. . . Minerals play an important role in widely differing body functions. For example, calcium and phosphorus form the sturdy crystals that give bone strength and durability. Iron is essential for blood formation and for carrying oxygen to the tissues in the hemoglobin molecule. And elements like zinc and manganese influence the action of many critical body enzymes concerned with metabolism.

Certain minerals are essential in human nutrition. In case you want to learn all 14: calcium, chlorine, cobalt, copper, fluorine, iodine, iron, magnesium, manganese, phosphorus, potassium, sodium, sulfur, zinc. Chromium, selenium, molybdenum, and other trace minerals may eventually be added to this list.

Minerals comprise about 4 to 5 percent of total body weight. You may be surprised to learn that a 150-pound man carries at least seven pounds of minerals in his body—including enough salt to fill a small salt shaker; iron for three hairpins; and enough calcium phosphate to chisel out a good-sized statuette.

Enough minerals are in the diet of any average American to keep you from worrying about a mineral lack. Some exceptions [are]: women may have a tendency toward iron depletion—especially during their childbearing years; iodine deficiency can develop in certain land-locked states unless it is supplied in drinking water or table salt; and certain special mineral supplements are sometimes prescribed by the doctor for pregnant women or chronically ill, elderly people.

Vitamins

. . . Why do we know vitamins are very important to human nutrition? Because when experimental animals—or poorly nourished humans—are maintained on a diet containing only fats, proteins, carbohydrates, minerals, and water, they get sick.

In fact, they die.

After years of nutrition research, the brilliant Polish chemist Casimir Funk found the reason: vitamin lack.

Vitamins are accessory food factors, with differing chemical structures, which are active in very minute quantities and are absolutely essential for life processes. Originally, chemist Funk extracted a white powder from rice that enabled him to cure beriberi; he thought the active chemical was an amine—hence the term "vital amine" which soon became vitamin. Actually, later research showed that Funk's magic white powder was vitamin B_1.

Vitamins have widely varying functions in the human body. To name a few:

— *Thiamine (B₁)*: plays an important role in the body processes that convert ingested sugar into energy . . . a lack causes beriberi;
— *Vitamin D:* controls the way in which the human body uses calcium for the proper formation of bones and cartilage . . . a lack causes rickets;
— *Vitamin A:* is part of visual purple, the retinal pigment that is so important for seeing objects in dim light . . . a lack causes night blindness. . . .

Vitamin supplements are sometimes prescribed for growing children, people on very strict diets or people with certain types of illnesses. But on the whole, nutritionists agree that there is no need for vitamin pills as long as you are eating a balanced diet. That's because those expensive vitamin pills are quickly excreted in the urine—simply because they're not needed!

Fats

. . . Together with proteins and carbohydrates, fats are one of the three basic foodstuffs. Fats are one of the important components of adipose tissue (translated: fat tissue) which is found just beneath body skin. But fats are also widely distributed in tissues such as brain, muscle, and bone marrow. Ounce for ounce, fat gives off more energy (9 calories/gram) when metabolized by the body than any other foodstuff—which is precisely why nutritionists refer to it as having "high food value."

Chemically fats are composed of a molecule of glycerol linked to one or more molecules of fatty acid.

Nutritionists further classify fats into three categories:

Saturated: each carbon atom is linked to two hydrogen atoms.

$$-\underset{\underset{H}{|}}{\overset{\overset{H}{|}}{C}}-\underset{\underset{H}{|}}{\overset{\overset{H}{|}}{C}}-\underset{\underset{H}{|}}{\overset{\overset{H}{|}}{C}}-\underset{\underset{H}{|}}{\overset{\overset{H}{|}}{C}}-\underset{\underset{H}{|}}{\overset{\overset{H}{|}}{C}}-$$

Monounsaturated: two adjacent carbon atoms lack a hydrogen atom each, and are linked by a double bond.

$$-\underset{\underset{H}{|}}{\overset{\overset{H}{|}}{C}}-\underset{\underset{H}{|}}{\overset{\overset{H}{|}}{C}}-\underset{\underset{H}{|}}{\overset{\overset{H}{|}}{C}}-\overset{\overset{H}{|}}{C}=\overset{\overset{H}{|}}{C}-$$

Polyunsaturated: There are two or more double bonds.

$$-\overset{\overset{H}{|}}{C}=\overset{\overset{H}{|}}{C}-\underset{\underset{H}{|}}{\overset{\overset{H}{|}}{C}}-\overset{\overset{H}{|}}{C}=\overset{\overset{H}{|}}{C}-$$

The body can form most acids from other foodstuffs, but it can't turn the trick for one of the polyunsaturates namely, linoleic acid. This is an "essential fatty acid" required for growth, reproduction, healthy skin and proper functioning of all parts of the body. It can be partially replaced by linolenic acid and is partially converted in the body to arachidonic acid.

In addition, the degree of fat saturation may be important in helping the body handle cholesterol. Saturated fats increase cholesterol concentrations in the blood. Polyunsaturated fats tend to depress blood cholesterol, and monounsaturated fats tend to have no effect at all. If the blood cholesterol level has an influence in causing heart disease — something most nutrition experts now suspect — the degree of fat saturation may be more than chemical jargon. . . .

Proteins

. . . You can picture protein molecules in terms of a long chain — where each individual link is an amino acid. For this reason, amino acids — of which there are twenty different types in the human body — are called the "building blocks" of protein. The actual chemical link from one amino acid to another in the protein chain is called a peptide bond. . . .

The body can form most of the amino acids from other foodstuffs; but it can't turn the trick for eight specific amino acids. These are called "essential amino acids" and must be present in certain minimal amounts in every diet. The basic eight: tryptophan, phenylalanine, lysine, threonine, valine, methionine, leucine, isoleucine. Tyrosine can replace part of the phenylalanine, and cystine can do some of methionine's work. In addition, infants require histidine.

Every balanced diet needs adequate protein in order to replace the body tissues which are constantly in the process of renewal. The requirements are much higher during periods of stress — such as fever, pregnancy, or chronic illness. Basically the body's need for protein is a need for the nitrogen present in the individual amino acids.

Most nutritionists agree that a daily protein intake of about one gram per kilogram of body weight (1 kilogram = 2.2 pounds) is quite adequate for a person receiving sufficient fats and carbohydrates to meet body energy requirements. For an average-sized adult, 70 to 75 grams of protein daily fills the bill. [Editors' note: Most nutritionists now agree that a daily protein intake of 0.8 grams per kilogram of body weight is sufficient for a person receiving sufficient carbohydrates and fats to meet energy requirements. This allowance is recommended for individuals consuming diets that provide most of the protein from animal sources such as milk, eggs, cheese, meat, fish, and poultry. The efficiency of protein utilization in the typical American diet is 70 to 75 percent. This means that the allowance of the average-sized woman and man of 44 and 56 grams, respectively, fits the bill.]

Carbohydrates

. . . Carbohydrates, too, are best pictured as long chains. In this case each link is a sugar molecule—like glucose or occasionally fructose—and therefore a large carbohydrate molecule (like starch) is just a string of smaller, simpler sugar building blocks. . . .

Remember! There is no nitrogen in carbohydrates—just carbon, hydrogen, and oxygen atoms.

The body derives energy from carbohydrates mainly by causing the conversion of the simple glucose molecule to carbon dioxide and water.

This chemical reaction is one of the most vital in biology—it is the single most important way in which the sugar in a candy bar or the starch in a potato is harnessed to swinging a tennis racket, walking up steps, or just having enough energy to breathe.

But sugar molecules do a lot more than just provide energy. In fact, sugars like ribose and deoxyribose are an integral part of the nucleic acid molecules that form genes. Genes control heredity, exert an important influence on all body metabolism and may play a key role in diseases like diabetes or cancer.

Selection 6 Making Nutrition Simple

Medcom

Editors' Introduction

Your body as a whole is a biological system. It contains a number of subsystems that can be studied at various levels of organization and include organs, tissues, cells (components of organs and tissues), and organelles (the minute structural components within cells). The cell is the basic unit of life—the smallest part of your

Source: Medcom, Inc., "Making Nutrition Simple," *Three Times a Day* (Englewood Cliffs, N.J.: Best Foods Corporation, 1970), pp. 6–11. Copyright, Medcom, 1970. Reprinted by permission of Medcom. Diagrams appearing in this article have been omitted here; for further information consult the original version.

body that has all the characteristics of life. Groups of similar cells acting together to perform a particular function are called tissues. There are various types of tissues: epithelial, connective, muscle, nervous, reproductive, and blood. Organs are made up of a number of tissues working together to perform a specific task. The most important organs include the brain, heart, lungs, kidneys, stomach, and the pituitary, adrenal, sex, and thyroid glands. These organs operate as parts of systems such as the digestive, circulatory, respiratory, excretory, or reproductive.

Cells, tissues, organs, and systems function reciprocally with the nourishment of the cells that make up these tissues and organs. The availability of nutrients for utilization by cells and tissues depends on interrelated processes involving many tissues and organs. These interrelationships depend on the following series of physical and chemical processes:

1. *Selection of an adequate diet*—a diet that will provide all the needed nutrients in proportions that best meet individual needs. The diet should include foods and beverages that contain the six classes of nutrients discussed in selection 5.
2. *Ingestion*—intake of food into the gastrointestinal tract.
3. *Digestion*—physical and chemical breakdown of food into simple nutrients in the form of glucose (from carbohydrates), amino acids (from proteins), and fatty acids and glycerol (from fats).
4. *Absorption*—taking in of simple nutrients by the intestine and their passage into the circulatory system.
5. *Transport*—movement of nutrients by the circulatory system to cells and tissues and transport of wastes from cells and tissues to the excretory system.
6. *Respiration*—delivery of oxygen to the blood and removal of carbon dioxide from the blood. The circulatory system is responsible for the transport of these gases.
7. *Metabolism*—chemical reactions involved in the use of nutrients within cells and tissues. Nutrients are used in one or more of the following ways: as sources of fuel energy, as body builders, or as body regulators.
8. *Excretion*—the removal of wastes, including end products of metabolism by the kidneys and skin, and materials that cannot be digested or utilized by the body through the intestines.

These processes are presented in a simplified form in the following reading.

How can you make nutrition simple? You can't, because nutrition is a highly complex biological science, often requiring a lifetime to master with expertise and demanding a bevy of scholastic disciplines.

But let's try anyway.

Basically, nutrition is intimately linked to what scientists call metabolism. And metabolism, simply, is the sum total of all the chemical and physical reactions that go on in every cellular nook and cranny of the body. Asking just how many such chemical processes are taking place in the body at a given time will only bring a whimsical smile to any nutritionist's face.

If you could define life in one word, metabolism would be a good choice. The body employs chemical metabolic "machines" to break down ingested food into the simple building blocks that eventually become bone, or muscle, or fingernails, or liver tissue. It saps the chemical energy out of food molecules and uses it as fuel—literally as sustaining fuel—to keep the body warm, to regulate the rate at which chemical reactions take place, and even to energize the processes that go into thinking. It creates the chemical protective mechanisms that kill foreign bacteria or viruses. And somehow, when these and other metabolic schemes are slightly out of kilter, people become ill—whether with a headache, the common cold, arthritis, or even cancer.

That's metabolism. You can see why scientists ally the word so closely to their definition of life. And nutrition provides the very chemicals that feed the metabolic fires.

That's nutrition. And that's why it just isn't simple.

Cell Energy

It helps to understand the complexity of the human body by first understanding the cellular basis of life. This biological theory was first announced in 1839 by two highly disciplined German scientists, Matthias Schleiden and Theodor Schwann. Their theory, still around today, is useful as a starting point in understanding nutrition: "The fundamental unit of life in all of nature's living organisms is the cell, and all the complex biological phenomena peculiar to living things are in reality the integrated expression of basic cellular phenomena."

It is impossible to summarize the limitless chemical actions and interactions that cells perform in maintaining your body. For example, cells or collections of cells digest food and absorb it into the bloodstream. Red blood cells carry life-sustaining oxygen to every region of the body. Cells of the kidney excrete potentially harmful waste products. Reproduction cells ensure perpetuation of the species.

Basically, each cell is a miniature factory provided with both a source of energy—food—and the managerial talent—chemical reactions—to direct output—energy—into efficient production.

Even though a cell is a minute drop of protoplasm which you

could easily crush between your fingertips, it is capable of breaking down the chemical bonds of fat, protein, and sugar and extracting from them the energy which can empower you to shovel snow, play a game of tennis, or dash 100 yards with a football.

. . . If a simple sugar molecule were placed in a combustion chamber, it would be broken down into smaller molecular units of carbon dioxide and water; and in addition, the cleavage of the chemical bonds present in the original sugar molecule would be associated with the release of energy for body functions. The body has many of these miniature combustion chambers constantly breaking the chemical bonds in food.

ATP—Miracle Molecule

. . . Think of ATP as a storage tank, an energy storage tank, not unlike a tank of compressed natural gas used to light a stove.

Chemically, what happens is this.

The adenosine molecule is sequentially linked to three phosphate groupings. The links between the third phosphate group and the second, and between the second phosphate group and the first, are called high-energy phosphate bonds. This simply means that to make adenosine diphosphate (ADP) from adenosine monophosphate (AMP) and to make adenosine triphosphate (ATP) from adenosine diphosphate requires a heavy input of energy; it also means when the trend is reversed—namely, ATP goes to ADP and ADP goes to AMP, large amounts of chemical energy are released.

Now watch how smart nature is.

As fatty acids, amino acids, or sugar molecules are metabolized by the body into carbon dioxide and water, the rupturing of the chemical bonds in these basic foodstuffs releases a large amount of energy. Ordinarily this energy would come off as heat. But the body isn't a boiler. It needs the energy to do other things—like walking, or breathing, or thinking—and it needs the energy at just the right time.

Enter AMP—a beautifully simple, deceptively ingenious biological innovation. The energy liberated by burning foodstuffs is used—or stored, really—hooking phosphates to adenosine by sequentially converting AMP . . . to ADP . . . to ATP. Now, energy-rich ATP can be stored in the cell. When the demand comes for energy input—presto—ATP is converted into ADP and large amounts of chemical energy are released. The kind of energy for example that permits your eyes to move across this page . . . or permits your respiratory muscles to sustain breathing . . . or permits the liver to form biliary juices . . . or the endocrine glands to manufacture delicate hormones.

Remember the relationships. Body cells break foodstuffs down into carbon dioxide, water, and energy . . . the energy is stored in ATP . . . and the ATP ultimately gives the stored foodstuff energy to support vital metabolic processes in the body.

Digestion begins the instant food is placed in the mouth. The incisor teeth rip food into smaller pieces, canines get a firm grip on the smaller morsels, and bicuspids and molars grind the mixture into a semisolid lump—the food bolus.

At the same time salivary glands provide moisture that mixes with the bolus and facilitates swallowing. There are a few weak digestive enzymes in the saliva, too, but they don't play a very significant role in starting the chemical breakdown of foodstuffs.

After swallowing, food passes down the esophagus into the stomach. Here the 35 million tiny gastric glands located in the stomach lining begin secretion of acidic gastric juice. Gastric juice contains just the right proportions of hydrochloric acid and the enzyme pepsin to initiate the process of protein digestion — namely, conversion of the large protein molecules into smaller chains of amino acids, called peptides.

Alternate contraction and relaxation of the stomach wall soon converts the semisolid bolus to a semiliquid material called chyme; over the period of an hour or so chyme is gradually propelled by rhythmic muscle contractions — called peristalsis — through the lower-most portion of the stomach into the small intestine.

As far as digestion is concerned, the small intestine is pretty much where the action is. In fact, the small intestine is the one part of the digestive tract that you just can't live without.

Anatomically, it looks somewhat like a long garden hose (20 to 25 feet long and one-half inch in diameter) and is divided into three parts: first, the *duodenum*—about 12 finger-breadths in length (in Latin, *duodeni* means 12 each) which is wrapped around the pancreas and receives both the pancreatic and bile secretions; next, the *jejunum*—which extends from the duodenum into the third segment, the *ileum*. The latter two comprise all but about one foot of the small intestine.

In the duodenum the pancreatic digestive enzymes begin to break proteins and peptides into simple amino acids . . . complex carbohydrates into simple sugars . . . and fats into glycerol and fatty acids. These are moved into the jejunum and ileum by intestinal peristalsis where— together with minerals, water, and vitamins—they pass through the delicate mucous membrane lining cells into tiny digestive tract blood capillaries that carry the basic nutritional substances to every cell and organ in the body.

Soon the small intestinal contents pass from the ileum into the colon, or large bowel, in the lower right portion of the abdomen. Again, peristalsis moves the liquid material gradually on its way—up the ascending colon, across the transverse colon in the upper portion of the abdomen, then down the descending colon on the left side, and on into the rectum. During this transit, increasing amounts of water are absorbed back into the bloodstream—which accounts for how the liquid material of the small intestine eventually becomes transformed into the solid, formed stool.

Very few important digestive processes occur in the colon and rectum. They function mainly to store the bowel contents and to permit conservation of water from the liquid intestinal material.

Summed up it comes to this. The smooth interaction of digestive enzymes . . . intestinal bacteria . . . peristalsis . . . and complex intestinal wall absorptive mechanisms permit food to be broken down—or degraded—into the basic foodstuffs of water, minerals, vitamins, fatty acids, sugar, and amino acids. After that, it's up to another aspect of metabolism—namely, synthesis—to rebuild these basic blocks into body tissue.

Using the Products of Digestion

You've already learned that the end products of digestion—fatty acids, amino acids, and sugar—can be burned for energy; the liberated energy, in turn, is stored in the magical ATP molecule.

But what about the other aspect of the story. How do the basic building blocks get reconverted into body tissue? . . . They undergo a process of building up from smaller integral parts called synthesis. In a way, an oversimplified way, it's the reverse of digestion. With the important difference that now the molecules are tailor-made for the part they play in each cell. If, for some reason, the diet is deficient in an essential amino acid or an essential fatty acid, there will be defects in the newly synthesized molecules . . . and eventually a breakdown in the metabolic machinery.

Where the Minerals Work

Minerals, besides their own metabolic tasks, are also interrelated in human physiology to supply a number of needs. Zinc, manganese, magnesium, copper, and cobalt are required for the proper operation of many key intracellular enzymes, and in some instances actually appear to be part of the enzyme molecule.

Iron is an essential part of hemoglobin which carries oxygen in the red blood cell, and is also found in myoglobin, the oxygen-binding pigment located in muscle. Calcium forms the bulk of bones and teeth, helps blood clotting, controls the excitability of the nervous system, exerts an effect on the heartbeat, and activates several enzymes. Phosphate is closely linked to calcium in bones and teeth, is a vital part of the energy-storing ATP molecule and is involved in fat and carbohydrate metabolism. Sulfur is abundant in cartilage, tissue proteins, and liver bile. Sodium and chloride, the constituents of ordinary table salt, are the chief minerals in blood plasma and extracellular fluid and are the dominant minerals controlling the distribution of body water. Potassium is the chief intracellular mineral, and proper ratio of intracellular potassium to extracellular sodium is absolutely essential for virtually every life-sustaining process taking place in the body tissue. Iodine is part of the thyroid hormone. Fluorine, beneficial in the prevention of tooth decay, is often added to dentrifices and drinking water for this purpose.

Where Vitamins Work

Vitamins can best be described as metabolic catalysts involved in many vital biochemical processes. If vitamins are present in sufficient quantity, metabolic machinery runs smoothly. If there's a vitamin deficiency, chemical reactions slow down or may come to a complete halt.

Vitamin A: Necessary for normal growth and development. Part of visual purple; important in rod vision of retina. Maintains integrity of epithelial tissue throughout the body.

Some Food Sources: Margarine, yellow vegetables, fruits, egg yolk.

Vitamin D: Helps absorption of calcium and phosphorus from intestine. Helps calcification process important in bone formation.

Some Food Sources: Irradiated milk (or with vitamin D added), fish liver oil.

Vitamin E: Helps regulate intracellular oxidation of lipids.

Some Food Sources: Vegetable oils, margarine.

Vitamin K: Needed for normal blood clotting.

Some Food Sources: Leafy green vegetables.

Vitamin C (ascorbic acid): Participates in a variety of cellular metabolic functions. Helps maintain intercellular matrix of bone, cartilage, and dentine.

Some Food Sources: Citrus fruits, berries, melons, tomatoes, green peppers, leafy green vegetables (easily destroyed by cooking).

Vitamin B₁ (thiamine): Essential for normal metabolism of carbohydrates to supply energy. Enters into almost every aspect of cellular functioning.

Some Food Sources: Lean pork, whole or enriched cereals, peanuts, legumes.

Vitamin B₂ (riboflavin): Essential part of enzyme systems involved in energy transfer.

Some Food Sources: Milk, leafy vegetables, legumes, enriched cereals.

Vitamin B₃ (niacin): Essential adjunct of enzymes involved in energy transfer and carbohydrate utilization. Can be partially replaced by the essential amino acid, tryptophan.

Some Food Sources: Lean meats, fish, poultry, milk, legumes, peanuts.

Vitamin B₆ (pyridoxine): Essential part of enzyme systems involved in protein metabolism and utilization of essential fatty acids.

Some Food Sources: Lean meats, milk, legumes.

(pantothenic acid): Part of co-enzyme A molecule, which functions in many metabolic reactions.

Some Food Sources: Lean meats, egg yolk, peanuts, potatoes.

(folic acid): Needed for the formation of red blood cells.

Some Food Sources: Leafy green vegetables, legumes, cauliflower.

Vitamin B₁₂ (cyanocobalamin): Necessary for normal red blood cell synthesis and healthy nervous system.

Some Food Sources: Lean meats, milk, fish, eggs.

(lipoic acid, biotin, inositol, PABA): Included in B-complex group of vitamins; role in human nutrition and daily requirements less well established than other members of B-complex group.

Calories and Obesity

Excess calories, for practical purposes, are the single cause of obesity. To understand how your body converts calories into fat, again think of your body as a machine. The food you eat is fuel . . . fats, proteins, and carbohydrates that are digested and then absorbed into the blood stream. In the tissues they are further broken down into small molecules which provide the units needed for rebuilding and repairing tissues used up in meeting daily energy requirements. Some days when you exercise a lot, or are sick, the extra energy you burn comes from the body fat tissues you have in reserve.

But if you eat the same amount daily, and exercise too little, the body builds a surplus of energy in the form of fat. One pound of fat is about 3,600 calories. Hence, if you eat 100 more calories a day than you are burning up, you are gaining about 10 pounds of excess weight a year. You must modify calorie intake according to the amount of energy you burn.

Selection 7 Guides for Good Eating

National Dairy Council
Alice L. Tobias

Editors' Introduction

Foods vary in their nutrient composition. Some have a high nutrient density—that is, the concentration of vitamins, minerals, and proteins is high in relation to the food's energy (caloric) value. For example, broccoli (along with other green and yellow vegetables and fruits) is rich in vitamins and minerals, yet it does not contribute excessive calories. Milk provides protein and minerals and such vitamins as vitamin A and vitamin B_2 (riboflavin). In addition, vitamin D is provided by fortified milk. Milk contributes many important nutrients in comparison to its calories. By contrast some foods are high in caloric value but contribute little in the way of other nutrients. These foods are commonly referred to as junk foods. Although soft drinks, candy bars, and other concentrated sweets are high in caloric value, they carry only insignificant amounts of vitamins, minerals, and proteins. Similarly, alcohol provides calories but none of the essential nutrients.

The availability of food alone does not insure adequate nutrition. The Ten State Survey (1968–1970), the First Health and Nutrition Examination Survey (HANES, 1971–1972), and observations by physicians, nutritionists, and nurses indicate that not all North Americans are well nourished. Vitamins C and A, iron, and calcium are among the nutrients that are most often lacking in the diets of some people in our population. Poor nutrition can also be the result of an excessive intake of nutrients. The diets of many North Americans have an excessively high caloric content.

How can you be sure you are getting all the necessary nutrients? In order to obtain all the nutrients required for good health, it is best to eat a varied diet. In 1943, the Basic 7 was used as a guide for selecting an adequate diet. In 1956, the seven-group

plan was replaced by a simpler, less detailed four-group plan
called the Basic 4, which is shown in the following section. The
Basic 4 was designed so that people with no scientific knowledge
could select an adequate diet by including certain classes of food in
their diets. These plans are compared in table 7.1.

A varied diet includes whole grain and enriched breads and
cereals; vegetables and fruits; milk and its products; legumes; and
small amounts of fish, poultry, meat, eggs; as well as a small
amount of oil and margarine. The Basic 4 is still widely followed,
however, it is not the only food plan for a nutritionally adequate
diet.

Both food plans were designed as teaching tools for people
with typical American food patterns. Because people have varying
food needs and habits, no single plan can work for everyone.
Other cultures have developed food plans to meet needs under a
variety of environmental and social conditions. These plans also
provide an adequate diet. In fact, within the United States there
are cultural and ethnic groups that do not conform to the Basic 4.
The combinations of food found in some of the diets that depart
from the standard American diet may also be regarded as following sound principles of nutrition. Rice and beans, for example, are
such a combination. As we shall learn, some food combinations
can be explored as a basis for more ecologically responsible eating
patterns.

Be aware that the recommendations for servings under the

Table 7.1 Comparison of Basic 7 and Basic 4 Food Plans

Food Group	Basic 7	Basic 4
Milk and milk products	Children, 3–4 cups Adults, 2 cups	Children, 3–4 cups Adults, 2 or more cups
Fruits and vegetables		4 servings
Green and yellow vegetables	1 serving	
Citrus fruit or raw cabbage	1 serving	
Potatoes, other vegeta- bles and fruits	2 servings	
Meat, poultry, fish, and eggs and other high- protein alternatives	1 serving 1 egg (at least 4 per week)	2 or more servings
Bread and cereal prod- ucts (enriched or whole grain)	3 servings	4 or more servings
Butter or fortified margarine	The equivalent of 2 tablespoons	(Assumed in the diet if above are met)

Basic 4 may lead to abuses such as overnutrition in terms of excessive caloric consumption and excessive consumption of animal protein. Many people misinterpret guides such as "two or more" servings of meat, fish, poultry, eggs, or high-protein alternatives to mean that if two is good, then more than two must be even better. This interpretation is not true. Excessive consumption of calories may lead to obesity. Excessive consumption of food — even nutritious food — may have adverse effects on health and negative ecological ramifications.

If you want to know more about your pattern of eating and whether your eating habits meet your needs, use the Basic 7 or Basic 4 to increase your knowledge of the nutritive value of food. In addition to providing a check on your eating habits, these guides can teach you more about nutrient sources and the role of nutrients in your body. A Self-Check on Your Diet in the following selection provides a guideline to determine if the foods you are presently selecting provide you with all the needed nutrients in the proper amounts.

A Recommended Daily Pattern*

The recommended daily pattern provides the foundation for a nutritious, healthful diet. The recommended servings from the four food groups for adults supply about 1,200 calories. Table 7.2 gives recommendations for the number and size of servings for several categories of people.

Nutrients for Health**

Nutrients are chemical substances obtained from foods during digestion. They are needed to build and maintain body cells, regulate body processes, and supply energy. About fifty nutrients, including water, are needed daily for optimum health. If one obtains the proper amount of the ten leader nutrients in the daily diet, the other forty nutrients will probably be consumed in amounts sufficient to meet body needs. One's diet should include a variety of foods because no *single* food supplies all the fifty nutrients and because many nutrients work together. When a nutrient is added or a nutritional claim is made,

* Source: "A Recommended Daily Pattern," adapted from *Guide to Good Eating. Copyright,* © 1977 National Dairy Council. All rights reserved. Reprinted by permission.

** Source: "Nutrients for Health" adapted from *Guide to Good Eating.* Copyright, © 1977 National Dairy Council. All rights reserved. Reprinted by permission.

Table 7.2 A Recommended Daily Pattern

Food Group	Recommended Number of Servings				
	Child	Teenager	Adult	Pregnant Woman	Lactating Woman
Milk	3	4	2	4	4
1 cup milk, yogurt, or calcium equivalent					
1½ slices (1½ oz) cheddar cheese*					
1 cup pudding					
1¾ cups ice cream					
2 cups cottage cheese*					
Meat	2	2	2	3	2
2 ounces cooked, lean meat, fish, poultry, or protein equivalent					
2 eggs					
2 slices (2 oz) cheddar cheese*					
½ cup cottage cheese*					
1 cup dried beans, peas					
4 tbsp peanut butter					
Fruit-vegetable	4	4	4	4	4
½ cup cooked or juice					
1 cup raw					
Portion commonly served such as a medium-sized apple or banana					
Grain (whole grain, fortified, enriched)	4	4	4	4	4
1 slice bread					
1 cup ready-to-eat cereal					
½ cup cooked cereal, pasta, grits					

* Count cheese as serving of milk or meat, not both simultaneously.

nutrition labeling regulations require listing the ten leader nutrients on food packages. These nutrients appear in table 7.3 with food sources and some major physiological functions.

A Self-Check on Your Diet*

For each food component category in table 7.4, give yourself one (1) point if you met your daily needs and ½ point if you eat only some of the amount you need. Leave a blank if you have not met this requirement.

* Source: "A Self-Check on Your Diet" developed by Alice Tobias for the Annual Food and Nutrition Fair at Herbert H. Lehman College of The City University of New York.

Table 7.3 Nutrients for Health

			Some Major Physiological Functions		
Nutrient	Important Sources of Nutrient	Energy Supplied	Build and Maintain Body Cells	Regulate Body Processes	
Protein	Meat, poultry, fish Dried beans and peas Egg Cheese Milk	Supplies 4 calories per gram	Constitutes part of the structure of every cell such as muscle, blood, and bone; supports growth and maintains healthy body cells	Constitutes part of enzymes, some hormones and body fluids, and antibodies that increase resistance to infection	
Carbohydrate	Cereal Potatoes Dried beans Corn Bread Sugar	Supplies 4 calories per gram Major source of energy for central nervous system	Supplies energy so protein can be used for growth and maintenance of body cells	Unrefined products supply fiber—complex carbohydrates in fruits, vegetables, and whole grains—for regular elimination; assists in fat utilization	
Fat	Shortening, oil Butter, margarine Salad dressing Sausages	Supplies 9 calories per gram	Constitutes part of the structure of every cell; supplies essential fatty acids	Provides and carries fat-soluble vitamins (A, D, E, and K)	
Vitamin A (retinol)	Liver Carrots Sweet potatoes Greens Butter, margarine		Assists formation and maintenance of skin and mucous membranes that line body cavities and tracts such as nasal passages and intestinal tract, thus increasing resistance to infection	Functions in visual processes and forms visual purple, thus promoting healthy eye tissues and eye adaptation in dim light	

Table 7.3 Nutrients for Health (continued)

Nutrient	Important Sources of Nutrient	Energy Supplied	Some Major Physiological Functions	
			Build and Maintain Body Cells	Regulate Body Processes
Vitamin C (ascorbic acid)	Broccoli Orange Grapefruit Papaya Mango Strawberries		Forms cementing substances such as collagen that hold body cells together, thus strengthening blood vessels, hastening healing of wounds and bones, and increasing resistance to infection	Aids utilization of iron
Thiamin (B$_1$)	Lean pork Nuts Fortified cereal products	Aids in utilization of energy		Functions as part of a coenzyme to promote the utilization of carbohydrate; promotes normal appetite; contributes to normal functioning of nervous system
Riboflavin (B$_2$)	Liver Milk Yogurt Cottage cheese	Aids in utilization of energy		Functions as part of a coenzyme in the production of energy within body cells; promotes healthy skin, eyes, and clear vision
Niacin (B$_3$)	Liver Meat, poultry, fish Peanuts Fortified cereal products	Aids in utilization of energy		Functions as part of a coenzyme in fat synthesis, tissue respiration, and utilization of carbohydrate; promotes healthy skin, nerves, and digestive tract; aids digestion and fosters normal appetite

Mineral	Food sources	Function	
Calcium	Milk, yogurt Cheese Sardines and salmon with bones Collard, kale, mustard, and turnip greens	Combines with other minerals within a protein framework to give structure and strength to bones and teeth	Assists in blood clotting; functions in normal muscle contraction and relaxation, and normal nerve transmission
Iron	Enriched farina Prune juice Liver Dried beans and peas Red meat	Aids in utilization of energy Combines with protein to form hemoglobin, the red substance in blood that carries oxygen to and carbon dioxide from the cells; prevents nutritional anemia and its accompanying fatigue; increases resistance to infection	Functions as part of enzymes involved in tissue respiration

Table 7.4 A Self-Check on Your Diet

Food Component	Function	Losses in Food Processing or Preparation	Necessary Daily Intake	Comments
Carbohydrates	To supply the energy needed for body functions and muscular exertion (Carbohydrate rich foods should be the major source of energy in your diet.)		7–8 servings or more, depending on calorie requirement, of grains, legumes, fruits, and vegetables	
Protein	For the growth, maintenance, and repair of body tissues and for the production of enzymes and hormones		2 servings of fish, poultry, meat, or 1 serving of fish, poultry, or meat and 2 servings chosen from milk, yogurt, egg, beans, or nuts; or (for vegetarians) 4 servings chosen from milk, yogurt, cheese, egg, beans, or nuts	Vegetarians must remember to complement or supplement plant proteins. The following are examples of complementary protein mixtures: grains with dried beans or wheat germ; dried beans with grains or wheat germ; nuts and seeds with dried beans, wheat germ, or grains; grains; dried beans, and nuts and seeds with milk, yogurt, cheese, or eggs.
Fat	To supply the one fatty acid you must get from food (linoleic acid); prolongs digestion time of a meal, gives a feeling of fullness after a meal	Linoleic acid is destroyed by overheating or prolonged cooking.	Oil, margarine, butter, well-marbled meat, and nuts	The essential fatty acid is found in vegetable oils and nuts.

Nutrient	Function	Stability	Food Sources	Comments
Water	To promote chemical reactions in the body (All chemical reactions take place in water.)		5–6 glasses of fluids (such as water, beverages, soups)	
Fiber	To assure the proper functioning of the digestive tract and to make the stool soft, preventing constipation	Removed from refined and highly processed foods	Fruits, vegetables, and whole grains	
Vitamin A	For growth and maintenance of the skin and the interior linings (epithelial tissues) of the mouth, eyes, ears, and the respiratory, digestive, and urinary tracts (Vitamin A is part of visual purple, a substance in the eye, which is necessary for proper night vision.)	Stable to heat at ordinary cooking temperatures	1 serving chosen from liver, dark green leafy vegetables, carrots, sweet potatoes, winter squash; or 4 servings chosen from milk, cheese, apricots, tomatoes	Excessive amounts may be toxic. A diet high in fruits and vegetables will not cause toxicity because these foods are rich in carotene, the precursor rather than the active form of vitamin A. Use of mineral oil as a laxative decreases absorption.
Vitamin D	To control the absorption of calcium and phosphorus into bones	Stable	Fish liver oil, vitamin D fortified milk	Excessive amounts may be toxic, possibly causing calcium to be deposited in various organs of the body.
Vitamin E (tocopherol)	To act as an antioxidant protecting vitamins A and C and the membranes of cells from rapid destruction	Removed by refining cereals and flour; freezer storage causes some destruction	Vegetable oils (except coconut), nuts, seeds, whole grains, green leafy vegetables, wheat germ	The requirement for vitamin E increases with increased consumption of polyunsaturated vegetable oils.

Table 7.4 A Self-Check on Your Diet (continued)

Food Component	Function	Losses in Food Processing or Preparation	Necessary Daily Intake	Comments
Vitamin K	For the formation of the factors that make blood clot	Stable under ordinary cooking conditions	Green vegetables, liver, egg yolk	Prolonged use of anticoagulants such as dicumarol can cause a deficiency. Can be manufactured in the intestine by bacteria so we are not completely dependent on dietary sources. Aspirin and certain antibiotics decrease bacterial synthesis.
Vitamin B Group				
Vitamin B₁ (thiamin)	To promote the release of energy from starches and sugars; to help maintain a healthy central nervous system	Destroyed if baking soda is added to the water when cooking vegetables; destroyed by overheating and prolonged heating	1–2 servings of wheat germ, yeast, or pork; or 4 servings chosen from whole grains, or enriched cereals, fish, and lean meat	
Vitamin B₂ (riboflavin)	For steps in the release of energy from starches and sugars	Exposure to ordinary daylight causes considerable loss (Milk in a glass bottle left standing on a doorstep in direct sunlight loses 50–70 percent of its riboflavin.)	1 serving chosen from whole grains, or enriched cereals, fish, lean meat, poultry, milk, cheese, yogurt, dried peas, or beans	
Vitamin B₃ (niacin)	To promote steps in the release of energy from starches and sugars needed for the conversion of glucose to		1–2 servings of liver, yeast, or wheat germ; or 4 servings whole grains or enriched cereals, protein foods	

Vitamin	Function	Stability / Loss	Food Sources	Remarks
Vitamin B₆ (pyridoxine)	glycogen (the body's storage form of carbohydrate) To help in the utilization of protein such as the synthesis of nonessential amino acids and in the conversion of amino acids into substances that can be used as a source of energy	Considerable loss in the refining of cereal and bread; other refined or processed foods are much lower in vitamin B₆ than the original food	2–3 servings chosen from wheat germ, meat, yeast, milk, whole grains	Substantial increase in need during pregnancy and when taking oral contraceptives
Folic acid (folacin)	For the formation and renewal of body cells; particularly important in the production of red blood cells	Considerable loss in processing and in cooking; easily destroyed when small pieces of vegetables are overcooked	1 serving of liver or green leafy vegetables	Increase in need during pregnancy and when taking oral contraceptives
Vitamin B₁₂ (cobalamin)	For the formation and renewal of body cells; particularly important in the production of red blood cells	Significant loss in processing procedures	1 serving of meat, fish, poultry, or cheese, egg, or yogurt	There is no plant source of vitamin B₁₂ so strict vegetarians must supplement their diet with vitamin B₁₂.
Pantothenic acid	For the release of energy from carbohydrates, fats, and proteins; needed for the utilization of other vitamins, especially riboflavin	Considerable loss in refining cereals and grains; unstable in heat; significant loss in canning	Most diets provide adequate amounts. The best sources are organ meats such as liver, most fish, eggs, legumes, milk, wheat germ, peanuts, poultry	
Biotin	To assist in the synthesis of fatty acids and the release of energy from carbohydrates and fats	Unstable in alkaline solution and when exposed to heat	Wheat germ, peas and beans, nuts, milk, egg yolk, whole grains	Eating large amounts of raw eggs may cause a deficiency, because egg whites have an antibiotin factor (cooking destroys this factor).

Table 7.4 A Self-Check on Your Diet (continued)

Food Component	Function	Losses in Food Processing or Preparation	Necessary Daily Daily Intake	Comments
Vitamin C (ascorbic acid)	For the synthesis of collagen, the cementing material that holds body cells together; helps keep blood vessels and capillaries strong; aids in the absorption of iron and the utilization of folic acid	Very susceptible to destruction during processing and cooking because it is so water soluble and easily oxidized	1 serving of orange, grapefruit, mango, papaya, broccoli, acerola, brussels sprouts; or 2 servings chosen from strawberries, tomatoes, melon, dark green vegetables, cauliflower, or cabbage	Excessive amounts, over 1 gram, for a prolonged period, may produce kidney stones.
Calcium	Acts in cooperation with phosphorus to build and maintain bones and teeth; plays a part in muscle contraction and relaxation and blood clotting		2–3 servings milk, yogurt; or 1 serving (2–3 ounces) hard cheese	
Phosphorus	To form and maintain bones and teeth; to facilitate all reactions involving energy		2–3 servings milk, cottage cheese, yogurt; or 1 (2–3 ounce) serving hard cheese	Many nutritionists believe that a calcium-to-phosphorus ratio of 1:1 results in the best absorption of calcium. The current ratio is 1:3. The high phosphorus content of soda pop and phosphorus-containing substances in processed food contribute to the low calcium-to-phosphorus ratio in the diet. This imbalance may

Nutrient	Function	How lost	Food sources	Comments
Iron	As a component of the hemoglobin molecule in red blood cells (Hemoglobin carries oxygen to the cells of the body.)		2–4 servings lean red meat, soy beans, whole grains, and enriched or fortified grains, dark green vegetables	be a factor in the development of bone abnormalities in middle and old age.
Magnesium	To regulate cardiac, skeletal, and nervous tissue function; to facilitate the snythesis of protein	Processing of food often results in high losses	1–2 servings of nuts, wheat germ, or shell fish; or 4 or more servings chosen from whole grains, fruits, vegetables	Alcoholics have an increased need.
Zinc	As a component of insulin; to facilitate the synthesis of protein; to promote growth and wound healing	Lost in the milling of grains; easily destroyed by heat and long storage	Meat, liver, eggs, seafood, and whole grains	The typical American diet may not provide optimal amounts of zinc.
Iodine	To make thyroxine, a hormone that regulates the rate the body uses energy	Lost in refinement	Iodized salt, kelp, saltwater fish (Content in food varies with soil content of iodine.)	

Guide to serving sizes in chart (check chart for number of servings recommended): meat, fish, chicken—3 oz.; meat, fish, chicken—3 oz.; hard cheese—3 slices; cottage cheese—¾ cup or 6 oz.; eggs—one; milk or yogurt—1 cup or 8 oz.; fruits or vegetables—½ cup; grains—1 slice bread, ½ cup cereal, or ½ cup rice, bulgar wheat, millet, etc.; wheat germ—¼ cup; yeast—2 tablespoons.

Guide to dark greens: Dark green vegetables include spinach, kale, collard greens, broccoli, beet greens, chicory, endive, Chinese cabbage, and parsley.

Guide to other nutrients: Other food components used by the body that are supplied in adequate amounts if a variety of foods listed in this chart are eaten include chloride, copper, fluoride, manganese, potassium, sulphur, sodium, and water.

SCORE:

Above 20 = Excellent (Your good nutrition should bring you good health.)

15–20 = Good (You are doing something right but should learn to select a better diet.)

10–15 = Poor (Your eating pattern falls in the danger zone.)

Below 10 = Warning (See a professional nutritionist. Your health is at stake.)

Selection 8 The Requirements of Human Nutrition

Nevin S. Scrimshaw
Vernon R. Young

Editors' Introduction

Nutrition allowances are recommendations for the amounts of nutrients that healthy individuals should consume each day. They reflect differences in need based on physiological factors such as age, sex, rate of growth, and health (including pregnancy and lactation—breast-feeding). The allowances do not take into account variations in need arising from infections, metabolic disorders, or chronic diseases. Dietary standards such as the RDA, Recommended Dietary Allowance (see the appendix), should not be confused with *individual* requirements. Such standards as RDA serve rather as broad-based goals for good nutrition. Recommended allowances for specific nutrients are based on the average requirement of healthy, representative segments of the population. A margin of safety is added above the average requirements of sampled individuals to cover the needs of most individuals in the population.* The allowance for energy is treated differently than the allowances for specific nutrients; it estimates the average need of the population. Energy intake should be adjusted by the individual to maintain desirable weight in relation to age, sex, height, and physical activity.

The unique requirements of each individual are the result of the specific interaction of many genetic and environmental factors. These factors include cultural food patterns, nutrient composition of specific foods, and individual ability to adapt to any given diet. Therefore, it is difficult to determine the exact dietary requirements for any one person.

Recommended allowances give acceptable daily nutrients and as such are meant to serve as guides in planning well-

---

* The margin of safety is generally 2 standard deviations (2 SD) above the average requirements.

Source: From Nevin S. Scrimshaw and Vernon R. Young, "The Requirements of Human Nutrition," *Scientific American* (September 1976):51–64. Copyright © 1976 by Scientific American, Inc. All rights reserved. Reprinted with permission. Charts appearing in this article are not included here; for further information consult the original version. Tables appearing in this article are included in appendix A of this text.

balanced diets for groups of people. Slight deficits or overages may balance out from day to day. However, when the intake of one or more nutrients is consistently below two-thirds of the RDA, there is a possibility of a nutritional problem. Such preliminary information about nutritional status must be confirmed by health care professionals using a variety of assessment techniques, including data based on information obtained through the diet history, clinical examination, anthropometric measurements, and laboratory and biochemical tests.

The original RDAs have undergone periodic revisions every five to six years; the latest revision was published in 1980. The RDA will be revised again in the future as more scientific information becomes available. To insure the possibility of the existence of presently unrecognized nutritional needs, the RDA should be provided from a wide variety of foods.

Nevin S. Scrimshaw and Vernon R. Young show the difficulties in establishing broadly applicable nutrient requirements in the following reading.

Human beings lack the biochemical machinery to manufacture a variety of carbon compounds required for the formation and maintenance of tissues and for the metabolic reactions that sustain life. These compounds, which all animal cells and organisms must obtain preformed from the environment, together with a number of mineral elements, are termed the essential nutrients. Over the past few million years of evolutionary time the competitive struggle to obtain them in sufficient amounts has favored the emergence and dominance of the human species and has profoundly influenced man's social and cultural ascent. At the same time man's inability to manufacture the essential nutrient compounds has exposed him to deficiency diseases that continue to threaten hundreds of millions of people in today's world.

How did the diverse nutritional requirements of animals, including man, evolve? A significant clue was provided some thirty years ago when the pioneering studies of George W. Beadle and Edward L. Tatum of Stanford University with the red mold Neurospora demonstrated that gene mutation can bring about alterations in the needs of cells and organisms for an external supply of compounds. Like all other plants, Neurospora normally requires no vitamins or amino acids for its metabolism and growth; it makes them itself. When Beadle and Tatum exposed the mold cells to X-rays, however, the resulting mutations caused a loss in the cells' ability to synthesize vitamins such as thiamine, pyridoxine and para-aminobenzoic acid and the amino acids histidine, lysine, and tryptophan.

Evolutionary biologists now believe a similar series of mutations occurred in the remote past to give rise to the nutrient-synthesizing deficiencies of animals. The earliest forms of life appear to have been simple bacteriumlike organisms that were capable of manufacturing all the compounds they needed from mineral salts, nitrogen, simple compounds of carbon and, of course, water. This ability entailed the storage of an enormous amount of genetic information, and cells that could reduce the metabolic costs of replicating and maintaining genes gained a selective advantage. With natural selection favoring mutations that eliminated the "unnecessary" enzymatic synthesis of readily available nutrients, primitive forms of life evolved and ultimately developed into animal cells.

When the first single-cell animals appeared about a billion years ago, they lacked a number of the biosynthetic pathways found in plant cells, notably the photosynthetic pathway that enables a plant to convert the energy of sunlight into the energy-rich compounds that drive the metabolism of cells. All the animal species that subsequently emerged from these ancestral beginnings had similar deficiencies, but they survived by obtaining the energy and nutrients they needed from external sources. For example, plants have retained the ability to make all the twenty amino acids found in their proteins from simple carbon and nitrogen compounds, whereas animals depend on their diet to supply about half of these amino acids.

An interesting and quite recent evolutionary development of nutritional significance is the inability of certain animals to synthesize ascorbic acid (vitamin C). I.B. Chatterjee of the University College of Science in India has estimated that some 350 million years ago the capacity for synthesizing this vitamin arose in amphibians, but that a gene mutation about 25 million years ago in a common ancestor of man and other primates led to a loss of the enzyme L-gulono oxidase, which catalyzed the terminal step in the conversion of glucose to ascorbic acid. Linus Pauling has suggested that the loss of this pathway was selectively advantageous in that it freed glucose for energy use by the body. In any case the mutation was not lethal because the missing compound was present in the food of the mutant animals. Their evolution could thus continue.

Man's need to obtain an adequate supply of essential nutrients through his diet not only is a part of his biological evolution but also has shaped his social evolution. It has been suggested that the migration of human groups to the northern regions of the earth was slowed by the limited amounts of ascorbic acid in the foods available in those areas during the long winter months. Moreover, man's dependence on an adequate supply of nutrients meant that he initially had to be a hunter and gatherer, which circumscribed his cultural development. With the domestication of the cereal grains and other plants, along with a limited number of animal species, he was able to organize a stable way of life and secure the essential nutrients without foraging over substantial areas. This freed his energies for new kinds of social, economic, and artistic activities.

At least forty-five and possibly as many as fifty dietary compounds and elements are now recognized as essential for a human being to live a full, healthy life. Plant and animal foods cannot, however, be directly utilized by the cells of human tissues. The nutrients contained in foods are released by digestion, absorbed in the intestine, and transported to the cells by the blood. As long as the overall diet supplies all the essential nutrients, the cells and tissues of the body are capable of synthesizing the many thousands of additional compounds required for life.

Since the body is dependent on a regular supply of nutrients, intricate biochemical mechanisms have evolved to regulate the availability of the nutrients to the cells so that the organism can adjust to a wide range of intakes. Those nutrients that have been acquired in excess of cellular needs are handled by catabolic pathways that bring about their breakdown. The breakdown products are then eliminated in the urine, bile, sweat, and other body secretions so that they do not accumulate and reach toxic levels.

The importance of regulating nutrient levels is dramatically illustrated in certain human diseases. In the genetic disorder known as maple-syrup-urine disease infants cannot adequately metabolize the branched-chain amino acids (leucine, isoleucine, and valine). In another genetic disorder, phenylketonuria, the enzyme for breaking down the amino acid phenylalanine is lacking. Both conditions cause a buildup of amino acids in the blood and the tissues, particularly the brain, leading to cell death and mental retardation. The management of patients with these diseases consists of special diets containing a low level of the offending nutrient.

Another example of the accumulation of nutrients to toxic levels is hemochromatosis, a severe form of liver disease usually resulting from a combination of high iron and alcohol intakes that give rise to an excessive accumulation of iron in the liver. Vitamins A, D, and K are also toxic in high concentrations. Hypervitaminosis from an excessive dietary intake of vitamin A, usually from the misguided use of high-potency vitamin pills, results in thickening of the skin, headaches, and increased susceptibility to disease.

In the other hand, if the nutrient intake is so low that it is insufficient to meet the normal needs of cells, changes occur within the cells and tissues that act to conserve the limited supply. These changes may involve a more effective absorption of nutrients from the intestine and the activation of biochemical mechanisms that enhance the retention of the nutrient once it is inside the body. If the dietary intake continues to be inadequate, these metabolic adaptations break down and deficiency disease rises above the "clinical horizon," with characteristic symptoms that can lead to disability and death.

In addition to essential nutrients the body needs a supply of energy, that is, energy-rich compounds whose energy content is measured in calories. The assessment of the quantitative requirements for calories and the essential nutrients is clearly of great practical importance in human nutrition. The task is far more difficult than is generally realized. In animal husbandry the minimum needs of the animal for individual nutrients can be judged in relation to certain productive functions, such as rapid growth in meat-producing animals, high milk yield in dairy cows, and maximum fleece production in sheep. The nutrient requirements of the human organism cannot be defined as readily because its well-being is more difficult to measure. What are the appropriate yardsticks? Maximum physical fitness and disease resistance would seem to be logical criteria for assessing the requirements for individual nutrients, but because we cannot quantify physical well-being as precisely as we can the growth of experimental animals, we must seek more objective measures.

Some nutrients or their breakdown products are excreted daily in the urine, feces and sweat and are lost through the shedding of small amounts of skin and hair. For the body to remain in metabolic equilibrium the total gain of a nutrient in food must equal the total loss. Therefore by measuring the intake required to balance the amount lost daily by the body it is possible to estimate the minimum metabolic need for a given nutrient. For example, nitrogen, a characteristic and relatively constant component of protein, is measured to determine protein needs. The metabolic-balance approach has also been followed in measuring the requirements for calcium, zinc, and magnesium, but it is not suited to nutrients that are oxidized and whose carbon is eliminated in the respired air, such as fats and vitamins. For those nutrients the requirement can be estimated by determining the minimum amount of the nutrient that prevents the onset of subclinical deficiency disease, although the technique has its methodological and ethical restrictions.

Even when the metabolic-balance method is applicable, it does not provide information on where in the body the nutrient is being retained or utilized; overall nutrient balance might be achieved with a given intake of the nutrient being examined, but this does not prove that the tissues are functioning optimally and that health will be maintained. In addition it is difficult to carry out balance studies for prolonged dietary periods; such studies call for sophisticated facilities and a team of trained workers. The need to carefully control nutrient-intake levels requires that the daily menu be monotonous. Losses in the urine and feces (and ideally in sweat, skin, and hair as well) must be assayed quantitatively, which means additional inconvenience for the subjects and technical problems for the investigators, particularly when the subjects are infants, young children, or elderly people. For these reasons metabolic-balance studies are usually of short duration: a week or less in children and two or three weeks in adults. The long-term nutritional and health significance of these brief study periods has not been critically determined, so that the adequacy of our current estimates of nutrient requirements, which have been based on short-term studies, is uncertain. This is not a satisfactory state of affairs.

In the Department of Nutrition and Food Science at the Massachusetts Institute of Technology, working with Edwina E. Murray as research nutritionist and several physician graduate students, we have been able to complete a series of long-term metabolic-balance studies with highly motivated and cooperative students. These subjects have adhered to monotonous diets and have followed strict regimens for the complete daily collection of urine and feces for periods lasting up to 100 days, a significant increase over the usual fourteen- to twenty-one-day balance period.

In one study six volunteer subjects lived on a diet providing protein at a level equal to the safe practical intake recommended by the 1973 Joint Food and Agriculture Organization–World Health Organization Expert Committee on Energy and Protein Requirements. By the end of three months metabolic measurements on these subjects indicated that there were decreases in lean body and muscle mass and/or changes in liver metabolism. These results strongly suggest that short-term metabolic balance studies are not sufficient as the sole criterion for assessing human protein requirements and that the current recommendations for dietary protein intake for large population groups are inadequate. Although our own balance studies have involved experimental diet periods significantly longer than those employed for the FAO–WHO estimates, the fact remains that the experimental subjects are few in number and are confined to privileged American males, and that the duration of the study is still limited.

For some of the essential nutrients none of these approaches has been followed, and only vague epidemiological data are available. Here we must depend mainly on data obtained in animal experiments and extrapolate the results cautiously to humans, or attempt to assess how much well-nourished groups consume and consider that as an adequate intake level.

The many difficulties faced in determining the amounts of

nutrients required by an individual are compounded by the problem of determining the variation in the requirements of that individual over a period of time, and with the variation encountered among individuals. It is easy to establish that physiological states such as growth, pregnancy, and lactation call for greater amounts of most nutrients than those needed by healthy adults for maintenance alone. It is harder to measure the subtle changes in requirements that occur in the aging adult, a problem often complicated by the cumulative effects of both acute and chronic diseases that can affect requirements for nutrients by interfering with their absorption or utilization.

Knowledge of nutrient requirements in infants and in young children is also on uncertain ground. There is a tendency for investigators to regard such individuals as little adults and, with a small allowance for their growth, to extrapolate their requirements proportionately by weight from studies of older individuals. This approach does not take into account changes in the metabolic activities of cells and in the rates of nutrient turnover with age. For body protein, studies in our laboratory demonstrate high rates of turnover in newborn infants that diminish rapidly during the early weeks and months of infancy. Thereafter the decline is less rapid, but on a whole-body basis it probably continues with the passage of time during the adult years. Although protein requirements are not determined entirely by metabolic-turnover rate, the direction of change in the requirements for total dietary protein is the same as that for body protein turnover.

There is also variation in nutrient requirements among individuals of the same age, sex, and physiological state because of the interaction of genetic and environmental factors. The important variation in nutritional requirements is the one that is due to the actual expression of genes in the individual, rather than the potential expression of genes under ideal circumstances. For example, in Japan there has been an increase in the height of adults over the past 30 years, when a progressively greater proportion of the full genetic potential was expressed as dietary and environmental conditions improved.

One problem in knowing the appropriate variation to assign to nutrient requirements in normal individuals is the lack of data on the populations of different countries. In a study at MIT we have given students a protein-free but otherwise adequate diet for twelve days in order to estimate the minimum level of nitrogen excretion, known as the obligatory loss. The statistical means of this urinary nitrogen value were significantly higher than those found subsequently for university students in Taiwan, who were studied under comparable conditions by P.-C. Huang of the National Taiwan University College of Medicine. Whether this disparity is due to genetic differences or to environmental and experimental factors is currently undetermined, but the fact of the difference appears to be indisputable. The nutritional significance of this observation is not fully known, but it emphasizes the great need for a larger number of comparative studies on nutrient metabolism and requirements in populations of differing geographic, cultural, and genetic backgrounds.

Nutrient requirements also depend on a variety of environmental factors that may be physical (for example, average ambient temperature), biological (the presence of infectious organisms and other parasites), or social (physical activity, the type of clothing worn, sanitary conditions and personal hygiene, and other patterns of behavior). Environmental factors can influence nutritional status by directly modifying dietary requirements or by their effects on the production and availability of food and on its consumption.

The major dietary factors influencing nutrient requirements are threefold. The first is that the form of a nutrient in food may have a significant effect on its degree of absorption and utilization. For example, the relatively low efficiency of the absorption of iron from vegetable foods is a major factor in the total iron intake required by human beings. Ferrous iron (reduced iron, as in ferrous sulfate or finely divided elemental iron) is more effectively absorbed than ferric iron (as in ferric chloride or iron pyrophosphate). Even ferrous iron, however, is absorbed less efficiently when it is ingested in combination with phytates and oxalates, which are found in leafy green vegetables and the whole grain, unleavened bread of North Africa and the Middle East. The iron found in meat (heme iron) is much better absorbed than iron of vegetable origin, and small amounts of red meat markedly improve overall iron absorption.

The second major factor affecting nutrient requirements is that the presence or absence of one nutrient frequently affects the utilization of another. For example, when dietary protein intake is deficient, the two proteins that play a role in the transport of vitamin A retinol-binding protein and prealbumin) are not made by the liver in adequate amounts. The esterified form of the vitamin remains stored in the liver, unavailable to the other body tissues. Signs of vitamin A deficiency may then appear, in spite of the fact that the intake of the vitamin (or of its precursor, beta-carotene, which is present in plant foods) would be sufficient if protein nutrition were adequate.

The third factor is the presence in the human large intestine of bacteria that live on organic molecules not absorbed in the small intestine. In the course of their metabolic activities these bacteria manufacture vitamins that their human host absorbs; it is a symbiotic, or mutually beneficial, relationship. Vitamin K, a deficiency of which causes failure of blood clotting, is synthesized in this way, as are small quantities of some of the B vitamins.

The factors influencing the adequacy of dietary protein for an individual may be even more complex. In the first place, the normal requirement is not for protein per se but, depending on the individual's age, for some nine or ten essential amino acids in adequate amounts and appropriate proportions. Whether an amino acid is utilized for the synthesis of new protein or is degraded for its energy content (a wasteful process) depends on a number of factors. First, each of the essential amino acids must be present simultaneously in the intracellular pool for protein synthesis to proceed. If a given amino acid is present only in a limited amount, the protein can be formed only as long as the supply of that amino acid (called the limiting amino acid) lasts. If one essential amino acid is missing from the pool, the remaining ones cannot be stored for later synthesis and will be catabolized for energy.

The level of nonprotein calories in the diet is also important. If it is high with respect to need, the ingested protein is spared from breakdown to meet energy requirements, but the individual tends to become obese. If it is low, some of the protein will be preempted to meet energy requirements and will not be available to fulfill the actual protein needs of the body. It is sometimes mistakenly believed that it is not worth improving the protein content of a diet if caloric intake is deficient. Our studies of young adults indicate that some improvement in protein retention is achieved even under circumstances of deficient energy intake. Adequate nonspecific sources of nitrogen are also needed so that the nonessential amino acids and other metabolically important nitrogenous compounds can be synthesized in the body.

Various proteins differ in their essential amino acid concentration and balance. A nutritionally "complete" protein source such as meat, eggs, or milk supplies enough of all the essential amino acids needed to meet the body's requirements for maintenance and growth. A low-quality or nutritionally "incomplete" protein such as the zein of corn, which lacks the amino acids tryptophan and lysine, cannot support either maintenance or growth. A somewhat less inferior protein such as the gliadin of wheat provides enough lysine for maintenance but not enough for growth. Plant proteins usually contain inadequate amounts of one essential amino acid or more. Lysine and threonine levels in cereals are generally low, and corn is also deficient in tryptophan. Legumes are good sources of lysine but are low in the sulfur-containing amino acids methionine and cystine; leafy green vegetables are well balanced in all the essential amino acids except methionine.

In spite of these shortcomings of individual foods it is possible to devise meals containing acceptable proportions of essential amino acids by combining proteins from several sources. In general, cereals that are deficient in lysine are complemented by legumes that are deficient in methionine. Every culture has evolved its own mixtures of complementary proteins. In the Middle East wheat bread, which lacks adequate levels of lysine, is eaten with cheese, which has a high lysine content. Mexicans eat beans and rice, Jamaicans eat rice and peas, Indians eat wheat and pulses, and Americans eat breakfast cereals with milk. This kind of supplementation, particularly in infants and growing children, only works, however, when the deficient and complementary proteins are ingested together or are ingested separately within a few hours.

Acute or chronic infections or other disease processes that cause decreased gastrointestinal function increase the need for dietary protein, because less of it will be absorbed. Trauma, anxiety, fear, and other causes of stress have an even more pronounced effect in altering protein requirements. Stress results in an increase in the catabolism of muscle protein with respect to synthesis, leading to the transport of amino acids away from muscle and peripheral tissues to the liver, where they are converted to glucose for energy purposes. This process creates a deficit in the protein content of the body, which must be compensated for by increased protein retention during the recovery period.

With any infection, even immunization with live-virus vaccines, there is a loss of appetite that leads to a decrease in food intake. The metabolic consequences of acute infections have been most extensively documented by William R. Beisel and his collaborators at the Army Medical Research Institute of Infectious Diseases. The first changes are increased synthesis of antibodies and other proteins characteristic of acute illness, followed by catabolic responses that result in increased losses of nitrogen (from body protein), vitamin A, vitamin C, iron and zinc, and probably other nutrients as well.

Disease may also directly upset the mechanisms controlling the metabolism of essential nutrients, thereby altering dietary nutrient requirements. The conversion of vitamin D into its metabolically active form, for example, depends on the activities of the liver and the kidneys. If the kidneys are diseased, the normal utilization of the vitamin is compromised. It is for this reason that many individuals suffering from kidney disease show skeletal abnormalities similar to those seen in rickets, a disease of vitamin D deficiency. When these patients are given a synthetic form of the active derivative of the vitamin, they show a marked improvement in health.

The absorption of nutrients is reduced whenever the gastrointestinal tract is significantly affected by acute or chronic infections, by a high concentration of intestinal parasites or by malaria (which interferes with the mesenteric circulation). Chronic infections and parasitic infestations are also capable of increasing nutrient requirements in other ways. Even with a diet that would otherwise be adequate iron-deficiency anemia can develop as a result of the intestinal blood loss associated with hookworm, schistosomiasis, and certain protozoal infections. In northern European countries where the eating of raw fish commonly leads to heavy infestations of fish tapeworm, vitamin B_{12} deficiency disease (anemia and neurological damage) often develops in affected individuals because the parasite has a particularly large requirement for the vitamin.

For these reasons young children in developing countries who are subject to intestinal, respiratory, and other infections that increase nutrient requirements, and who at the same time have a poor diet, are particularly likely to develop acute nutritional disease. The ideal public health approach would be to eliminate the infections rather than to provide the extra amounts of nutrients these conditions require, but that is frequently not possible because of a lack of resources or for social reasons.

All these sources of variation in nutrient requirements make it impossible to generate precise values for nutrient requirements in either individuals or population groups. Instead nutrient allowances must be viewed statistically, on the assumption that individual variation in a nutrient requirement is distributed in a bell-shaped curve above and below the mean requirement for that population group.

It is not practical to attempt to arrive at nutritional recommendations sufficient to cover 100 percent of a population, because this would require far more nutrition than is necessary for most people. There will always be a few normal individuals in a population, two or three per 100, who need more of a nutrient than can be recommended in a practical dietary allowance, and a smaller number at the extreme tail of the bell curve, two or three per 1,000, whose metabolic abnormalities significantly increase their requirements. Finally, recommended daily allowances (RDAs) are intended only to cover healthy individuals and are often not adequate for people suffering from acute or chronic diseases.

The major limitation to the practical use of RDAs is that they are based on data from small and possibly unrepresentative samples that have been extrapolated to populations of all types. In developing countries, where a large fraction of the population is likely to be suffering from disease, children have a greatly reduced weight and height for their age because of the combined effects of repeated infections and malnutrition. As a result body size of adults is also small. For them the age-specific nutritional figures derived from well-nourished populations may be unnecessarily high and estimated caloric requirements may be excessive. It is therefore preferable to calculate allowances for adults in developing countries on the basis of kilograms of body weight.

Per-kilogram allowances are not sufficient, however, for children whose growth has been stunted by malnutrition and disease. Such allowances will be too low for maximum catch-up growth and will perpetuate the existing poor nutritional state of the children. A compromise in countries where nutritional dwarfism among children is common is to estimate the specific requirements of children on a per kilogram basis and add a modest extra allowance for catch-up growth.

When acute infections are prevalent in a population, extra allowance must be made for the individual during recovery, although because of reduced food intake during the acute phase of the illness and increased retention of some nutrients in depleted individuals, the overall food requirements of the group suffering from infections may be little affected. Increased dietary allowances may nonetheless be needed to compensate for continuing high nutrient losses or for the impaired absorption associated with intestinal-parasite load and chronic disease.

In sum, recommended allowances cannot serve as an absolute indicator of the adequacy of a given intake for a given individual. They can justifiably be applied only to a reasonably healthy population. In spite of their limitations, however, estimates of caloric requirements and recommended allowances for essential nutrients must be supplied. They guide the design of diets for individuals, the evaluation of the relative adequacy of diets for populations, the content of nutrition-education programs, and the planning by government of nutrition-intervention programs.

There is no area of human health in which research is more urgently needed than the nutritional requirements of representative human populations over the full range of both health and disease. Clearly an adequate knowledge of the amount and kinds of food required by man is essential for food and nutrition policy planning and will be of major importance for the generations ahead.

Part II

Population Pressures
and the Food Supply

In the previous selections we established that the world's peoples live in an ecosystem of fixed-sum resources. For all populations other than humankind, numbers increase when the food supply is plentiful. Among human groups, when there are too many mouths to feed, the population is reduced to the life-supporting capacity of the habitat. In this way, natural forces act to maintain equilibrium. In modern times, technological advances have upset this balance.

In recent times, the human population has been increasing with great rapidity. Each new mouth to feed on the planet makes new demands on available resources. Now, as in the past, two major environmental factors have influenced population growth. One is the availability of food and other means of subsistence; the other is what Thomas Malthus (1766–1834), the British economist and pioneer in population studies, called "natural restraints." By this term he meant such things as disease, famine, war, crime, and natural disasters. Overpopulation means more people than the environment can support. Disease, famine, war, crime, and natural disasters occur to limit and reduce population density to a number that the environment is capable of supporting. In modern terms we would say that the global ecosystem is overstressed and that these "natural restraints" act to restore equilibrium.

Human population growth throughout most of history has undergone a slow, gradual increase. Three major technological breakthroughs have influenced population growth. These are the tool-using revolution, the agricultural revolution, and the scientific-industrial revolution. Each of these revolutions was followed by a surge in human population that lasted for several centuries. The first two lasted a few centuries and were followed by a period of equilibrium.

The scientific-industrial revolution began in 1650 and still continues. Since the beginning of the industrial revolution, there has been a population explosion of unparalleled magnitude. Medical advances and public health measures have reduced infant mortality, and life expectancy is more than seventy years in some countries and on a world average is between forty and fifty years. If this rate of growth continues, the population will increase tenfold within 230 years. The limited amount of arable land, fresh water, fuel, capital, and other renewable and nonrenewable resources, combined with increased pollution that destoys potentially useful resources, will set limits on the world's means of subsistence. Perhaps an increase in efficiency of food production to tenfold or even twentyfold can be achieved but not without a substantial reduction in the standard of living to which the industrialized nations have become accustomed.

What will happen in the not-so-distant future, if the population continues to double at shorter and shorter intervals? At present, there are no more frontiers. We live in a world of fixed-sum resources, and there is no place to turn to seek more. At this writing, space exploration is a distant, but not too realistic, immediate possibility for the human population. We must seek solutions on our home planet. We must face the fact that, unlike the pioneers and immigrants who settled a new world, there is no more unexplored territory to offer land and unexploited resources that will support an expanding population.

Will humankind recognize this problem and voluntarily limit population growth, or must we wait for Malthusian restraints to reduce our numbers back to a population density that the environment can reasonably support? Georg Borgstrom, a world authority on the food problem, has coined terms referring to the *Hungry World* (HW) versus the *Satisfied World* (SW). This polarization is the basis of many economic and political problems in the world today.

In the Hungry World the pressure of population growth is now being felt. However, it is not a problem that the Satisfied World can continue to ignore if the developed nations wish to maintain their present standard of living. An objective examination of the facts suggests that we may have to reexamine our present standard of living that relies on energy-intensive (hard) technology. We may have to consider a return to a labor-intensive (soft) technology that takes advantage of the human-energy resources inherent in human populations.

In the selections that follow, we will examine the fundamental problem of population pressures and their relation to the food supply. As we shall see, the ratio of population to food is a pivotal issue for maintaining equilibrium in our global ecosystem.

Selection 9 The Population Explosion and the Food Supply

Donella H. Meadows et al. for the Club of Rome

Editors' Introduction

The number of people in the population is constantly changing. We gain new individuals by birth and lose members by death. Population growth occurs when the number of births exceeds the number of deaths in a given period.

The global population has grown at an increasingly rapid rate in recent times. This accelerated growth has been referred to as the *population explosion* and has frequently been pointed to as a major factor in the increased global demand for food. Consider the following statistics. In 1650 the world population numbered about 0.5 billion and was growing at the rate of 0.3 percent annually. It, therefore, took 250 years for the population to double. In more recent times, population has been growing at the rate of 2 percent annually. In March 1980, the world population had reached 4.5 billion. At this rate of growth it will double in approximately thirty-five years.

It took more than a million years for the world's population to reach a billion. The second billion was added in 120 years, the third in 32 years, and the fourth in 15 years. Can such growth continue indefinitely? The Club of Rome, an international research team composed of scientists, educators, humanists, industrialists, and national and international civil servants, indicates that it cannot. How did this research team arrive at this conclusion? They studied human ecology and isolated five major interrelated human activities that they believed would, in the long run, affect the limits of population and technological growth. They built these into a world model. The factors included were:

— *Human population*—the number of people;
— *Industrial output*—the amount of goods and services produced per capita per year;

Source: Adapted from *The Limits to Growth: A Report for The Club of Rome's Project on the Predicament of Mankind*, by Donella H. Meadows, Dennis L. Meadows, Jørgen Randers, William W. Behrens III. A Potomac Associates book published by Universe Books, New York, 1972. Reprinted by permission. Figures and complete notes and references appearing in this article are not included here; for further information consult the original version.

- *Agricultural production*—the food produced per capita per year;
- *Nonrenewable resources*—the fraction of nonrenewable resources retained each year;
- *Pollution*—wastes that are the result of the production of the other four factors.

Using systems analysis and computer-simulation techniques to analyze their world model, the Club of Rome members prepare graphs to explain the data they have gathered. In the case of population, graphs show the net population (net births minus net deaths) over a regular interval of time. Such graphs show dramatically that population exhibits *exponential growth*. This means that a doubling of population takes place at shorter and shorter intervals.

The Club of Rome projected that, by the year 2000, there would be a rapid decline in the available natural resources and this sharp drop would cause a sharp drop in food production and industrial output. According to these projections, the human population will continue to grow for a short period of time and then rapidly decline as the fall in industrial output and food production prevents humankind from obtaining the basic necessities of life from the environment. In the following excerpt, the impact of exponential growth on the global ecosystem is carefully explored.

The Nature of Exponential Growth

. . . A quantity exhibits *exponential* growth when it increases by a constant percentage of the whole in a constant time period. A colony of yeast cells in which each cell divides into two cells every ten minutes is growing exponentially. For each single cell, after ten minutes there will be two cells, an increase of 100 percent. After the next ten minutes there will be four cells, then eight, then sixteen. If a miser takes $100 from his mattress and invests it at 7 percent (so that the total amount accumulated increases by 7 percent each year), the invested money will grow much faster than the linearly increasing stock under the mattress. The amount added each year to a bank account or each ten minutes to a yeast colony is not constant. It continually increases, as the total accumulated amount increases. Such exponential growth is a common process in biological, financial, and many other systems of the world.

Common as it is, exponential growth can yield surprising results—results that have fascinated mankind for centuries. There is an old Persian legend about a clever courtier who presented a beautiful chessboard to his king and requested that the king give him in return one grain of rice for the first square on the board, two grains for the second square, four grains for the third, and so forth. The king readily agreed and ordered rice to be brought from his stores. The fourth square of the chessboard required eight grains, the tenth square took 512 grains, the fifteenth required 16,384, and the twenty-first square gave the courtier more than a million grains of rice. By the fortieth square a million million rice grains had to be brought from the storerooms. The king's entire rice supply was exhausted long before he reached the sixty-fourth square. Exponential increase is deceptive because it generates immense numbers very quickly.

A French riddle for children illustrates another aspect of exponential growth—the apparent suddenness with which it approaches a fixed limit. Suppose you own a pond on which a water lily is growing. The lily plant doubles in size each day. If the lily were allowed to grow unchecked, it would completely cover the pond in thirty days, choking off the other forms of life in the water. For a long time the lily plant seems small, and so you decide not to worry about cutting it back until it covers half the pond. On what day will that be? On the twenty-ninth day, of course. You have one day to save your pond.

It is useful to think of exponential growth in terms of *doubling time,* or the time it takes a growing quantity to double in size. In the case of the lily plant described above, the doubling time is one day. A sum of money left in a bank at 7 percent interest will double in ten years. There is a simple mathematical relationship between the interest rate, or rate of growth, and the time it will take a quantity to double in size. The doubling time is approximately equal to 70 divided by the growth rate, as illustrated in table 9.1.

Models and Exponential Growth

Exponential growth is a dynamic phenomenon, which means that it involves elements that change over time. In simple systems, like the

Table 9.1 Doubling Time

Growth Rate (% per year)	Doubling Time (years)
0.1	700
0.5	140
1.0	70
2.0	35
4.0	18
5.0	14
7.0	10
10.0	7

bank account or the lily pond, the cause of exponential growth and its future course are relatively easy to understand. When many different quantities are growing simultaneously in a system, however, and when all the quantities are interrelated in a complicated way, analysis of the causes of growth and of the future behavior of the system becomes very difficult indeed. Does population growth cause industrialization or does industrialization cause population growth? Is either one singly responsible for increasing pollution, or are they both responsible? Will more food production result in more population? If any one of these elements grows slower or faster, what will happen to the growth rates of all the others? These very questions are being debated in many parts of the world today. The answers can be found through a better understanding of the entire complex system that unites all of these important elements.

Over the course of the last thirty years there has evolved at the Massachusetts Institute of Technology a new method for understanding the dynamic behavior of complex systems. The method is called system dynamics. The basis of the method is the recognition that the *structure* of any system—the many circular, interlocking, sometimes time-delayed relationships among its components—is often just as important in determining its behavior as the individual components themselves. . . .

Dynamic modeling theory indicates that any exponentially growing quantity is somehow involved with a *positive feedback loop*. A positive feedback loop is sometimes call a "vicious circle." An example is the familiar wage-price spiral—wages increase, which causes prices to increase, which leads to demands for higher wages, and so forth. In a positive feedback loop a chain of cause-and-effect relationships closes on itself, so that increasing any one element in the loop will start a sequence of changes that will result in the originally changed element being increased even more. . . .

Suppose $100 is deposited in [a bank] account. The first year's interest is 7 percent of $100, or $7, which is added to the account, making the total $107. The next year's interest is 7 percent of $107, or $7.49, which makes a new total of $114.49. One year later the interest on that amount will be more than $8. The more money there is in the account, the more money will be added each year in interest. The more is added, the more there will be in the account the next year causing even more to be added in interest. And so on. As we go around and around the loop, the accumulated money in the account grows exponentially. The rate of interest (constant at 7 percent) determines the gain around the loop, or the rate at which the bank account grows.

We can begin our dynamic analysis of the long-term world situation by looking for the positive feedback loops underlying the exponential growth in the five physical quantities we have already mentioned. In particular, the growth rates of two of these elements—population and industrialization—are of interest, since the goal of many development policies is to encourage the growth of the latter relative to the former. The two basic positive feedback loops that account for exponential population and industrial growth are simple in principle. We will describe their basic structures. . . . The many interconnections between these two positive feedback loops act to amplify or to diminish the action of the loops, to couple or uncouple the growth rates of population and of industry. . . .

World Population Growth

. . . In 1650 the population numbered about 0.5 billion, and it was growing at a rate of approximately 0.3 percent per year. That corresponds to a doubling time of nearly 250 years. In 1970 the population totaled 3.6 billion and the rate of growth was 2.1 percent per year. The doubling time at this growth rate is thirty-three years. Thus, not only has the population been growing exponentially, but the rate of growth has also been growing. We might say that population growth has been *super* exponential; the population curve is rising even faster than it would if growth were strictly exponential. . . . In a population with constant average fertility, the larger the population, the more babies will be born each year. The more babies, the larger the population will be the following year. After a delay to allow those babies to grow up and become parents, even more babies will be born, swelling the population still further. Steady growth will continue as long as average fertility remains constant. If, in addition to sons, each woman has on the average two female children, for example, and each of them grows up to have two more female children, the population will double each generation. The growth rate will depend on both the average fertility and the length of the delay between generations. Fertility is not necessarily constant.

There is another feedback loop governing population growth. . . . It is a *negative feedback loop*. Whereas positive feedback loops generate runaway growth, negative feedback loops tend to regulate growth and to hold a system in some stable state. They behave much as a thermostat does in controlling the temperature of a room. If the temperature falls, the thermostat activates the heating system, which causes the temperature to rise again. When the temperature reaches its limit, the thermostat cuts off the heating system, and the temperature begins to fall again. In a negative feedback loop a change in one element is propagated around the circle until it comes back to change that element in a direction *opposite* to the initial change.

The negative feedback loop controlling population is based upon average mortality, a reflection of the general health of the population. The number of deaths each year is equal to the total population times the average mortality (which we might think of as the average probability of death at any age). An increase in the size of a population with constant average mortality will result in more deaths per year. More deaths will leave fewer people in the population, and so there will be fewer deaths the next year. If on the average 5 percent of the population dies each year, there will be 500 deaths in a population of 10,000 in one year. Assuming no births for the moment, that would leave 9,500 people the next year. If the probability of death is still 5 percent, there will be only 475 deaths in this smaller population, leaving 9,025 people. The next year there will be only 452 deaths. Again, there is a delay in this feedback loop because the mortality rate is a function of the average age of the population. Also, of course, mortality even at a given age is not necessarily constant.

If there were no deaths in a population, it would grow exponentially by the positive feedback loop of births. . . . If there were no births, the population would decline to zero because of the negative feedback loop of deaths. . . . Since every real population experiences both births and deaths, as well as varying fertility and mortality, the dynamic behavior of populations governed by these two interlocking feedback loops can become fairly complicated.

What has caused the recent superexponential rise in world population? Before the industrial revolution both fertility and mortality were comparatively high and irregular. The birth rate generally exceeded the death rate only slightly, and population grew exponentially, but at a very slow and uneven rate. In 1650 the average lifetime of most populations in the world was only about thirty years. Since then, mankind has developed many practices that have had profound effects on the population growth system, especially on mortality rates. With the spread of modern medicine, public health techniques, and new methods of growing and distributing foods, death rates have fallen around the world. World average life expectancy is currently about fifty-three years and still rising. On a world average the gain around the positive feedback loop (fertility) has decreased only slightly while the gain around the negative feedback loop (mortality) is decreasing. The result is an increasing dominance of the positive feedback loop and the sharp exponential rise in population. . . .

What about the population of the future? How might we extend the population curve . . . into the twenty-first century? . . . we can safely conclude that because of the delays in the controlling feedback loops, especially the positive loop of births, there is no possibility of leveling off the population growth curve before the year 2000, even with the most optimistic assumption of decreasing fertility. Most of the prospective parents of the year 2000 have already been born. Unless there is a sharp rise in mortality, which mankind will certainly strive mightily to avoid, we can look forward to a world population of around 7 billion persons in thirty more years. And if we continue to succeed in lowering mortality with no better success in lowering fertility than we have accomplished in the past, in sixty years there will be four people in the world for every one person living today.

Growth in the World System

. . . Population cannot grow without food, food production is increased by growth of capital, more capital requires more resources, discarded resources become pollution, pollution interferes with the growth of both population and food.

Furthermore, over long time periods each of these factors also feeds back to influence itself. The rate at which food production increases in the 1970s, for example, will have some effect on the size of the population in the 1980s, which will in turn determine the rate at which food production must increase for many years thereafter. Similarly, the rate of resource consumption in the next few years will influence both the size of the capital base that must be maintained and the amount of resources left in the earth. Existing capital and available resources will then interact to determine future resource supply and demand.

The five basic quantities, or levels—population, capital, food, nonrenewable resources, and pollution—are joined by still other interrelationships and feedback loops that we have not yet discussed. Clearly it is not possible to assess the long-term future of any of these levels without taking all the others into account. Yet even this relatively simple system has such a complicated structure that one cannot intuitively understand how it will behave in the future, or how a change in one variable might ultimately affect each of the others. To achieve such understanding, we must extend our intuitive capabilities so that we can follow the complex, interrelated behavior of many variables simultaneously.

. . . [Here] we describe the formal world model that we have used as a first step toward comprehending this complex world system. The model is simply an attempt to bring together the large body of knowledge that already exists about cause-and-effect relationships among the five levels listed above and to express that knowledge in terms of interlocking feedback loops. Since the world model is so important in understanding the causes of and limits to growth in the world system, we shall explain the model-building process in some detail.

In constructing the model, we followed four main steps:

1. We first listed the important causal relationships among the five levels and traced the feedback loop structure. To do so we consulted literature and professionals in many fields of study dealing with the areas of concern—demography, economics, agronomy,

nutrition, geology, and ecology, for example. Our goal in this first step was to find the most basic structure that would reflect the major interactions between the five levels. We reasoned that elaborations on this basic structure, reflecting more detailed knowledge, could be added after the simple system was understood.

2. We then quantified each relationship as accurately as possible, using global data where it was available and characteristic local data where global measurements had not been made.

3. With the computer, we calculated the simultaneous operation of all these relationships over time. We then tested the effect of numerical changes in the basic assumptions to find the most critical determinants of the system's behavior.

4. Finally, we tested the effect on our global system of the various policies that are currently being proposed to enhance or change the behavior of the system.

These steps were not necessarily followed serially, because often new information coming from a later step would lead us back to alter the basic feedback loop structure. There is not one inflexible world model; there is instead an evolving model that is continuously criticized and updated as our own understanding increases. . . .

The Purpose of the World Model

In this first simple world model, we are interested only in the broad behavior modes of the population-capital system. By *behavior modes* we mean the tendencies of the variables in the system (population or pollution, for example) to change as time progresses. A variable may increase, decrease, remain constant, oscillate, or combine several of these characteristic modes. For example, a population growing in a limited environment can approach the ultimate carrying capacity of that environment in several possible ways. It can adjust smoothly to an equilibrium below the environmental limit by means of a gradual decrease in growth rate. . . . It can overshoot the limit and then die back again in either a smooth or an oscillatory way. . . . Or it can overshoot the limit and in the process decrease the ultimate carrying capacity by consuming some necessary nonrenewable resource. . . . This behavior has been noted in many natural systems. For instance, deer or goats, when natural enemies are absent, often overgraze their range and cause erosion or destruction of the vegetation.

A major purpose in constructing the world model has been to determine which, if any, of these behavior modes will be most characteristic of the world system as it reaches the limits to growth. This process of determining behavior modes is "prediction" only in the most limited sense of the word. . . .

Selection 10 The Dimensions of Human Hunger

Jean Mayer

Editors' Introduction

To the Satisfied World the Hungry World seems far away. Yet considering the world as a global ecosystem brings shocking facts to our attention. Estimates indicate that one person in eight in the world today is hungry. Most of these people live in the poor, less developed regions of the world. Projected growth curves for population and food production, as shown in the previous selections, indicate that in the future food may become even more scarce. Technology has increased the life span of many people in this part of the world, and longer-living adults produce more children. However, technology has not kept pace with the demand for food.

In Africa, Asia, the Far East, the Near East, and Latin America vast numbers of people suffer from both hunger *and* malnutrition. The term *malnutrition* refers to a deficiency (too little), excess (too much), or imbalance in nutrients. Malnutrition also includes *undernutrition,* which refers to a lack of calories or a *caloric deficit.* It also includes the across-the-board nutrient inadequacy that accompanies the caloric deficit. In general, people who live in areas where the food supply is uncertain suffer from a variety of illnesses caused by a deficiency of nutrients and low calories.

Severe deficiencies of necessary nutrients cause serious disease. The most prevalent health-related problems on a worldwide basis are protein-calorie malnutrition, iron deficiency anemia, goiter (the enlargement of the thyroid gland due to iodine deficiency), and blindness resulting from vitamin A deficiency.

From the moment of conception, nutrition is important to the developing human being. Fetal nutrition is related to the health of the newborn baby. From birth to old age, human growth and development follow stages in a predictable series called the *life cycle*. In general, because of the characteristic demands made at specific life-cycle stages, nutrition needs can be predicted within a fairly broad range. Pregnant women, infants, and children to the age of six are most vulnerable to malnutrition. Each of these stages in the life cycle involves a period of rapid growth that influences the well-being of the coming generation. During rapid growth at any stage, energy and nutrient stores are quickly depleted. The body uses them to support the growth of new tissues.

We will consider protein in some detail because (1) it is the single nutrient that most likely will be deficient on a worldwide basis and (2) a deficiency of this nutrient has a devastating effect on the development of children. In the poor, developing, over-populated countries, protein-rich foods containing essential amino acids (found in milk, eggs, meat, fish, poultry, legumes, and nuts) are not readily available. Often the total food consumption is so inadequate that the small amounts of protein consumed are used as an energy source. When the caloric content of the diet is inadequate to meet minimum requirements, protein is used as a source of energy and, therefore, the protein becomes unavailable for its special function in building and repairing body tissues.

Protein-calorie malnutrition (PCM) is by far the major cause of infant and childhood mortality and morbidity in the Hungry World. Moderate forms of this disorder lead to retarded growth and development as well as impaired learning capacity. At least 50 percent of the children in developing countries suffer from moderate protein-calorie malnutrition. In tropical and sub-tropical countries, millions of children suffer from PCM of such severity that—even with treatment—they die.

The population growth in developing areas with the great-est nutritional problems is double that of developed areas with relatively plentiful food. Other factors complicate this situation and contribute to the high incidence of malnutrition in de-veloping countries. One of the most important is poverty—inade-quate money to buy sufficient foods and/or to buy foods that have high nutrient density. Other significant factors include lack of education about what constitutes an adequate diet, the limited kinds of foods that are readily available, and dietary habits that are severely limited by cultural and religious taboos.

The inability to apply modern agricultural technology and to fund agricultural research results in inadequate food production and distribution. The unequal distribution of food, arable land, fertilizer, and other resources necessary for the production of food among and within countries also greatly contributes to the food deficit and occurrence of malnutrition in developing countries.

Jean Mayer, president of Tufts University and a world-renowned nutritionist, has devoted much of his career to identifying national and international nutrition problems, studying them, and developing proposals for their solution. In the following reading he has demarcated the problem of human hunger in both humane and scientific terms.

Famine, fearsome and devastating though it is, can at least be attacked straightforwardly. A famine occurs in a definable area and has a finite duration; as long as food is available somewhere, relief agencies can undertake to deal with the crisis. Malnutrition, on the other hand, afflicts a far larger proportion of mankind than any famine but is harder to define and attack. Only someone professionally familiar with nutritional disease can accurately diagnose malnutrition and assess its severity. Malnutrition is a chronic condition that seems to many observers to be getting worse in certain areas. In one form or another it affects human populations all over the world, and its treatment involves not mobilization to combat a crisis but long-term actions taken to prevent a crisis—actions that affect economic and social policies as well as nutritional and agricultural ones. In the background always is the concern that too rapid an increase in population, combined with failure to keep pace in food production, will give rise to massive famines that cannot be combated.

The statistics with which the public is bombarded are of little help. What is the layman to make of statements that a billion people suffered from hunger and malnutrition last year, that 10 million children the world over are so seriously malnourished that their lives are at risk, that 400 million people live on the edge of starvation, that 12,000 people die of hunger each day, and that in India alone 1 million children die each year from malnutrition? If the world's food problem is to be brought under control, and I believe it can be, we must first draw conceptual boundaries around it and place it in a time frame as we would a famine.

First, then, just what is the chronic hunger of malnutrition and how widespread is it? The first part of the question can be answered with assurance; the second, in spite of the statistics cited in the preceding paragraph, is really a matter of informed guesswork.

Malnutrition may come about in one of four ways. A person may simply not get enough food, which is undernutrition. His diet may lack one essential nutrient or more, which gives rise to deficiency diseases such as pellagra, scurvy, rickets, and the anemia of pregnancy due to a deficiency of folic acid. He may have a condition or an illness, either genetic or environmental in origin, that prevents him from digesting his food properly or from absorbing some of its constituents, which is secondary malnutrition. Finally, he may be taking in too many calories or consuming an excess of one component or more of a reasonable diet; this condition is overnutrition. Malnutrition in this sense is a disease of affluent people in both the rich and the poor nations. In countries such as the U.S. diets high in calories, saturated fats, salt, and sugar, low in fruits and vegetables and distorted toward heavily processed foods contribute to the high incidence of obesity, diabetes, hypertension, and athero-sclerotic disease and to marginal deficiencies of certain minerals and B vitamins. Bizarre reducing diets, which exclude entire categories of useful foods, are self-inflicted examples of the first two causes of malnutrition. The nutritional diseases of the affluent are not, however, the subject of this article. In areas where the food supply is limited the first three causes of malnutrition are often found in some combination.

In children a chronic deficiency of calories causes listlessness, muscle wastage and failure to grow. In adults it leads to a loss of weight and a reduced inclination toward and capacity for activity. Under-nourished people of all ages are more vulnerable to infection and other illness and recover more slowly and with much greater difficulty. Children with a chronic protein deficiency grow more slowly and are small for their age; in severe deficiency growth stops altogether and the child shows characteristic symptoms: a skin rash and discoloration, edema, and a change in hair color to an orange-reddish tinge that is particularly striking in children whose hair would normally be dark. The spectrum of protein-calorie malnutrition (PCM, as it is known to workers in the field) varies from a diet that is relatively high in calories and deficient in protein (manifested in the syndrome known as kwashiorkor) to one that is low in both calories and protein (manifested in marasmus).

Although protein-calorie malnutrition is the most prevalent form of undernourishment, diseases caused by deficiencies of specific vitamins or minerals are also widespread. It is true that the prevalence of certain classic deficiency diseases has decreased drastically since World War II. Beriberi is now rare and pellagra has been essentially eradicated, at least in its acute form; rickets is seen mostly in its adult form (osteomalacia) in Moslem women whose secluded way of life keeps them out of the sun, and scurvy is unlikely to be seen except in prisoners who are not provided with enough vitamin C. In contrast, blindness caused by the lack of vitamin A occurs with particular frequency in India, Indonesia, Bangladesh, Vietnam, the Philippines, Central America, the northeast of Brazil, and parts of Africa. In remote inland areas (central Africa, the mountainous regions of South America and the Himalayas) goiter, the enlargement of the thyroid resulting from a deficiency of iodine, is common. The World Health Organization estimates that up to 5 percent of such populations are afflicted with cretinism, the irreversible condition caused by iodine deficiency in the mother before or during pregnancy. From 5 to 17 percent of the men and from 10 to 50 percent of the women in countries of South America, Africa, and Asia have been estimated to have iron-deficiency anemia.

The human beings most vulnerable to the ravages of malnutrition are infants, children up to the age of five or six, and pregnant and lactating women. For the infant protein in particular is necessary during fetal development for the generation and growth of bones, muscles, and organs. The child of a malnourished mother is more likely to be born prematurely or small and is at greater risk of death or of permanent neurological and mental dysfunction. Brain development begins *in utero* and is complete at an early age (under two). Malnutrition during this period when neurons and neuronal connections are being formed may be the cause of mental retardation that cannot be remedied by later corrective measures. The long-term consequences, not only for the individual but also for the society and the economy, need no elaboration.

Growing children, pound for pound, require more nutrients than adults do. A malnourished child is more susceptible to the common childhood diseases, and illness in turn makes extra demands on nutritional reserves. In addition many societies, still believing the old adage about starving a fever, withdraw nourishing foods from the child just when he needs them most, thus often pushing him over the borderline into severe malnutrition. So common is the cycle of malnutrition, infection, severe malnutrition, recurrent infection, and eventual death at an early age that the death rate for children up to four years old in general and the infant mortality rate in particular serve as one index of the nutritional status of a population as a whole. For infants less than a year old the death rate is about 250 per 1,000 births in Zambia and Bolivia, 140 in India and Pakistan, and 95 in Brazil (for all its soaring gross national product). The rate in Sweden is 12 per 1,000 births; in the United States the average is 19, but in the country's affluent suburbs the rate equals Sweden's, whereas it rises to about 25 in the poor areas of the inner cities and as high as 60 for the most poverty-stricken and neglected members of the society: the migrant farm workers.

How reliable the figures for the developing nations are, however, is another matter. In most instances statistical reporting is as underdeveloped as the rest of the economy. Deaths, particularly of one-day-old infants, often go unreported. In all probability the rates are higher than the ones I have cited.

More precise nutritional assessments are attempted in two ways. One is to construct a "food balance sheet," which puts agricultural output, stocks and purchases on the supply side and balances them against the food used for seed for the next year's crop, animal feed, and wastage and hence derives an estimate of the food that is left for human consumption. That amount can then be matched against the United Nations Food and Agriculture Organization's tables of nutritional requirements to obtain an estimate of the adequacy of the national diet.

This method has a number of drawbacks. For several reasons it tends to result in underestimates. One is that it is difficult to estimate the agricultural production in developing countries with any degree of accuracy. Farmers have every incentive to underestimate their crop: they may be able to reduce taxes and the obligatory payment of crops (often as much as 60 percent of the harvest) in rent to the landlord. Second, the foods included in the balance sheet tend to be the items that figure prominently in channels of trade: grain, soybeans, and large livestock. Other farm products—eggs, small animals, fruits, and vegetables—vital to a good diet but grown for family consumption or sold locally are almost impossible to count and so are ignored.

On the other hand, the balance-sheet method has certain tendencies toward overestimates. For example, it is extremely difficult to estimate the postharvest loss of crops to insects, rodents, and microorganisms. The loss is known to be close to 10 percent for the U.S. wheat crop and is probably higher for other crops, even with the advanced technology available. In some tropical countries the loss can run as high as 40 percent. For all these reasons figures on food production do not provide a particularly accurate index of the amount of food actually available for consumption or the types of food actually consumed, and they make no attempt to differentiate patterns of consumption within a population. They do, however, provide rough estimates of the state of nutrition by regions. . . .

The second way of estimating the degree of malnutrition within an area is to extrapolate from data compiled from hospital records and cross-sectional surveys. Statistics on illness, however, tend to be as unreliable as mortality statistics. The criteria for admission to a hospital on the basis of malnutrition vary from country to country; the records from rural areas may be sparse; the poor, among whom malnutrition and its related conditions are most likely to be found, are the least likely segment of the population to seek medical help, and if they do seek such help, the condition may then be so far advanced that the diseases associated with malnutrition, such as infantile diarrhea and pneumonia, may claim all the physician's attention, so that he misses or ignores the underlying cause.

Projections based on the results of seventy-seven studies of nutritional status made among more than 200,000 preschool children in forty-five countries of Asia, Africa, and Latin America place the total number of children suffering from some degree of protein-calorie malnutrition at 98.4 million. Percentages ranged from 5 to 37 in Latin America, from 7 to 73 in Africa, and from 15 to 80 in Asia (excluding China). These surveys, however, did not employ standardized procedures. In some of them clinical assessments were made and in others the children were measured against international weight tables. Thus, although the general indications of such studies are useful, figures derived from them are rough at best. In order to assign reliable figures to the degree of hunger and malnutrition in the world today we would need large-scale surveys that included both clinical examinations based on an established definition of malnutrition and individual consumption surveys that determine the amount and types of food eaten and the distribution of food within each family unit.

Even if the figures derived by these methods are doubtful, the situation they reflect is clear. In my judgment it would seem reasonable to set the number of people suffering from malnutrition at 500 million and to add to that another billion who would benefit from a more varied diet. The largest concentration of such people is in Asia, Southeast Asia, and sub-Saharan Africa. Clinical surveys and hospital records indicate that malnutrition wherever it exists is severest among infants, preschool children, and pregnant and lactating women; that it is most prevalent in depressed rural areas and the slums of great cities; that the problem is lack of calories as much as lack of protein; that (except in areas where the people subsist largely on manioc or bananas) where calories are adequate protein tends to be adequate too, and that although a lack of food is the ultimate factor in malnutrition, that lack results from a number of causes, operating alone or in combination. A nation may lack both self-sufficiency in food production and the money to buy food or to provide the farm inputs necessary to increase production; the poorer members of the population may lack income to buy the food that is available, and regional factors, such as customs in child-feeding and restrictions on the movement of supplies, may prevent the food from getting to the people who need it most.

On the basis of these findings one can divide the nations of the world into five groups. The first group consists of the industrialized nations, where food is plentiful but pockets of poverty persist. Here governments are able to deal with problems of malnutrition through food assistance to the poor, nutrition and health programs, and nutrition-education programs. The chief members of the group are the United States, Canada, the nations of Western Europe, Japan, Australia, New Zealand, Hong Kong, and Singapore.

The second group consists of the nations with centrally planned economies, where whatever the economic philosophy the egalitarian pattern of income distribution together with government control of food supplies and distribution have seemed in the past few years to insure the populations against malnutrition due to hunger. In this category are mainland China, Taiwan, North Korea, South Korea, North Vietnam, and South Vietnam. In the third group are the nations of the Organization of Petroleum Exporting Countries (OPEC), whose overall wealth is undeniable but whose pattern of income distribution does not ensure that this wealth will benefit the poor. Fourth is a group of countries in Asia, the Near East, Central America, and South America that are already self-sufficient or almost self-sufficient in food production at their present level of demand. The demand, however, is impeded by an uneven distribution of income that is reflected in malnutrition in large segments of the population. Brazil, for example, has the highest economic growth rate in the world, but malnutrition is rampant in the northeast and widespread in the shantytowns surrounding the large cities.

The fifth group includes the nations the UN designates as "least developed." They have too few economic resources to provide for the people in the lowest income groups. Many of the countries are exposed to recurring droughts, floods or cyclones; some are ravaged by war. All twenty-five of the least developed nations are poor in natural resources and investment capital.

Looking back today, it seems incredible that in 1972 it appeared the world might soon, for the first time, be assured of an abundant food supply. The new wheat varieties of the "green revolution" had taken hold in Mexico and northwestern India, and the new varieties of rice developed in the Philippines promised a high-yield staple crop for the peoples of Southeast Asia. The harvest from the seas was still rising spectacularly (from 21 million metric tons in 1950 to 70 million in 1970—a steady increase of about 5 percent per year, outstripping the world's annual population increase of 2 percent). The worldwide production of grain was rising by an average of 2.8 percent per year, and there were substantial reserves in the form of carry-over stocks held by the principal exporting countries and of cropland held idle in the United States under the soil-bank program. The prospect was so rosy that the FAO suggested in 1969 that the food problems of the future might be those of surplus rather than shortage.

Although two sudden and short-term simultaneous crop failures in a number of areas and the sharp rise in oil prices were the immediate cause of the food crisis of 1972–1974, it has since become clear that four long-term factors that had been building up quietly for a long time were in any case about to alter the hopeful situation permanently. (The first short-term reversal, a reduction of crops in several parts of the world because of unfavorable weather in 1972, gave rise to a second: the massive purchases of grain by the U.S.S.R. that eliminated American reserves and caused the international prices of wheat, corn and rice to rise sharply. Moreover, the increase in oil prices effectively put the green revolution out of the reach of such countries as India, Pakistan, and Bangladesh, which are poor in petroleum and other resources and have gone about as far as they can in increasing yields with traditional methods of farming. The increase in oil prices also dislocated the economies of the wealthy nations, reducing their contributions to international aid.)

Even though the situation is less serious now than it was in 1974, it is more precarious as a result of the long-term factors. The primary long-term factor is the growth of the human population: 80 million people per year, the equivalent of the population of the United States every thirty months. Moreover, the population is growing most rapidly in the areas that are experiencing the greatest nutritional difficulties.

In considering the effects of population growth, however, one must bear in mind the phenomenon known as the demographic transition. It is the process whereby societies move from a stage of high birth and death rates to one of low birth and death rates. Usually the decline in death rates precedes the decline in birth rates by from one generation to three generations. On both sides of the transition the result is a stable level of population. The developed countries have made the transition or are well along in it; the developing countries are now making the transition but have traveled varying distances through it.

Alongside the inequality in population growth as a long-term factor affecting the food supply is an even greater inequality in the patterns of producing and utilizing food. It appears to be historically inevitable that as people or societies become wealthier their consumption of animal products increases. This means that more of their basic foodstuffs (grains, legumes, and even fish) that could feed human beings directly are instead fed to domesticated animals such as cattle and chickens. The efficiency of the conversion of plant food into animal food varies with the animal product but is in no case higher than the level of about 25 percent attained in milk and eggs.

The net effect of this trend is that rich countries consume far more food per capita than poor ones. For example, it has been estimated that in China each person is adequately fed on 450 pounds of grain per year; 350 pounds are consumed directly as cereal or cereal products and 100 pounds are fed to domesticated animals. In the United States the average individual consumes more than 2,000 pounds of grains per year; 150 pounds are eaten directly (as bread, pasta, breakfast cereal, and the like) and the rest, more than 90 percent of the total, is fed to animals.

The third source of pressure on the world's food supply has been the diminishing effectiveness of the fishing industry, an important source of protein for many poor nations. In 1970 and 1971 the total catch remained steady at about 70 million tons. It dropped abruptly in 1972 to less than 55 million tons. The reasons for the decline are overfishing and pollution.

Finally, it has become apparent that the "miracle" of the green revolution requires more time, more work, and more capital than was thought in the first flush of enthusiasm. . . . In sum, the situation as it exists today is precarious but manageable, barring some catastrophe such as a massive crop failure in the Untied States, which is currently the granary of the world.

What of the future? Let us first consider three advances that could be made in dealing with famine. Their common aim is to sight and attack incipient famines in an early stage of development.

The first requirement is an early-warning system. It would employ weather satellites, economic indexes (such as the movement and amounts of food in a region), and clinical indicators. One of the most sensitive clinical indicators is provided by the charted weight and growth curves for children in the most vulnerable socioeconomic sectors of a society.

The second requirement is a permanent small international organization that would keep track of such information for every region and monitor it for any sign of an impending emergency. The agency would maintain manuals on how to proceed against disaster and famine, would hold periodic training sessions for key people from each nation, would draft contingency plans (listing likely requirements and sources of food, medicine, transportation, and personnel) and would explore such matters as stockpiling essential supplies and setting up alternative systems of distribution. In an emergency the organization would stand ready to assist a national relief director.

The third requirement is an adequate grain reserve, distributed strategically around the world. It would serve as a standby supply for nearby countries while grain shipments intended for them were diverted to the stricken area. This arrangement might not avert a famine, but it would prevent one from becoming a major disaster.

Several things can also be done to deal with malnutrition. For the next few years it will be necessary to continue to provide food relief where it is needed. The least developed countries may require special assistance in the form of food distribution and feeding programs for some years to come. Those nations should also be helped to develop methods to increase their ability to store food and to distribute it to vulnerable areas in times of emergency.

Simple and inexpensive programs are available to eradicate certain diseases of malnutrition, and they should be instituted. The blindness resulting from a deficiency of vitamin A can be prevented with two injections per year of 100,000 units of the vitamin, at a cost of a few cents per person. Goiter can be prevented by the iodization of salt, also at infinitesimal cost.

In the intermediate term (the next 15 years or so) the goal must be to make the developing nations independent in their food supply. The fish catch appears to have stabilized at the 1970 level. The production of animal foods that compete with human beings for grain should be reduced. (Grazing animals, which utilize land that cannot be cultivated and crops that cannot be eaten by human beings, are another matter.) The development of new foods is still in the future. The only sure resource is the green revolution, which still has the potential of doubling or tripling yields in some areas.

Therefore it is important to begin immediately the construction of fertilizer plants, preferably right at the source of supply (the flare gas around the Persian Gulf and in Nigeria, for example) or in the needy countries. The task should be furthered by international assistance and by oil sold by the OPEC nations at concessional prices.

Another step, which entails something that Americans do well, is to help the food-deficit nations set up agricultural research and extension services, with the aim of adapting the green revolution to a tropical, labor-intensive agriculture and of assisting the small farmer to obtain an increased yield while maintaining a varied production of small animals, fruits, and vegetables so that he is not dependent on large tonnages of one crop for an adequate income. Such countries can also be helped to develop ways of protecting a crop once it is harvested and of establishing an indigenous food industry that can package and distribute the food. A system of international credit that favors the small farmer and the small businessman and promotes a more equitable distribution of income and opportunity should be established. Finally, an international system of weather forecasting should be activated so that future crop failures will not come as a surprise.

These actions will buy time for the next twenty-five years. If the population of the world is then between 6 and 7 billion, as seems likely, new sources of food will have to be at hand—on the dinner table, not in the development stage. Unfortunately the nations that will need the new foods the most desperately have neither the financial resources nor the technological skill to do the necessary research, and the nations that do have these things have so far felt no urgency about doing it. The objectives of the research should include the intensive development of aquaculture, the establishment through genetic techniques of new species of animals (such as the beefalo) and of grazing animals that can utilize forage more efficiently, the domestication of some wild animals, the development of one-cell microorganisms as food and the direct synthesis of food from oil. Work on all these objectives should now be under way.

To sum up, we know who is hungry, if not precisely how many people are affected. We also know why. Economists often say that expanded food production will solve the problem. Social reformers maintain that the need is for more equitable distribution. The evidence shows that we must and can have both.

Selection 11 Starvation

Ellen S. Parham

Editors' Introduction

At this moment at least 1 million people are so hungry that many are suffering from starvation. They are the victims of the world food crisis described in the previous selections.

North Americans (citizens of Canada and the United States) live in countries where food is readily available. For the most part we eat in response to our appetite rather than in response to hunger. Dr. Jean Mayer has called appetite a response to complex sensations that make us aware of the desire for food and the anticipation of palatable food. These sensations are pleasant or at least not unpleasant.

The only personal experiences most of us have had with hunger are the slight twinges or stomach contractions that we feel on those occasions when a meal is skipped or delayed. Our discomfort is temporary. It is relieved in a relatively short period of

Source: Adapted from Ellen S. Parham, "Starvation," *Journal of Home Economics* 67, no. 6 (November 1975):7–11. Reprinted by permission of the American Home Economics Association. Notes and references appearing in this article have been omitted here; for further information consult the original version.

time. It is not comparable to the chronic hunger that becomes a way of life for the millions who habitually go for days without a full meal. They live in near famine conditions when there is not enough food available for them to meet minimum human needs. They are forced to subsist on diets that are deficient in caloric content. Moreover, the inadequacy of energy intake is complicated by shortages of other nutrients. Dr. Mayer describes this type of hunger as the complex of unpleasant sensations that is felt after prolonged deprivation that compels a person to seek, work, or fight for immediate relief by the ingestion of food.

When chronic hunger is severe, it results in a state of starvation. The term *starvation* refers to the level of caloric deprivation that, if permitted to continue without suitable amounts of food, will eventually lead to death. Loss of weight and the wasting of vital tissues occurring in an effort to meet the energy requirement needed for survival are characteristic features of starvation.

In the following reading Dr. Ellen S. Parham, a registered dietitian, professor of home economics, and nutrition educator, describes the physical, mental, social, and moral deterioration that occurs in humans in response to their need for physiological survival. She uses the words *hunger* and *starvation* interchangeably in describing these debilitating effects. Her article is based on the accounts of those who have experienced starvation, the experiences of those who have worked in hunger-relief efforts, and research reports on the limited number of controlled studies available.

For most of us in the Western world, real hunger is beyond our experience or imagination. It is difficult for us to relate hunger statistics—often tabulated for us in highly impersonal form—and predictions of future famines to our experience of life.

Hunger: Physiological Effects

When there is a calorie deficit, the body adjusts to or compensates for that deficit by breaking down adipose (fatty) tissue to satisfy the body's primary need for energy.

In most adults of normal weight, this breakdown of adipose tissue can continue for from forty-five to fifty days before death ensues. A healthy nonobese adult can lose up to 25 percent of body weight without endangering life, and some persons have survived losses of 50 percent of their initial weight. Greater losses than this are likely to cause death.

Although most of the body's cells can use fat (or fat's metabolic products, ketones) for energy, certain bodily processes require glucose. Because the body's carbohydrate stores are depleted after only a few hours without food, body proteins become the main source of glucose and eventually of energy.

Because the body's fat supply cannot last forever, eventually all the adipose tissue is lost and the skin hangs loosely over a gaunt frame. Because of the protein loss described, vital body tissues atrophy: the heart of a starved person is about one-half normal size. Circulatory difficulties develop and heart failure may cause death. The endocrine glands also atrophy, producing a deficiency of their hormones. Only the brain is spared in the body's relentless search for energy.

The lining of the intestinal tract changes from a lush, velvety surface of tremendous absorptive capacity to a paper-thin tissue resembling pigskin. As it is this surface that absorbs nutrients, what little food is available may not be absorbed by this pigskin-like tissue in a starving individual. Often, the result is a devastating diarrhea that frequently accompanies death, especially in infants and children.

On the other hand, that same pigskin-like intestinal surface can also cause extreme constipation. Both the diarrhea and the constipation are frequently worsened by the nature of the foods that *are* available.

Many starved persons also suffer from fluid retention (edema) because of upsets in the body's balance of proteins, fluids, and electrolytes. This edema, which may mask tissue atrophy, is responsible for the classic protruding abdomen of a starving child. Sometimes, however, in contrast to edema, there is extreme dehydration, especially in children with diarrhea.

As the system's energy supply decreases, the body begins to make certain adjustments to compensate for the loss. In early starvation, there may even be improved efficiency of nutrient absorption and decreased excretion of nutrients. As body weight is lost, the rate slows at which cells use energy, thus decreasing calorie needs and lowering the body temperature.

A starving person is therefore very sensitive to cold. The lowered body temperature of the starving may then mask fever symptoms of the diseases that frequently accompany famine—malaria, tuberculosis, and infective gangrene of the mouth.

Sexual Function and Reproduction

Starvation undoubtedly depresses sexual function and reproduction. The extent and nature of its depressive effect is difficult to determine exactly, however, because of the lack of controlled studies and because sociological factors frequently complicate observations of famines.

Although the chronically undernourished usually have high birthrates in comparison to well-fed populations that practice family planning, acute starvation reduces the number of conceptions and live births. As many as 60 to 70 percent of young women in a famine have amenorrhea (absence, or abnormal stoppage, of menstruation).

The Minnesota Experiment, a controlled observation of young men living under semistarvation conditions, reported a decrease in the men's sperm viability and in their excretion of 17-ketosteroid—an indicator of the extent of male sex hormone production.

During World War II, a number of American men in Japanese prison camps who had been underfed developed breast enlargement, apparently because their diets had caused failure of the liver to inactivate the estrogens also normally produced by males. This phenomenon has not been reported in other famine conditions.

Females usually survive famine better than males, perhaps because of lower calorie needs, freedom from heavy work, adaptation resulting from amenorrhea, their favored position in society, or, for those with children, from some maternal instinct to survive.

Babies conceived and delivered by undernourished mothers frequently have low birthweight and a reduced chance for survival. The prognosis for these babies is highly related both to their mothers' prepregnant condition and to the severity and duration of their mothers' starvation.

A comprehensive follow-up study of children born or conceived during the Dutch famine winter of 1944–45 found that the fetus was most vulnerable during the third trimester.

The milk produced by undernourished mothers is of generally high quality but, after the infants are about six months old, it is seldom of adequate quantity. Because little other food is available, the infant slowly starves as the mother's milk production dwindles. Too weak to cry and barely able to suck, the infants can only lie quietly, without movement.

Growth and Development

Growth requires energy—but so does survival, which takes precedence. When the body has only enough energy to survive, physical growth is severely retarded and sexual development is delayed.

There is some evidence that "catch-up" growth can occur when a liberal food intake is again available. On the other hand, after the first two years of life, the brain loses nearly all of its capacity to grow in size.

For babies to have a normal number of brain cells, not only must they have received adequate nourishment during their first few postnatal months, but their mothers also must have had adequate nutrients during their pregnancies. Infants who die of undernutrition during their first year of life may have as few as 40 percent of the normal number of brain cells. Undernourished infants who survive do not acquire normal brain size even when they receive normal nourishment again.

The relationship of reduced brain size to intelligence is not entirely clear. Although malnourished children frequently have reduced mental capacity, it has not so far been possible to separate nutrition effects from those of heredity, infection, and sensory deprivation.

The twenty-year study of the Dutch famine in the winter of 1944–45 showed that the hunger had been without effect on the mental performance, physical stature, or general health of the young men whose prenatal life included that period — with one exception.

That exception was the increased frequency of central nervous system anomalies — including spina bifida (a defect in the bone surrounding the spinal cord), hydrocephalus, and cerebral palsy. This effect had apparently been the result of nutritional deprivation plus some other stress — possibly infection.

The numbers affected were small. The investigators believed that prenatal brain-cell depletion had probably occurred but had not resulted in mental dysfunction. The human body is remarkably resilient. It usually gives the brain top priority in satisfying its energy needs over all other bodily systems.

Those at greatest risk in famines are young children and old persons. Children have the combined needs for growth and maintenance and have limited body stores. Unlike the aged, however, they are often given high priority in food distribution.

The starved appear to age at an accelerated rate. A thirty-five-year-old man may look eighty; he feels and acts old. His loss of adipose tissue is largely responsible for his aged appearance, and the slowing of his body processes and metabolism causes him to feel and behave as an aged man. There is no evidence of a real change in the aging process.

The Importance of Nutrient Stores

People survive famines by using the nutrient stores in their bodies to eke out the little food available. Body tissues are consumed as energy "fuel," but vitamins and minerals are made available to the body in the process. Because these substances are already in the blood, the normal digestion and absorption processes are not required.

The most likely famine victims are those who, for most of their lives, have had inadequate diets; they seldom have significant nutrient stores. Those who survive seem to do so because their bodies have had a long adjustment to low-nutrient intakes and because they have developed immunity to the many infectious diseases usually accompanying famine.

Although the nutrient-deficiency diseases of scurvy, rickets, and beriberi have been associated with some famines, vitamin and mineral deficiencies are usually minor problems for the food-relief administrator compared with the population's energy deficit.

[Hunger:] Behavioral Effects

When well-fed Americans imagine how starvation feels, we imagine extreme hunger pangs. Indeed, in starvation's early stages, there is extreme hunger, and food becomes an overwhelming preoccupation.

A study of the sixteen survivors of the 1972 Andes crash relates the young men's planning of a fantastic restaurant, their contest for the best original menu, their extensive list of their favorite eating places. Food completely replaced sex as a conversational topic. However, they finally had to outlaw all food-related conversation because it had increased their discomfort.

Children of the African Ik tribe, which has suffered slow starvation for years, play very elaborate games involving mud food. The children often end their game by eating their mud concoctions or small pebbles as make-believe food.

Usually, however, appetite maintenance depends on food consumption. As starvation proceeds and large amounts of body weight are lost, appetite dwindles and the starving person may even reject food. When near death from starvation, some become euphoric and feel they no longer need food.

The starving move as little as possible, an adaptive behavior that seems to conserve energy. The young men in the Minnesota Experiment found even routine exertion extremely taxing. There is dizziness or fainting when a starving person moves quickly to a vertical position, but this becomes less of a problem as starvation continues because the person can no longer make rapid movements.

Most persons experience unpleasant personality changes after enduring hunger for some time. They are no longer rational or objective, and their moods oscillate from high to low without recognizable cause. They lose interest in sexual activity.

In spite of their apparent lack of response to their environment, their senses seem to be sharpened. They have increased sensitivity to sound. Although their intelligence remains the same, they lose the ability to concentrate and their motivation to learn.

There seems to be wide variation among individuals in the will to survive. Members of the Donner expedition, stranded in a high pass of the Sierra Nevadas during the winter of 1846–47, are examples of this. Sturdy (but unattached) young men took to their beds — not even rising to remove their companions when they died — and surrendered to death.

But the parents of young children struggled for miles on frozen bleeding feet in a desperate effort to find help. Histories of famines include some remarkable tales of heroism. These are the exceptions, however; most people respond to hunger in far less noble fashion.

[Hunger:] Social Effects

These behavioral changes among individuals naturally bring about changes in social relationships. As the weight losses of the Minnesota volunteers approached 20 percent a very serious degree of civil disorder and strife developed. Weight losses beyond the 20 percent level, however, usually produce a decline in such behavior as the weakened individual slips into a state of apathy.

The basic human response to starvation seems to be survival at all costs. There is an initial attempt to protect the weak, but as conditions worsen, social behavior deteriorates and family ties break.

This phenomenon is dramatically demonstrated by members of the Ik tribe. The tribe once had the usual ties within families and villages to support the young and old. After several years of starvation, however, the "survival of the fittest" has become the major behavioral guideline. At the age of three, children are turned out of the family hut to fend for themselves. The hunters who would once have brought their catch home to share with pride now gorge themselves in hiding. It is quite acceptable Ik social behavior to take food away from weaker Iks, even from their mouths.

Hunger sends human beings tumbling down Maslow's hierarchy of human needs to the very bottom level—physiological survival. Humanity's higher needs—for security, a sense of belonging, status or esteem, and self-realization—have little relevance.

We have even seen this effect among well-fed Americans. Remember the response to the rumor of a beef shortage a few years ago?

Starvation Is a Slow Process

The threat of a food shortage causes people to engage in an activity that will obtain food—prostitution, theft, selling their children, or migration.

When people are hungry, they are forced to slaughter their domestic animals, which for a short time provide a high-protein diet, usually of more animal protein than the family has ever had before. When this abundance comes to an end, not only is the meat gone but also the source of milk or eggs or the cash those bring. The family pets are usually the next to be sacrificed.

Persons able to do so roam far in search of food. Although that reduces the number to be fed in a famine area, it also uses up calories, spreads diseases, interferes with crop planting, and causes the abandonment of the sick or immobile.

In the past, some food-relief measures have taken the form of work programs, which encourage self-help but also increase calorie expenditures and benefit only those strong enough to work. Workers often must walk miles to the work location.

Throughout human history, famine has been accompanied by cannibalism, although not all starving people have resorted to such measures to assuage hunger. It is most likely to occur in an acute, rather than a chronic, starvation situation and where it is clear that there are no alternatives if one is to survive. The taboo against eating human flesh is probably the strongest dietary taboo in most cultures, and it is not easily overcome. People in Western societies who have survived starvation by eating their dead companions have met extreme public criticism after their rescue.

Hunger Is Rarely the Only Burden

Seldom is deprivation of food the only stress the starving person has to bear. Famine is a sibling of war. Famine also brings too little of everything else besides food—too little water, soap, heat, or shelter. Donner expedition diaries, for example, tell of being in the bitter cold for three weeks without dry clothing—clothing in which lice and fleas flourished to torment the wearers and their babies.

The body's need for water is more acute than its need for food, and precious human energy must often be expended in famines in obtaining a safe supply, scarce even—or perhaps especially—in flood situations.

Relocation centers for the starving, with barely room to move and few or no sanitary facilities, are seldom much of a haven and are often breeding grounds for famine's companions—bubonic plague, cholera, smallpox, and the like, The relocated are often bewildered, floundering helplessly without the sustaining ties of the extended family or a means of livelihood. Many try to return to their homeland, even though the famine continues there.

Implications

Chronic hunger has profound effects on all aspects of a people's existence. Hungry people cannot be expected to behave as though they are well fed. This is especially true with regard to rational and objective planning and to working for their own future. By necessity, their concern is with surviving this day. Any famine-relief programs must cope with the realities of immobility, apathy, and resentment.

Hunger is ugly. The well-fed world would prefer to ignore its existence. However, the next few decades will involve a mighty struggle between the world's population and its resources. Hunger will be there. Perhaps in understanding the personal side of hunger, home economists and nutritionists can take an active role in the battle.

Selection 12 Breast-Feeding in Ecological Perspective

Alice L. Tobias
Patricia J. Thompson

Editors' Introduction

Oliver Wendell Holmes said that "the breasts were more skillful at compounding a feeding mixture than the hemispheres of the most learned professor's brain." Interestingly, human breast milk is one of the most undervalued natural food resources in the Satisfied World. The decline in maternal nursing has complex cultural and economic roots, but the effects on infant well-being are significant. Breast-feeding may contribute to the prevention of illness and perhaps even obesity in later life. According to nutritionist Alan Berg, "It is surely strange that while scientists explore such exotic forms of protein as bacteria and pond weed, the most biologically adapted, consumer-tested home food for infants is neglected because of indifference and inadequate understanding."

In 1979 the American Academy of Pediatrics began a campaign to encourage mothers to breast-feed their babies and to counsel mothers who encounter problems in this area rather than have them switch to formula-feeding.

The mother is the child's first environment. Prenatally, her health and level of nutrition influence the health and nutritional status of her baby. In mammals, evolution has provided a continuing source of protection in mother's milk so that the helpless human infant is less vulnerable to the external environment.

Good nutrition is essential for normal health and development throughout the life cycle, but it is especially critical during the first weeks and months of life. The infant needs food in order to provide enough energy and nutrients (1) to carry on vital internal processes, (2) for general activity, and (3) to support rapid growth involving the creation of new body cells and tissues. The infant's rate of growth is normally faster during the first year than at any other time in life. This rapid rate of growth explains why nutrient requirements are so high per unit of body weight during this stage of the life cycle.

Mother's milk provides the baby with optimal nutrition, increased resistance to infection, and important psychological benefits. Mother's milk is usually capable of meeting all the infant's nutritional needs for the first four to six months of life, except for vitamin D and possibly iron and vitamin C. Even after the introduction of semisolid food, breast milk can serve a major role in providing adequate nourishment. For example, it can usually be relied upon to supply up to three-quarters of the child's protein needs from the sixth to the twelfth month of life. It can provide a significant proportion of the total protein requirement for some months beyond this period. Furthermore, in many developing countries high-quality protein sources (foods containing all the essential amino acids) are expensive and scarce. Prolonged breast-feeding in these areas is vitally necessary. The child is quite often dependent on it, since mother's milk often represents the only protein source containing all the essential amino acids.

Cultural Perspective

Viewed historically and cross-culturally, breast-feeding has been the accepted means of feeding infants. In some societies, elaborate myths and rituals have developed to reinforce the tradition of breast-feeding. In Jordan and other Arabic societies, small water-rounded stones are believed to have special powers to enhance lactation, and stones from "the grotto of milk" are worn by expectant and nursing mothers. In Japan, women make special offerings in shrines—a practice they believe will bring more breast milk.

Among some American Indian tribes, clay and herbs were rubbed over mothers' breasts, and nursing mothers were warmed in heated pits and fed the reproductive organs of animals in the belief that this ritual would improve lactation. In the African Ndebele culture in Zimbabwe Rhodesia, women who have given birth are fed with inkovi, a souplike concoction made from the juices of a melonlike plant. The nursing mothers receive encouragement and assistance in breast-feeding from the older women in the extended family. For several months after giving birth, mothers' activities center around feeding the baby.

In spite of the traditional support of breast-feeding, there has been a significant decline in the practice in many developing countries. Dr. Derrick B. Jelliffe, an authority on infant nutritional problems in developing countries, has long opposed unnecessary bottle feeding. Discouraging breast-feeding among mothers who would otherwise happily and successfully breast-feed their infants is a policy that needs to be seriously reconsidered.

Increased urbanization and modernization and the emergence of new social values and roles have paved the way for the acceptance of artificial feeding procedures. Foreign manufacturers of baby foods have capitalized on this period of transition to expand their markets. Massive sales campaigns and advertising programs are aimed at semiliterate mothers who sincerely wish to improve their children's chances for health and longevity. Women are persuaded to abandon breast-feeding in favor of prepared formulas—a more complex, less economic, and frequently less healthful method. Mothers prepare the formula under unsanitary conditions, and children are exposed to communicable diseases before they have had a chance to build up immunities to such things as unboiled water. Household sanitation and refrigeration for prepared formula are lacking. Mothers who are too poor to purchase sufficient quantities of formula dilute it in futile attempts to stretch the supply. The result is increased malnutrition and infant death caused by too early weaning and improper and inadequate bottle-feeding.

The expense of infant formula to a poor family is extraordinary. For many the cost of properly feeding one child exclusively on formula may represent as much as 30 percent or more of the total family income. A properly nourished mother can feed herself and her infant for considerably less money and at virtually no risk to their health. Is it possible to overcome the mother's almost magical faith in infant formula and reverse this trend? Can governments in low-income countries encourage maternal nursing through a nutrition-education campaign aimed at convincing mothers that human milk is safe, sanitary, ready-made, simple, and inexpensive? Unhappily, in the light of current economic and political realities, governmental efforts to control infant-formula advertising and aggressive marketing practices have been largely ineffective.

Modern Perspective

There has also been a decline of breast-feeding in the developed countries of the Satisfied World—but for different reasons. According to Dr. Samuel Fomon, a pediatrician and expert in infant nutrition in the United States, only 30 percent of American women breast-feed their infants for even one week and only 15 percent for as long as two months.* He believes that the fact that women who breast-feed are in the

---

* Samuel Fomon, *Infant Nutrition,* 2d ed. (Philadelphia: W.B. Saunders, 1974) pp. 474–75.

minority discourages other women from even considering breast-feeding. Moreover, many women in developed countries work and pursue other interests and activities outside the home. It may be necessary for mothers to be separated from their infants for nine or ten hours at a time, and therefore breast-feeding may not be feasible. In addition, oral contraceptives seriously interfere with success in breast-feeding.

Many cultural and aesthetic factors enter into the decision not to breast-feed. As a consequence, when breast-feeding is no longer the norm in a country, women are generally inept at offering advice and encouragement to their sisters, daughters, and friends who may wish to breast-feed. Without widespread personal and social sanctions, the woman who encounters difficulty in breast-feeding may become tense and frustrated. If she turns to a physician for advice and support, she may find that even the doctor has little interest or experience in encouraging the practice. In fact, the doctor may recommend discontinuing breast-feeding rather than attempt to deal with the problems presented by the mother. Some physicians have begun to change their approach to this problem.

In some parts of the Satisfied World, among young, environmentally conscious mothers, breast-feeding is again gaining acceptability. These mothers, convinced of the natural superiority of breast milk, are overcoming pressures to abandon the practice. They point also to the savings in food resources and in energy utilized to prepare manufactured formula. Can this be the wave of the future in a world beset by shortages of food and energy resources? The problem is worth serious consideration and widespread discussion.

Selection 13 Malnutrition in Early Childhood: An Ecological View

J. Cravioto
E.R. DeLicardie

Editors' Introduction

A nutritional disease occurs when one or more nutrients are unavailable to perform metabolic activities and a disability, a

Source: Adapted from J. Cravioto and E.R. DeLicardie, "Malnutrition in Early Childhood," *Food and Nutrition* (FAO Quarterly), vol. 2, no. 4, 1976. Figures and complete notes and references appearing in this article are not included here; for further information consult the original version.

defect, or even death results. Success in the prevention and control of a nutritional disease is dependent on an understanding of the *ecology of malnutrition*. This term refers to the many factors that work together to produce a nutritional disease. It includes conditions that exist within the individual, the host; the relative lack of a nutrient, the agent; and the quality of the surrounding conditions, the environment.

The person who suffers from malnutrition is called the *host*. Age, sex, physiological and pathological status, habits and customs, genetic background, and psychological characteristics and reactions are known as *host factors*. They affect the individual's nutrient requirements and also affect the extent to which the nutrients can be utilized by the individual. For example, the physiological state of a person during pregnancy, lactation, or growth makes increased demands for nutrients. Other physiological states such as infection, gastrointestinal disease, certain metabolic diseases, and parasite infection also increase the nutrient requirements and may compound the course of malnutrition.

In developing countries many children suffer from repeated bouts with infections. These infections precipitate and aggravate nutrient inadequacies. Malnourished children who contract infections have reduced ability to combat diseases. Malnutrition and infection are synergistic—that is, they work together to produce a combined effect that is more severe than either would produce alone. In developing countries, deaths attributed to childhood diseases (such as measles) are really the result of the child succumbing to the combined effects of the infectious disease and the nutritional disorder. If these children were adequately nourished, these childhood diseases would not ordinarily be fatal.

The primary cause of a nutritional disorder is called the *agent*. This term refers to the relative lack of one or more nutrients for utilization by cells and tissues. Carbohydrates, fats, proteins (including the essential amino acids), vitamins, and minerals must all be present in sufficient quantity to function in one or more of the following roles: as sources of energy, as building materials, and as body regulators (as previously discussed in selections 5, 6, and 7).

Nutritional deficiencies usually occur when the quantity and quality of the diet is inadequate. *Quantity* refers to getting enough food to meet energy requirements. The term *quality* denotes getting enough proteins, vitamins, and critical minerals.

Biological, physical, economic, political, and sociocultural factors that influence nutritional status are referred to collectively as the *environment*. Any factor in the environment that interferes with the intake of an adequate diet, that increases the requirement for nutrients, or that interferes with the availability and utilization of nutrients increases the host's susceptibility to malnutrition.

As previously noted, nutrition is part of humankind's biological environment along with other major elements such as infectious-disease agents and the plants and animals that are the basis of the food chains that support life. The food supply is dependent on the physical environment, which includes such elements as the geography, land, soil, water, minerals, and climate as well as methods of agricultural production and distribution. The environment also includes the economic and political system as well as the power structure. These factors have a profound influence on the administrative policies governing the distribution of food and on the distribution of resources necessary for agricultural production. The economic structure will also influence the average income per person. Income affects the individual's food-buying power as well as the ability to purchase land and other resources necessary for agricultural production.

Educational attainment, a socioeconomic factor, is related to nutritional status. Education is necessary to obtain the skills needed to secure employment, to provide an understanding of what constitutes an adequate diet, and to obtain the knowledge and skills necessary to prepare food in a manner that will permit the preservation of nutrients. The sociocultural aspects of the environment also include the population distribution and food habits and customs. The population in a given area will influence the amount of food available per person, especially when the total food production does not keep up with the growth in population. Social customs, taboos, and superstition are major determinants of food intake and may limit the intake of an adequate diet.

Poverty and ignorance are among the principal causes of malnutrition throughout the world. Lack of available food, overpopulation, lack of education, antiquated agricultural methods, widespread health problems, unequal distribution of food, land, and capital within and among countries, and increasing urbanization are also major causes of malnutrition in developing countries. Since poverty and ignorance are the major causes of malnutrition, let us briefly explore some of their ramifications. In developing countries the typical annual income of the average family is 10 percent or less than the average per capita income of Americans. This less-than-marginal income severely limits the ability to purchase food and other means of subsistence; food must compete with the other necessities of life.

In rural areas the majority of people are either landless tenant farmers or farmers who must make a living from meager land, water, and other agricultural resources. They are unable to obtain the land, capital, machinery, and fertilizers needed to improve their standard of living. Because their standard of living is so hopeless, they often migrate in large numbers from rural areas to urban centers despite the fact that unemployment and underemployment among the poor in urban centers are usually very high. Furthermore, their lack of education is a great handicap in urban centers. They lack the skills necessary to get jobs. Lack of education and ignorance not only hamper the ability to find employment but also result in the unwise use of whatever limited money is available for food. Poor food choices lead to an inadequate diet. Those who are ignorant about the principles of nutrition are also particularly susceptible to food faddism and substitutions and may refuse to eat available nutritious food.

As the previous discussion illustrates, each element in the environment does not operate independently. All environmental factors are intertwined and act together to constitute a complex or a composite—an environment acting as an ecological unit. With humankind, they form an ecosystem. By studying the ecosystem we can identify problem areas and plan programs that will be more effective in combating malnutrition.

In recent years, there has been an increasing interest in the ways through which environment can affect man. Growth and development have become a major topic of interest for an increasing number of persons and institutions dealing with social, political, and economic policies. This, in turn, has led to the consideration of unfavorable environment as an important factor in the life of the individual from the time of conception to socially functioning adulthood.

Among the many features of the child's environment, nutrition has been accepted almost as a prerequisite for optimal growth and development. Nowadays nobody denies that a diet adequate in quantity and quality is a relevant factor in the life of man and, perhaps, the most ubiquitous factor affecting growth, health, and development. Since inadequate nutrition is a characteristic of social, cultural, and educational deprivation, it has become essential to define through research the relationship between malnutrition and such manifestations as depressed levels of intellect and elevated rates of school failures and learning disabilities, and the interaction of this negative influence with other adverse social, cultural, and educational circumstances affecting the child.

It is of the utmost importance to realize that even if at first appearance nutrition is primarily related to physical environmental factors such as climate, weather, topography, and geological structure, and to the biologic component of human environment represented mainly by its food chains, the primordial determinant of the nutritional status of a population is the social environment.

Malnutrition at the community level is a man-made disorder characteristic of the underprivileged segments of society. This is particularly true of the preindustrial societies, characterized by a social system which consciously or unconsciously creates malnourished individuals generation after generation through a series of social mechanisms such as limited access to goods and services, limited social mobility, and restricted experiential opportunities at crucial points in life.

The understanding of malnutrition in man thus requires an ecologic frame of reference in which the social, psychological, and cultural aspects of human behavior are appropriately related to the biological nature of man and to the physical environment in which he lives. Nutrition is above all an important focus on organized human behavior.

Nutritional inadequacy in preindustrial societies and in underprivileged segments of affluent societies is manifested by a series of disease states, which, although usually affecting a large proportion of those populations, are particularly prevalent in the vulnerable groups: infants and young children, and lactating and pregnant women. This is due to the influence of the social milieu on individuals whose physiological requirements for nutrients are the highest.

The Nature of Malnutrition in Infancy

The ecologic nature of malnutrition—in particular of its most prevalent expression on a worldwide basis, protein-calorie malnutrition in young infants—can be [conceptualized as] . . . a series of [pathways] . . . constructed with data obtained from studies of several communities in central Mexico, Central America, South America, and Africa.

[The first pathway is composed of] . . . the influences that operate in a society in which systematic application of modern technology is minimal or absent: a sector of the population would have a low purchasing power as a result of a limited income, and since the total income (measured as the rate of conversion of energy into consumption goods) is barely enough to cope with the minimal necessities of life, lack of surplus or reserves will limit investment in environmental sanitation. This in turn will maintain, in the group, traditional concepts on health and disease. This unscientific concept of the role of food in the production of disease is one of the main determinants of the pattern of distribution of available food within the family according to age and gives as a net result a reduction in the type and amounts of food that the infant is allowed to consume. This ultimate step would then be responsible for malnutrition. . . .

A second pathway, initiated by the lack of surpluses, proceeds to pressures for early school-leaving as an attempt to increase the purchasing power of the family unit. A consequence of this would be illiteracy, or at least a diminished opportunity for receiving adequate information, which establishes a feedback mechanism for technological backwardness and for the persistence of primitive concepts on health and disease.

Early school-leaving would in turn result in society giving adulthood status and role to a group of individuals at an earlier age than would be the case had they remained as pupils. This leads to the increased probability of marriage at a younger age to an equally uneducated spouse and the procreation of a larger number of children, with the further probability of inadequate child care, increased frequency of illness, and malnutrition.

A third pathway has at least two different starting points. One could be considered as a branching at the level of the persistence of primitive conceptions of health and disease which results in insufficient awareness of the hygienic requirements of the child. This, through a chain of unsanitary conditions in the community and in the home, would lead to a higher frequency of infectious processes in the child which directly or indirectly produce malnutrition. A second starting point is the link between inadequate child care in the large uneducated family and the poor personal-hygiene cycle just described. The increased morbidity would increase expenditures in health services, acting thus as a feedback mechanism for low purchasing power.

The possibility that malnutrition may result in suboptimal functioning of the individual makes it necessary, within this context, to consider the role of food and feeding in several dimensions. The first one, which may be called a physiological dimension, has as a unit of measurement the nutrient and its function to provide chemical substances to the organism for growth, maintenance, and metabolic regulation.

The second dimension of food may be considered as psychophysical. Its unit of measurement would be the foodstuff, which through its organoleptic characteristics would provide the organism with a variety of stimuli (such as texture, color, aroma, flavor, temperature). In this context a foodstuff presented at the table as two different kitchen preparations having the same nutrient and caloric content would, in fact, appear as if two different foods were offered to the individual.

Finally, the third food dimension may be considered as psychosocial in nature. Its unit of measurement would be the meal time. The functions of food in this context are, on the one hand, to aid in symbol formation through the value family and society attach to food as a form of reward or punishment, as an identifying characteristic of an ethnic or subcultural group and so on. On the other hand, the meal time provides opportunities to demonstrate, clarify, and practice role and status at the family and at the community level. Who is waited on first? Who sits at the place of honor at the table? Who is served the choice bits?

It seems easy to visualize that food deprivation in young children represents not only a shortage of nutrients necessary for the increase in body mass but also a deprivation of sensory stimuli and of social experiences. Is it surprising that children who suffered food deprivation in early life show at later ages a lower mental, physical, and social performance as compared to those who were not deprived?

The presence of malnutrition in conjunction with a high prevalence of other potential conditions of risk for maldevelopment makes it difficult to determine the contribution which the malnutrition per se may be making to the inhibition of growth and development. The problem is particularly complicated as it relates to mental development, because of the varying degrees at which the central nervous system is vulnerable to damage at different ages. Thus, not only the fact of malnutrition, but *the time of life at which it has been experienced* must be taken into account, if the relation between exposure and outcome for the central nervous system and mental development is to be assessed.

The assessment of the developmental consequences of serious malnutrition experienced during infancy and the preschool years can rarely be fully evaluated at the time of the damage. This is particularly true when one wishes to assess the consequences of malnutritional exposure to such functions as intellectual ability, school achievement, and later social and economic competence. For the assessment of these consequences, a considerable gap in time must elapse between the periods in which the functions to be evaluated can be examined meaningfully.

This gap in time permits the operation of many environmental factors other than the fact of prior malnutrition to influence the course of the child's developing competence. For the effect of the nutritional variable to be assessed, the influence of these intervening events must be determined and related to outcome.

It would be wrong to think that the gap in time between the nutritional damage and the assessment of complex nervous system functions is to be lamented. Clearly, the effect of malnutrition on the developing nervous system is unlikely, except in rare cases, to be fully manifested by changes in simple reflex and adaptive behavior.

Many years ago, Lashley[1] demonstrated in his animal experimentation that as much as 20 percent of the rat cerebral cortex could be extirpated without demonstrable consequences for simple maze learning. However, Maier,[2] using the same species, showed that as little as 3 percent of destroyed tissue demonstrably affected more complex learning performances. Thus, lags in developmental differentiation or even distributed lesions produced in the nervous system by malnutrition would be expected to manifest themselves at varying distances in time from the age of the primary damage.

At these later ages, when more complex demands for integration are made, opportunities for increased sensitivity in the assessment of consequences exist. A time gap in the assessment of consequences, therefore, is essential if the full force of the potential damage is to be measured. However, the existence of a time gap does make it necessary to know and to account for the influence of social and other variables on the course of development during the intervening period.

Consequently, our interpretation of the role played by malnutrition in the production of disorders of growth and development is complicated by the presence of contaminating variables. These variables include infection, social disadvantage, and the complexities introduced by both the time of life at which malnutrition was experienced, and the dates at which more sensitive evaluation of its consequences for adaptive functioning may take place.

Some Consequences of Early Malnutrition

Mortality due, directly or indirectly, to protein-calorie malnutrition is manifested in preindustrial societies as an excess of deaths over the rate for the same age group in a society in which malnutrition is not prevalent. In other words, if, from the mortality rate in children from one to four years of age, one subtracts the corresponding rate observed in a similar age group living in a society in which malnutrition is not prevalent, one can reasonably assume that an important proportion of the excess of deaths can be ascribed to malnutrition. For example, in Mexico in 1967 the preschool-age mortality rate was 9.2 per thousand children; for the same year the preschool mortality rate in the United States was 0.9 per thousand. Thus, a major factor in the difference of 8.3 deaths per thousand preschool children could with confidence be attributed directly or indirectly to malnutrition. . . .

Besides the loss of human capital due to the excess of deaths produced by malnutrition, malnourished children suffer more severe infectious episodes than their well-nourished counterparts. Gordon et al.[3] have reported that the incidence of diarrhea in the rural area of Central America during the period from February 1961 to June 1962 was 22.9 percent in well-nourished children and 40.0 percent in severely malnourished children of the same age. Vega-Franco and associates[4] have documented that the frequency and severity of bacterial complications in measles in children below five years of age increased in direct proportion to the severity of malnutriton; total duration of sickness is thus increased making treatment more expensive, besides the higher risk of death due to a process generally benign in a well-nourished population.

The consequences of malnutrition in young children are not confined to the economic losses due to the higher risk of death. The awareness that in vast regions of the world the majority of school-children and adults have had at least one episode of malnutrition early in life makes it imperative to try to disentangle from the complex mesh of negative influences which characterize the world of disadvantaged children the particular contribution which malnutrition may make to the development of the lower mental performance characteristic of this segment of the population. . . .

Possible Mechanisms of Action of Malnutrition on Mental Performance

In attempting to define a causal linkage between insufficient dietary intake and subnormal mental functioning, at least two possibilities should be considered. The first one would postulate that nutrient deficiency affects the intellect by directly modifying the growth and biochemical maturation of the brain.

In favor of this explanation are the reports from investigators in Chile, Mexico, and Uganda, who have found a reduction in brain size and cell number in children who died from severe malnutrition.

The second hypothesis considers that malnutrition in children does not need to produce structural lesions of the central nervous system to affect intellectual competence, behavior, and learning. Three possible indirect mechanisms are postulated:

1. *Loss of learning time.* Since the child was less responsive to his environment when malnourished, at the very least he had less time in which to learn and had lost a certain number of months of experience. On the simplest basis, therefore, he would be expected to show some developmental lags.

2. *Interference with learning during critical periods of development.* Learning is by no means simply a cumulative process. A considerable body of evidence exists which indicates that interference with the learning process at specific times during its course may result in disturbances in function that are both profound and of long-term significance. Such disturbances are not merely a function of the length of time the organism is deprived of the opportunities for learning. Rather, what appears to be

important is the correlation of the experiential opportunity with a given stage of development, the so-called critical periods of learning. It is possible that exposure to malnutrition at particular ages may in fact interfere with development at critical points in the child's growth course and so provide either abnormalities in the sequential emergence of competence, or an undesirable redirection of the developmental course.

3. *Motivation and personality changes.* It should be recognized that the mother's response to the infant is to a considerable degree a function of the child's own characteristics of reactivity. One of the first effects of malnutrition is a reduction in the child's responsiveness to stimulation and the emergence of various degrees of apathy. Apathetic behavior in its turn can function to reduce the value of the child as a stimulus and to diminish the adult's responsiveness to him.

Thus, apathy can provoke apathy and so contribute to a cumulative pattern of reduced adult-child interaction. If this occurs it can have consequences for stimulation, for learning, for maturation, and for interpersonal relations, the end result being significant backwardness in performance on later, more complex learning tasks. It has been shown that experimental animals subjected to stimuli deprivation have a significant reduction in number and size of cells in the cerebral cortex.

Apart from whether or not insufficient nutrient intake per se can cause mental subnormality, it is evident that children who have survived the severe forms of malnutrition show alterations in intellectual performance and learning ability which clearly place them at a higher risk of failure to profit from school exposure.

Early Severe Malnutrition and Risk of School Failure

In a preindustrial society in which staying in school imposes a real sacrifice on the part of the parents and other members of the household, the demand for leaving school to contribute to the familial purchasing power may be a social mechanism which prevents the child from being classed as backward. Instead it casts him in the role of the victim whose sacrifice is necessary, almost indispensable, for the survival of the family group. It is conceivable that through this mechanism the self-esteem of these individuals may be sustained, since the self-concept, that is, the individual as he is known to himself, is the result of the reactions that other persons have to his behavior and of the expectations of others about his behavior. To remain in school could lead to a series of failures which would create a negative self-image which, in turn, would produce a self-concept in which the individual would have to define himself as incompetent. To abandon school, on the other hand, is to conform to the expected pattern of behavior, to take the role and status of a victim and thus to avoid a series of failures. Motivation to complete a fairly good number of school years, for example the national norm, would be markedly reduced under these circumstances.

It has been observed that children who were malnourished in infancy, or belong to families where food is not abundant, tend to develop anxiety about food. It is understandable that if a child is worried about what or when he will eat next time, his attention and motivation for learning will be reduced, limiting his probability of profiting from the school experience. Even if the child has good mental equipment, if his motivation is low, he will not learn early what the school expects of him. He may be forever handicapped or he may be another member who could not progress because his sacrifice was a need of his society.

Recently, Richardson and co-workers have examined the scholastic achievement of school-age children who suffered severe malnutrition in early life.[5] Efficiency in reading, writing, and arithmetic abilities as well as the teacher's evaluation of school performance was lower in survivors of malnutrition and in their siblings when compared to that of peers attending the same school grade. Teachers judged the survivors of malnutrition as lower in school performance level, with poor ability in the school tasks and giving a higher frequency of school problems. The school grade attained by the survivors of malnutrition was below the grade attained by both siblings and schoolmates of the same chronological age.

It is apparent from all that has been said that children who survived a severe episode of chronic malnutrition are at a higher risk of failure to profit from the cumulative knowledge available to their socio-economic group. Survival from severe malnutrition may constitute the event that starts a developmental path characterized by psychological defective functioning, school failure, and subsequent subnormal adaptive functioning.

At familial and societal levels, the ultimate result of this chain of events is what in an ecological sense could be called a "spiral" effect. A low level of adaptive functioning, lack of modern knowledge, social custom, infection, or environmental insufficiency of foodstuffs produce malnutrition which gives a large pool of survivors who come to function in suboptimal ways. Such survivors are themselves more at risk of being the victims of their poor socioeconomic environment, being less effective than otherwise would be the case in their social adaptations. In turn, they will choose mates of similar characteristics and may rear children under conditions and in a fashion fatally programmed to produce a new generation of malnourished individuals.

It is obvious from the consideration of unequal distribution of malnutrition among the various socioeconomic groups of society that its consequences are interacting with the negative impact of all the other factors present in those subsegments of the population which interfere with the optimal functioning of the individual. It is apparent that many questions, particularly those related to a causal relationship between nutrient deficiency and mental development, remain to be answered, but it is clear that the available knowledge leaves no doubts about the strong association between the antecedent of malnutrition in infancy and suboptimal performance at school age. It is also obvious from the review that the consequences of early malnutrition will be greatest when, after rehabilitation, the child continues to live in an environment in which both social and nutritional circumstances will continue to be poor and noxious for his growth and development.

Notes

1. K.S. Lashley, *Brain Mechanisms and Intelligence* (Chicago: University of Chicago Press, 1929).
2. N.R.F. Maier, "The Effect of Cerebral Destruction on Reasoning and Learning in the Rat," *Journal of Comparative Neurology* 54(1932):45.
3. J.E. Gordon, M. Guzman, W. Ascoli, and N.S. Scrimshaw,*La Enfermedad Diarreica en los Países en Desarrollo*, Discusiones técnicas XIV Reunión del Consejo de la OPS, Publicaciones Cientificas, no. 100 (1964), p. 14.
4. L. Vega-Franco, *Ecología de la Desnutrición y su Repercusión Socioeconómica en México*, en A. Cuellar, ed., *Nutrición y Pediatría* (México, D.F.: Soc. Mex. de Ped., 1964).
5. S.A. Richardson, H.G. Birch, and M.E. Hertzig, "School Performance of Children Who Were Severely Malnourished in Infancy," *American Journal of Mental Deficiency* 77(1973):623.

Selection 14 Eating in the Dark

Senate Select Committee
on Nutrition and Human needs

Editors' Introduction

In the last few years malnutrition has surfaced as a public concern in Canada and the United States. There was a time when many health professionals considered malnutrition a significant public health concern only in countries where the food supply was

Source: From U.S. Senate, Select Committee on Nutrition and Human Needs, report to 93rd Congress, 1st Session, Washington, D.C., 1974. Figures and tables appearing in this article are not all included here; for further information consult the original version.

limited. Before 1968, when several reports on hunger and malnutrition among the poor in the United States came into national focus, few politicians or citizens saw a need for major efforts to change the pattern of food consumption in North America.

Today malnutrition clearly does exist in Canada and the United States. As in less technologically developed countries, malnutrition is the result of poverty, ignorance, misinformation, the uneven distribution of food supplies, and the overprocessing of food. The Ten State Survey (1968–1970), and HANES—Health and Nutrition Evaluation Survey—(1971–1972) in the United States, and Nutrition Canada (1970–1972) have disclosed a number of nutritional problems in these affluent countries.

Many people, especially those in low income and minority groups, were found to be malnourished. The most commonly observed dietary inadequacies were deficiencies of iron, vitamin A, and vitamin C. Dietary inadequacy in vitamins A and C does not necessarily identify malnutrition, but it is highly suggestive of nutritional risk. The term *nutritional risk* refers to factors that increase a person's chances of developing malnutrition. A high incidence of iron-deficiency anemia was observed in menstruating and pregnant women, infants, and young children. Iron-deficiency anemia is a form of malnutrition.

The growth of poor children under the age of six was below the standard norms in a number of areas in Canada and the United States. The differences in growth rate between low-income children and other children in the same ethnic and geographical area appeared to be related to the caloric content of the diet. Evidence suggests that poor children who do not get as much to eat as other children in the same ethnic group and same geographical area also do not grow as fast. Protein intakes were generally adequate and often excessive. However, protein-calorie intakes were frequently low among teenage girls.

Nutritional problems were by no means confined to these groups. In fact, the average American is more likely to be overfed than underfed. Obesity was a major problem in all age, sex, socioeconomic, and ethnic groups studied. Obesity is the result of excessive calories and lack of physical activity. Under these circumstances, weight is gained because the caloric intake of the diet exceeds individual caloric expenditure.

When the term *malnutrition* is applied to North Americans, it usually refers to the excessive intake of calories, fat, saturated fat, salt (sodium), and cholesterol and to their relationship to the development of certain chronic diseases. These diseases include heart disease, high blood pressure (hypertension), and diabetes mellitus. Saturated fats contain long-chained fatty acids that carry the maximum possible number of hydrogen atoms. In general, animal fats tend to be saturated fats. Unsaturated fats contain fatty acids that lack four or more hydrogen atoms and have two or more double bonds. Most vegetable oils are polyunsaturated fats. Cholesterol is a substance found in the fatty portion of animal foods and foods of animal origin.

Recent research indicates that the excessive consumption of fat, saturated fat, cholesterol, and calories in the diet is a contributing factor in the development of arteriosclerosis and coronary heart disease. The term *arteriosclerosis* refers to the hardening of the inner layer (intima) of the arterial walls. The disease results in the reduction of the blood flow through the vessels. The obstruction of the blood flow is life threatening because oxygen and the food supply to body cells are curtailed. Atherosclerosis is a type of arteriosclerosis characterized by the patchy thickening of the intima as a result of cholesterol deposits. The arteries are particularly affected at branching points. These diseases are among the leading causes of death in Canada and the United States.

The United States Senate appointed the Select Committee on Nutrition and Human Needs, and the following selection is an excerpt from the testimony before that committee.

One in three men in the United States can be expected to die of heart disease or stroke before age sixty, and one in six women. It is estimated that 25 million Americans suffer from high blood pressure and that about 5 million are afflicted by diabetes mellitus. These diseases have been directly related to overconsumption of certain foods.

At the same time, millions of Americans are not receiving the nutrients they need. The Department of Health, Education, and Welfare's Health and Nutrition Evaluation Survey (HANES) reported in 1974, for example, that significant numbers of children are deficient in iron. The highest incidence of this learning-impeding deficiency was found among black children, ages one to five, above the poverty line, where 22 percent were affected. Protein deficiency was found to increase with age, hitting hardest among whites age forty-five to fifty-nine, where 15 percent of the sample was found affected.

The consequences of malnutrition both through the over- and underconsumption of nutrients is expensive not only in terms of human suffering and wasted potential, the monetary cost is staggering. . . .

In a paper prepared for the select committee in 1969, *Economic Benefits from the Elimination of Hunger in America*, Barry M. Popkin, of the Institute of Research on Poverty at the University of Wisconsin, made the following estimates of economic benefits that might flow from eliminating malnutrition among the poor . . . :

- *Education*—Improved nutrition improves learning, prevents an interruption of cognitive development, and increases the ability to concentrate and work ($6.4–19.2 billion).
- *Physical performance*—Improved nutrition increases the capacity for prolonged physical work, raises the productivity of workers, and increases the motivation to work ($6.4–25.8 billion).
- *Morbidity*—Improved nutrition results in higher resistance to disease and lowers the severity of disease ($201–502 million).
- *Mortality*—Improved nutrition decreases fetal, infant, child, and certain types of maternal mortality ($68–157 million).
- *Intergenerational effects*—Improved nutrition makes healthy mothers who have healthy children. Also, better educated parents lead to better educated children ($1.3–4.5 billion).

It is clear that poor nutrition is a major public health problem in the United States. Its cause is rooted in our habits and our economic system, and it is a problem greatly aggravated by ignorance.

The Diseases of Overabundance

Testifying at the National Nutrition Policy hearings, Dr. William E. Connor, cochairman of the select committee's panel on nutrition and health, reported:

> The vast majority of Americans suffer from overabundance of food. The changed ecology of our land . . . has led to a whole new spectrum of diseases in which nutritional factors either play the prime etiological role or else are highly contributory to the development of the given disease state, that is coronary heart disease, obesity, and so on.

He presented the following list of primary or contributing dietary factors in some of the most widespread diseases.

1. *Coronary heart disease*—An excessive amount of cholesterol, saturated fat, and calories in the diet.
2. *High blood pressure*—Dietary salt and excessive calories contributing to obesity.
3. *Diabetes mellitus*—Excessive calories with associated obesity (also high dietary-cholesterol and saturated-fat intakes may predispose to the vascular complications of diabetes).
4. *Obesity*—Excessive calories and lack of physical activity with the result that caloric intake exceeds caloric expenditure.
5. *Dental caries*—High intake of sugar.
6. *Liver disease*—Excessive usage of alcohol.

Table 14.1 shows the 10 leading causes of death in the United States, with the diet-related illnesses noted.

Table 14.1 Death Rates for the Ten Leading Causes of Death, United States, 1972

Rank and Cause of Death	Death Rate	Percent of Total Deaths
Diseases of heart*	361.3	38.3
Malignant neoplasms, including neoplasms of lymphatic and hematopoietic tissues	166.6	17.7
Cerebrovascular diseases*	100.9	10.7
Accidents	54.6	5.8
Influenza and pneumonia	29.4	3.1
Diabetes mellitus*	18.8	2.0
Certain causes of mortality in early infancy	16.4	1.7
Arteriosclerosis*	15.8	1.7
Cirrhosis of liver*	15.7	1.7
Bronchitis, emphysema, and asthma	13.8	1.5
All other causes	148.9	15.8
All causes	942.2	100.0

Note: Table 14.1 is based on 10 percent sample of deaths; rates per 100,000 population.

* Nutrition-related causes

These illnesses, even though they are related to the overconsumption of certain foods, are not peculiar to any one income level. . . . the HEW Health and Nutrition Evaluation Survey (HANES), shows that obesity, one of the nation's major health problems, is suffered almost equally at almost all income levels.

Experience in other nations as well as our own indicates that a general reduction of certain foods in the diet is likely to lead to improved health. . . . there is a greater incidence of death from heart disease in the more affluent nations where the intake of cholesterol is higher.

European experience during World Wars I and II offers further evidence that reduction in consumption can be healthful. . . .

[A] . . . Swedish report gave the following advice "as regards average diets in Sweden"

— The fat content should be reduced . . .
— The consumption of sugar and sugar-rich products should be reduced by at least a quarter.
— Saturated fat should as far as possible be replaced by polyunsaturated fats.
— The consumption of vegetables, fruit, potatoes, dairy products with a low fat content, fish, lean meat, poultry, bread and other cereal products should be proportionately increased in accordance with proposals from the National Institute of Public Health.

The diet is very similar to the "alternative" diet for reducing fat and cholesterol consumption recommended by the select committee's panel. . . .

Undernutrition

The underconsumption of nutrients, the other half of the nation's nutrition problem, is widespread, and it affects many of those also afflicted by diseases just mentioned. Dietary deficiencies may affect stamina, outcome of pregnancy, learning ability, growth and susceptibility to illness.

The 1965 Household Food Consumption Survey, conducted by the Department of Agriculture, found insufficient dietary intake of vitamins A and C, B₆, thiamine, riboflavin, iron, and calcium among significant numbers of its sample population. The Ten State Nutrition Survey, directed by HEW and gathering data from 1969 to 1970, also found substantial nutrient deficiencies, as did the most recent nutrition survey, HANES. The preliminary HANES report, based on data gathered between 1971 and 1972, found great deficiencies in nutrient intake, especially among persons below the poverty level. . . .

While nutrient deficiencies strike at most income levels, the forgoing figures show that the poor are at greatest nutritional risk. This was also a finding of the Household Food Consumption Survey and the Ten State Survey, which said:

> persons with lower income, with lesser parental education, blacks, Spanish-Americans, and persons from low-income areas tend to have a higher prevalence of multiple deficiencies.

Other Factors Affecting Nutritional Health Status

Perhaps the most significant factor affecting the composition of the American diet is food prices. Food prices rose 43 percent between September 1972 and September 1975. This rapid increase has led families to trade down on the food scale, for instance from meat to beans, causing an increase in the prices of staples. At the same time, shoppers are reported to be buying less convenience foods and returning to basics.

Another significant factor is the shift to eating more meals away from home. Between 1971 and 1974 the percent of personal income spent on meals away from home rose from 3.4 to 3.5 percent, and the trend is expected to continue.

An HEW internal report on nutrition, written in 1971 . . . said that changing patterns of consumption have "made obsolete some of the food fortification and improvement practices initiated by regulations over the last twenty to thirty years. . . ."

Still another factor is the change in composition of foods and the use of food additives. In many cases, we possess inadequate knowledge of food compositions, and we are unable to measure its impact. . . .

Various curative and biological control preparations, increasingly being introduced into the market, also affect nutritional health. For example, use of contraceptive steroid pills may affect vitamin B_6 nutrition.

Nutrition Knowledge

In spite of the evidence relating nutrition to health, the obvious changes in eating habits and in food itself, Americans have almost no access to a means of measuring their individual nutritional health.

Although there is ample evidence of widespread nutrient deficiency and imbalance, the average medical examination does not thoroughly inquire into the nutritional status of the patient. The rate for heart attack among men from thirty-five to forty-four years is five times greater when the blood cholesterol level is over 260 mg percent than if it is under 200 mg percent, yet how many men know their cholesterol level? Iron deficiency anemia is widespread among children and can affect learning; but how many mothers know the iron status of their children? . . . the medical profession has been extremely slow to take nutrition seriously. Doctors and nutritionists consulted in the preparation of this report said uniformly that nutritional evaluation in most physical examinations is done in a cursory fashion, if at all; that no uniform standards are currently being applied in nutritional assessment; and that doctors generally do not follow up on prescribed diet changes even though experience indicates that the importance a physician attaches to a diet is a major factor in its success. Possibly the most striking evidence of the medical profession's disdain for nutrition, however, are the findings of malnutrition in hospitals.

Filling the Vacuum

The vacuum in individual and collective nutrition knowledge leaves the field open for "painless" diet plans and fraudulent reducing devices. It also allows the food industry through advertising to guide diet choices toward the most profitable foods and toward ever-increasing food consumption. . . .

Not only do television networks find great economic advantage in food advertising, they would find considerable economic peril in running ads attempting to counter heavy consumption of the foods found related to health problems. A television executive said in an interview he was free to run nutrition spots showing the virtues of eating nutritious foods that would be alternatives for food such as candy but that pressure from advertisers would not permit spots advising reduced consumption of foods containing high levels of cholesterol or sugar.

Selection 15 Changing Public Diet

Beverly Winikoff

Editors' Introduction

In the United States efforts have begun to develop strategies for combating hunger and malnutrition. The Senate Select Committee on Nutrition and Human Needs issued a policy statement declaring that "All citizens shall have access to an adequate and safe supply of food and ability to identify, select, and prepare an optimal diet irrespective of social or economic status." The following four ideas were among the proposals for accomplishing these goals.

Income maintenance. Millions of Americans are poor. Approximately 25.5 million individuals, 13 percent of the population, are living in poverty. Far too many Americans still find it hard to obtain a nutritionally adequate diet as well as other basic essentials of life. The provision of cash payments in the form of income maintenance rather than food stamps and commodity distribution would mean that the family itself becomes the major determinant of how much money is spent on food.

Special nutritional and home management consideration for vulnerable groups. Certain segments of our population are particularly vulnerable to malnutrition. They include pregnant and nursing women, infants, children of all ages, and teenagers, as well as the elderly and ill. It was urged that special efforts be made to assess the nutritional status of people in these groups, to identify special problems, and to provide those individuals in need

Source: Adapted from Beverly Winikoff, "Changing Public Diet," *Human Nature* (January 1978):60–65. Reprinted with permission from *Human Nature* Magazine. Copyright © 1978, Human Nature, Inc. Tables appearing in this article are not included here; for further information consult the original version.

with remedial services including nutritious meals, nutrition counseling, rehabilitative services, and home management counseling.

A comprehensive nutrition education program. The recommendation for a comprehensive nutrition education program envisions formal nutrition teaching in schools from early years through advanced instruction in universities. Less formal methods of nutrition education would be carried on in communities to create public concern for the nation's nutrition problems, to foster understanding of nutrition, to disseminate information regarding food programs, and to promote better food habits.

Nutritional counseling as an integral aspect of preventative and remedial health care. Many types of nutrition problems contribute to poor health and disability with accompanying loss of productivity. Since many problems require dietary modifications for prevention and treatment, the provision of nutrition services (particularly nutrition counseling) is needed as a built-in part of health care. Nutrition services should also be built into and provided at community health care centers, hospitals, and other social and health care institutions for ambulatory populations as well as in- and outpatients.

Significant nutrition-related problems include obesity, nutrition-deficiency diseases (especially iron-deficiency anemia), dental disease, infant mortality, chronic health care problems (including diabetes mellitus), and cardiovascular disease. The major dietary problems appear to be related to the *affluent diet*— that is, the overconsumption of food, meaning too many calories, too much fat, too much sugar, and increasingly too many calories from sugar and alcohol.

In the following reading Dr. Beverly Winikoff, a nutritionist and medical doctor, suggests ways to realize the goals set forth by the policy statement of the Senate Select Committee on Nutrition and Human Needs.

"An apple a day keeps the doctor away" is probably the most familiar expression of the influence of diet on health. But Americans, as a group, have not succeeded in keeping the doctor away. The medical man and his assistants, his drugs, his machines, and his hospitals are steadily consuming more of our money, our time, and our thoughts.

Over 70 percent of all deaths in the United States in 1973 were casued by diseases linked to the composition of our diet, including high levels of fat, sugar, and salt. The leading causes of death, heart disease and stroke, are strongly related to the types of food we eat and overeat. If we could eliminate these disorders, we would add eighteen years to a baby's life expectancy, according to Leonard Hayflick of the Children's Hospital Medical Center in Oakland, California. Eliminating cancer, he estimates, would increase a baby's life expectancy by only two years.

In some sense we must have neglected to eat the aggregate apple. Our daily diet has been so distorted that it no longer protects us from the medical man's attentions. Over the last century—even over the last generation—our eating habits have changed markedly. As a society, we have embraced new and untested eating patterns.

According to conventional nutritional wisdom, efforts to significantly alter a community's pattern of eating are hopeless. The importance of dietary preferences to societies and individuals—rice to most Asians, tortillas to Mexicans—suggests that eating habits are difficult to change. But the idea of an "immutable diet" is a myth and it has become a barrier that frustrates efforts to think rationally about the American diet. On the other hand, if we can understand why we eat the way we do, we may be able to use governmental influence and industrial creativity to improve our eating patterns.

History proves that diet can undergo both rapid and major change with easy, even eager, community acceptance. Corn is not indigenous to East Africa, but it has become the major staple in large areas of that region in only a few generations. Sweet cola beverages are accepted, even coveted, from the Amazon jungles to the Russian steppes despite the absence of local traditions regarding soft drinks. In the United States, yogurt, traditionally a food of Balkan and eastern European herdsmen, is a nutritional craze and serves in various forms as a substitute for ice cream, mayonnaise, and sour cream.

If these examples disprove the myth that people refuse to change the way they eat, they also give grounds for believing that problems caused by dietary patterns can be attacked logically and effectively.

But these and other dietary changes have occurred for reasons more pressing and personal than the exhortations of professionals. Before we can develop a public policy on nutrition, we need to identify the influences behind dietary alterations, the implications of these changes, and the impediments to revisions of diet.

Eating habits that may link the way we eat to the way we die include: (1) an increase in the percentage of calories derived from fat; (2) an increase in refined-carbohydrate consumption, mainly sugar; (3) an increase in the amount of protein from animal sources; (4) an increase in salt intake; (5) a decrease in the consumption of foods containing crude fiber, especially fresh fruits and vegetables.

Since 1909, according to the U.S. Department of Agriculture, the caloric intake of each American has decreased slightly, but the amount of fat consumed has increased by 25 percent. Although the share of calories derived from protein has remained relatively constant, the quantity of protein derived from animal sources—particularly beef—has risen considerably. This means that with their protein, Americans are served a hefty helping of the saturated fats and cholesterol suspected of being causes of heart disease.

Carbohydrate consumption has decreased by approximately 25 percent, but the sources of starch and sugar have changed remarkably. Between 1909 and 1913, Americans ate 68 percent of their carbohydrates in the form of complex starches—fruits, vegetables, and whole grains—and 32 percent as sugar. By 1976, only 47 percent of dietary carbohydrates came from complex carbohydrate sources and 53 percent came from sugar. The consumption of refined sugar rose from an average of 76.7 pounds per person in 1909 to 102.4 pounds per person in 1971. Much of this increase was due to the popularity of soft drinks: consumption per person nearly doubled between 1960 and 1975. Every American, according to the U.S. Department of Agriculture, drinks an average of 221 sixteen-ounce cans of soda a year.

If what we eat has changed, so has the way we prepare it. Accustomed to shortcuts, we obtain more and more calories from processed foods, with a significant increase in the cost of nutrients. Each American ate more than 400 pounds of unprocessed fruits and vegetables and less than 100 pounds of processed produce in 1929; in 1971 each of us consumed approximately 300 pounds of processed and 250 pounds of unprocessed fruits and vegetables.

These trends are worrisome for two reasons. One is that as we eat more processed foods and obtain more calories from sugar and fat, the burden of providing the vitamins and minerals necessary to maintain health falls to a more limited range of foods. We leave ourselves less leeway to choose a diet that satisfies nutritional requirements. Women of childbearing age have particular difficulty in obtaining enough iron. More serious is the relationship between present dietary patterns and the major fatal diseases. High-fat, high-cholesterol, refined-carbohydrate foods combined with a tendency toward sedentary behavior have markedly increased the number of obese Americans. Fully one-third of our population is overweight to a degree that will diminish life expectancy.

Because obesity is associated with hypertension and increased blood-cholesterol and blood-sugar levels, it increases the risk of a person's having coronary disease, hypertensive illness, stroke, or diabetes. Using data from the long-term Framingham study of heart disease, investigators predicted that a 10 percent increase in weight among men between thirty-five and fifty-five years of age would increase the incidence of coronary disease by 30 percent, while a weight loss of the same amount would decrease it by 20 percent. Other illnesses linked to what we eat are: high blood pressure (salt); dental caries and possibly the kind of diabetes that begins in adulthood (sugar); colitis and perhaps some cancers (low-fiber foods). In living the "good life" represented by rich, sweet foods, we expose ourselves to increased health risks.

If we are concerned about the way we eat as adults, we should be doubly concerned about the way we feed the next generation. Nutritionists emphasize breast-feeding in developing countries because of significant economic, psychological, hygienic, and immunologic advantages, but they ignore the same benefits in industrial societies in favor of prepared formulas, which are more expensive but socially acceptable.

The pattern of artificial feeding from birth and the introduction of solid foods too early in life is particularly ominous. The combination produces babies that grow bigger and fatter—and do so faster—than breast-fed babies. These pleasingly plump infants are two to three times more likely to be obese as adults than average-weight and lightweight infants. Given the health problems associated with obesity, we are not serving the next generations well by feeding babies for plumpness, as we do penned livestock.

Judging from the way most Americans eat, one might suppose that they are unaware of the relationship between diet and health; this is not so. A Harris poll conducted early in 1977 revealed that people were surprisingly knowledgeable about good nutrition. Three out of four people polled were concerned with cholesterol and considered it important to limit the amount they ate. Two out of five thought that they would be healthier if they included more fish, fruit, and whole grain bread in their diet. Approximately the same number believed they would be healtheir if they consumed less white bread, coffee, butter, salt, sugar, and soft drinks. Over one-quarter said they should include fewer eggs in their diet, and close to one-half recognized that too much salt is related to hypertension.

But these nutritionally informed people did not act on the facts they knew, and further questioning revealed frequent misconceptions of the implications of these facts. They grossly underestimated the chances that they themselves might contract any of the common killing diseases. A clear majority viewed it as unlikely that they would ever have diabetes, heart attacks, stroke, high blood pressure, or any of the major types of cancer, which in combination kill about two out of every three Americans.

Many of those polled misunderstood the seriousness of major diseases and believed that cures exist where none do or that major breakthroughs would occur in their lifetimes. One-third believed that 60 percent of lung-cancer victims survive their illness, whereas in reality 90 percent die from the disease within five years of diagnosis.

Even when given nutritional information people are not persuaded to change their diet. Many health campaigns have failed because their messages induce fear: Act in certain ways, or suffer horrible consequences. In an essay on behavioral change, Judith Henderson and Allen Enelow of the University of the Pacific in San Francisco noted that techniques that arouse fear are "disastrous unless accompanied by specific recommendations for action."

Unfortunately, much health advice is vague, difficult to understand, and moralistic. The public, even when willing to follow the guidelines, is often unsure what to do. Messages about eating foods from the seven—or four—food groups, and admonitions to reduce cholesterol or saturated fats are among the most confusing. Poorly expressed educational advice goes unheeded while commercial messages make their points clearly and often humorously, demanding simple action: Buy a particular product.

Information on health is received and used together with many other environmental influences. In this sense, individual nutrition does not depend so much on medical advice as on the response to incentive systems at all political and social levels. When social and economic pressures conflict with factual information, the former usually prevails. If nutritional facts are to affect American choices of food, the lessons of science must be integrated into the incentives of the socioeconomic system.

These forces make it hard to act on health recommendations. We are exposed to barrages of commercials for soft drinks, sweet snacks, high-fat foods, cigarettes, and alcohol. The government subsidizes tobacco production with price supports. There are candy machines in our schools and cigarette machines in our offices.

In 1970, the lunches served to schoolchildren were rated as even higher in saturated fats than the average American diet. And we can assume that lessons learned in the lunchroom are stronger determinants of eating habits than rules taught in the classroom.

Until 1972, federal law prohibited the sale of milk products in which highly saturated fat was replaced by vegetable oils. When the law was overturned, the Department of Agriculture imposed artificially high prices on such milk products.

These government actions, which are contrary to good nutrition, may be inadvertent or may result from a lack of coordination or from the failure to evaluate their potential effect on health. Too often the government assumes—erroneously—that nutrition is affected only by policies specifically labeled "health."

In reality, nutrition is influenced by decisions—or lack of them—in almost every area of governmental concern, including agriculture, taxes, budget, land use, and import-export regulations. Nutrition is also affected by industrial decisions regarding food production, transportation, processing, and marketing. All these, in turn, are affected by various government regulations. In effect, the government sets out the national buffet.

When we fail to consider the impact on nutrition of these government decisions, we doom efforts to improve general health because we fail to promote other opportunities to eat the "apple a day" that keeps the doctor away. It is illogical to run to a doctor to be told that we are eating apples from the wrong tree or to be carried to the hospital once we have poisoned ourselves with too many of the wrong apples. In nutritional terms, prevention of illness should mean keeping people out of the medical care system.

The need to explore the nutritional impact of policy decisions in areas outside of medicine could be answered by the establishment of an agency designed to deal with nutrition. Such an office was proposed in 1975 by the Senate Select Committee on Nutrition and Human Needs.

In February 1977 the same committee released "Dietary Goals for the United States," the first federally sponsored document relating the overall pattern of diet to the health problems of the American people. The report examines the problem of the American diet not merely from a medical perspective but as part of the total system of food production. It also attempts to reverse disease patterns by suggesting a number of changes consumers might make in food selection and preparation.

The document culminates in logical, but in some ways timid, recommendations for government action; they do not address the problem as forcefully as does the analysis itself. The emphasis is on money for public education, money for the Departments of Agriculture and Health, Education and Welfare to develop food-processing techniques, and money for nutritional research—none of which would directly affect the structure of the American diet.

The committee's strongest recommendation is for expanded regulations governing the labeling of food products. The report advocates that the printing of percentage and types of fat, percentage of sugar, milligrams of salt and cholesterol, calorie content, and additives on all food packages be compulsory so that an individual can more easily choose a diet low in saturated fats, cholesterol, and sugar. Current nutritional labeling is voluntary for most products and identifies only the nutrient categories found in the Recommended Daily Allowances (protein, fat, carbohydrates, and certain vitamins and minerals).

One way to attain the dietary goals set by the Senate committee is to create incentives that will encourage consumers to demand and industry to produce nutritionally valuable foods. The baby-food industry is a case in point. Acknowledging popular concern over obesity in infants, Beech-Nut ceased adding sugar to its fruit juices for babies in 1976.

According to a Beech-Nut spokesman, sales doubled. In January 1977 Beech-Nut stopped adding salt to all its products because of concern over hypertension, and reduced or eliminated the remaining sugar and sweeteners. Sales rose about 20 percent in four months.

The vast networks of federal, state, and local institutions that buy and prepare food provide an opportunity to influence the diet of large segments of the population. Building nutritional specifications for fat, sugar, salt, and cholesterol into purchasing regulations for food served in prisons, schools, hospitals, and employee cafeterias would force private industry to produce nutritionally superior food products. Encouraging the sale of nutritionally sound items in vending machines would induce new creativity in production, packaging, and marketing.

The $5.5 billion spent by the federal government on food-supplementation programs, such as food stamps and the Women, Infants and Children's (WIC) Feeding Program, protect people against hunger, but they have had little impact on the usual American dietary patterns. Food stamps simply allow almost 18 million low-income Americans to stretch their food dollars to satisfy their personal preferences. The WIC program, designed to supply food to infants and pregnant and lactating women with inadequate nutrition, has been beset by administrative confusion and inconsistencies, and has never set uniform guidelines that would encourage a general upgrading of nutrition. The program has also neglected an opportunity to promote breast-feeding while providing mothers with free prepared infant formula.

If we are to create significant consumer demand for more nutritionally sound food, we need to assess the influence advertising exerts on our selection of foods. A recent study by Lynne Masover and Jeremiah Stamler of Northwestern University Medical School analyzed food advertising on four Chicago television stations. It found that on weekdays over 70 percent, and on weekends over 85 percent, of such advertising promotes products believed to be detrimental to health: foods high in fats, cholesterol, sugar and/or salt. A report prepared by Richard Manoff, an advertising executive, suggested that more than 50 percent of the money spent on television food advertising touts items closely linked to the most significant risk factors in the American diet. The Senate Committee on Nutrition labeled this estimate conservative since the calculations did not include the advertising of sugared cereals, cake mixes, meat products, eggs, butter, and cheeses.

Several aspects of food promotion need to be carefully evaluated:
1. Advertised food items are presented as if they were in competition with other foods or food groups, and the tenor of advertising communicates, implicitly or explicitly, that the advertiser's product is necessary to good health. A corollary of such messages is that the more of

the product consumed, the better for the consumer's health. Americans are already faced with having to limit their consumption of calories if they are not to become overweight, so it seems inadvisable to urge increased consumption, particularly of foods with questionable nutritional value.

2. Advertising emphasizes the positive without mentioning the negative. Eating eggs, for example, is a low-cost way of getting extremely high-quality protein, but it is also a good way to consume extra cholesterol. "Who should eat eggs?" and "How many should be eaten?" are questions that need careful examination, but for answers the egg industry is not the best source.

3. Classification of foods in advertising can be misleading. Products better described as snacks or candy are advertised as children's breakfast cereals. These sugar-coated tidbits often lack the protein and vitamins a child needs in the morning and encourage a fondness for sweets.

4. Some new products are publicized as alternatives to more nutritious foods. Stuffing is urged as a replacement for potatoes, although it substitutes a processed product made of white bread crumbs for a low-calorie, high-fiber, unprocessed vegetable containing minerals and vitamins. It is not a good trade-off for health.

We should seriously consider whether food should be promoted over television. Although this idea raises thorny questions, public debate over the issues involved would at the least be educational.

Just as industries might be induced to promote healthful products in the marketplace, the existing systems of preventive care could also foster better eating habits. Nutrition, most concerned professionals acknowledge, is a neglected area of medicine. As a beginning, all group medical facilities could be encouraged to offer nutritional services so that physicians could refer patients to these services as they would to other specialists. As medical costs rise we might find it economical to pay for keeping people well. The professional who spends time trying to prevent disease by persuading a patient to change his diet deserves fees similar to those given professionals who attempt to cure the sick by prying, poking, testing, and cutting.

As one way of fighting obesity in young children, obstetrical services could encourage breast-feeding, a superior way of feeding babies for which there is no commercial advocate. Since education alone is not completely effective, we might try to foster an environment in which working mothers can nurse their infants as easily as mothers who stay at home. This could be accomplished through day-care centers in offices or flexible working hours for nursing mothers. These arrangements may appear far from the concerns of nutrition, but they are not. If people are to make decisions that will improve their health, we should make those options easier to choose. People cannot be expected to swim against commercial and socioeconomic currents.

The goal of national health policy should be to minimize illness by structuring a national environment that fosters well-being. Because we are certain that the kinds and amounts of food people eat affect their chances of having a heart attack or a stroke or diabetes, influencing diet through education, advertising, and agricultural policy has become as critical a determinant of health as the most sophisticated medical hardware.

Selection 16 Isn't There Anything Left to Eat?

Jean Mayer

Editors' Introduction

Many people in our society are motivated to eat sensibly for better health. The American consumer has become health conscious, diet conscious, nutrient conscious, and additive conscious. Thus we have a population eager to be informed but unable to distinguish fact from fiction. How did this inconsistency come about?

The development of the food assembly line from farmer to consumer and the development and promotion of new foods led to many questions. For example, what is the nutritional and health value of such convenience foods as TV dinners, pop tarts, and instant breakfast? Moreover, the entire food supply has become a matter of concern. The climate is now ripe for the "surefire" answers of the food faddists. The scientific world is often misinterpreted by the media. Many popular books and articles about nutrition have appeared, and old ones are gaining a new reading public. Such popular books and articles often raise the expectations of the public to unreasonable levels without benefiting either the public or the science of nutrition. The rhetoric and pamphleteering of amateur food zealots exaggerate the

Source: Adapted from Jean Mayer, "Isn't There Anything Left to Eat?" *Family Health* Magazine, February 1971. Reprinted with permission *Family Health* Magazine, February 1971©. All rights reserved.

hazards of certain dietary factors. They often do this for the wrong reasons and produce unfounded fears in certain sectors of our population. Some preach the return to the good old days when we relied only on natural foods, meaning unprocessed foods free of additives. The term is sometimes used interchangeably with the term *health foods*. The term *organic foods* refers specifically to foods grown in soil treated with natural fertilizers and free of additives and pesticide residues. All food is organic, however, and consumers must be careful not to be misled by this term into believing that foods labeled "organic" are nutritionally superior.

Why are the "good guys" seldom quoted? In this article world-famous nutritionist Jean Mayer expresses an understanding of the concerns of the average citizen and responds to them. He conveys his message by using the device of *expansio ad absurdam*—that is, by stretching nutritional claims to the point of absurdity. Reassuring the consumer about the overall safety of the American food supply, he offers the public a number of common-sense recommendations for the selection of safe and nutritious diets.

There used to be a popular joke about how everything that is fun in life is illegal, immoral, or fattening. In today's more complicated times, the literal-minded would feel compelled to add "or bad for your heart, liver, lungs, genes, brain, and bones."

It isn't just the nasty habits, such as smoking and drinking, you innocently acquired before you knew the facts. The problem is that you can't even do the things necessary to life without endangering life. At least you can't if you believe all the toxicologists, ecologists, consumer-protection groups, food crusaders, research scientists, and various other professional and amateur improvers of the quality of living. You can't breathe deeply in certain places at certain times; you mustn't exercise too strenuously or too little; and reproducing your own kind is fraught with genetic peril. Most terrifying of all is sitting down to a good meal.

An intelligent man who reads the papers, keeps up with current science, and takes life at all seriously must eye each plateful or glassful critically, with the following statements in mind (but without any means whatever of distinguishing "true" from "false" from "exaggerated"):

— *Cow's milk*—Its fat will cause heart disease; its lactose can make you blind. Contains DDT.
— *Mother's milk*—Contains so much DDT that, if bottled, it would not be permitted to cross state lines.
— *Eggs*—High in cholesterol; could give you a coronary.
— *White bread, spaghetti, macaroni, etc.*—Made of flour deficient in

nutrients. Most vitamins and minerals removed by milling, and only a few restored through the "enrichment" process.
— *Whole wheat bread*—Much the same, but has a few more nutrients. Also may retain more pesticides.
— *Brown rice*—Same as whole wheat bread. And also high in mercury.
— *Meat*—High fat content will give you heart disease. Contaminated by estrogens, which are carcinogenic and interfere with sex function. Lower in nutritive value, since animals are fed devitalized, chemically grown feeds.
— *Sausages and lunch meats*—Same as above. High in nitrates, nitrites, and other dangerous chemicals.
— *Fish*—Contaminated with mercury, DDT, and other toxicants.
— *Shellfish*—Veritable "Typhoid Marys" and source of infectious hepatitis. Contaminated with oil and pesticides.
— *Breakfast cereals*—Contain either "empty calories" or fill you up with "synthetic chemicals." Added sugar may promote diabetes.
— *Butter, hydrogenated vegetable fats*—Raise your blood cholesterol, give you heart disease.
— *Polyunsaturated oils*—Rumored to cause multiple sclerosis and cancer.
— *Vegetables and fruits*—Contaminated by pesticides, some of which are related to nerve gas.
— *Water*—Full of chemicals, including fluoride, which will harden your skull and soften your brain.
— *Coffee*—Promotes diabetes and coronaries. Keeps you awake nights.
— *Ice cream*—High in fat (heart disease) and in sugar (empty calories, diabetes), possibly flavored with cancer-causing chemicals.
— *Salt*—Promotes high blood pressure.
— *Liver*—A veritable repository of DDT, parathion, and artificial estrogens.
— *Cheeses*—Full of heart-threatening fat and cholesterol.
— *Yogurt*—Makes rats blind (if they eat nothing else).
— *Canned foods*—Devitalized, low in nutrients, filled with chemical preservatives and antioxidants.
— *Frozen foods*—Changes in store and home-freezer temperatures will bring about "bacterial infestation."

Obviously, a good deal of the above is nonsense, either because the proposition was untrue to start with or because its truth is carried to a ridiculous extreme. But if taken literally, the groans of the overweight, tying their shoes in the morning, would soon be replaced by the cry, "Isn't there anything left . . . to eat?" Nutritionists know there is. More than ever. And this nutritionist offers the following suggestions:

— Eat a *varied* diet. The greater your choice of foods, the less chance you will miss out on essential nutrients.
— Eat as many unprocessed foods as you can: meat, fish, milk, eggs, fruit, and vegetables. Eat fresh foods in season. Wash them well before serving.
— But remember that canned and frozen vegetables and fruits are useful foods that enable you to provide a varied and balanced diet when fresh goods are out of season. A variety of processed products—including fruits, juices, and vegetable soups—can help counterbalance our usually inadequate intake of the vitamins and minerals they contain.
— "Convenience foods" are fine. But your family will eat better if you prepare the food yourself. The simpler the preparation, the better the nutrition.
— Meat (beef, pork, poultry) provides protein, trace minerals, and certain vitamins, such as B_{12}. Choose leaner cuts. When eating, trim fat. Liver and organ meats are particularly lean. Bacon is relatively expensive and fat; if you must have bacon, Canadian bacon is leaner and nutritionally superior. Poultry is high in protein, low in fat.
— Fish and shellfish are high in protein, minerals, and polyunsaturated fat.
— White bread is a low-fat food. One slice has no more calories than a hard-boiled egg. If you prefer whole wheat or wheat germ bread, by all means have them. Do not discount enriched bread and bakery products. They are lower in some trace minerals and vitamins, but contain essential nutrients such as iron, which you may not get elsewhere.
— Milk and cheese are still the major sources of calcium. They contain many essential nutrients, including protein and vitamin B_2 (riboflavin). They do contain fat. But before you switch to relatively fat-free skim milk, try to cut down on other fats that do not contribute as much to nutrition, such as hydrogenated vegetable fat, bacon fat, and so forth.
— Eggs are a near-ideal food for many people, and particularly children, adolescents, and pregnant or lactating women. But middle-aged people with high cholesterol levels should limit their intake to about three eggs a week.
— Although there is still a great deal we do not know about fat, it seems reasonable, in cooking, to replace saturated (hard) fats with polyunsaturates such as safflower, corn, peanut, cottonseed, or fish oils. Actually a diet lower in fats of all kinds is a good idea.
— Go easy on the salt. It tends to accelerate blood pressure. As an alternative, use more spices, vinegar, and lemon juice.
— Although I set out to be reassuring about our diet, there is nothing

good I can find to say about sugar. The argument that "it is a source of calories and we need calories" is specious. True, the calories are present. But the nutrients are not. The difference between a good and bad diet is how much of the nutrients you get with the calories. Unfortunately, sugar is everywhere: soft drinks, candy, ice cream, baby-food vegetables, fruit juices, canned fruit in heavy syrup, and so on, to the point where the average American adult consumes about 100 pounds a year. At best, sugar is a necessary evil, making certain nutritious foods more palatable. We could lessen the evil by cutting down on its use. If you *have* to have sugar, brown sugar at least contains some trace minerals.

Carefully read labels on jars and cans. These should become more informative as to ingredients and caloric content as the recommendations of the White House Conference on Food, Nutrition, and Health are put into effect.

Despite all the confusing hoopla to the contrary, remember that our rich and varied agriculture and advanced food technology make it possible to prepare a highly nutritious diet for your family. Modern sanitation has practically eliminated any danger of disease-carrying organisms in foods. The fluoridation of water has cut down on dental caries to a striking extent. As for pollutants, they are carefully monitored not only by federal and state agencies, but also by many scientific and industrial organizations.

We should all continue to press for expanded investigation of environmental risks, for the development of more nutritious processed foods and drinks, and for more informative labeling. But we should also try to distinguish between real problems, unsupported claims, and the mouthings of food cranks. Otherwise there may soon be a national tendency to eat nothing but bean sprouts and alfalfa sprouts, which a few faddists have already undertaken to survive on.

Part III

Technological Impact
on the Food System

To the urban consumer, agriculture is a remote concept, and the series of events required to put food on the table is only vaguely perceived. Many who have never seen a farm think of farming as a romantic or idyllic existence close to nature. Such views are unrealistic and potentially divisive. Economic systems are based on food production, distribution, and consumption. In simple societies most of the population is involved in some way with food getting. In complex societies, however, the food supply involves a myriad of interlocking skills, technologies, and services. This makes our present food-production system vastly more complicated than in previous times.

The food system is no longer a natural self-restoring ecological system. Instead, it has become an economic and technological one that often damages the environment on which it depends. Its operations are not always clear to the consumer, except when they result in higher prices in the marketplace or when concern over contamination or adulteration of the food supply is discussed in the mass media.

In part I the man-food continuum was explored in ecosystem terms. We saw how what Joseph Wood Krutch has called "the great chain of life" works in interlocking pathways to maintain equilibrium so that each species can survive in its own ecological niche. Only the human species, as a consequence of its capacity to adapt through technology, can survive in the widest possible variety of environments—from inhospitable to abundant.

In part II we explored the magnitude of the food-population problem. In part III we examine the role of technology and its impact on the food-production system. We also explore the fact that we may be reaching the "limits of growth" described in selection 9. Certainly, modern agricultural and industrial technology has made great strides toward increasing the earth's capacity to sustain a growing human population, but they have also disrupted the water and nutrient cycles of the biosphere. Some optimists believe that scientific and technological innovations will permit us to overcome these problems and that the solution to possible ecocatastrophe lies in finding the *right* technical solution or combination of solutions. They assume that human inventiveness can provide substitutes whenever resources are depleted and that improved technological efficiency can reduce projected levels of pollution. They believe also that improved technology can increase the availability of food through increased yields of crops per acre of land.

Many ecologists argue that without population control science and technology cannot meet the demand for food required by the world's burgeoning billions. The interlocking problems of agriculture, technology, and population growth are examined from various perspectives in the following selections.

Selection 17 Population: Quantity versus Quality

Shirley Foster Hartley

Editors' Introduction

In Africa, Asia, Latin America, and the Near East, vast numbers of people subsist on monotonous diets that fall into three typical patterns based on the staple food on which they rely. These three diets are (1) those based almost exclusively on cereals—wheat, rice, maize (corn), millet, oats, and rye; (2) those relying on tubers—potatoes, sweet potatoes, cassava, and yams; and (3) those based on tubers in combination with such fruits as bananas and plantains. Such diets are often inadequate in both quantity (calories) and quality (proteins, vitamins, and minerals). Although these staples are rich in certain nutrients, other protective foods must supplement them in order to provide adequate amounts and the right balance of protein (essential amino acids), vitamins, and minerals.

Most diets that are nutritionally adequate provide at least 10 to 12 percent of the calories from protein. Most commonly consumed foods contain protein, but the proportion and the

Source: Adapted from Shirley Foster Hartley, *Population: Quantity vs. Quality,* © 1972, pp. 121–42. Adapted/Abridged by permission of Prentice-Hall, Inc., Englewood Cliffs, New Jersey. Complete notes and references and some tables appearing in this article are not included here; for further information consult the original version.

quality of the protein vary greatly. Vegetable sources account for a major portion of the protein in the diets of people in less developed countries. Cereals are the major suppliers of protein not because they are a complete protein or contain it in the proportion required, but because they are eaten in such large quantities in comparison to other foods. A significant plant source of protein is legumes or pulses, such as navy beans, soybeans, black-eyed peas, nuts, and lentils. These nitrogen-containing vegetable protein sources provide a secondary source of protein in many under-developed countries. They have a higher protein content than cereal grains but are deficient in the sulfur-containing essential amino acid methionine. On the other hand they are rich in lysine, another essential amino acid.

Lysine is the limiting amino acid in many cereals. The term *limiting amino acid* refers to the essential amino acid in shortest supply relative to the other amino acids necessary for protein synthesis. When cereals and legumes are available in combination, the nutritional quality of the diet is greatly improved. When eaten together, they complement each other's amino acid deficiencies and have nutritional value as good as animal protein. This mutual reinforcement is called *protein complementarity*. However, the production of legumes on a worldwide basis is declining. Many experts fear that farmers are replacing these crops with new high-yielding varieties of wheat and rice.

The incidence of protein malnutrition is highest in the areas where the staples are tubers or tubers and fruits and there is little or no supplementation with grains, legumes, or animal products (eggs, milk, and cheese) to increase the quality of the vegetable protein. Tubers and fruits are very low in protein content. Most of the efforts to improve the world's food supply have concentrated on quantity—that is, producing enough food to meet caloric requirements. Few major achievements have been made in reducing the malnutrition that results from diets deficient in protein or vitamins and minerals.

In the less developed countries, there has been an increase of about 30 percent in agricultural productivity over the past two decades, constituting what has been called a *green revolution*. These gains, however, have been absorbed by the rapidly growing population. Food production per capita in these poor countries is barely holding constant at its present inadequate level.

In the following excerpt from her book *Population: Quantity vs. Quality*, Shirley Hartley discusses proposals for improving the quantity and quality of the diets of people in the less developed countries.

There are so many proposals to increase the world's food supply by applying present knowledge and research potential that I would like to survey these *possibilities* in light of the *probabilities* involved.

Imaginative thinking is certainly necessary, but suggestions that purport to solve the problems of the world without evaluating the practicality of implementing the proposed solution are irresponsible. Such schemes as layered farming in skyscrapers with special lighting systems need not be taken seriously, because the costs of construction and maintenance, on the scale necessary to provide added billions of persons with food, would be prohibitive.

We will attempt to determine the possibilities for agricultural improvements from expanding the acreage cultivated and/or increasing the yields per acre. There are problems in obtaining the necessary fertilizers, water, improved seeds, and trained manpower to facilitate such expansion and whether or not these can all be coordinated is an open question. Suggestions for increasing the food yields from the oceans and the possibilities of producing synthetic proteins and vitamins or making new combinations of these will also be explored.

Agricultural Improvement

An increase in the production of food from the land may be accomplished either by expanding the land area being used, by increasing the amount of food obtained from the land already cultivated, or by a combination of these two strategies.

Expansion of agricultural acreage. In the past, population growth was accommodated by the colonization of new land areas—North and South America, Australia, New Zealand, and even Siberia. The irrigation of arid regions as a means of expanding agricultural acreage has also been practiced over the centuries, but only recently has it found widespread use.

Population growth and the resultant need for land have increased so rapidly in recent years that most of the land which is readily cultivatable is already being used. Continued expansion of the land area on the scale of the past is, therefore, unlikely. Although the presently cultivated acreage is only about half of that classified as "potentially arable" (see table 17.1), the unused portion lies idle for good reasons. In most cases the necessary inputs of energy and investment are greater than anticipated yields. For instance, it is often suggested that the tropical rain forests of northern South America, Africa, and Indonesia could be used for agriculture. Indeed, the present heavy foliage would imply a fertile soil. There is also adequate water and plenty of sunlight. Yet whenever the overgrowth has been cut down and the soil cultivated, the returns

Table 17.1 Cultivated Land on Each Continent, Compared with Potentially Arable Land

| Continent | Area in Billions of Acres | | |
	Total	Potentially Arable	Cultivated
Africa	7.40	1.81	0.39
Asia	6.76	1.55	1.28
Australia and New Zealand	2.03	0.38	0.04
Europe	1.18	0.43	0.38
North America	5.21	1.15	0.59
South America	4.33	1.68	0.19
USSR	5.52	0.88	0.56
Totals	32.49	7.88	3.43

Source: United States Congress, Senate Committee on Government Operations, Hearing, *Population Crisis*, Part 2, January 31, 1968, p. 302.

have been disappointing. The soils are apparently extremely poor in quality and the areas are infested with insects and fungi. Crops may be harvested for only one, two, or sometimes three years before soil becomes "leached out," dried, and cracked—useless to man or beast. The work necessary to clear the land, therefore, has hardly been worth the short-term returns. The land is uncultivated now for good reasons.

Table 17.1 also indicates that virtually all of the potentially arable land of Asia is presently under cultivation. This is why many agricultural specialists refer to the region as "overdeveloped" rather than "underdeveloped." They suggest that, over time, the soils have been overworked and exhausted. In India, so many forests have been cleared that the land suffers from an inability to hold moisture. Thus the area alternates between extremes of parched soils and flooding. The recommendation that soils not be used every year lest they become exhausted apparently has some merit, but population pressure in many areas of the world will not allow the land an occasional recuperative year.

Increasing the yield per acre. There are many possibilities for raising the yields per acre of land, but most of them require the same high investments that would be necessary to expand the acreage in use.

First, yields can be improved simply by changing the particular crops grown. Sugar beets, if grown under the kind of intensive farming practices found in Northern Europe would seem to maximize the caloric yield per acre per year. Under these conditions, sugar beets could contribute three times the calories of wheat or twice the calories of rice per acre. If energy intake constituted the only nutritional requirement of human beings, the average person could live adequately by consuming

1.5 pounds of sugar a day. However, a person who consumes a diet consisting only of carbohydrates (sugar and starches) or fats will soon die. For proper functioning the body also needs proteins and amino acids, vitamins, and minerals, such as calcium, phosphorus, salt, iron, and iodine. Maximizing the yield per acre in either calories or protein content does not solve the world problem of how to feed the multiplying numbers of human beings.

Harrison Brown points out that although alfalfa is presently grown to supply protein in animal diets (and thus *indirectly* in the human diet), it could be used to supply protein *directly* in the human diet. . . . Clearly, the returns would be multiplied if alfalfa were consumed directly by human beings. One of the difficulties noted by Brown et al. is that:

> In order to use plant protein on a large scale as food for people, however, it would be necessary to devise methods by which the plant may be ground and the protein thus extracted into materials resembling meat, milk, eggs, and so forth. But these are merely technological problems and are certainly soluble. This modification of our food technology would permit us to supplement human diets with the needed amino acids at a fraction of the cost in acres that characterizes our present system.[1]

It would also be necessary to convince people that reconstituted alfalfa is something they *want* to eat. Not much is known about how to motivate people to eat what is good for them—whether they be poor or affluent.

The yield per acre varies in different geographic and climatic areas and under different types of cultivation the caloric and protein value per acre also varies according to the crops grown and the uses to which they are put. Increasing the yield of particular crops on particular acreage, in any geographic area is dependent upon maximizing the advantages of additional inputs of fertilizers, irrigation, improved seeds or animal breeds, and pest control. Adequate utilization of these inputs, furthermore, requires intelligent labor, trained in the technical skills necessary for quantity production. Perhaps in no other area is the Marxian theory of labor shown to be so clearly in error as in agriculture: additional output will not result from adding additional labor; rather increased production will come from added capital investment, including investment in improving the technological skills of human beings.

Land reform, the division of large landholdings (often with absentee landowners) into small, family-owned plots, may provide a greater incentive to farm workers to put more effort into improving yields. Sharecropping often reduces the incentives of both the landowner and the worker to invest in improved seeds, fertilizer, tools, and so forth. Subdivision of large landholdings is necessary in many parts of the world for a variety of reasons. By itself, it may provide increased motivation for the farm worker to increase productivity. If, at the same time, training in new methods, lending for the purchase of new seeds, fertilizer, and tools, or even cooperatively owned equipment are made available stepwise increases in yields may be expected. Land reform alone, however, cannot guarantee improvement. If population continues its rapid climb, small plots (such as five-acre parcels) might be subdivided among sons until the size of an individual unit will not even support a farm family at the subsistence level, much less allow for marketable produce.

Adding Necessary Inputs
to Increase Agricultural Output

If the potentially arable land of the earth is indeed twice as great as that presently cultivated and if yields per acre vary greatly from crop to crop, then the possibility of increasing the world's food supply must be great. What inputs are required to effect the necessary increases and how may they be obtained?

Fertilizers. These are made from nonrenewable materials. The manufacturing technology involved is not complex, but does depend heavily on energy sources for nitrogen fixation and, eventually, for phosphate treatment. Mining and transport are important; the tonnages distributed are large and involve global trade. Supplies of raw materials—potassium compounds, sulfur and sulfates, phosphate rock, limestone, natural gas or coal, and air (for nitrogen)—are adequate at present and for moderately increased rates of use. Increased fertilizer costs, however, would occur quickly if the needs of the less developed countries were to be met.[2] The production of fertilizer must increase more rapidly than in the past to meet the food crisis.

The phenomenal increase in food production in the United States since the First World War has actually occurred simultaneously with a reduction in acreage farmed and increased use of fertilizers. The Japanese and western Europeans use fertilizers even more intensively than U.S. farmers.[3]

The less developed countries together used 6.9 million metric tons of fertilizer—almost three times their own production of fertilizer—in 1968. One of the world's largest plants for manufacturing fertilizers is located in Sindri in India. Its annual production is approximately 350,000 metric tons, but this quantity is barely enough to grow food for the *annual* population *increment* of India! In other words, India would need an additional factory of this size every year simply to keep pace with the population increase. Yet it would require at least three to five years to build such a plant and to get it into final operation.[4] Table 17.2

Table 17.2 Fertilizer Needed to Increase Agricultural Production on Acreage Now under Cultivation in Asia, Africa, and Latin America by Percentages Indicated

Percent Increase in Agricultural Production	Tonnage of Plant Nutrients Needed (millions of metric tons)	Percent Increase in Fertilizer Usage	Capital Needed (million dollars)	Total Annual Cost to Farmers (million dollars)
	6*			1,300
10	11	80	2,500	2,400
26	19	220	6,500	4,200
43	28	370	11,000	6,200
63	40	570	17,000	8,800
100	67	1,000	30,500	14,800

Note: Asia does not include mainland China and Japan in this survey.
* Actual consumption in 1966.
Source: United States Congress, Committee on Government Operations (1968), p. 303.

indicates the amount of fertilizer needed to increase agricultural production on acreage now under cultivation in Asia, Africa, and Latin America. In order to increase the agricultural production of these areas by 43 percent (which might give the *present* populations an adequate diet), an initial capital investment of $11 billion would be needed. The total annual cost to farmers would then approximate $6 billion. However, by the time the plants were built, fertilizer produced and distributed, and additional crops grown, population increases would be significant. The less developed regions of the world are, in fact, doubling their population in about twenty years. In order to increase food production during that time by 100 percent, which would allow the same per capita rations as presently exist, would require a $30 billion investment in fertilizer alone, with an annual cost to the farmers of $14.8 billion.

[Georg] Borgstrom claims that by the end of this century the weight of the fertilizer that will require distribution around the world will exceed the total weight of the human race. Even so, that fertilizer would replace only about three or four key substances that crop lands require and not the whole range of nutrients that will have to be taken into account by then.

Irrigation. Irrigation will become even more important as the use of fertilizers increases. Sometimes irrigation alone can add an additional crop per year in warm climates. Water for irrigation may be drawn from three basic sources: underground supplies, freshwater rivers and lakes, and desalination of seawaters. All have limited applicability.

Wells are used around the world to retrieve water from underground. The capacity to pump water from below ground gives the illusion of an inexhaustible supply. When the amount of water pumped exceeds the amount replaced, however, the supply is reduced, the water level falls, and wells must be dug deeper. The process may be repeated until the water supply is exhausted or until the costs of pumping are prohibitive. The underground water table that has been tapped to irrigate the desert areas of Texas, Arizona, and southern California has dropped 100 feet since the irrigation began. The United States Geological Survey estimates that it would take 104 years to restore the groundwater to its natural level through natural replenishment, *if* it were not being pumped out in the meantime. Furthermore, saltwater is seeping into the continent from the ocean and filling the space evacuated by pumping out fresh water.[5]

The supply of river water can fluctuate widely; thus, for purposes of irrigation (and power), great dams have been built to hold back an adequate supply of water for the times at which it is needed. Again, the possibilities are not limitless: some rivers in the United States are already so "dammed" that salmon cannot get upstream to spawn; on some there are no more locations where new dams could be built. Furthermore, the estimated lifetime of a dam is from 30 to 100 years; it then fills with silt and becomes useless. Few people know that there was a little Aswan Dam, which was rendered useless in this way. The new, billion-dollar Aswan Dam will hold back the silt which used to be spread over the adjacent land each time the Nile River flooded and one of the richest river valleys in the world will lose its main source of fertility.

At present about 11 percent of the world's cultivated acres are irrigated by conventional methods. If the river waters of the world were conserved and distributed, it is estimated that it would ultimately be possible to irrigate 14 percent of the acreage now under cultivation (at current prices of water and of farm products). By building more expensive conventional irrigation projects, a maximum of 20 percent of the world's cultivated acreage could be served.[6] Thus fresh water is not available in sufficient quantity to supply more than one-fifth of the presently cultivated land, much less to supply the deserts and other "potentially arable" acreage.

The desalination of seawater is another possibility in the quest for increasing sources of fresh water. There are already a number of techniques or processes for removing the salt from seawater—all of them expensive. The problems of desalination are infinitely more complex than one would gather from reading a typical newspaper account. Cost, plant size, transportation, and salt disposal difficulties are among the problems that would need to be resolved before any widespread use of desalination would be feasible.

The cost of the reclamation of ocean water has been estimated at between $100 and $200 per acre-foot. To this must be added the cost of building canals and pipelines to distribute the water. Irrigation water in the United States presently costs approximately $10 per acre-foot delivered.[7] The cost of desalinated water for irrigation would be far more than the value of crops which could be produced. . . .

The water needs of the world are inflated further by population growth.

New seeds and breeds. The selective breeding of both plants and animals has allowed us to make giant leaps in the quantities of food produced.

> . . . To man's accomplishments in exploiting the plants and animals that natural evolution has provided, and in improving them through selective breeding over the millenniums, he has added in this century the creation of remarkably productive new breeds, thanks to the discoveries of genetics. Genetics has made possible the development of cereals and other plant species that are more tolerant to cold, more resistant to drought, less susceptible to disease, more responsive to fertilizer, higher in yield and richer in protein. . . .
>
> The results of man's efforts to increase the productivity of domestic animals are equally impressive. When the ancestors of our present chickens were domesticated, they laid a clutch of about 15 eggs once a year. Hens in the United States today average 220 eggs per year and the figure is rising steadily as a result of continuing advances in breeding and feeding. When cattle were originally domesticated, they probably did not produce more than 600 pounds of milk per year, barely enough for a calf. (It is roughly the average amount produced by cows in India today.) The 13 million dairy cows in the U.S. today average 9,000 pounds of milk yearly, outproducing their ancestors fifteen to one.[8]

New seeds, techniques, and knowledge are far from being utilized on a worldwide scale, however. The time lag between development and acceptance has been very long. It took nearly twenty-five years for hybrid corn to be accepted by farmers in the United States, where high incentives and technical manpower existed. The new high-yield varieties (HYV) have yet to be promoted and accepted among farmers on a wide scale. Furthermore, the seeds, fertilizers, pesticides, and agricultural techniques which produce stepwise increase in production in one geographical area cannot be simply transferred; they must be adapted to new locations.

Pest control. There is no way to adequately assess the amount of farm produce lost to pests. Between 10 and 25 percent of the total grain crops of India are estimated to be lost to insects, rodents, birds, monkeys, and cattle. Billions of rats, millions of monkeys, and between 225 and 280 million cows compete with human beings for rice and wheat. Yet when a proposal to reduce the numbers of sacred cows came before the Indian Parliament, 100,000 Hindus turned out to protest. The only war ever sanctioned by the pacifist Gandhi was for the reduction of the monkey population. The death of 10 million monkeys made little difference, however, since millions of new monkeys quickly replaced those that were killed. Tigers, leopards, and other natural predators of the monkeys had previously been eliminated as the forests were cleared in order to cultivate all available land.[9]

Other national groups that do not share the Hindu reverence for all forms of life have fewer problems with mammalian pests, but continuing problems with insects. Table 17.3 indicates the amounts of pesticides that would be needed to increase the agricultural production on acreage now under cultivation in Asia (except China and Japan), Africa, and Latin America. To double the agricultural production would require a sixfold increase in the tonnage of pesticides and an annual cost to farmers of $3.5 billion. In the next chapter we will discuss some of the problems caused by the use of certain pesticides.

Trained manpower. Many people assume that because almost anyone can grow flowers, fruits, or vegetables in a backyard garden, there is little technical training required for farming. Indeed, farmers are often classified as unskilled laborers. Yet, it is the scientific approach and

Table 17.3 Pesticides Needed to Increase Agricultural Production on Acreage Now under Cultivation in Asia, Africa, and Latin America by Percentages Indicated

Percent Increase in Agricultural Production	Tonnage Needed (metric tons)	Capital		Total Annual Cost to Farmers (million dollars)
		Manufacturing (million dollars)	Formulation and Distribution (million dollars)	
	120,000			580
10	150,000	70	40	730
26	220,000	200	110	1,060
43	300,000	380	200	1,460
63	420,000	630	340	2,040
100	720,000	1,240	670	3,500

Note: Asia does not include mainland China and Japan in this survey.

Source: United States Congress, Senate, Committees on Government Operations, *Population Crisis*, vol. 2 (Washington, D.C.: Government Printing Office, 1968), p. 304.

the application of its techniques that have made some farms productive while others stagnate.

Landownership patterns have little effect on productivity, without technical leadership. In Latin America and many parts of Asia, rich landlords with extensive holdings maintain a feudal system and collect rent, services, or shares of the harvest from peasant farmers. The landlords have little motive or desire to help the peasants. However, if governments seize large estates and divide them among peasants, the result is often *decreased* production. The new peasant owners lack the knowledge, money, and equipment to make the most of what they have acquired. Furthermore, these small bits of land become divided into inheritance or marriage dowry parcels to the point that the individual plots are so reduced in size that subsistence is about all that can be had from them. Land reform is desirable for social progress, but some authors assume it is the whole solution.

Agricultural education. Agricultural education has a long history in the Untied States. The Land Grant College Act was passed in 1862. Prior to World War II, one-third of all research money funded by the United States government went to agriculture.

In the countries which need them most, however, agricultural research specialists and technicians are not being trained in the numbers needed. . . .

The number of acricultural research workers per 100,000 persons active in agriculture in specific countries in 1960 is given in table 17.4. One reason for the shortage of trained manpower is that young people in food-deficit nations tend to decline an agricultural education; farming

Table 17.4 Agricultural Research Workers per 100,000 People Active in Agriculture, 1960

India	1.2
Philippines	1.6
Mexico	3.8
Pakistan	4.5
Thailand	4.7
Colombia	9.0
Iran	10.0
Argentina	14.0
Japan	60.0
Taiwan	79.0
Netherlands	133.0

Source: United States Department of Agriculture, *Changes in Agriculture in 26 Developing Nations, 1948–1963.* (Washington, D.C.: Government Printing Office, 1965), table 46.

represents a lowly occupation to them. Students fortunate enough to obtain an education abroad hold the same prejudice. In 1967–1968, 42 percent of the foreign students in the United States were studying engineering or humanities. Only 3 percent had chosen agriculture. Some nations (Egypt, the Philippines) now have an excess and underemployed group of university-trained persons, while lacking adequate trained manpower in agriculture. It is clear from table 17.4 that even if we could double or triple the number of research workers in India and the Philippines, it would still be difficult for individualized help to reach the millions of farmers.

Machinery. The tools in use by farmers range from the primitive digging stick and the hoe to very complex, sophisticated machinery. In the United States, according to Lenski:

> As Edward Higbee so dramatically describes in *Farms and Farmers in an Urban Age*, agriculture is rapidly losing its distinctiveness and more and more coming to resemble other forms of industrial activity. . . . In addition, those farmers who are surviving and prospering in the increased intense competition find themselves caught up in a network of business relationship, government controls, and financial transactions no less complex than those of their urban counterparts in the business world.[10]

By 1969 the total value of farm implements and machinery in the United States had reached over $32 billion. [According to the 1970 U.S. census,] farmers were spending $5 billion yearly for additions and replacements of machinery and equipment, and for motor vehicles for farm use. There is little possibility that the less developed nations will be able to meet these kinds of costs for advanced machinery.

Food from the Oceans

Present catch. In the search for means of increasing the world's supply of food, man has turned to the seas. The 1968 worldwide catch of fish, crustaceans, and mollusks was 58 million metric tons. The yield from the seas has been increasing at a faster rate than any other source of food. The annual rate of growth from the 1955–1957 average to the 1965–1967 average was 6.4 percent per year (see table 17.5). In fifteen years the total world catch almost tripled.

Even with the rapid increase in fishery products, the present totals contribute only about 2 percent of the caloric consumption of the world. At the same time, however, fish supplies valuable protein, equal to about 20 percent of the annual protein consumption of the world. . . . fish protein [plays a relatively minor role] in comparison to other animal and

Table 17.5 Estimated World Catch of Fish, Crustacea, and Mollusks

	Average Catch (million metric tons)							Change 1967 to 1968*	Annual Rate of Growth 1955–1957 1965–1967
	Average 1948–1952	1957	1960	1962	1965	1967	1968*		
Western Europe	6.31	7.59	7.71	8.21	10.24	11.26	10.97	−3%	3.4%
Eastern Europe and USSR	1.94	2.82	3.40	4.02	5.73	6.43	6.93	8	8.0
North America	3.50	3.80	3.79	4.15	4.04	3.78	3.97	5	—
Oceania	0.09	0.11	0.13	0.15	0.18	0.20	0.21	5	6.3
Latin America	0.63	1.36	4.73	8.62	9.43	12.71	13.48	6	26.0
Far East	6.85	10.30	11.81	13.04	14.52	16.41	18.04	10	4.8
Near East	0.35	0.39	0.40	0.44	0.52	0.49	0.53	8	2.5
Africa	1.20	1.98	2.20	2.52	3.04	3.62	4.10	13	5.8
World	20.90	28.40	34.20	41.20	47.70	54.90	58.20	6%	6.4%

Note: "World" does not include mainland China.

* Preliminary.

Source: United Nations, Food and Agriculture Organization, *The State of Food and Agriculture, 1969* (Rome: FAO, 1969), p. 13.

vegetable protein consumption. . . . But, although the supply is small, it has been growing more rapidly than world population.

A large part of the total catch, which has increased most rapidly in the Latin American nations, is being sold to the developed nations. And, a significant portion of that is fed to hogs and chickens rather than going directly (and more efficiently) to human consumption. Some of the fish meal so used is defined as inedible by humans, but could be used as a protein additive in other foods.

Fish products are consumed unevenly around the world. They make up a far larger proportion of both calorie and protein consumption in Norway and Japan than in many other parts of the world. India recently advanced to sixth place among the world's fishing nations. Most of the catch of the Asian countries is destined for local consumption. Yet, even if the total world catch could be used for India alone, it would not provide each individual inhabitant with more protein than the equivalent of one average herring a day.[11] The 1969 improved catch of 2 million metric tons for India yields about the equivalent of one herring per person per month.

Future possibilities. Oceanographers estimate that, with a massive investment in ships, by the year 2000 a maximum of 100 million metric tons of fish could be harvested from the oceans yearly without damaging future supplies. However, with the anticipated population increase, the per capita harvest in the year 2000 could average 8 *percent less* than at present.

Two problems threaten to reduce the maximum possible catches of the future. One is overexploitation: man has become such an efficient fisherman that numerous species are now in danger of becoming extinct. Another problem is oceanic pollution: the areas close to shorelines, where fish are in greatest abundance, are being polluted at an increasing rate.

Most of the ocean, approximately 90.7 percent of the surface, is a biological desert. It is only close to the shorelines and in a few areas where powerful upwellings bring nutrients to the surface that fish are abundant enough to be caught in quantity.

Although marine farming has a long history, the world has hardly begun to tap the potential of farming fish and shellfish. Man has the knowledge and experience to move beyond the primitive hunting and gathering of food in the sea. Especially as some of the high-demand species are in danger of overexploitation, we may expect and encourage the stocking and the farming of portions of the ocean. The numerous complications are for the most part known and resolvable with investments that are reasonable in relation to the expected returns.

However, the fish is a relatively inefficient converter of ocean plants to human food. It is estimated that 100,000 pounds of algae are necessary to produce about one pound of codfish.[12] There are numerous suggestions, therefore, that we might increase the ocean's yield of human food by moving down the food chain and harvesting smaller fish. Algae could even be strained from the ocean water directly by some mechanical means. However, a lot of straining would have to be done, since one cubic meter of seawater contains on the average only about one cubic centimeter of plant material.[13] Suggestions that algae cultivation (hydroponics) in huge tanks could produce forty tons of algae per acre per year have not been implemented because of the high investment required (from 10 to 100 times the investment in conventional agriculture) and because of the small likelihood that human beings would be interested in eating the "nasty little green vegetable." An attempt to sell algae tablets and candy is currently being made in Japan.

Although there are possibilities for continuing to increase the harvest from the oceans, there are limits to what is possible. And those limits may be reached before population growth comes to a halt.

Synthetic Proteins and Vitamins

Synthetic food. The chemical synthesis of food would seem to be a remote possibility. The human body requires chemical compounds that are complex and exceedingly various. Although scientists know how to use simple compounds as the starting materials for the chemical synthesis of the sugars, fats, amino acids, and vitamins necessary in the human diet, it is still a complicated chemical operation.[14]

During World War II the Germans manufactured synthetic fats from both coal and petroleum to feed to forced laborers. These fats did not conform to desirable standards of taste or safety. The petroleum-based fats retained a petroleumlike odor and were probably not fully metabolized by the human body. Although there has been a recent renewal of interest in the low-cost production of food from petroleum sources, some of the old problems remain. Furthermore, the world supplies of petroleum and coal are exhaustible and are in demand as energy supplies. Reserves will be driven far lower before atomic power comes into such widespread use as to reduce the demand for coal and oil. Further, chemical plants are themselves expensive and even if people would accept these sources of food, bulk distribution would remain a problem.

It would be possible to supplement diets with synthetically produced amino acids, which typically are lacking in the cereal diets of persons in underdeveloped areas. But the plan is not economically feasible. The cost is estimated at $40.00 per person, and would thus require half of the entire national income in many of the nations whose people need it most. Foreign aid is an unlikely source of funds for such a program, since the yearly cost of supplying this single food supplement to India alone would be about $22 billion.

Borgstrom[15] points out that even if it were economically, physically, and aesthetically possible to use synthetic foods, man cannot withdraw from a fundamental cooperation with nature. Man is dependent upon the green plant to pull carbon dioxide from the air and return it to the great carbon cycle of nature. Too many men destroying our green acres and poisoning the green plants of the ocean will destroy the air they breathe. The interrelationships of nature must be respected, which is one reason why the population problem is not merely a food problem.

Vitamins. Although the chemical synthesis and the widespread production and distribution of bulky foods remains impractical, vitamin production and supply is a different story. Harrison Brown et al. claim that it is possible to supply a human being with his required rations of vitamins, all synthetically produced, at a cost of between 25 cents and one dollar per year.[16] Vitamins, although complex and expensive to manufacture, are required by human beings only in minute amounts. The mass distribution of vitamins would be a reasonable minimal starting point for international agencies. Only a few billion dollars per year would be needed for a certain improvement in human health.

New Sources or New Combinations of Food

There may be food sources which human beings have not yet recognized. Many "filling substances" would not be used as food except in dire circumstances, and some not even then. Nevertheless, scientists continue to seek possibilities for increasing the supply of foods for human consumption.

It would be possible, though at present it is too expensive, to cultivate algae in water or even on petroleum or the sewage from our cities. The algae, after processing, could serve as food or could aid in the cultivation of yeast.

Grown on the wastes of human beings, the wastes from cane sugar production, or on the wastes from pulp factories, yeast could become an efficient and inexpensive source of protein. But, since yeast is not self-generating, it is as limited in supply as the waste matter upon which it grows.

Many of the new high-yield varieties of grains have lower protein content than prewar varieties. Research is now concentrating on developing and testing grain varieties with higher protein content as well as possible additives to enrich the present varieties.

Incaparina, a combination of corn, high-protein cottonseed meal, vitamin A, and tortula yeast (a source of vitamin B), was announced to the world in 1957 and was heavily promoted in a pilot project in Colombia. After more than ten years of determined effort and investment, however, the Quaker Oats Company is still losing money on the product. People apparently do not like its unaccustomed taste and texture.

A tasteless and odorless fish-protein concentrate has recently been developed for use as a food additive, especially for the hungry peoples of the world. It has the advantage of not interfering with the tastes and textures desired by the various peoples of the world. It can be unobtrusively added to the basic food, whether cornmeal, wheat, rice, or potatoes. In 1968 the world production of fish meal neared 10 percent of the total tonnage caught. Like the coarser fish meal, the protein concentrate can be produced from inedible fish or parts of fish. Like fish in general, however, the supply is limited. The processing factories also require investment funds, but the returns in value to the human diet are far greater than when the fish meal is fed to chickens and hogs. The later consumption of those chickens or hogs by human beings would provide only a fraction of the protein which could be derived from consuming the fish-protein concentrate directly.

If human beings were to accept these unconventional sources of food, they might also derive animal protein from species that are presently unacceptable for consumption. Some persons in the United States have come, like some Europeans, to regard snails as a delicacy. Some cultures utilize snake meat, caterpillars, and so forth. Should the Indian come to define beef cattle, rodents, and monkeys as food sources, he would simultaneously add several sources of animal protein to his diet and save a portion of the grains eaten by those animals. A cultural pattern thousands of years old is not likely to be readily changed, however. Waves of starvation have occurred at many times in human history when sources of food defined as unacceptable were in plentiful supply. The Ehrlichs[17] point out that the hungriest people are precisely those who recognize the fewest items as food.

Food and Population — The Wrong Problem

Although, as Malthus suggested, "ultimately" the human species cannot expand its numbers beyond the food supply, the precise quantity and quality of food considered necessary to keep human beings alive varies greatly according to the level of existence considered acceptable.

The skeletal human beings found in some German concentration camps had continued breathing on daily rations 800–1000 calories per person per day. Yet an average daily ration of 2300 calories is judged inadequate to provide normal levels of energy and working men require well over 3000 calories per day. Calories alone are not enough. Vitamins, minerals, and daily supplies of protein are all necessary for human health and development.

There is a great difference, then, in food requirements necessary for a "bare" existence and those required for a healthy, energetic life. Given a choice, most people would obviously choose the latter for themselves and for mankind. When the choice becomes a conscious one, as we come to understand how rising populations have been nullifying the advances in food production, it makes sense to match our control over deaths with birth control. The human capacity to plan ahead allows us to reduce births in order to improve the quality of life. We are not left to the self-steering aspects of nature in either death control or birth control.

If mankind had been content to let the death rate find its "natural level," there would not already have been such rapid population growth. Human beings have made the decision to manipulate nature and soon we will have to decide whether to maximize the numbers of bodies to be kept alive at some low level or whether to maximize the creative, aesthetic, and intellectual capacities of all—in contrast to those of only a small proportion of the world's people. It is not possible to maximize both the quantity and the quality of human beings.

Ours is a world divided. And, by whatever measure is used, the gap between the haves [SW] and the have-nots [HW] is widening.

After an examination of the effects of population growth on natural resources, we will review the extent of the economic gap between the developed and less developed nations. Whether in the economic or material realm, in food production, housing, medical care, or education, whatever gains are made in the "developing" countries are approximately nullified by population growth. The gains become insignificant in light of the more rapid gains of the slower-growing, advanced nations.

Summary

A survey of the past, present, and future food situation of the world can hardly result in an optimistic view of the race between population and food. Although world food production has actually been proceeding at a slightly more rapid pace than has population growth, the increases in the underdeveloped countries have been little more than equal to population increases.

The increased production in recent years was brought about by great effort on the part of all the nations of the world and with the cooperative efforts of the United Nations agencies and private foundations. The increases *could* have allowed all the people of the world to have improved and adequate diets. Thereafter, man's improved health, vitality, productivity, and energy presumably would have contributed to general improvements in living standards. But population increase has nullified almost all of the gains made.

The developed nations must share an increasingly greater portion of their production with the underdeveloped countries. But even complete sharing will not solve the problems as long as population continues to increase.

The so-called "green revolution" is partial and spotty. New seed strains are not usable under all geographic, climatic, and soil conditions. Millions of people need to cooperate in order to achieve a maximization of food production with present facilities.

The possibilities for future expansion of agricultural output typically require vast investments in trained manpower, tools, fertilizers, water, new high-yield seeds and breeds, and the control of pests. The more primitive the agricultural methods of a particular society, the more these additions are needed and the less likely that the people will be willing to accept the necessary changes.

New and strange food products are also likely to meet resistance, not only among peasant populations but even among highly educated persons.

No single solution is probable for the food-population problem. Every approach to improving the production and distribution of food needs to be facilitated, with the long-term preservation of the soil and waters of the earth in mind. Whether per capita food supplies improve or worsen, the people of the world will improve their total situation more rapidly if population is soon brought under control.

Notes

1. Harrison Brown, James Bonner, and John Weir, *The Next Hundred Years* (New York: Viking Press, 1957), p. 72.

2. Sterling B. Hendricks, "Food from the Land," in *Resources and Man: A Study and Recommendations by the Committee on Resources and Man of the Division of Earth Sciences, National Research Council with the cooperation of the Division of Biology and Agriculture* (San Francisco: Freeman, 1969), p. 73.

3. Jean Mayer, "Food and Population: The Wrong Problem?" in *Population Studies: Selected Essays and Research*, ed. Kenneth Kammeyer (Chicago: Rand McNally, 1969), p. 486.

4. Georg Borgstrom, *The Hungry Planet* (New York: Macmillan, 1965), p. 130.

5. Ibid., p. 418.

6. Harrison Brown et. al., *The Next Hundred Years*, p. 74.

7. Ibid. p. 75.

8. Lester R. Brown, "Human Food Production as a Process in the Biosphere," *Scientific American* 223, no. 3 (September 1970): 162–63. Reprinted by permission.

9. Georg Borgstrom, *The Hungry Planet*, pp. 121ff.

10. Gerhard E. Lenski, *Power and Privilege* (New York: McGraw-Hill, 1966), p. 383.

11. George Borgstrom, *The Hungry Planet*, pp. 121ff.

12. Harrison Brown et. al., *The Next Hundred Years*, p. 76.

13. Ibid.

14. Ibid., p. 77.

15. Georg Borgstrom, *The Hungry Planet*, p. 401.

16. Harrison Brown et. al., *The Next Hundred Years*, p. 78.

17. Paul R. Ehrlich and Anne H. Ehrlich, *Population, Resources, Environment: Issues in Human Ecology* (San Francisco: Freeman, 1970), p. 73.

Selection 18 The Food System: From Field to Table

D. Katz
M.T. Goodwin

Editors' Introduction

Our modern food system allows us to set tables with food of a variety and quality unrivaled elsewhere. Fresh strawberries are available in winter. Fresh, frozen, or canned broccoli is available year-round. Unexpected guests can quickly be served a full meal from freezer or pantry shelf. Supermarket aisles are stacked with more than 10,000 food items. Forty percent of these products were not there ten years ago. In spite of this dazzling array of food, most people today are not involved in food production: they are urban, and only 6 percent of our population works on farms.

When did this reduction in the number of farmers take place? How was it possible? Before the War Between the States, an American farmer could produce only enough to feed and clothe himself and three other people. By the time we entered the Second World War, the major agricultural revolution had begun. New

Source: Adapted from D. Katz and M.T. Goodwin, "The Food System—From Field to Table," *Food: Where Nutrition, Politics and Culture Meet*, an activities guide for teachers. Copyright 1976, Center for Science in the Public Interest, 1755 S St., NW, Washington, D.C. 20009. Reprinted by permission. Tables and figures appearing in this article are not included here; for further information consult the original article.

machines and farming methods made it possible for one farmer to feed himself and eleven others. Today's modern food system allows the farmer to feed himself and forty-five to more than fifty other people.

Major changes resulting from advances in the physical and biological sciences and from inputs of huge amounts of energy and capital enabled us to increase our yields per acre and to store, process, distribute, and market food with increased efficiency. Research, credit, mechanization, synthetic fertilizers, pesticides, hybridization, and animal feedlots have dramatically increased food production. As these changes came about, farming became big business, or *agribusiness*. With the shift from small diversified farms to large, more specialized production, the family farm became obsolete.

Today, a complex network for the storage, processing, and distribution of foods and sophisticated advertising and merchandising techniques make it possible to offer the consumer a veritable cornucopia of traditional and new foods. As a consequence, giant corporations now control many aspects of the food system. These corporations have expanded by means of horizontal integration, diversification, and vertical integration. The consequences of these changes will become clear as Katz and Goodwin describe the modern American food system.

The modern supermarket, where most Americans shop, is a dizzying array of more than 10,000 food items that come from all over the world. Forty percent of items available today did not exist ten years ago; more than 60 percent are new since World War II. Contemporary Americans do their hunting and gathering in the vast aisles of the supermarket; accurate reading of signs, labels, and prices are the skills that have replaced knowledge of the seasons, of terrain, of nature.

. . . [S]tudents learn about the food chain; humans eat meat or fish (which have eaten smaller animals, grains, or grass) and therefore are at the "top" of the food chain. Some food energy is lost at each step of the chain.

Today's food supply involves a "new food chain," consisting of the processing, handling, transporting, storing, and merchandising of food before it reaches the table. Like the food chain of nature, each step consumes energy. In 1970 every calorie of food energy required about nine calories of energy.

The food industry is a giant: the fourth largest industrial user of energy, the employer of about one-seventh of the working population, a complex network with its parts spanning the globe. How many of us know where our food comes from, how it gets to us, and what processes it passes through on the way?

The food system consists of:

Sources of food. Farmers, ranchers, fishermen. In the past, single-family farms comprised most of this sector—from a small truck farm to a 5,000-acre wheat farm in Nebraska. For the last decade 50,000 to 100,000 farms, however, have folded each year. The family farmer, though demonstrated a more efficient producer by government studies, is retreating from the farm as government and corporate policies favor large corporations.

Farm marketing. About 120,000 persons who assemble, buy, sell, or handle the products of farms and other food producers. This sector of the food industry employs feedlot operators, creamery operators, and grain operators.

Food processing. About 1.7 million people are employed canning, freezing, refining, transforming, and manufacturing food. Prior to 1940, few foods were highly processed in the United States. In general, food manufacturers simply used processing techniques that were practiced in the home, such as shelling peas, and canning fruits and vegetables. In the last three decades, food production and marketing have undergone revolutionary changes, resulting in major changes in the American food supply. Simulated foods, formulated foods, textured vegetable proteins, and meat analogs (imitation meats) now fill up much of the supermarket shelf.

Transportation. An engineer on a freight train bringing cattle or grain from the western states, a trucker carrying a load of oranges to Minnesota, and a flight crew delivering pineapples from Hawaii are among the more than 600,000 workers employed in transporting food. Transport of foods to faraway markets is critical to today's food system. Most transporting is done by truck.

Scientific research. The USDA, food companies, and many state universities employ food and agricultural scientists, engineers and marketing experts to create the products and develop processing techniques desired by the food industry. In the last thirty years research has sought to increase efficiency (larger crop yields, more easily shipped vegetables) and minimize costs. Research to improve nutritive value, taste, or to lower retail prices and help small farmers, has been too often neglected.

Chain and wholesale distribution. This link gathers food from farmers and processors throughout the nation and the world and provides the storehouses that stock the country's retail stores. Large retail chains and cooperatives (societies of supermarkets) often own their own warehouses.

Retail distribution. Food stores: supermarkets, mom and pop stores, "convenience" stores. Small mom and pop stores and local supermarket chains have been replaced in most parts of the country by mammoth chains, regionally or nationally known, that dominate over 50 percent of the market. Small grocers have been unable to compete with large, powerful chains which are vertically integrated, possess giant advertising budgets and the "deep pockets" to withstand and buy out even the most efficient, productive competition.

Feeding the public. Restaurants have become a growing part of the food system as more and more Americans eat out. One in three meals is currently eaten away from home. Franchised restaurants, serving a limited menu of convenience foods, proliferate; eating out to many means a choice between Burger King, McDonald's, Taco Bell, and Kentucky Fried Chicken.

The Structure of the Food System

A small number of hands own and control today's food system, resulting in "economic concentration." The food industry is moving closer to a system "integrated" from field to table. . . . enormous power shared by a very few corporations.

Both representatives of the food industry and its critics recognize that structural changes in the industry have greatly affected prices and quality of food. Industry lauds these structural changes, maintaining that growth and profits stimulate individuals and companies to explore new ideas, increase efficiency, and improve products. The growth of corporations testifies, they claim, to superior products, efficient production, and responsive manufacturing and marketing strategies. Growth is a result of better service, resulting in still better service and consumer savings.

Critics maintain that consumers rarely see these savings. Expansion actually allows the corporations greater control of the market; the lack of competition enables them to manipulate and increase prices and enjoy excessive profits. . . . Unrestrained growth of food corporations does not result from superior products or efficient production, but from favorable government policies, effective political pressures, and other advantages of bigness. Smaller firms, which may produce a good quality, reasonably priced item are squeezed out not by the superior products of corporate giants, but by unfair marketing advantages and political and economic clout.

Corporations expand in three major ways: [First,] horizontal integration is a company's capturing of a greater share of the market for its product. This growth may come through internal expansion (expanding production or building additional plants) or by external expansion (acquiring other businesses which manufacture the same product). If there are two banana growers on an island, and one buys the other, horizontal integration through external expansion occurs. The result of extensive horizontal integration is monopoly or oligopoly (shared monopoly).

[Second,] diversification is another method of expansion. A firm acquires businesses that manufacture other products. If our island banana grower buys a mango farm, it diversifies its business. The Campbell Soup Company, well-known for its canned soups, also produces Swanson frozen prepared foods, Franco American products, Pepperidge Farm baked goods, Godiva chocolates, and other food products for retail sale. Borden Foods, well-known for its dairy products, also manufactures Aunt Jane's pickles, Bama jellies, Campfire marshmallows, Cracker Jacks, Drake's cakes and snacks, Frosted Shake, Kava instant coffee, None-Such mincemeat, Old London potato chips, ReaLemon reconstituted lemon juice, Sacramento tomato juice, Wise potato chips and Wyler soup and drink mixes. According to Jim Hightower,

> The independent firms that are being merged into large corporate structures are not failures, not inefficient competitors on the verge of folding. Quite the contrary, they are being bought by the giants precisely because they are competitive, innovative, and exhibit favorable growth potential. Frequently the companies that are bought are the leading producers of their respective products.

[Third,] vertical integration involves a firm buying control of as many steps in the production and marketing of its products as possible—from growing the raw product to retail sale. Our hypothetical banana grower buys his own crate-making factory, and purchases banana boats for transport. A grocery store chain such as Safeway processes its own ice cream for sale; a chicken processor such as Holly Farm raises its own chickens, and markets them in its own chicken restaurants; these are examples of vertical integration.

Horizontal integration, vertical integration, and diversification help a firm acquire a larger share of the market for its products. Monopoly or shared monopoly (oligopoly) is widespread in the U.S. economy as a whole, and in the food industry.

What are the consequences of monopoly or oligopoly? According to Dr. H. Michael Mann, Director, FTC Bureau of Economics, "Monopolies and concentration within industry may cost the nation as much as 6 percent of the gross national product (GNP) — that is, some $60 billion yearly." More specifically, monopoly frequently leads to:

— Price fixing, or the more subtle form of administered pricing (whereby prices are set by leader companies and are not based on responses to supply and demand);
— Excess profits, despite inefficiencies and wastes resulting from a lack of competition;
— High advertising costs — As much as 20 percent of the sales dollar is used to advertise products that have few real differences, aside from labels;
— Suppression of technological innovation;
— Barriers to entry — New competitors face roadblocks put up by concentrated industries; raising large advertising funds and finding distribution outlets is difficult.

Who is regulating the food industry? Three government agencies bear most of the responsibility: U.S. Department of Agriculture (USDA), Food and Drug Administration (FDA), and Federal Trade Commission (FTC).

USDA's functions include agricultural and economic research, soil conservation, forestry, inspections, grading, federal feeding program, and, above all, maintenance of farm incomes.

USDA has overemphasized the economics of production while not adequately protecting the family farmers' livelihood or insuring the availability of nutritious, low-cost food to all Americans. In the last two decades, 50,000 to 100,000 farms have disappeared each year; the nutritional status of Americans has also been declining. In 1955, 50 percent of Americans had an adequate diet while in 1965 only 40 percent of Americans had adequate diets, according to USDA surveys. Both poor farmers and consumers have been losing while large farmers and corporations are benefiting from USDA policies.

Too often USDA policies serve the profit motives of industry. While consumer groups are recommending that Americans reduce meat consumption, USDA is actively promoting the beef industry; USDA has worked in tandem with the agrichemical industry's promotion of pesticides and inorganic fertilizer; what little nutrition education USDA has done has been carefully geared not to conflict with industry viewpoints. The cooperation between USDA and industry is not surprising since many USDA officials were formerly food industry executives. Earl Butz, [former] secretary of agriculture, was . . . [once] director of Ralston Purina; Clifford Hardin, his predecessor as secretary, became vice president and director of Ralston Purina after leaving his USDA post. USDA-sponsored agricultural research is largely directed towards industry needs — and the research of today shapes the food of the future.

While USDA monitors the quality of agricultural products (and slightly processed foods like milk), FDA monitors more processed foods. FDA is charged with insuring food safety and honest labeling of food. It evaluates the safety of food additives. The agency has moved very cautiously in regulating the food industry. It has worked traditionally on the basis of voluntary compliance and self-regulation within the industry rather than mandatory or legal enforcement. A relatively low budget and consistent staff crossovers between FDA and industry (in 1973, twenty-two of fifty-two top officials had worked for regulated industries or organizations that cater to these industries) reinforce FDA's lenient treatment of the companies it theoretically regulates.

The FTC is authorized to prevent "unfair methods of competition"; to prevent dissemination of unfair advertisements; to prevent monopolistic practices; and to enforce truthful labeling, as well as other duties. The agency has done much useful research concerning economic concentration in the food industry, but litigation has been exceedingly slow, while our future food supply continues to be shaped daily by large, monopolistic corporations.

And what does the future look like? If present trends continue, the food industry will be dominated by a few giants; vertically integrated conglomerates will control food from field to table; government and private industry will be geared to the marketing needs of these firms; the family farmer will disappear along with ma and pa grocery stores and independently owned restaurants.

As for the food itself, processing is much the trend. In 1975 Alexander Schmidt, Commissioner of FDA, predicted that by 1980 two-thirds of food consumed will be prepared outside the home. A USDA publication states, "The processor is guided by the wants and desires of the consumer and the consumer's demand for food is shifting from raw commodities to more sophisticated products." But with advertising so able to create "wants," "desires," and "demands," it is more and more difficult to distinguish between what consumers really want and what industry, armed with slick advertising, imposes on them.

Critics see the trend towards highly processed foods as another indication that profit is the food industry's paramount concern. One company can't sell a tomato, for example, for much more than another company. But process it into ketchup, add spices and a fraction of a cent of flavor, and bottle it; call it barbecue sauce; advertise it; tout its brand name, and higher and higher profits can be made because the product seems unique.

The next step is to create synthetic ingredients which simulate the taste of tomatoes, and bypass the real vegetable and its difficult handling altogether. We live in an age of simulated foods, formulated foods, textured vegetable proteins, and meat analogs. Few of these products provide low-cost nutritional advances for consumers, but they do represent additional profit for food companies.

Decisions that greatly affect our food supply are made daily. Who is making these decisions? Are decisions based on people's needs or corporate profit schemes? Do we want a homogenized food system shaped and controlled by the profit needs of fifty giant corporations? Or, can we provide for present and future food needs with a rational, human policy based on the needs of all the citizens of this nation and the world? What can each one of us do in our community to insure a fair outcome in this fight?

Selection 19   On the Trail of a Steer: From Birth to Burger

William Serrin

Editors' Introduction

The urban consumer is relatively divorced from the facts of farm life and food production. The availability of food in abundant variety in supermarkets, restaurants, and at fast-food outlets is taken for granted. A number of interlocking social, economic, technical, and political factors contribute to the cost and quality of the food supply. The following selection helps to detail how beef prices are arrived at—and why they are hard to change.

How Prices Get That Way, and Why They're So Hard to Change

Early on the evening of June 26, in the backyard of Robert and Susan Mandell's house in Montvale, N.J., the hamburgers were sizzling on the gas-fueled barbecue grill. It was the final chapter of a saga that had begun two and a half years before on a farm in Missouri.

What follows is the story of an Angus-Hereford steer and the industry that prepares it for market, from feeding farm to slaughterhouse to butcher. Along the way, the article explores the role of a publication

Source: Adapted from William Serrin, "On the Trail of a Steer, from Birth to Burger," *New York Times*, December 10, 1978, Sec. 3, pp. 1, 10–11. © 1978 by The New York Times Company. Reprinted by permission.

called The Yellow Sheet in determining prices, a controversy over beef grading—and how an animal that initially sold for 35 cents a pound ended up selling for as high as $3.49 a pound.

More than 40 percent of the average family's food budget goes for meat, and Americans have been eating more and more of the stuff. Beef consumption, for example, rose from 63 pounds per capita in 1950 to 93.2 pounds in 1977. The price of beef has had its ups and downs during that time, keeping pace with the size of the nation's cattle herds, but of late it's been soaring—consumer beef prices for October were up more than 29 percent over October 1977—and has become a major target of President Carter's anti-inflation moves.

The supply of beef, however, changes according to a cycle imposed not by presidents but by natural patterns of gestation and digestion. Even if cattlemen were to decide to increase their herds, and there is no clear indication that they are so inclined, the effect would be three to four years in the making. Meanwhile, the size of the herds continues to decline, exacerbating the upward price pressure caused by inflation's impact on industry costs.

February 1976

Off in a corner of a cold, bleak pasture on the Missouri plains a cow dropped a wet, wobbly male calf. She licked it clean; in a few moments, she had it on its feet. It weighed about 80 pounds and was black save for a white face—a cross between an Angus and a Hereford.

Don Gretzinger, fifty-five years old, runs a cow-calf operation on 3,400 acres near Urich, Mo. He maintains 650 cows of his own and pastures 290 for a Kansas City cattle company. He carries about thirty bulls. He's never calculated—as he says, "Never put a pencil to it"—just how much a pound it costs him to put weight on his cattle, but he knows profits and losses. He's had both.

He recalls buying land at $50 an acre when he got out of the service after World War II; now land in this part of the state is worth at least $500 an acre. He also recalls buying cows at $500 and then watching their value drop to $150.

The Angus-Hereford born this day was castrated at one to two months, weaned at about six months, kept on the farm a total of nine months until it weighed about 450 pounds. It was then loaded on a truck for the trip to the Kansas City Livestock Exchange for the first in a series of ownership changes that would lead, inevitably, to the slaughterhouse.

At the exchange, the steer was purchased by Raymond Neth, a cattle feeder known as a "backgrounder." Mr. Gretzinger received $35 a hundred pounds, or somewhat more than $150. His farm, with its rich grasslands, was well-suited for the initial phases of the cattle-raising process, but economically, it lacked the size and scale required for the next, more rapid weight-gaining stage.

Summer 1977

Broad in the neck and shoulders, strongly muscled, thick in the rear, the steer at about sixteen months of age was something like a high school guard or tackle working on the blocking sled. But shorter—four feet—and more than a bit heavier at 650 pounds.

Ray Neth, fifty-four years old, his three sons and his brother, Howard, maintain about 1,600 cattle on 2,100 acres of pasture fifteen miles northeast of Liberty, Mo. In addition to the pasture—with its Kentucky bluegrass plus brome and fescue—they keep 300 acres for hay for winter feed. The hay sits, not in stacks, but in six-foot-high oval bales like giant Shredded Wheat behind one of the farmhouses.

The cattle on the Neth farm are allowed to eat all the grass they can plus a bit of grain. Grass puts the weight on more slowly, but it's cheaper; the grain is necessary because when the calf is sold to a feeder, the final stage before slaughter, it will be put on "full feed," a grain diet, and it must be able to take to the grain immediately. (The final feeding operation was out of Ray Neth's reach, Missouri not being one of the major corn-producing states.)

The Angus-Hereford was gaining weight at the rate of one and a quarter to one and a half pounds a day. As fall approached, it neared its selling weight, for the next stage, of 700 to 800 pounds. One morning, in company with others of the Neth herd, it was trucked back to the Kansas City Livestock Exchange and led into a weather-grayed, rickety cattle pen.

For Ray Neth as for other backgrounders, the timing is all. Will his cattle be at peak weight when the beef market is peaking, too? The Angus-Hereford was at 733 pounds when it was sold to the Kanasas City Livestock Company for $308, or $42 a hundred pounds. After subtracting the original $150 purchase and the cost of feed (the steer gained about 300 pounds at 6 cents a pound, or $18 altogether), trucking and other expenses, Mr. Neth figured he made about $35 to $40 net on the steer.

Lee Throckmorton, a founder of the livestock company, thought that was good money, but then, he was the buyer—and within hours he'd be the seller.

"People not in the business," says Mr. Throckmorton, who has been in the business for some 30 years, "don't understand anything about meat. They think we pick steaks off trees, like peaches."

As a buyer, Mr. Throckmorton picks steers from his customary place in the first tier of seats in the sale barn of the Kansas City exchange.

He spends hours each day watching cattle being guided into the show ring with the help of a long, thin whip. Even when he talks to clients on the cream-colored telephone plugged in at his feet, his eyes seldom wander from the auction.

When the cattle from Ray Neth's farm had appeared, Mr. Throckmorton joined the bidding. The slightest movement of his left hand was like a clarion call to the auctioneer down below. Other buyers were wiggling fingers, waving hands. The bids, but not the identities of the bidders, poured forth in the auctioneer's spiel.

Mr. Throckmorton had a particular client in mind when he bought Ray Neth's steer. Each fall, Mr. Throckmorton gets a telephone call from Lemoine Moll, a farmer outside Shannon, Ill., with a request to buy about 800 head of cattle. Mr. Throckmorton had been handling Mr. Moll's order for several years, though the two men had never met, and he knew what his client wanted: As many Angus-Hereford crossbreeds as possible, because he felt they put on weight best—the rest Angus and, if necessary, some Herefords. He wanted the cattle at about 750 pounds, and he wanted them to take quickly to grain feed.

Between September and November, Mr. Throckmorton and his partner, Harold Schmidt, purchased 798 cattle for Mr. Moll. Of course, the prices they paid, and the prices at which they were sold to Mr. Moll, varied. But on average, Mr. Moll—"Bill" as he is known—paid $44.70 a hundred pounds, out of which came the $2.10-a-head commission to Mr. Throckmorton's company and trucking costs of $9.62 a head.

June 18, 1978

The Angus-Hereford born on the Missouri plains almost two and a half years before was now weighing in at better than 1,000 pounds. During the past eight months Mr. Moll had carefully brought it along, starting with chopped corn stalks, then chopped ears of corn including the cobs—a gradually enriched diet. The feed was also sprinkled with soybean meal for added protein. The goal: a weight gain of two to two and a half pounds a day.

Lemoine Moll is a sophisticated farmer who lives in the town of Shannon and commutes five miles every morning to his 800-acre spread in a pickup truck. He keeps careful records, and he knows where every dollar goes. In 1977, he marketed 814 steer, which he'd bought at an average of $39.75 a hundred pounds and sold at $39.04 a hundred pounds. As he figured it up, he lost $45,226.69 on his cattle operation for the year.

"You can lose some money, you can make some," Mr. Moll said. And 1978 looked to be a making year.

The beef business operates on fairly regular cycle. When prices are favorable, or when ranchers and farmers expect that prices will become favorable, they expand their herds. It take several years—sixteen to twenty-four months for a heifer to be born, to mature and be bred; nine months for gestation; thirty months for the calf to be ready for market. When the beef supply outstrips demand, prices fall, ranchers begin to sell off heifers instead of holding them for breeding, cows are sold off and the extra meat going to market further depresses prices.

In 1975, the number of cattle was a record 131.8 million, but by January 1, 1978, that figure had dropped to 116.3 million. Meanwhile, Americans had continued to increase their beef consumption—going as high as 93.2 pounds per person in 1977.

Mr. Moll was benefiting. Through late spring he had sold 701 steer in nine batches for prices ranging from $53.50 a hundred pounds to $62, the highest he'd received in all his twenty-five years as a farmer. Then, on May 31, Mr. Moll heard that at the Joliet Livestock Exchange, where he markets his cattle, the price had hit a record $62.75 a hundred pounds. Mr. Moll had another seventy-three steer to sell, including the Angus-Hereford from Missouri, and Mr. Moll was pleased.

Then, on June 2, President Carter announced that the government would allow an additional 200 million pounds of imported beef into the country—the purpose being to lower the price of beef in general and hamburger in particular. Six days later, the United States Department of Agriculture released its periodic report on the number of cattle being fed in seven western states; the number, according to the USDA, was up more than 12 percent from early in the year. Prices started dropping.

Late on this sunny morning of June 18, as his wife was preparing the noon meal, Bill Moll was on the telephone, calling friends in the business including Bob Miller, a Shannon neighbor who buys and sells cattle on commission. What did they think of the market? The consensus: Bad and getting worse. Mr. Moll immediately called a trucker, and before the day was over the seventy-three cattle were headed down route 80 toward Joliet, 135 miles away.

What, Mr. Moll was asked, do you hope to get for your cattle? "Oh, maybe 58," Mr. Moll said. "Maybe 58 and a half." Bob Miller, his neighbor, would represent him at the stockyards.

June 19, 1978

At 7:30 A.M., truck fumes mingled with the odor of manure; cattle bellowed and bleated, moving to the shouts and whistles of handlers; sparrows and pigeons darted about the pens and back to their nests in the rafters under the metal roof.

Bob Miller had flown down to Joliet in his Cherokee 235. A tall, jocular forty-three-year-old, he started out in the commission business at the Chicago stockyards, moved shop in 1971 when the Chicago yards were closing, a victim of the increasing decentralization of the beef market.

Now he was chatting with a handful of farmers, who had come to watch their animals being sold, and some buyers. Early in the morning, when temperatures are in the sixties, say, and the sun is still shining, with good prices still a possibility, there is a feeling of good humor and camaraderie. As the hours pass, as the temperatures rise and the prices fall, unpleasantness sets in.

"Tempers can flare pretty good," Mr. Miller said, though grudges aren't generally kept. "You've got to get along with the buyers. If you don't, they're not going to buy cattle from you."

Once the business day starts, the chief actors don't mix. The farmers talk among themselves, only very occasionally speaking to commission men and almost never to buyers. Nor do buyers talk to them. "That's just the way it is," said Cal Clark, a small, weathered buyer from Illini Beef Packers Inc., a major Midwest slaughtering and beef marketing company.

Just after 7:30 A.M., Mr. Miller and Mr. Clark began walking the aisles of the stockyard. Occasionally they'd stop to allow Mr. Clark to examine the cattle, checking the way they walk, their rib coverage, the amount of fat around the eyes. He was trying to figure their yield—how many pounds of meat they'd produce once they were slaughtered. In other words, as he walked along, Mr. Clark did not see *live* cattle, but cattle already hanging on hooks in Illini Beef's cooling room, 135 miles to the west in Joslin, Ill.

Mr. Clark operates under instructions from Edward C. Olsson, director of procurement for Illini Beef, who is in telephone and radio communication each morning with sixteen buyers across eastern Iowa and western Illinois. The company slaughters 1,400 to 1,500 animals a day and likes to have a two-day supply on hand or scheduled for shipment. Each buyer like Mr. Clark receives a daily order, subject to change at any time, to buy so many cattle at a price not to exceed a given figure.

Along with 70 to 90 percent of the packers and wholesalers in the American meat business, Illini bases its bids upon a four-page publication known, because it is printed on yellow paper, as The Yellow Sheet.

Published from a century-old, refurbished brick townhouse on the near west side of Chicago, The Yellow Sheet began in October 1923, after—as its president, Lester I. Norton, seventy years old, tells the story—some meat packers asked the people who ran *National Provisioner* magazine to set up a monitoring service for hog prices. The packers, Mr. Norton said, were spending too much time trying to find out what prices their competitors were paying, and, because of federal antitrust laws, they could not ask each other, at least legally. *National Provisioner* began to report beef prices just before World War II.

Each day, beginning at 7:45 A.M., four reporters get on telephones and begin calling packers and wholesalers around the country to determine what prices are being paid for beef products. Throughout the day, the figures are dispatched to the company's clients, by telegram or by special delivery.

The Committee on Small Business of the United States House of Representatives has held hearings on The Yellow Sheet, amid charges that it performs a price-fixing function and, moreover, fabricates a large percentage of the prices it reports. In October, the committee issued a report charging that the free market in the meat industry had deteriorated and was close to being eliminated. The committee's chairman, Representative Neal Smith, Democrat of Iowa, has introduced a bill that would license all meat-price services like The Yellow Sheet and would authorize the secretary of agriculture to explore whether the government should establish a national pricing system.

Mr. Norton denies the charges and professes to be unruffled by the whole business: When meat prices get high, he says, it's traditional to kick The Yellow Sheet around a little. Mr. Norton emphasizes that his publication does not list prices of live cattle; that doesn't, however, prevent companies like Illini Beef from using The Yellow Sheet's carcass prices to determine what they'll pay for live cattle.

On Friday, June 16, the sheet's closing price for slaughtered beef was $90.50 a hundredweight. At the opening of the market on Monday, June 19, Mr. Olsson of Illini Beef instructed his buyers, including Mr. Clark at Joliet, to pay no more than that figure—by translating from a steer's live weight to its slaughtered, or carcass, weight. Thus, once he decided that a steer would dress out at, say, 63 percent, he could figure that his bid for the live animal should theoretically not be above $57.02. But figuring in the cost of trucking (43 cents a hundred pounds) and the fact that cattle bids are made in quarter-dollar increments, Mr. Clark knew his real top bid this nineteenth day of June could be only $56.50.

As he moved through the aisles of the Joliet stockyards, Mr. Clark and Mr. Miller played out a time-honored game.

"How much you want for these, Bob? They sure don't look that damn good."

"Dammit, Cal, those are superb cattle. Damn superb cattle."

"C'mon, Bob. Stop toying with me. I know my business."

Then the two would laugh and continue their walk, They had passed Mr. Moll's cattle several times and Mr. Clark had looked them over. He had bought from Mr. Moll in the past and he knew they were likely to be good cattle.

At 9:02 A.M. Mr. Clark bid $56.50 a hundred pounds for Mr. Moll's seventy-three cattle. Mr. Miller had hoped for more, but the market seemed to be falling, and he accepted the offer. Yardmen began herding the cattle, including the Missouri-born Angus-Hereford, out of the pens to the scales at the back of the cattle shed. They weighed in at 86,432 pounds, an average of 1,184 per steer, and were loaded on trucks for the trip to the slaughterhouse.

Meanwhile, Mr. Miller continued to sell cattle until just before noon. The market had kept dropping, closing at $55 a hundredweight. Now it was time for a daily ritual—the call to the farmer-clients to tell them the prices at which their cattle had been sold. The commission men sat at a bank of telephones in the exchange office, a modern building in the middle of the yards. For the commission men, it is not always a happy ritual.

Mr. Moll took the news stoically. He'd hoped for better than $56.50. Mr. Miller agreed it wasn't the best, but what can you do?

That evening, Mr. Moll sat on a davenport in his living room and toted up the results of his cattle operation for the year. The 798 animals that Lee Throckmorton had bought for him in Kansas City had cost $261,465, which he'd borrowed from the First State Bank of Shannon at 9 percent interest.

How would it work out in terms of a single steer, he was asked—in terms, say, of an Angus-Hereford born on Joe Gretzinger's farm in Missouri. Mr. Moll broke it down this way: $327.66 for purchase; $192.38 for feed; $33.57 for management and overhead; $15.11 for interest on the loan; $2.73 for processing and medicine; $2.33 for its share of the loss caused by the death of four fellow steers.

By the time the steer was ready to be sold, it represented an investment by Mr. Moll of $573.77. Add to that the $2 a head for Bob Miller's commission plus the cost of trucking the steer to the stockyards, feeding it there and insuring it. Mr. Moll figured that for his six months' labors he had made a profit of $62.73 on the steer. For the whole batch of 798 cattle, which he'd sold at different times and at different prices, Mr. Moll said he'd realized a net profit of $86,875—an annual return of about 6.5 percent on his investment.

It was the first time in three years, he said, that he'd be making money on his cattle operation.

June 20, 1978

The Illini Beef Company in Joslin is the largest packer east of the Mississippi River. Last year, it said, sales were $218 million; net profit was $614,000. Employment was 525. In a typical week, the plant slaughters 7,250 cattle.

At 7:46 A.M. on this June day, a young blond man smoking a Marlboro stood to the side of the giant, white-faced Angus-Hereford from Missouri and fired a gunlike device, sending an eight-inch-long pin into its forehead and ending its life. Another worker inserted a hook beneath the bones and sinews of a rear foot, and the dead steer, blood pouring from its giant body, was lifted high into the air.

At 7:52 A.M., the steer's throat was slit. At 8 o'clock a worker cut a small piece of hide in the shape of a tab, like that on a cereal box; a roller-like machine seized the tab, and within four minutes the steer's hide was off. Two minutes later, the head was removed, almost simultaneous with the stripping out of the tongue. Just 25 minutes after the fatal device was fired, the steer had been turned into a carcass and by-products.

The carcass was on its way to the cooling room; the by-products were speeding on conveyer belts toward secondary processing. The hide was dropped to the basement into a vat of brine, start of curing. Skull, hooves, bone, hair, moved toward a combination crushing machine-cooking vat — eventually to become fertilizer or soap.

In spite of its mission, the Illini plant is scrupulously clean and largely odorless — a far cry from the early days of the century when Upton Sinclair's *The Jungle* helped pave the way for the passage of the Pure Food and Drug Act. There are eleven government men on duty in the Illini plant. Dennis Breen, the plant manager, feels that's too many, that his industry still labors under a false public impression. As he puts it, during the course of a tour of the facility, "This is no 'Jungle.'"

Last summer the General Accounting Office issued a study hauling the beef grading system over the coals. It is a voluntary program on the part of meat packers, who pay a fee to have Agriculture Department-trained employees do the grading. The GAO charged that the prime and choice labels were in error 20 percent of the time, that the errors were often made in favor of the meat packers, and that some retailers were placing their own labels on ungraded meat, sometimes using the word "choice" on these labels. The Agriculture Department agreed with some of the findings, and reported that it was preparing to add 240 trained graders to its current nationwide force of 400.

June 21, 1978

At 7:10 A.M., the beef carcasses — including the two parts, known as sides, that were the Angus-Hereford from Missouri — are moving on hooks out of the twenty-five-degree cooling room toward the grading room. William Benner, forty-eight years old, who has been grading cattle for the federal government for eighteen years, was waiting. As the carcass approached, an Illini employee made an incision at the eighteenth vertebra, exposing what is known as the rib eye. Mr. Benner inspected it for color, texture, marbling. He studied the cartilage on the carcass to determine its age. He noted the quantity of fat in the kidney, heart and pelvis. The entire process took fifteen seconds.

The government authorizes four grades of beef quality (prime, choice, good, and standard) and gives five grades of meat yield, ranging from grade one for the leanest to grade five for the fattest. Mr. Benner judged the Angus-Hereford to be grade three choice—the grade most cattle farmers aim for since Americans tend to prefer some fat on their meat.

The slowly swinging carcass was then pushed along to the end of the grading room where Terry Carstens sat waiting. He decides what customers will receive which carcasses.

The Illini company has what amounts to a standing order for three truckloads of beef a week from an Englewood, N.J., wholesaler, Richard H. Lubben. Mr. Lubben was known to have exacting standards, and Mr. Carstens thought the Angus-Hereford would meet them. He attached a paper ticket to the carcass, labeled "Lubben, Englewood, N.J.," and sent the meat along to the end of the line.

On Monday, June 19, The Yellow Sheet had reported that the typical price for a grade three choice animal was $87 a hundred pounds; there were no price quotations on Tuesday, because the paper had decided there'd not been enough sold to warrant a quotation. Now, on Wednesday, Illini salesman Tim Hughes was going by the Monday quotations in his telephone talk with Mr. Lubben.

"We'll ship you one truckload today, Rich," Mr. Hughes said. "At $87 a hundredweight." Mr. Lubben agreed. That meant the company would receive $649.63 for the meat from the Angus-Hereford, about $25 less than what Mr. Moll had been paid. But that figure left out the by-product.

The tongue, for example, went to the Sweigert Sausage Company, a subsidiary of Illini Beef, to be made into salami or bologna. The intestines would be made into sutures or tennis racket strings. The lung and spleen were bought by the Kal Can Company of Columbus, Ohio, to be turned into pet food.

Based on USDA figures for that week, the only available guidelines, the by-products of the Angus-Hereford sold for about $64. That gave Illini a gross profit of $39.52 on the animal, and an anticipated net of about $7.14.

At 11 A.M., the carcasses chosen for Mr. Lubben were being loaded into a refrigerator truck trailer on forklift trucks. The trailer holds fifty-five carcasses, about 40,000 pounds of beef. At 12:30 o'clock the doors of the truck were closed and secured with a metal loop and lock.

At 4 P.M. Helmut Altenhain, a small, wiry trucker from Dunmore, Pa., pulled his truck cab into the Illini Beef shipping yard. He backed it up to the refrigerated trailer, and was hooked up. Then he set off—up the Illinois tollpike, down I-294 at Chicago, and on to New Jersey and Mr. Lubben's offices 923 miles away.

June 23, 1978

In a second-story office overlooking the loading dock of Richard H. Lubben & Sons Wholesale Meat, in Englewood, N.J., the boss was seated at his desk. It was 4:30 A.M. "The meat business is a tough business," Mr. Lubben, forty-eight years old, was saying. "You have got to put in a lot of hours and have a lot of money."

Mr. Lubben supplies chain stores such as Shop Rite, specialty butcher shops and restaurants such as Laurent in New York City, Boulderberg Manor in Tomkins Cove, N.Y., and the Casa Hoffbrau in Emerson, N.J. Ed Mosier, operator of the B&M Meat Market, is an old customer and a good friend who is looking for quality. "I'm sending that Illini steer to Ed Mosier," Mr. Lubben said. The price: 98 cents a pound.

Outside, on Englewood Avenue, Mr. Altenhain is sleeping in his cab. He had arrived at midnight. By 6 o'clock he was awake and ready to join Mr. Lubben for breakfast at a nearby cafe. There Mr. Altenhain sang a sad song of the expenses a trucker faces. He can gross $35,000 in a year, Mr. Altenhain said, but given such costs as engine overhauls, net only $8,000. On the previous day's run, he figured to net less than $200.

Back at Mr. Lubben's plant, Mr. Altenhain smashed the lock on his truck with a hammer, and the unloading began. The carcass of the Angus-Hereford was placed on a meat hook and transported on a conveyer system into the plant. Meanwhile a Lubben truck had backed up to the loading dock; its floor was covered with brown butcher paper to receive slab after slab of the meat.

Mr. Lubben had paid $649.68 for the carcass of the Missouri steer, plus $26.18 for trucking, or $675.86. He sold the 738-pound carcass to Mr. Mosier, the butcher, for $723.24. (The carcass had shrunk 8.7 pounds during the trips from the slaughterhouse to Lubben's, as cattle do on every trip they take, alive or dead. Mr. Lubben must absorb this shrinkage.) Thus Mr. Lubben grossed $47.38 on the steer, and he figures he will net $15.

It was light now, about 7:05 A.M., as two young workers jumped onto the Lubben truck: "Hustle up," Mr. Lubben said. "Don't waste time." They moved off, driving briskly up Kinderkanack Road toward Park Ridge, N.J.

"It should have been graded prime," Mr. Mosier said. He was standing in the back room of his shop, looking admiringly at a large piece of meat from the hindquarter of the steer from Missouri. A worker had just put it down on the butcher block while the rest of the animal was being hung in the cooler to age.

Only about two-thirds of a carcass — 492 pounds in the case of this steer — can be marketed as beef. The remainder, consisting of fat and bone, are sold, generally, to a rendering firm. Or a meat market man could make a few extra dollars by leaving extra bones on meat or grinding some of the fat into hamburger. Mr. Mosier said that wasn't his style.

His shop serves the largely upper income area of Park Ridge and Montvale, in the northern part of the state. At a meat market like his, Mr. Mosier said, he tries to mark meat about 22 percent above what he paid for the carcass. The forequarter is marked up perhaps 32 percent, the hindquarter perhaps 18 percent — more kinds of cuts can be obtained from the forequarter, he explained. Mr. Mosier hoped to sell the carcass of the steer from Missouri for $882.35, or $1.79 a pound. His prices this day ranged from $3.49, for porterhouse steak, to $1.39 for hamburger. The remainder of the carcass he would sell to a rendering company for $8 total. Mr. Mosier said he would net about $35 on the carcass.

At 7:59 o'clock, the first pieces of meat from the steer, eight sirloin steaks, were placed in Mr. Mosier's meat case; London broil and ground chuck following in fast order. Ten minutes after the store opened at 8 o'clock, the first customer arrived. At 9:23 o'clock, Susan Mandell walked in; she is field director with David-Petersen Associates Inc., of 747 Third Avenue, New York City, which performs marketing and advertising surveys. Mrs. Mandell, who lives in nearby Montvale, has shopped at Mr. Mosier's market for two and a half years. She acknowledges that the prices are high there, but she says the quality of meat makes it worthwhile. Meat bought here, she said, does not cook away.

At 9:46 o'clock, Mrs. Mandell made the first purchase of meat from the Missouri steer — two pounds of ground chuck, specially cut for her, made from the neck and tenderloin, at $1.99 a pound.

June 26, 1978

Early on this still sunny summer evening in Montvale, Bob Mandell, had the barbecue going in the backyard of the large, single-family home. He and Susan had invited a friend, Dr. James Diehl, a surgeon, to join them. Mr. Mandell was almost done broiling the ground chuck when his wife started setting out the salad, fresh corn on the cob, potato chips, and soda. An hour later, the meal was over. The meat, everyone agreed, had been excellent.

Selection 20 Tracing Elements Through the Food Chain

U.S. Department of Agriculture

Editors' Introduction

Living organisms require many inorganic elements—commonly referred to as minerals—for their normal life processes. These elements function in plants and animals as building materials and/or as regulators of chemical reactions. Minerals have demonstrable functions in the human body. They are often classed either as macronutrients or micronutrients, on the basis of how much of the mineral is found in the body and how much of the mineral is needed in the diet. Calcium, phosphorus, potassium, sulfur, chlorine, sodium, and magnesium are considered macronutrients. Iron, iodine, fluorine, zinc, copper, chromium, selenium, cobalt, manganese, molybdenum, vanadium, tin, silicon, and nickel are known as micronutrients, or *trace elements*. We do not know the role many of these trace elements play in human life processes. Moreover, minute amounts of aluminum and arsenic are found in the human body, but there is no proof they are essential to life.

Research teams, including soil scientists, plant physiologists, biochemists, and animal nutritionists are busy studying dozens of trace elements in the food chain as they pass from soil to plants to animals. These scientists hope one day to control the levels of these elements in the food chain so they will more closely parallel the dietary requirements of humans. They are focusing on the following concerns.

First, does the soil in certain geographical areas produce crops that lack some of the trace elements essential for animals and humans? These elements may not be essential for the normal growth of plants but may be essential for the normal functioning of some animals and/or humans.

Second, once scientists have identified deficiencies of trace elements in plants and animals other questions arise: What is the best way to overcome the deficiency? Should they prevent or treat these nutritional diseases by adding trace elements to the soil? to the crops? Should they administer nutrient supplements to livestock? Physicians and nutritionists are enthusiastic about the

Source: From U.S. Department of Agriculture, Washington, D.C., April 1970.

possibility of applying information gained from these research efforts in developing innovative techniques and preparations that can be used in the prevention and treatment of human nutritional problems.

In the past many people living in inland areas of the United States, where the soil is lacking in iodine, suffered from the iodine-deficiency disease manifested by an enlarged thyroid, known as *goiter.* This condition can be prevented through the practice of iodizing salt. The use of this product has significantly reduced the incidence of goiter in the United States.

At present, most cases of iron-deficiency anemia seem to be due to the poor availability rather than the absence of iron in food sources. Although many foods of vegetable and animal origin contain iron, the absorption of iron is much poorer from vegetable sources than from animal sources. The incidence of iron-deficiency anemia is very high among people who rely on plant, rather than animal, foods to meet their protein needs. Preliminary findings from animal experiments indicate that when the amino acids lysine and/or histidine are added to vegetable proteins, the efficiency of absorption is enhanced. However, a word of caution should be added: Before histidine or lysine can be used in the prevention and treatment of iron-deficiency anemia and protein-deficiency syndromes, the use of the amino acids should be tested for their effectiveness under clinical conditions.

In the following selection, scientists explain how they pursue such nutritional detective work.

A physician swabs a frail, young patient's arm with alcohol before injecting a measure of soluble iron.

A soil scientist studies the results of tests to determine the iron content of soils and food crops growing on those soils.

What is the connection between physician and soil scientist? They both are combating iron-deficiency anemia, probably the world's most widespread nutritional disorder. Like scientists of many disciplines, they are concerned with trace elements and their effect on human health. This interest is growing because of recent findings by the Agricultural Research Service and medical science that show, for example:

— Iron absorption can be increased greatly in laboratory animals by combining it with the amino acids histidine or lysine.
— Zinc aids in healing wounds in some cases following injury or surgery. It also affects animal reproduction.
— Selenium can be added to soils to eliminate deficiencies in sheep that cause white muscle disease in their lambs.

— Cadmium in excessive amounts can lead to high blood pressure in people.

These and similar findings are of direct interest to soil scientists, plant physiologists, biochemists, and animal nutritionists at the U.S. Plant, Soil, and Nutrition Laboratory, Ithaca, N.Y. The laboratory is operated by ARS in cooperation with Cornell University. Scientists there are studying dozens of trace elements in the food chain—from soil to plant to animal. Their challenge: Can we control the levels of these elements in the food chain so that they better parallel the needs of consumers?

This Agricultural Research Service laboratory is literally a miniature Scotland Yard when it comes to detecting elements in soil samples, and in plant and animal tissue. There, scientists have at their fingertips such sophisticated detection equipment as:

— Atomic absorption spectrophotometer to analyze plant and blood samples for such elements as magnesium, calcium, chromium, and cadmium.
— Isotope counter to trace radioactive elements through the plant cycle—from soil to plant to animal—and within a plant or animal.
— Gas chromatograph to identify unknown substances in various materials under study.

In fact, such equipment is largely responsible for the increased success scientists are achieving in determining the part trace elements play in plant and animal life.

"We must know the movement of micronutrients from the soil to plants—and into the animal or human food chain," says Dr. W.H. Allaway, who directs the laboratory. Equipment such as the isotope counter has helped determine what happens to different trace elements when they are added to soils.

Fortunately, plants provide an effective barrier against several trace elements that could be poisonous to animals. These include arsenic, iodine, beryllium, fluorine, nickel, and vanadium. Plant growth would cease or be greatly depressed before these elements could accumulate to levels that would be dangerous to man or animals.

It is possible, on the other hand, for plants to grow at normal or near-normal rates and still contain enough selenium, cadmium, molybdenum, or lead to be harmful in feed or food.

It is also possible for feed and food plants to grow normally even though they do not contain enough of certain elements to meet the dietary requirements of some animals. These elements include cobalt, chromium, copper, iodine, manganese, selenium, and zinc.

Two challenging questions facing the staff at the U.S. Plant, Soil, and Nutrition Laboratory, then, are these: Do the soils in certain areas produce crops lacking in some elements that are essential to animals and man, even though not required by plants? Are there potentially harmful minerals in the plants from certain areas?

Deficiencies of trace elements are not new. To illustrate this point, Dr. Allaway tells the story about Indian Chief Chocorua, who, as the legend goes, put a curse on the people of Saco River Valley, New Hampshire, for taking his land. The so-called "curse," which fell upon the cattle, was actually a cobalt deficiency of the soils in the valley. Cattle refused to eat; they became anemic, weak, and emaciated. Many died.

This cobalt deficiency has since been overcome by animal scientists. Their modern-day cure for Chief Chocorua's "curse" came as cobalt salt in the form of salt licks or feed supplements. Fertilizers containing trace amounts of cobalt are also applied to pasture soils. ARS scientists helped resolve this problem by mapping areas of cobalt deficiency in the eastern United States.

Once agricultural scientists have found a plant or animal deficiency, questions then arise: What is the best way to overcome the deficiency? Should we add the trace element to the soil? To feed crops? Or as a treatment to livestock?

Iron: Present but Unavailable

But what if the element is present but tied up chemically and unavailable? This is the case of iron, required by both plants and animals. If deficient in soils, it can be added effectively as a soil treatment or in sprays on food or feed crops. Either way supplies the crop with its needs. Why, then, do we hear so much about "iron-tired blood" in humans?

Dr. Darrell Van Campen, a biochemist at the Ithaca laboratory, explains it this way: "In most cases, a deficiency of iron in plants or animals is due to its poor availability. We add a soluble form of iron to the soil or plant, and this takes care of the crop need."

But if food crops contain iron, why do people suffer from iron deficiencies?

"The reasons for poor iron utilization by individuals aren't really known," Dr. Van Campen says. "We do know that iron-deficiency anemia is very high among peoples in low-protein areas. This is true particularly where protein needs are met primarily by plant rather than animal protein."

Following this lead, Dr. Van Campen began studying amino acids, the structural units of proteins, and their effect on the utilization of iron by laboratory rats. There are about twenty amino acids in most proteins.

Some of these are good iron chelators—that is, they have the ability to combine with iron in a form that is soluble and can be absorbed into the bloodstream.

The results with the amino acids, histidine and lysine, were both dramatic and graphic.

When iron alone was injected into rats, only 5 percent was absorbed into the bloodstream in three hours. If lysine was added to the iron solution, about 50 percent of the iron was absorbed in the same time; if histidine was added to the iron, the absorption exceeded 75 percent in three hours.

These results were obtained by injecting radioactive iron and the amino acids directly into a tied-off section of intestine. . . . In another approach, radioactive iron and histidine were given to rats through a stomach tube. Histidine given in this manner also increased the absorption of iron but not as much as the injections.

Dr. Van Campen is highly enthusiastic about these results and their implications. He stresses, however, that before histidine or lysine can be used to increase the absorption of iron, "they should be tested for effectiveness under clinical conditions and the effectiveness compared to that of other methods of treating iron-deficiency anemia."

But these approaches suggest treatment—a dose of soluble iron as a treatment against anemia. What of a cure? In fact, what about a cure for deficiencies of both iron and protein?

ARS scientists already have developed protein food supplements for use in countries where the supply of protein, especially animal protein, is limited. Peoples in these same countries also suffer from iron-deficiency anemia. Further research may demonstrate that adding histidine or lysine to these protein food supplements at levels needed to provide maximum absorption of iron will serve to solve the problem of both iron deficiency and protein deficiency.

Zinc: New Roles in Life

Zinc, like iron, can be "present but unaccountable" in the diets of animals. For this, and other reasons, scientists have renewed interest in the part zinc plays in human health. It is known that zinc has a role in healing following wounds and surgery, that zinc affects animal reproduction, and that zinc may be beneficial in counteracting detrimental effects of cadmium.

Coupled with these nutritional and health needs is concern over the availability of zinc. The decline in the use of galvanized metals in plumbing systems, oddly enough, has decreased the amount of zinc available to animals and humans. Zinc deficiency in plants is becoming more widespread so its availability in food and feed crops is probably declining. Even of more concern, however, is the fact that zinc is less available in plant proteins than in animal proteins. And plant proteins in human foods far exceed the use of meat as a source of protein in underdeveloped parts of the world.

It is in this climate that Dr. Jean Apgar, a biochemist at the Ithaca laboratory, is studying the role zinc plays in the reproduction of rats.

While trying to raise rats on a soybean meal diet, Dr. Apgar discovered that the females had a difficult time in reproduction. Soybean meal contains zinc but in a form that is unavailable, a fact learned in the 1950s by animal nutritionists in hog-feeding experiments.

Dr. Apgar observed that pups born to female rats on zinc-deficient diets died shortly after birth, and the females themselves underwent excessive stress and bleeding. Addition of zinc to the diet enabled the females to deliver normally and to raise litters successfully.

Even when Dr. Apgar fed adult rats an adequate zinc diet up to breeding time, and then took them off zinc, the same problems arose. "They became so zinc-deficient in the twenty-one days required for pregnancy that delivery of the pups took as much as twenty-four hours," she said. (Two hours is normal for the rat.) "Sometimes the females died. And even if they managed to deliver, the young hardly ever survived."

When Dr. Apgar fed female rats a zinc-deficient diet for three weeks and then attempted to breed them, only a small number mated. And of those that did mate, very few were able to carry the pregnancy through the full twenty-one-day term.

What are the implications for humans? Dr. Apgar said that very little is known about the incidence of zinc deficiency in humans, partly because there are no very good tests for zinc deficiency. And when tests are made on laboratory animals, there is little correlation between the level of zinc in the blood, hair, or urine and the development of zinc deficiency in the animals.

"It is possible that marginal zinc deficiencies do occur in people but are not detected," she says. "This is particularly likely when you consider that rats, sheep, and cattle store zinc in very limited amounts. An animal becomes deficient very quickly after zinc is removed from the diet. Zinc requirements also seem to be higher than was previously thought."

Dr. Apgar considers it possible that the female rat's need for zinc in reproduction has a counterpart in woman. However, all that is known at this time is that the level of zinc in the blood goes down during human pregnancy. And it is lower after delivery in the blood of women on plant diets than in the blood of women eating some animal protein.

Selenium: Necessary but Toxic

Each trace element has its own distinct complexities. But selenium, perhaps better than any, illustrates the very narrow margin between too little and too much.

Dr. Allaway keeps his hand in as a working scientist, besides directing the laboratory. He, Earl Cary, and Joe Kubota are working on selenium. "Even though selenium is essential to animal life—in very small amounts—it is more poisonous than arsenic," he says, "and is less abundant in the earth's crust than gold."

The margin between too little and too much selenium in feed for cows and sheep is critically narrow—less than one-fifth an ounce in a ton of hay. Too much selenium causes growth of the animals to be depressed, hooves to break off, and hair to fall out; too little results in white muscle disease in calves and lambs. At levels higher than one-fifth of an ounce per ton, cattle and sheep may die.

This is a major reason why deliberate additions of selenium to foods or animal feeds are prohibited in the United States. Injections of selenium are permitted, however, to prevent white muscle disease in lambs and calves.

The Ithaca lab has developed a map of the United States showing regions where feed crops are deficient in selenium and regions where crops contain adequate amounts. . . . They did this by collecting and analyzing over 3,000 samples of forages, and making use of information from earlier studies of selenium content of wheat and feed grains.

As the map took shape, one thing became obvious. The shipment of feed grains from the west central United States to the Northeast has helped meet the selenium needs of dairy cattle and poultry in selenium-deficient areas of the Northeast.

But what about treating soils with selenium? Would the resulting crop contain enough of the trace element to prevent white muscle disease in lambs and calves?

To find out, scientists at the Ithaca laboratory teamed up with scientists of the Oregon Agricultural Experiment Station in a study on an Oregon alfalfa field known to be deficient in selenium. Half of the field was treated with selenium; the other half was not treated.

Over half of the lambs born to ewes fed alfalfa from the untreated part of the field developed white muscle disease. Twenty percent of these died. In contrast, none of the lambs born to ewes fed alfalfa from the treated portion of the field got white muscle disease. Meat from these lambs did not contain selenium at levels toxic to people.

The research didn't end there, however. It was important to know what happened to that portion of the selenium applied to the Oregon field and not used by the alfalfa. Only abut 2 percent of the selenium was taken up by the alfalfa crop in the first 3 years after application. The rest remained in the soil. Would it be available to other crops? And was there a possibility that it could be taken up in amounts that would be toxic?

The scientists tackled these questions by "tagging" a number of different soils with radioactive selenium, growing alfalfa on them for a year, and hunting for the selenium that was left in the soils. It turned out that most of the selenium left in the soil was in one of two forms, both of which are quite inert and unavailable to plants. Application of selenium to the soil, therefore, may have a place in future efforts to improve the quality of feed crops.

Magnesium: Its Complex Interactions

Overcoming a deficiency in plants or animals often isn't as simple as adding selenium to the soil or cobalt to a cow's diet. ARS Soil Scientist D.L. Grunes will attest to that. He is working with a complex magnesium deficiency that affects lactating cattle, primarily.

The malady is grass tetany, often called "grass staggers" because animals develop stiff legs and give the appearance of staggering. In late stages of the disease, the animal may fall down, have convulsions, and die. The level of magnesium is low in the blood of affected animals. Grass tetany has caused losses of more than 10,000 cattle in California and Nevada in recent years.

Dr. Grunes, who is working with state and ARS scientists in California, Georgia, Idaho, Nevada, and North Dakota, points out that grass tetany strikes as a result of a combination of several interacting conditions:

— When a cow is lactating and losing magnesium to her milk;
— When a cow is grazing cool-season grasses (crested wheatgrass, ryegrass, wild rye, and tall fescue, for example);
— When the weather is cool, most often in early spring but also in the fall;
— When the content of grasses is high in certain organic acids, such as trans-aconitic acid;
— At times when a cow's diet is high in potassium and nitrogen;
— And recently in southeastern states when cows grazed pastures that had been fertilized heavily with chicken litter.

Despite these complex interactions, Dr. Grunes feels, "We are well on the road to determining how cattlemen can eliminate grass tetany."

In Nevada, for example, cooperating scientists induced tetany in lactating cattle by causing them to ingest equal parts of potassium chloride and organic acids. These compounds obviously interfered with metabolism and the use of magnesium by the cattle.

Affected cattle usually recover from grass tetany if they are injected with calcium-magnesium gluconate in the first few hours after symptoms occur. "The problem with this treatment," Dr. Grunes says, "is one of timing. If treatment is delayed eight to twelve hours after the first symptoms occur, chances of recovery are slight. And cattlemen, particularly those with range cattle, don't visit their herds that frequently."

What, then, do the scientists feel is the solution? Dr. Grunes hopes soon to be able to come up with a formula—based on weather reports—that can be used to warn stockmen against grazing certain pastures. That is why it is important to pinpoint precise cool-weather temperatures and all grass species that influence the disease.

Challenges: Many and Complex

In summary, scientists at the U.S. Plant, Soil and Nutrition Laboratory feel many questions remain unanswered—both with trace elements now under study and those they hope to study. Here are some of the challenges, element by element:

— Zinc—Can we manage our soils and our food crops in ways that will provide people with the essential zinc they need in their diets?

— Selenium—Can we control the level of selenium in soils, crops, and animal feeds at a level that will prevent selenium deficiencies in animals without any danger of selenium toxicity?

— Magnesium—Can we supply magnesium from soil to plant to animal in amounts that will prevent grass tetany in cattle, sheep, and goats?

— Chromium—How much chromium is there in food plants? Can we increase this amount to protective levels? Are there any adverse side effects from increasing chromium content of food plants? (Chromium has been found to help, along with insulin, in the prevention of diabetes in older people.)

— Cadmium—If cadmium, as many medical authorities believe, leads to high blood pressure in people, can we develop soil management practices that will reduce the amount of cadmium in foods?

Complicating the problem is the fact that some cadmium enters food from polluted air and some from the soil. How much cadmium is given off, for example, in the exhaust of vehicles powered by diesel engines traveling our highways? How much of this cadmium then is taken up by crops growing along highways?

J.F. Hodgson, ARS soil scientist at the Ithaca laboratory, will conduct research to find some of the answers. His preliminary studies indicate that there may be very important differences in the cadmium concentration in plants growing on different soils. These differences are related more to the parent rocks and the natural processes of soil formation than to differences in pollution of the soils with cadmium from fuels or other man-made sources.

In general, Dr. Allaway feels that information on trace elements eventually will become a routine part of the diagnostic techniques used by the medical profession. When a patient is examined by a diagnostician, a sample of blood will be taken and analyzed for a number of different trace elements. The patient will then be treated to adjust the levels of trace elements to a "desired range."

"The challenge facing agricultural scientists," Dr. Allaway points out, "is to develop a food supply that has uniform or standardized amounts of trace elements for the major types of food. In some cases, it may be possible to control trace-element levels in food so that people will receive the desired amounts of these elements through the food they eat. With the more stubborn trace elements, it may be necessary to provide supplements. Overdosage in the supplements is less likely if we know the precise levels of trace elements in the major food types."

Selection 21 Case Study: Tragedy and Triumph of a Michigan Farm Family

Judith Ramsey

Editors' Introduction

A primary concern of all American consumers is the safety of the food supply. Because of the complexity of the food-production system, an unintentional additive entering the system may have long-range toxic effects. The ability of the federal Food and Drug Administration to have thorough and sound sampling, testing, and notification procedures to monitor the safety of our new food

Source: From Judith Ramsey, "The Tragedy and Triumph of a Michigan Farm Family," *Family Circle*, January 9, 1978. Copyright © 1978, the Family Circle, Inc. Reprinted by permission.

system is critically important. As pointed out in selection 18, the food-production system consists of the processing, handling, transporting, storing, and merchandising, as well as the growing and raising, of food. At any place along this new food chain, food may be contaminated with toxic substances. Those who work in our food system—from farmers to factory workers in chemical fertilizer- and pesticide-manufacturing operations—are especially vulnerable to contamination by industrial chemicals. These are considered unintentional additives in our food and represent a potential threat to all consumers. In the following case study Judith Ramsey shows us the links in a long chain of events that spell tragedy for one family in this case—but in the future, for how many?

When the red feed-delivery truck from the Farm Bureau Services in Falmouth, Mich., turned down her driveway, Lois Zuiderveen, a pleasant-looking woman of thirty-nine, saw it from the kitchen window of her white frame farmhouse and continued preparing lunch. Her husband, Gary, was out in the main barn, cleaning out the stalls. In the summer, his herd of black-and-white Holsteins grazed in the surrounding pastures, but at this time of year the cattle were in the barns and the fields were covered with the first coating of snow.

Without giving any thought to the delivery, the rugged, powerfully built farmer took an attentive look at his milking cows, who were clustered around the bunk feeder, contentedly munching their haylage and silage. . . .

Stopping at the calves' barn, Gary patted the head of a four-week-old calf. The poor little wet-muzzled fellow had been through a siege of pneumonia. Now he seemed to be responding nicely to antibiotics. Gary remembers thinking to himself, "Thank God, he's the only sick one in the bunch."

Three-Generation Farm

A proud and fiercely independent man of forty-two, Gary loved dairy farming despite frequent hardships of bad weather, disappointing crops and occasional calf deaths. Like so many of the other Falmouth farmers of Dutch descent, he faced life with a strong mixture of religious conviction, stoicism, and friendly humor. So did his seventy-five-year-old father, Cody, who, with Gary's mother, Nettie, lived in the small green house next to Gary and Lois's. Cody still took care of the young calves. Gary's own son, Gary Lee Jr., nineteen, was in his second year of agricultural studies at Michigan State University and came home each weekend to lend a hand with the milking and other chores. Lori, [16], the older daughter, who by her father's own admission was a "first-rate milker," helped with the evening milking after school. Daughter Sandy, twelve, also did her share. The farm, valued at a high six figures, supported three generations of Zuiderveens and would support a fourth when Gary Lee graduated, returned to Falmouth (population 300), married Mary, the pretty student nurse he had been dating and started his own family.

Cows Begin to Sicken

The next morning followed the usual routine. Up at six, Gary headed for the barn to milk the cows, a two-hour procedure. As soon as the gates to the milking parlor were open, the cows, who could wander at will, filed in and took their places in the stalls—usually in the same order every time. They stood placidly eating the feed while Gary and Ted, the hired hand, attached the milkers to their swollen udders.

Soon the fresh milk was coursing through pipelines into a huge refrigerated bulk tank in an adjoining room. Production averaged fifty pounds a day for each cow—an excellent yield. Every noon a truck picked up the milk at the Zuiderveen farm and took it to a plant in Detroit. There, mixed with milk from hundreds of other dairy farms, it would be homogenized, pasteurized, and bottled. By the following morning, it would be delivered by truck to retail stores as far east as Pennsylvania and as far south as Ohio.

This morning, Gary noticed that the cows had eaten very little of the new feed. The farm raised all its own animal feed, but at the Farm Bureau Services where Gary had it ground, a supplement was mixed in. Puzzled, Gary tasted a bit of it himself, but it seemed all right to him. Since cows are unpredictable and often finicky creatures, reacting to the slightest change in diet or weather, he didn't think much about it. He assumed that when they got hungry enough they would eat it. Indeed, in the days that followed, the cows did consume the feed while they were being milked, but not at their usual rate. While it normally took them twelve days to finish off five tons, there was still one-third of the feed left at the end of twenty days. As a safeguard, Gary asked the Farm Bureau Services' local co-op manager to check a sample of the feed. The official tasted it, as Gary had done, and said it seemed all right. The feed apparently was never tested.

As autumn merged into winter, however, the Zuiderveens' milk cows became not only finicky but unmanageable. Instead of walking calmly into the milking parlor twice a day, most of them would clump irritably in the doorway and refuse to enter. In fact, Gary and Ted had to drive them inside. Also, a considerable number of them were suffering from intermittent diarrhea. And there was an outbreak of respiratory infections among the new calves; they were moping about with dripping, ulcerated eyes and runny noses.

Insidiously at first, though their numbers grew each week, the Zuiderveens' animals sickened. Some of the milkers developed mastitis, an inflammation of the mammary tissue. Others showed signs of a liver ailment. Still others developed swollen joints or lameness, causing Gary to wonder whether they had contracted some sort of infection.

By mid-January, milk production on the Zuiderveen farm had fallen off from fifty to thirty-four pounds per cow a day, a large enough drop to cut into profits. No one was more perplexed than the veterinarian, Dr. Alpha Clark, who now was making frequent visits to the farm. One day when he was treating a sick cow, he scratched his head and said, "Gary, you're certainly having a run of bad luck and I can't figure out why. It beats me."

The Farm in Trouble

A visible pall hung over the family. Everything the Zuiderveens had ever worked for or cared about was tied up in those animals. Gary was reluctant to discuss his problems with his friends and neighbors. If he had, he would have discovered that several of them, including his good friends Roy and Marilyn Tacoma, who lived four miles down the road, were having similar difficulties with their cattle: an unusual incidence of respiratory infections, mastitis, liver symptoms, and unexplainable deaths.

In May, 1974, Gary and Lois read a newspaper account of an accidental poisoning involving dairy cows in Fremont and several other communities 150 miles to the south. A number of cattle had been fed contaminated feed purchased from a local mill which contained a chemical toxin called polybrominated biphenyl, or PBB, as the newspaper article referred to it. The PBB had been produced by Michigan Chemical Corp. in St. Louis, Mich., and mixed in cattle supplement at a Farm Bureau Services plant near Battle Creek. Gary says he would have questioned Farm Bureau Services in Falmouth about where they obtained their supplement, but he received a letter from them assuring him that his supplement had not been contaminated.

About that time, Gary and Lois heard that Rick Halbert, a farmer who lived in Battle Creek, also had ailing cows that had been poisoned by a chemical toxin. After many sensitive, expensive and time-consuming tests, the culprit had been found to be PBB, the same chemical that had contaminated the cows in Fremont. But the feed purchased by Halbert was supposed to contain magnesium oxide, which some farmers add to the feed of their cows. Apparently PBB had been mixed with Halbert's feed instead of magnesium oxide. Since Gary had not bought magnesium oxide to mix with his cattle feed, he presumed his feed was free of PBB. Yet Gary could not quite get rid of his suspicion that the feed had been tainted by something.

That August of 1974 was a terrible time for Gary. Besides caring for the sick cows, who were not producing enough milk to pay for their keep, he had to harvest the hay and corn. Gary, who formerly could haul hay all day without any effort, now tired easily.

In the evenings, Gary was finding it increasingly difficult to relax. When he went to bed he would fall into a troubled sleep filled with nightmares of maimed and dying animals, only to awaken feeling groggy and out of sorts. He also was bothered by unexplained stiffness in his joints and ankles, but since these symptoms were vague and came and went, he ignored them. None of the Zuiderveens ever consulted a doctor unless they were literally flat on their backs with a high fever or a serious injury.

Family's Weird Symptoms

Meanwhile, Lois, who for several years had been working two days a week in the hardware department of Ebel's General Store, was finding her job more tiring. She began to have stomach troubles. Even Gary Lee, who never got sick, was complaining of aching joints and weird sensations as though his head were disconnected from his body. Looking back now, Gary and Lois don't understand how they could have been so blind, how they could have ignored so many obvious clues.

Of all the Zuiderveens, Lois took their misfortunes the hardest. She realized that their herd had virtually lost its productive capacity. Even if some of the milking cows were to recover and give a reasonable amount of milk again, many of them had already proved to be sterile or had lost their calves at freshening. From the time she had been a little girl growing up on a nearby farm, Lois had been involved with livestock and crops: the cycles of animal birth and death, the sweet reawakening of the land every spring and its subsequent harvest. Dairy farming was not a business to her, it was a way of life. "It's all we know and all we want to do."

In her own soft-spoken way, Lois was the anchor of the Zuiderveen family. She imparted the values she and Gary shared—industriousness, thrift, honesty and religious spirit—to their children. Even Gary often turned to her for advice when things got tough. Now, for the first time, there was nothing she could do to help except to offer comfort.

Subtly at first—it was hard to pinpoint when it started—Gary began having trouble with his eyes. There were brief periods when objects weren't in focus; their edges became blurred. But since the fuzziness would disappear after a few minutes, he did nothing about it.

One morning while Lois was preparing pancakes, Gary gazed absentmindedly out the window. Right before his eyes, an elm tree that was about 50 feet away seemed to recede in the distance so that it appeared to be 100 feet away. Gary blinked twice and stared again. Suddenly the tree was back in its proper place. Shaken and confused, Gary wondered whether he had imagined the entire experience. Without saying anything to Lois, he went out to the barn. The cows seemed to be having eye problems, too. Some of them were blundering about, bumping into the barn siding as though they couldn't see what was in front of them.

During the second week in September, the Zuiderveens learned from Alpha that the state public health department had quarantined the herd of a neighbor of theirs when it was discovered that some of their cattle were contaminated by PBB in amounts over the allowable level, which at that time had been arbitrarily set by the Food and Drug Administration at one part per million in animal tissue. This meant that the neighbor could no longer sell his animals, although he could continue to sell their milk. By now, the Zuiderveens were convinced that their herd had been poisoned; it seemed the only possible explanation for the deaths and disorders among their cattle and perhaps even for some of the mysterious ills that they themselves were suffering.

Later that month, Alpha telephoned the state of Michigan's Department of Agriculture and requested that they draw samples from the bulk milk tanks of farmers with suspicious herds to determine how widespread PBB contamination was in their area. He gave them the Zuiderveens' name and about a dozen others. An inspector did come to the Zuiderveen farm and took milk samples for analysis. No report was ever issued to them.

Strange Lab Reports

In October of 1974, at Alpha's urging, Gary agreed to take two of the ailing cows to a diagnostic laboratory in Lansing for pathology study—an analysis of fat tissue to determine the cause of illness. A ten-week-old calf and an eight-year-old cow were selected. On the way, the calf died. Gary requested that the tissue samples be tested for the presence of PBB. A report came back from the lab that the calf was "nondetect," which meant that no traces of PBB had been identified in its tissues. The cow had .05 parts per million of PBB, which was not then considered significant (although by today's revised standards it is above allowable levels).

Upon learning the news, both Gary and Alpha were mystified. It just didn't make sense. If they were to accept the lab report at face value, it would mean that their animals' symptoms could not be caused by

PBB—yet their herd bore a remarkable resemblance to those contaminated herds some of their neighbors had. Unwilling to accept a verdict based upon only one laboratory analysis, Gary sent off eight more tissue samples from different cows to a lab in Lansing used by the Michigan Department of Agriculture. Weeks later, the report came back: no cow had registered more than trace levels of PBB.

By this time, the cows were in even worse shape. When Gary went to the barn each morning for the milking, he was confronted by a pathetic sight: emaciated, lame, and wheezing cows with a lackluster appearance. Their hides were matted and coarse, and they wandered about forlornly, just picking at their feed.

Even more upsetting, the young calves had no resistance to disease and had repeated colds, coughs, and pneumonia, from which many of them never recovered. Their rib cages heaved with labored breathing and their mouths in some instances gaped open. Several times Gary stayed up until early morning trying to save a dying calf caught in a losing struggle for life. Normally a dairy farmer will lose four or five calves a season, but Gary and his father lost over thirty calves that winter.

Whenever Gary telephoned Alpha Clark's house to ask him to come over and treat a sick cow, he would be told by his wife that he was out on call. Alpha confided to Gary that he was being run ragged, rushing from one farm to another, administering to ailing animals. At night, the jangling of the telephone disturbed his sleep, sending him out to the cold barns in response to cries of help from frantic farmers.

In November, in response to public pressure, the federal government lowered the allowable amount of PBB in livestock from 1.0 per million to .3 per million parts in body tissue. Financial aid was provided by Michigan Chemical and Farm Bureau Services to some of the farmers with quarantined herds.

That winter of 1974–75 Lois's symptoms worsened. If she sat in a chair for a long time, her neck would become sore and stiff and it was uncomfortable to turn her head. She got frequent headaches that seemed to radiate from the back of her head forward. Never one to display weakness, she often burst into tears when she was alone. And she had begun to worry about Lori, who was experiencing blurred vision and headaches. Sandy, the more exuberant one, seemed depressed. She often missed school and her grades dropped. She complained that her fingers sometimes felt stiff and painful, making it hard for her to hold a pencil and to take notes in school.

Gary was now convinced that there was definitely something in the ground feed they had fed their animals in November 1973, even though local and state officials told them they were mistaken. In March he selected another cow for pathology study. This time, he decided not to depend on one laboratory's analysis; splitting the samples, he sent half to two commercial labs in Ann Arbor. When the results came back, the first lab was nondetect, but the other found PBB in concentrations of .07 and .08 in different sites on the animal's body.

In the weeks that followed, Gary sent tissue samples from eight cows taken from different sites on each animal to different labs. The discrepancies among the reports were wild. One cow, for example, tested over quarantine level at two labs but had trace levels at a third. And levels in the same animal varied widely depending upon the site from which they were taken. What was even more strange, some of the most debilitated animals registered as having the lowest levels of PBB, whereas some of the healthiest-looking ones had among the highest levels.

Details Are Revealed

Along in April, the details of the PBB error at Michigan Chemical broke in the newspapers. According to the different reports, it would appear that the magnesium oxide manufactured by the company and used as feed supplement was sold under the label Nutrimaster and packaged in brown paper bags. Michigan Chemical also made the fire retardant known as polybrominated biphenyl (PBB), which was also sold in brown bags with its name—Firemaster—stenciled on them.

The newspapers reported that one day in mid-1973 some bags of Firemaster were inadvertently loaded on a truck carrying Nutrimaster and sent to the Farm Bureau Services' modern plant near Battle Creek. There at the plant, an unknown amount of Firemaster was mixed with feed supplement and sold to farmers across the state, who fed it to their livestock. Also, residual traces of PBB in the feed mills and grain elevators had contaminated additional feed and feed supplement. Ultimately, hundreds of thousands of Michigan cows, hogs, and chickens were affected.

So there it was. Because of a tragic mix-up, the Zuiderveen dairy business was virtually shut down, the herd that they had developed for years was ruined, the family who had drunk the milk and eaten the meat of the contaminated cows was suffering from bizarre medical symptoms.

Because it had not been studied extensively, the case against PBB had not been conclusively proved. Yet there was enough damning evidence to make Gary stop and ask himself: Why had it taken so long for public officials to sound the alarm? Why had so many months gone by before the cause of the contamination was discovered—or admitted?

Finally, several of the many samples from the Zuiderveen herd came back over the quarantine level, which meant that their herd would be quarantined. Told by the Farm Bureau that they would be reimbursed only for the animals with PBB over the quarantine levels, Gary objected strongly. He felt that all of his cattle—regardless of their measurable PBB levels — were contaminated. In fact, some that measured low levels of PBB were the sickest. (Even though many other farmers in his predicament had kept selling their meat, Gary had taken his cattle off the market in January 1974, which meant a further loss of income.) He pointed out that before it was known how widespread the PBB poisoning was, some farmers had been reimbursed for their entire herds. He argued that he could no longer afford to feed the contaminated cows, nor did he have the money to replace them.

One day in May, when young cattle normally are frolicking in the greening pastures, Gary's father, Cody, came dejectedly into the Zuiderveen house at lunchtime. "Gary, I found another dead calf when I went to the barn this morning. I guess I'm too old to take care of them any more. I wish you'd take over." He turned away so Gary wouldn't see that his face was wet with tears. That summer was even worse than the one before; the Zuiderveens felt overwhelmed by their losses.

In the fall, Gary decided his situation was so complicated that he'd better get a lawyer. He contacted Paul Greer, a Fremont lawyer whose own herd had had to be destroyed because of PBB contamination, and a Grand Rapids lawyer named Gary Schenk. The two attorneys agreed to represent the Zuiderveens on a contingency basis and to start suits against Michigan Chemical and the Farm Bureau Services.

Meanwhile a pressing problem faced Gary Zuiderveen: what to do about their contamined cattle, including those he would normally have sold by now. Winter was approaching; the heifers would have to be moved to the barn and would be consuming $300 worth of feed a week. Heavily in debt, the Zuiderveens were carrying huge bank loans and had spent money on account at the stores in town. And they had mortgaged most of their farm equipment. There seemed to be no choice except to shoot some of the animals they had bred and proudly raised, and yet neither the state nor the defendants in the lawsuit, Farm Bureau Services and Michigan Chemical, would take on this heartbreaking task for them.

Eighty Cattle Are Destroyed

It was a grim day in November 1975 when Gary, his son, and his nephew Kenny gathered at the pasture lot where the heifers were kept. Eighty cattle were destroyed that day, each one shot quickly in the head. The men returned to the barn with heavy hearts. In two days the carcasses were frozen stiff and soon covered by fresh snow, which acted as a natural preservative.

The following March, the Zuiderveens were notified by the Department of Natural Resources that the frozen carcasses would be collected by a local contractor and taken to Kalkaska, the burial ground designated by the state for PBB cattle so that the decomposing bodies would not contaminate the grazing land. The Zuiderveens later learned that approximately 30,000 cattle were buried there.

It was finally recognized that PBB was a statewide problem. Continuing newspaper coverage and TV accounts made many Michigan residents afraid to consume local milk and meat products and certain enterprising store owners advertised that they sold beef from other states and cheese from Wisconsin.

On April 20th, after months of negotiations, the Farm Bureau notified Schenk and Greer that they were willing to meet the Zuiderveens' terms for a settlement. The money only covered the cost of replacing their cattle. With money borrowed from the bank, which kept extending their credit, the Zuiderveens had purchased some cows that were to be the foundation of a new herd. The settlement in no way covered the losses incurred by the virtual shutdown of milk production for two years, nor the cost of cleaning up the barns, nor the vet fees, or research expenses. "But it allowed us to hold on to the farm and go back into business," says Gary simply.

There was one more ugly decision to be made: Should they sell the remaining cattle who were below the quarantine level, as many state and local officials were encouraging them to do, or should they destroy them, incurring further financial losses? Gary brooded over the matter for several days before deciding that he had no choice; he could not live with himself if he sold PBB-contaminated meat to other people, meat that his own family wouldn't touch.

During the third week of April, the Zuiderveens rented a bulldozer and dug a hole on the far eastern corner of their property. For many years to come, that land would not be used for grazing. It took two days and the help of several friends to destroy another 170 cows. When it was done, Gary Lee and his father looked at each other with a mixture of sorrow and relief.

In the months that followed, the new herd seemed to adjust well to their home. But the Zuiderveens' perplexing medical problems, though less severe, persisted, and some new ones developed. Gary, who by now looked ashen and drawn, still had episodes of eye trouble; a reddish rash on his legs, which had broken out earlier, then disappeared for a while, now reappeared. His coordination was poor. Lois was so exhausted and upset, it was often all she could do to keep from crying. Her joints ached so much that it was difficult for her to even lift a roasting pan or pot of potatoes from the stove.

In November 1976 the Zuiderveens were asked to participate in a health survey to determine the effects of PBB on people who had been exposed to it. They agreed to undergo a day of tests at Kent Community Hospital in Grand Rapids in the hope that some light would be shed on their medical difficulties. The survey, which would involve more than

1,200 Michigan residents and take many months to evaluate, was being conducted by a team of medical scientists headed by a leading authority in the field of industrial medicine and industrial pollutants, Dr. Irving Selikoff of New York City's Mount Sinai.

Along with other participants, the Zuiderveens filled out dozens of pages of medical and personal questions before undergoing a five-hour physical exam. They were given blood and urine tests, sophisticated lung and kidney tests, chest X-rays and a special physical examination with emphasis upon skin and joint problems.

As they waited to be called for various tests, family after family compared their PBB experiences.

"PBB was in the soil from the manure," said Gerald Woltjer, who bought his farm five days before PBB was identified in the feed. "It was in the stream that runs through my property. Healthy kittens that drank the cows' milk sickened and died five months later. Even frogs, opossums, and field mice were dying. Worse yet, my family became ill, with the same symptoms that the cows had—losing their hair and sleeping all the time."

Chris and Donald Rehkophf said that they had moved to Brewster, Wash., after they were forced to shoot their contaminated herd, and they, too, had developed medical problems. Their first child, a girl, had died at six weeks. "She was sick and jaundiced the whole time, but the doctors couldn't figure out what caused her death," Rehkophf sighed. "Thorin, who was born the next year, had a constant round of jaundice while we lived in Michigan; he's not been sick half as much since we moved."

One thirty-five-year-old man admitted that he had to stop driving his car because he kept dozing off at the wheel and had much severe memory difficulties that he kept getting lost in towns he had known all his life. Several farmers said they had been plowing crooked furrows for months after they drank milk and ate meat from their contaminated cows.

From 6,000 tubes of blood and urine taken from the participants and from more than 40,000 pages of questionnaires, the Selikoff team hopes to find some answers to the perplexing questions of just how toxic PBB is to people. Unfortunately, because the medical problems of the participants peaked some time in 1975 and then started to abate, the effects of PBB may not be known for years.

The preliminary report issued for the group strongly suggested a pattern of ills not essentially different from what Gary, Lois, and their children experienced: visual disturbances, joint pains, memory difficulties, excessive fatigue, wounds that wouldn't heal, diarrhea, abdominal pain, and other gastrointestinal problems. Neurologic disorders were found in 37 percent of the people; 27 percent had painful or swollen joints unrelated to age. Many of the sufferers were in their thirties or forties when disorders such as arthritis and weakness are ordinarily uncommon. Skin problems, including a form of acne caused by chemical substances related to PBB, were found in 21 percent of the participants, and 16 percent complained of abdominal pain, diarrhea and other GI problems. In special tests on a few individuals, the Mount Sinai team found strong evidence that PBB might interfere with the body's normal immunological defense system against disease, including cancer. When Gary Lee and his pregnant wife, Mary, learned this, they wondered whether PBB might have some untoward effects on their unborn baby.

Today, although the Zuiderveens still seem to be more prone than formerly to colds and infections, most of their symptoms have abated, and the farm is more than paying for itself again. Milk production is averaging a good 17,000 lbs. per cow per year. Of fifty-three calves, only two have died.

Despite the air of normalcy about their lives, the Zuiderveens know they will never be the same. They have been stressed, pushed to near bankruptcy, praised, blamed, and exposed to publicity. Gone is their former faith in government and regulatory agencies. They firmly believe that if this PBB disaster could happen in Falmouth, it could happen anywhere unless more stringent precautions and safety regulations are enforced.

What remains, what has never been destroyed, is the Zuiderveens' faith in God and in themselves. "Listen," says Gary today, "what we can be proud of is that we endured, that we built ourselves back to where we were. Whatever happens now, even if we have more medical problems, we'll deal with them the best we can—one at a time."

Selection 22 The Technological Impact on the Food Supply

Eleanor Meyerhoff
Alice L. Tobias

Editors' Introduction

Human beings have shown remarkable inventiveness in applying technology to nature's bounty. From the simplest hand process to the most complex machinery, foods have been mashed, ground, flaked, and pounded to create new textures and forms. Every culture has its own typical way of preparing foods and has created identifiable national dishes. Modern technology has created a range of options for the consumer that represent a mixed blessing. Can convenience be the only criterion for selecting foods? Is something lost in the translation when too many hands make light work? How much nutrition is sacrificed for the sake of eye or taste appeal? How vulnerable has the consumer become to the blandishments of manufacturers' advertising the latest or the newest product? In the following selection the authors compare traditional with industrialized technology and suggest some ways in which the average consumer needs to be informed of the degree to which technology may have impaired the nutritional quality of the food supply.

North America has long had a love-hate relationship with technology; Canadians and Americans enjoy the comforts and conveniences technology provides while they condemn its impact on their social and physical environments. Nowhere is their ambivalence more evident than in their attitudes toward food technology.

Who disputes the fact that science and technology have increased food productivity to the extent that Canada and the United States supply not only their own needs, but can, and do, offer assistance to other countries in need of food? "But," critics may ask, "at what cost?" Chemical fertilizers, pesticides, and herbicides pollute rivers and lakes and endanger wildlife. Mechanization of farm operations and the large-scale irrigation of farmlands increase demands on energy sources and strain an ecosystem in which water plays a fundamental role while the continuous use of chemical fertilizers adversely affect the physical and chemical balance of the soil.

Today's affluent life-styles, the entrance of more women into the work force, and the breakdown of traditional family meal patterns encourage the use of easy and convenient prepackaged, processed foods, and offer the luxury of selecting from a variety of foods at any season of the year. Few people realize, however, that the abundance of our food supply and all its luxuries and conveniences have been purchased at a price. The price is industrialization of the food system that replaced human workers with machinery. One consequence of this technological change is the decline of farm populations and an increase in urban populations and urban problems. The convenience of highly processed foods is purchased at the expense of valuable nutrients and home-cooked flavors. Natural texture, taste, and aroma are replaced with artificial color, flavor, and even a smell to simulate natural food. Preservatives are added to extend shelf life.

Thanks to technology, consumers have more food available than ever before, and they pay comparatively less for it than they did twenty-five years ago. The price includes all the built-in "maid service" features in our modern food supply—frozen foods, baked products, and other processed foods. If we assess each food item in our pantries, are there some we would be more willing to pay for in terms of disposable income than in terms of their long-term ecological and social consequences?

Grains

Grains are probably humankind's first engineered food, dating back to the neolithic discovery of their energy-giving kernels. Cereal grains could be transported and planted wherever they were needed. They could be mashed into a paste with water, baked on heated stones, and thereby transformed into a compact, portable food supply. Civilizations built on the stability of grain supplies soon developed milling, refining, and leavening techniques. Bread making became one of the first technologies established in early times.

From the beginning, the urge to refine cereal grains was associated with upward social mobility. Only the nobility could afford the painstaking hand labor involved in stripping rough dark bran from the creamy white endosperm. But as industrialization developed, milling became a large-scale operation; white flours and cereals became available to all at modest prices. Degermination soon followed and became standard practice to prevent rancidity during storage. Chemicals were added to insure softness and to prevent molding. Artificial colors and flavors were added to improve appearance and taste. A consequence of this technology was to provide a greatly weakened *staff of life* whose effects did not become significant until the middle of the twentieth century. In 1941, the effect of relying on refined grain products was shown by the poor nutritional status of army recruits. This discovery gave final impetus to the establishment of federal enrichment programs that mandated the return of some of the nutrients removed in milling processes. Not all the nutrients were restored. Those nutrients that were restored were not restored in the proportions in which they were removed. Nutritionists still advocated whole grain cereals and flours in a varied diet. Bread and cereal manufacturers, however, were enchanted with the ideas of enrichment and fortification with additional nutrients. They used such technologically inexpensive additives as advertising gimmicks to increase sales.

Earlier in the century, G.H. Kellogg and C.W. Post had perfected the technology of producing precooked cereals from rice, oats, wheat, and corn. These grains were flaked, popped, and shredded. They could be sprinkled with sugar and, with milk poured over them, eaten cold. These foods rapidly replaced homemade porridges and gruels as standard breakfast fare. The addition of vitamins and minerals now joined new flavors and shapes in the marketing competition among cereal companies. Packaging became important. Games and toys and giveaways became part of cereal companies' marketing strategies. After the development of television, cereal manufacturers could beam advertising directly to children. Precooked cereals increased in numbers and in variety of shapes, artificial colors, artificial flavors, and imaginative names. Highly sugared breakfast cereals not only replaced conventional precooked cereals in breakfast patterns but became popular snack foods.

When the health food movement of the 1960s was established, whole grain cereals and flours developed social status and soon moved from health food stores to supermarkets. Bakers and cereal makers who had advertised and profited from enrichment and fortification programs jumped on the "natural" whole grain and fiber bandwagon. As with enriched products, competition for sales produced products with questionable amounts of sugar (this time introduced in the form of honey) and products with fiber newly introduced from sources not usually used for food. Consumers must learn to pick and choose carefully from many products in order to assure that breads and cereals provide all the nutrients of whole grains without unnecessary additives that provide only cosmetic effects at increased cost.

Milk Products

Milk, which is highly perishable, was the first food subjected to preserving techniques designed to conserve its food value in palatable form. Almost all primitive societies that use milk for food have developed techniques for making cheese or fermented milk products. Fluid milk was successfully preserved in cans in the nineteenth century. Later, pasteurization made fresh milk a safer and more easily distributed product. Today, new procedures using ultrahigh temperatures are giving fluid milk the shelf life of any other canned food without changing its flavor or texture. Modern dehydration techniques have made dried skim milk as stable as flour. Fortification with vitamin D has virtually eliminated rickets in the United States. The addition of vitamins A and D to skimmed milk products has made such foods valuable additions to the low-fat diet. On the whole technology, including animal breeding, has improved both the quantity and quality of milk. Milk products, however, are another story.

Processed cheeses are pasteurized not for safety, but to maintain their bland flavor. In addition to pasteurization, cheese foods and cheese spreads require stabilizers and emulsifiers to hold their added moisture content. Artificial colors are added even to natural cheeses.

The traditional fermentation of milk by which it is converted to yogurt, for example, gives it a flavor and consistency that is conducive to its use as an accompaniment to fresh fruits and vegetables. Modern processes that add sugars, preserves, stabilizers, artificial colors, and artificial flavors have changed yogurt into a highly sugared snack and dessert food. Even ice cream has become a hodgepodge of chemicals as a result of our technological ability to produce more varieties of flavor and texture. The more varied the flavors and textures, the more numerous the additives. It has been estimated that at least 1200 different stabilizers, emulsifiers, neutralizers, artificial flavors, and artificial colors can now legally be used in its manufacture.*

Artificial or imitation milk and products such as coffee lighteners, whipped toppings, and cream substitutes are prepared with saturated fats along with other additives; the saturated vegetable fat in most cases has a higher saturation ratio than actual milk fat. Margarine, however, may be made with vegetable fats containing far less saturated fats than butter and is always fortified with 15,000 IU units of vitamin A. Since the vitamin A content of butter varies with the seasons, and artificial colors are added to both margarine and butter, the engineered margarine is considered to have more health-giving properties than butter. In terms of flavor and consistency, however, butter remains in favor with many gourmet cooks.

Fruits and Vegetables

Not too long ago, winter in North America meant many months when only root vegetables, cabbages, and dwindling supplies of apples were available to add variety to family meals. Sun drying was a traditional form of food preservation. Pickles and preserves varied the menu with colorful condiments. Today, technological advances in transporta-

*Rodger P. Doyle and James L. Redding, *Complete Food Handbook* (New York: Grove Press: 1976).

tion, storage, packaging, and processing provide us with a year long supply of fresh, frozen, and canned fruits and vegetables. The technology that brings consumers this continuous supply of fresh greens, citrus fruits, and other unseasonable items is directed mainly at maintaining the attractive appearance and marketability of the produce even at the expense of its nutritive value and sometimes, even, its safety.

The nutritive value of fruits and vegetables that are picked when immature and unripe and then artificially ripened during transit or in storage is significantly lower than the value of those allowed to ripen in field or orchard. Fruits and vegetables are bred to sustain harvesting and packing trauma rather than to increase nutritive value. The use of growth hormones to produce attractively large fruits has been linked to birth defects.

Pesticides left on the surface of fresh fruits and vegetables can penetrate to the interior during long periods of storage. Wax and paraffin coatings originally designed to preserve moisture are also used solely to improve appearance. In some products, such as tomatoes and apples, the coatings are hard to detect. They are often unknowingly ingested, although some medical authorities claim they are possible carcinogens.

Thanks to technology, processed fruits and vegetables are now closer in nutritive value to fresh produce than ever before. Picked at the peak of ripeness, fresh fruits and vegetables are promptly canned or frozen in factories adjacent to farmers' fields. Processed at the height of their nutritive value, they are also spared long storage periods with consequent loss of nutrients and increased pesticide penetration. New techniques of flash freezing and vacuum canning are further reducing nutrient losses and improving the texture and flavor of processed fruits and vegetables. But, like Dr. Frankenstein, technological geniuses cannot leave well enough alone. Instead of being simply and honestly preserved, fruits and vegetables are now enhanced with sugar, salt, artificial flavors, and other additives that diminish their nutritive value when compared to fresh produce. Fruit drinks, punches, and ades that are diluted fruit juices loaded with sugar, artificial colors, and artificial flavors and fortified with vitamins appear next to whole juices on supermarket shelves. Synthetic fruit drinks and powders that contain additional stabilizers and antioxidants are widely advertised as substitutes for genuine fruit juices. Technology has made these artificial products so sweet and their flavors so concentrated that many people no longer recognize and enjoy the natural flavor of freshly squeezed fruit juices.

Meat and Alternate Sources of Protein

In 1905 the muckraking author Upton Sinclair described in his book *The Jungle* the dehumanizing conditions created by industrialization of the meat industry. Little has changed since then—except that the same mechanization technology has been extended to poultry and egg production. Computer printouts control the development of livestock from insemination to presentation in the supermarket showcase. Efficiency and cost control have become the final spurs to any change. Meats are precut and packaged not only for the consumer, but also for the retailer and the wholesaler. Canned and frozen meat and poultry entrées are available in a variety of gourmet and TV dinners.

The modern food system has increased yields and cut costs, particularly for poultry and eggs. Genetic engineering has tailored poultry products to meet the convenience needs of busy consumers. Fowl, capons, geese, and ducks are found only in specialty butcher shops. In the supermarket, the commercially profitable broiler is promoted as the all-purpose chicken for every culinary purpose. Breeding for smaller size, freezing, packaging in parts, and developing specialty items such as turkey chopped meat and turkey frankfurters have turned that twice-a-year holiday bird into a reasonably priced, readily available, nutritious substitute for beef.

Moral and ethical concerns have been raised about our meat production system, particularly about the use of grains to fatten animals while millions starve throughout the world because of a lack of grain. Serious questions have also been raised about the danger to the consumer of using antibiotics to control animal diseases and of using growth hormones to increase their size and weight.

Government inspection guarantees the absence of organisms that cause disease in fresh, canned, and frozen meats. However, meat products may contain equally harmful additives. Smoked and cured meats are prepared with nitrates and nitrites, the long-term effects of which have been questioned by medical investigators and nutritionists. While most of the meat industry resists change, a few processors are successfully producing and marketing products free of nitrates, nitrites, and artificial colors. Local school nutrition committees, composed of parents, teachers, students, and lunchroom managers, are providing the major demand for these products.

Critics point out that the meat industry uses technology creatively to scrape or chop every bit of meat from animal bones. It then reforms those scraps into simulated meat cuts. Shouldn't it also be able to direct its technology toward developing alternate methods of preservation that would maintain the desirable characteristics of the processed meat without the use of potentially harmful additives? Perhaps the American consumer needs heightened consciousness concerning the "meat mystique" that supports the technology through purchase of the look-alike meat products.

In recent years, the correlation between meat consumption and heart disease has spurred many people to look for other sources of protein. Along with committed vegetarians, the general public is experimenting with combinations of complementary vegetable proteins such as those found in legumes and grains. A favorite American legume, the peanut, has gained new favor as an important source of protein, especially when combined with whole grain bread in a sandwich and served with milk. Peanut butter has traditionally been made of plain ground-up peanuts. Machine processing has increased its smoothness and creaminess. In addition, it has been homogenized to prevent the separation of its oil after standing. In addition to peanuts, peanut butter may now contain up to 10 percent sweeteners, salt, and hydrogenated fats. Peanut butter products that look like peanut butter may use fanciful names and be subjected to high-pressure advertising to promote nutritionally inferior products that actually contain fewer peanuts. These products are extended with artificial flavors, artificial colors, preservatives, and large amounts of sugars and saturated fats—all of which detract from their nutritional desirability.

Unfortunately, soybeans, the legumes that come closest to meat in protein value, rank lowest in palatability. The increase in the production of soybeans as a source of vegetable oil turned technological ingenuity to the conversion of its remaining soy residue to acceptable, edible forms. The result was soy flour, soy-protein concentrate, and isolated soy protein. Used with animal or other plant proteins, these soy derivatives can act as moisture retainers, binders, emulsifiers, and stabilizers while also enhancing the protein value of both plant and animal protein. Further technological development makes possible the production of a material spun from isolated soy protein that can be fashioned into lookalike meat analogs, or substitutes. Consumers now, if they wish, may buy imitation cubes of chicken, ham, and beef and imitation bacon strips and sausages. Unfortunately, these products are often served to unsuspecting consumers in restaurants or fast-food and takeout operations. Meat analogs are expensive to produce, but not as expensive as the "real thing." Furthermore, they require large numbers of additives in their preparation. Many think technological expertise should be concentrated on making the natural soybean a more palatable and convenient product that can be used along with limas, pintos, navy beans, and other legumes that are staples in the American diet.

The food system is especially suited to the development of what has come to be known as "appropriate technology"—technology that supports values that enhance the quality of life without degrading the inner or outer environment. Consumerists, health activists, and environmentalists have been highlighting technological abuses in the food system with encouraging results.

Health food stores featuring unprocessed foods have become

permanent installations in many communities, and health food sections are prominent in most supermarkets. Foods in the health food section of stores may seem more expensive than familiar processed foods, although in some cases they may not be more nutritious. However, they do spotlight the fact that in addition to convenience, many more consumers are concerned that foods be safe and promote health. As the popularity of health foods increases, food companies stress the health-enhancing qualities of their products in other supermarket areas. Margarines high in polyunsaturated fats are on the dairy shelves. A burgeoning variety of seeds are now found in the nut sections. Safflower and safflower oil appear on the shortening shelf. More legumes and whole grains are placed among the dried foods. An increasing assortment of whole grain products and breads are found in the cereal and bread departments.

Fresh produce markets, spurred by the new interest in locally grown, tasty fruits and vegetables, are flourishing in urban areas. However, in some areas, the buildup of suburban housing developments has occurred at the expense of prime farmland. Ethnic and farmers' markets, urban communes, and food co-ops are increasingly providing alternate sources of fresh foods. Supermarket chains with policies that permit the purchase of local produce in season are finding that they are a competitive asset.

In early 1977 when the Exploratory Project for Economic Alternatives proposed the preservation of existing farmlands and the development of new farms near urban centers, many considered it an impractical but laudable vision. Nevertheless, within the same year Suffolk County on the outskirts of New York City enacted legislation and appropriated funds to purchase development rights to local farmlands in order to keep them as working farms in the greater New York metropolitan area.

Demand is growing for the public to be part of the decision-making process in matters that involve its health and well-being. If the technology of food is to provide for humane ends, the participants must have an understanding of the alternatives based on knowledge. Abuses have continued in the past because of ignorance, misinformation, and the delusion that all progress is for the best.

The technology of mass communication has proven a potent force in the service of food for profit, but radio, television, newspapers, magazines, and books can be employed by governmental and educational agencies to promote sound food and nutrition practices. The fifteen-second radio and television spots sponsored by the Food and Drug Administration are demonstrating that advertising is as powerful a force in disseminating information as it is in marketing products.

The highly competitive food industry is sensitive to consumer demands. Until now, the demand has been viewed as a demand for more convenience. As Magnus Pyke prophetically pointed out, the trend toward greater convenience in foods would not continue indefinitely. Time, he said, is only worth saving if there is a more attractive use to which it can be put. Eating and the process of preparing foods to eat are two such attractive occupations, he noted.*

Modern family relationships emphasize the sharing of home responsibilities. They have encouraged home food preparation in what *Time* magazine (December 1977) called the growth of "The Cooking Craze." As Pyke predicted in reaction to standardized, tasteless, engineered foods, individuals, couples, and families are now emphasizing quality foods and fresh products in their cooperative meal preparation. Serving homemade, unprocessed foods has become a new opportunity for creativity and originality and has many economic and health implications for the concerned consumer.

Agricultural and food-processing technology exists only as a reflection of the existing social, political, and economic system. The way individuals choose to order their values and priorities, and the support they give political actions that implement those values, can turn technology to the support of goals that reflect a respect for the humanistic qualities of life.

Such social forces, coupled with knowledge and translated into political action, can result in governmental standards and regulations that will improve the quality of the foods that are currently produced and processed primarily for profit and convenience.

*Magnus Pyke, *Technological Eating* (London: Murray, 1972), p. 92.

Selection 23 The Green Revolution: Some New Perspectives

Don F. Hadwiger

Editors' Introduction

As we saw in selection 18, the industrialized form of the green revolution has been a conspicuous feature of the U.S. agricultural system since the 1930s. The green revolution was born in the

Source: Adapted from Don F. Hadwiger, "The Green Revolution: Some New Perspectives," *Change*, November 1975, pp. 36–41, 62. Reprinted with permission from Vol. 7, #9, *Change* Magazine ©, New Rochelle, N.Y.

research laboratories of the land-grant colleges that were established by the Morrill Act of 1862 "to teach such branches of learning as are related to agriculture and the mechanic arts." Thus, a system of state-supported agricultural and technical schools dealing in applied science as contrasted with the pure science of the eastern establishment schools was begun. In the land-grant colleges agricultural science, nutrition science, and home economics flourished and combined to make a significant impact on the production of food and the American family's food storage, preparation, and purchasing habits.

In 1887 the Hatch Act authorized the establishment of agricultural experiment stations. The Adams Act of 1906 set up agricultural experiment stations at the land-grant colleges. In 1914 the Smith-Lever Act established the Extension Service as part of the land-grant college system. The county-extension agent took the new knowledge developed in these research institutions to local farmers and their families. In combination, these institutions contributed to the revolutionizing of the American family farm and its shift toward large-scale production by corporate owners, or agribusiness.

Like any social institution, land-grant colleges are the focus of study and criticism, especially because of the shift in emphasis from a people-oriented perspective to one geared to corporate profit. The consumer only sees these issues in the form of less palatable fresh produce developed by food scientists to be more durable, slower ripening, or more easily transported food products, for example, the "hard tomatoes" mentioned in the following reading. Beyond the question of personal preference, what are the large-scale social, health, and aesthetic consequences of technological tampering with nature's bounty? Can new technologies developed for an industrialized farm system be exported to less developed countries? The answer, as Don Hadwiger points out, is not simple.

"The real hotbeds of world revolution," confided a spokesman for the land-grant colleges, "are the agricultural college research laboratories." It was an admission full of both pride and the realization that the life of a revolutionary becomes less comfortable when others realize what he is doing.

The agricultural colleges have been making a quiet revolution for years in a setting of conventional campus communities. Agricultural science has transformed food and its production. It has made the family farm perhaps irrevocably obsolete by introducing new strains of capital-

and energy-intensive farming. The vast arsenal of technology developed primarily at the land-grant colleges has provided the means for historic advances in agricultural "productivity" and "efficiency."

However, as production has increased, so has criticism. A nascent consumer movement has begun to ask whether, for all the visual changes in our food, it is any safer or more nutritious than it was. Others have noted that while the green revolution has kept supplies of rice and wheat rising with the world's population, more and more of the food supply finds its way to the bellies of the affluent. Still others have wondered if corporate agriculture, combining maximum productivity with minimum employment, can be adapted to those poorer nations where what is needed is both more food and more jobs.

At the heart of such criticism lies the agricultural research estab-lishment, for the policies that affect the massive food industry—from the packaging of tomatoes at A&P to the price of tea in Sri Lanka—are tied closely to the research laboratories in the land-grant colleges. So adept at genetic and environmental manipulation, this establishment seems to have been itself manipulated by a congeries of interests not wholly outside its control. Despite the potential of the agricultural scientists for easing—or exacerbating—the world food shortage, their institutional and sociological biases have not always been in full accord with a commitment to humanitarian goals.

The great collective achievement of the land-grant colleges is the "agricultural revolution," one of whose spectacular manifestations is the train of busy machines that crosses a commercial farm. Nowadays, the farmer may sit in a lofty, air-conditioned, glass-walled cab with carpeted floor and ceiling, working a bank of levers and buttons as he listens to country music. Implements drag behind, each spread wide, each sporting unique combinations of hoses, wheels, discs, and tanks, hissing chemi-cals into the soil while also stirring and seeding it. Here is a product of many subsystems, as complex and integrated as those that support a spaceship.

Agricultural scientists have taken charge of evolution, and to a large extent also of the environment in which growth occurs. Their systems import tons of food for plants and animals, attack insects, diseases, weeds, and other hostile organisms, deliver the output from the farm, and automate the whole endeavor to the point where cropland the size of a county might be handled by fifty or so master farmers.

The man-made systems that underlie agriculture are continually challenged by nature, but scientists have struck back aggressively. When one of the thousands of serious animal scourges hits the United States, animal scientists seem always to find a weapon—vaccine, antibiotic, chemical spray—and they may even pursue the disease to its foreign habitat, as our navy once pursued the Barbary pirates. Their preventive medicine keeps hogs and cattle healthier than humans.

Entomologists are ganging up on damaging insects that were once barely kept at bay. They are trapping southern cotton's old nemesis, the boll weevil, in early planted cotton plots where they release sex attractants to confuse breeding, then sterile males to cause breeding failures. "Technology is now available to eliminate the boll weevil," says the U.S. Department of Agriculture, and cotton congressmen, whose influence, like the boll weevil's, is in decline, can take satisfaction that the funds they poured into boll weevil research have paid off, even though farmers in the South now seem to prefer raising soybeans.

While agricultural scientists have been shaping their systems, however, they have themselves been shaped by an effective political system put together by commercial farmers during this century.

Agricultural research is conducted primarily at fifty-five state agricultural experiment stations. These research agencies are located within the colleges of agriculture at the land-grant universities, where research is interwoven with the training of new agricultural scientists. The land-grant colleges were founded under the Morrill Act of 1862 with the express function of teaching better farming practices. The "experiment stations" or research arms were created under the Hatch Act of 1887, but today receive only about a quarter of their funds from the federal government, with the rest coming from the states and private sources. There are, in addition, six research agencies within the Department of Agriculture, a large proportion of whose scientists are stationed on university campuses. And agribusiness corporations, while developing brand products in their own laboratories, receive considerable assistance from the publicly subsidized researchers.

Agricultural research is a highly decentralized activity. Individual researchers or teams of researchers receive funds for projects with rather vague titles that would presumably allow researchers some degree of freedom. But in fact, the mission of the research institutions is quite constrained. They have been integrated into a social and political system that has shaped their growth and function and determined the careers and values of the researchers. As a result, the agricultural colleges have departed considerably from their original purpose of providing research and education for small farmers. The common farmers were never great champions of education and research to begin with, and the great farmers' mass movements of the nineteenth century seem largely to have ignored agricultural education. But the colleges finally did become politicized with the creation of the county extension agent under the Smith-Lever Act of 1914.

These county agents were supported by state, local, and private as well as federal funds, and were supervised by the land-grant colleges.

Their function was to "extend" college research findings to local groups of innovative farmers in farm bureaus, usually organized by the agent himself. The farm bureaus affiliated as a national organization in 1919, and the county agents continued for many years to serve the American Farm Bureau Federation as grass-roots organizers. The bureau became a national lobby, instrumental in developing three complementary strategies that together gave producers firm control over land-grant agricultural research, indeed, control over all agricultural policy.

The first of these strategies was a coalition of commodity interests (producers and processors of a farm product like wheat, cotton, or sugar), organized around the congressional agriculture committees. It asserted control over congressional decisions, and its leaders acted as permanent secretaries of agriculture supervising quotidian [day-by-day] administration. Committee members tended to represent one-commodity districts. Each major commodity had its own subcommittee, and even a federal bureau or two. Farm policy was, in effect, commodity policy— an amalgam of commodity programs put together by the committees, the general farm organizations, and the secretary of agriculture. . . .

A second strategy was to solicit farmer electoral support for commodity programs, in presidential elections and the few two-party congressional races.

The third strategy was administrative cooptation—giving rural power groups control over state and local branches of federally subsidized agencies—giving the Farm Bureau, for example, control over state and local extension services. In the state legislatures, commercial farmers exercised leverage because the states provided matching funds for research and extension. Representatives of the commercial farmers and agribusiness firms sat on college advisory boards.

This political subsystem is still a principal sponsor of agricultural research, though its strength is diminishing for several reasons. Farmers as voters have become a tiny minority. Cotton is going out as the commodity that mobilized the rural South. The conservative heads of the congressional agriculture committees were defeated in their battle against the food stamp program (now the largest single item in the Department of Agriculture budget). The department itself has been on the defensive during recent decades. The agricultural research establishment, which before World War II received almost half of all federal research funds, is now a minor claimant. And the number of scientist-years within the agriculture experiment stations has suffered a decline during the past decade.

Meanwhile the clientele of agricultural research has changed, as functions have been transferred from the farm to the large agribusiness firms that furnish the inputs and process the outputs. The colleges, of course, are understandably reluctant to change the image of a small-farmer clientele; the National Association of State Universities and Land-Grant Colleges recently reported on agricultural research in a publication entitled "People to People," and the extension service defined itself in a report called "A People and a Spirit." But at a recent national conference to consider future agricultural research priorities, the list of invited participants was top-heavy with representatives from agribusiness.

Service to big firms has come about gradually and with little or no soul searching. In fact, agricultural researchers were always proponents of growth, helping innovative farmers obtain profits (capital) and technology for expansion. Today, most of our farm production comes from a relatively few advanced farmers, while the others—still the majority—together produce comparatively little. The colleges have long been important, too, in training the people and providing the technology for the development of agribusiness firms. In the agricultural system, bigness seemed the inevitable by-product of greatest efficiency and productivity—the unquestioned goals of agricultural research, at least until recently. "Productivity" refers to production per acre (which has doubled in the last four and a half decades), or production per man (the average U.S. farm worker now feeds fifty-two people as compared to a Russian farm worker who feeds only seven people); it also refers to total output (livestock outputs per animal are up 130 percent in forty-five years). "Efficiency" refers to the blending of these elements to make a profit.

Many of the costs of attaining efficient production, however, are untallied and in some cases ignored. Farmers are squeezed by corporate suppliers and corporate purchasers, and sometimes the same corporation squeezes at both ends. Researchers trained to serve farmers have had to adjust to serving the corporations. The commercial agriculture system tolerates increased soil loss, chemical pollution of air, lakes, streams, and underground waters, destruction of wildlife, and dangers to the health and safety of those who work in agriculture as well as those who consume its products.

Agricultural scientists and administrators are increasingly cognizant of these costs, and a search is on for ways to alleviate them. But the face they present to the world is resentful of critics—both inside and outside the establishment—who have helped them evaluate the consequences of their revolution. Presumably, the research establishment fears criticism will detract from its public status, demean its self-image, threaten its relationships within the subsystem still its principal source of support, and urge upon it larger changes in values, structure, and associations than it is prepared to make at this time. Critics within the establishment are not appreciated, and outside criticism that cannot be dismissed as malicious, romantic, or uninformed is viewed as trivial in the context of agriculture's record of increased food production.

There remains a functional faith that society demands greater productivity. Secretary of Agriculture Earl Butz [was] an ebullient spokesman for this mentality. "The United States," he has said, "is still a young, vigorous, and growing nation," and he predicts 100 million more people by the year 2000. "As we expand to meet the needs of 300 million people at current consumption rates, we will have a new market each year for at least 500,000 beef cattle, 50,000 dairy cows, 1 million hogs, and 2.6 million hens. And that's just to keep even."

Secretary Butz gave further expression to the establishment view of itself and its critics in a speech to land-grant college administrators:

> Throughout history, land-grant colleges and state universities have identified with the business and professional life in the states. You have taught the technology of production. You have functioned to create useful knowledge and then you have translated that knowledge in such a way as to train useful people — people who could produce for society and serve the needs of society. With some notable exceptions, the demonstrations and disruptions of recent years have sprung from universities and from colleges within universities in inverse ratio to the production-orientation of that school. . . . We have, thank goodness, seen a trend away from such foolishness in recent years.

Butz urged administrators to let students know that "the public expects a substantial return in the form of allegiance to the American system."

Not all agriculture experts have been as wholeheartedly supportive of the status quo as has Mr. Butz, who was an agricultural college official and a board member of several of the largest agribusiness corporations at the time of the student demonstrations. Some farm economists had for years been pointing out that most farm program benefits went to the largest farms and were ultimately capitalized into the value of agricultural land. And land inflation, they noted, added nothing to productivity. A few rural sociologists had expressed anxiety about the social consequences of displacing farmers into the cities, long before the term "black ghetto" was invented. Some home economists were concerned about the diets of the rural poor. A research task force of land-grant administrators that met in the early 1960s suggested shifts in the distribution of agricultural research toward people-oriented problems like health, housing, nutrition, living standards, community services, and environment.

But not much happened as a result of inside studies. Existing research was retitled to fit into the people-oriented category. Some research being conducted for the lumber and housing industries, for example, was so reclassified. The extension services began to publicize those rare local projects serving low-income people or blacks—projects local staffers may have risked their careers to initiate and which even after being praised were not given the resources needed for expansion.

Outsiders have raised several issues more effectively. The black-led Poor People's Movement of 1968, which camped for several weeks on the mall outside Secretary of Agriculture Orville Freeman's office, demanded food and jobs. Black and civil rights leaders, by publicizing the conditions of rural blacks, supplied a sedimentation test that revealed that agriculture institutions were being used, on balance, *against* the interests of small farmers and farm workers. This was documented by reports from a presidential commission on rural poverty and from the U.S. Civil Rights Commission.

Another report, *Hard Tomatoes, Hard Times,* was issued by a group of young muckrakers headed by Jim Hightower and Susan DeMarco. They charged that "the tax-supported, land-grant complex has come to serve an elite of private, corporate interests in agriculture, while ignoring those who have the most urgent needs and the most legitimate claims for assistance." The term "hard tomatoes" referred to a thick-walled tomato developed by agricultural scientists so that tomatoes could be picked by a special machine. An economic analysis of the "benefits" of this machine concluded that it had displaced thousands of farm workers while returning large profits to manufacturers and those producers who could afford to buy it. The analysis also concluded that consumers as well as producers had benefited, but Hightower argued that tomato prices were no lower and that the new tomatoes were hardly edible.

Hightower's book was a combination of sarcasm about useless sociological studies, horror stories about the willingness of researchers to release findings despite hazards to the environment or to human health and safety, and angry lectures on the neglect of the rural poor. "The great majority of rural Americans," he wrote, "are strangers to these public laboratories that were created to serve them. When research does not ignore them, chances are it will work against them. If they do get help, it comes either in the form of a meager trickle that has been carefully sluiced and strained upstream, or in the form of irrelevant and demeaning sociological probes into their personal habits."

Hightower was astute in getting news coverage and in seeking legitimation through hearings before the Senate Labor Subcommittee on Migratory Labor chaired by Senator Adlai Stevenson. But agriculture college representatives were equally astute in winding down public and senatorial interest in the subject. Rather than being respectful and responsive, as they customarily were before the agriculture committees, they assumed a haughty stance. One official even distributed "hard" tomatoes to the chairman and the audience, claiming that they were tasty and consumers liked them. (In a subsequent national survey, consumers ranked tomatoes *lowest* in quality among *all* food items available in the grocery store.)

The principal spokesman for the land-grant schools, President Harry G. Caldwell of North Carolina State University, also came to the defense of agribusiness corporations. "Who is going to furnish the viable and reliable seed?" he asked. "Who the fertilizers? Who the insecticides? And when the crop is ready, who is going to buy it and store it and transport it and get it to market at a time and in a condition that makes it salable?" Implied in his questions is the answer to the question, Who are now the principal clients of the land-grant research establishment? Agriculture has in effect become like other production sectors, where large corporations are the main clients of training and research. The farm has become so relatively small a part of the total production process that the question of who will farm, still highly disputed, may not be important except on romantic grounds. President Caldwell took note that some critics of big agriculture "bring with their concern an ignorance, an innocence, and a romanticism that misses the point entirely."

Lack of realism exists on both sides. Although agriculture and research administrators are ready—though not always publicly—to accept the changed structure of agriculture and their new role in it, their defensiveness reveals a pathetic reluctance to confront the social and environmental consequences of their revolution.

But they have proved, on occasion, they can confront these issues in a constructive way—with outside support. Such support helped spur Congress to pass a Rural Development Act in 1972 to help small towns cope with the decline in their farming populations. The agricultural research establishment embraced rural development with considerably more enthusiasm than did the congressional agricultural appropriations subcommittees (which provided little more than token funding under the new law).

There are also abundant opportunities for new directions in research in farm production that have yet to be addressed with a sense of urgency and commitment, and in these cases it becomes clear that the weakening commodity coalition cannot be singled out for full blame. Although agricultural researchers have not ceased to be curious or to desire challenging problems, they have nevertheless become a mature and comfortable bureaucracy. They are slow to respond to new demands and are certainly not aggressive in seeking new missions and clienteles. They have been reluctant, for example, to think in terms of alternative agricultural systems, which might have a mix of different farming practices. They will have nothing to do with the organic farmers who regard themselves as the antithesis of the existing system. Organic farmers minimize the use of chemicals and of heavy-power tillage.

Land-grant scientists view the organic farmer as a modern version of the antiscience preachers. "The logic of arguing against machinery and fertilizer," President Caldwell exclaimed, "would take mankind back to primitive practices and to doomsday." In the eyes of his critics, however, President Caldwell's orthodoxy in support of the agribusiness establishment is itself a path to doomsday.

On the world scene, graver shortcomings of our technology are coming into public view. One is the fact that much of our research technology is committed to making our food luxurious, often at the expense of making it plentiful. It is a simple fact, borne out by production and trade statistics, that the world food shortage has been caused not by population growth in the developing countries but by increased per capita food consumption in affluent nations. We have switched to richer diets, like grain-fed beef. Indeed, the most ominous population growth is that of meat animals in the developed nations, especially beef cattle whose numbers in the United States alone have more than doubled in the last two decades.

The spread of luxurious diets in the developed nations may become a major cause of mass starvation among the world's poor, and certain aspects of agricultural technology may contribute to such an occurrence. Others, however, benefit the poor. Witness, for example, the "green revolution," which increased the production of wheat and rice in a number of hungry nations. Still, the producers who currently support agricultural research are primarily interested in research that increases food exports to dollar markets.

While research benefits have a mixed impact on world food supplies, their impact is more clearly perverse with respect to solving a larger problem—that of increasing the world's supply of agricultural jobs. India, Pakistan, Indonesia, Bangladesh, and other poor, heavily populated nations must find places for more rather than fewer farmers simply because the rural work force in those countries will grow faster than the number of nonagricultural jobs, even by optimistic estimates.

Neither the agricultural scientists nor the peasants can make the final decision for a developing country about whether a labor-intensive technology will be used or whether our own production system will be imposed. Such decisions are generally made by landlords and by the governments that depend upon them to siphon food from the country-side to the urban poor. Desperate governments, seeking food and imports to quiet their urban masses, thus seem by and large to be permitting the development of a mechanized, energy-intensive agriculture that increases the number of unemployed urban people to be fed while increasing the burden of imports. American policy and technology probably encourage these trends. Even the green revolution may have served merely as a reprieve for governments unable to make productive use of agricultural labor.

Developing countries need a different mix of labor and technology than we do. But developed nations have yet to find a synthesis that respects the interests of human beings involved in production, that protects the environment, and that accepts the possibility of new life-styles in agriculture. The research establishment may argue that such changes are for political institutions to bring about, not learning institutions (viz China). Unfortunately for that argument, the two have often interacted each to narrow the other's options.

How is the circle broken? In earlier periods, giants emerged from the scientific community, grasping public leadership to institutionalize a new ethic. Gifford Pinchot established the Forest Service. Hugh Hammond Bennett created the Soil Conservation Service. Seaman Knapp introduced demonstration farms. But no giant is yet visible within today's agricultural establishment. Those who are sent forth as its philosophers are as yet only conciliators and apologists.

Yet U.S. agricultural scientists are presumably as concerned as anyone about the welfare of the world's people—and are perhaps more frustrated than others by the perversity of systems. Although they cannot wholly control the impact of their technology, many of these scientists are searching for a better understanding of social and political environments and some envision research programs that will have a more constructive effect on the human condition.

The agricultural research establishment remains a ship full of riches, though long at the mercy of the prevailing winds of commercial agriculture interests, which have secured its public funding and have manipulated its outputs. New winds buffet this establishment—consumers, environmentalists, the media, some elected officials, enlightened insiders, and in the future, maybe, antithetical farmers and even a giant or two. But these have yet to form a coalition that can give agricultural research the breadth of perspective that a great research establishment ought to have.

Producers who want exclusive benefits have long known that public research expenditure is a good investment from their point of view. It is time to realize that it is also a potentially good investment from the point of view of those interested in spreading its benefits more equitably. In the meantime, the academic community should accept the responsibilities implicit in its position as a determinant of the world's food and job situation.

Scientists should insist on engaging in research that is worthy in their own eyes and insist on funding for it from new, as well as existing, sources. This could well mean a collective effort to corral national support for agricultural research. Moreover, they should free themselves from their present status as hired hands for the agricultural business. This will involve repudiation not only of grants for certain specific research areas and funds for graduate students, but also most travel money, which is perhaps the most corrupting influence in the scientific community. (Many agricultural scientists are in fact encouraged to seek travel money from private agribusiness firms.)

It is likely that each discipline has a few distinguished scientists who care about the impact of their work upon the world. The influence these people will have depends entirely on the degree to which others are keen enough to take their example. Unfortunately, such individuals have too often in the past been ignored or dismissed as eccentrics.

Finally, the various agricultural sciences should, as a discipline, devote more effort to formulating research strategies that maximize their contribution to world problems. Contrariwise, scientists should cease to take comfort from those who pass among them making light of these responsibilities; whose stock in trade must be crude humor ("Meat," quipped one agricultural school dean, "is good to eat.") rather than serious questions.

Selection 24 Mechanized Agriculture: Its Ecoenergetics and Environmental Impacts

William N. Richardson
Thomas Stubbs

Editors' Introduction

In classic studies David Pimentel and John and Carol Steinhart have discussed the input and output of farm production in terms of the dollar cost of energy used to provide food and the dollar cost of the food produced. Such calculations are exceedingly complex because hardly any food makes its way directly from the field to the table. Energy is used in the agricultural system to provide irrigation and farm machinery. Energy is also used to process,

Source: Courtesy William Norman Richardson & Thomas Stubbs: *Plants, Agriculture & Human Society,* Copyright © 1978 by W.A. Benjamin, Inc. Reprinted with permission. Complete notes and references appearing in this article are not included here; for further information consult the original version.

package, and store food for wholesale and retail distribution. All these energy costs are eventually passed on to the consumer and thus have an impact on food-purchasing behavior. For example, a typical breakfast includes orange juice from Florida, bacon from a Midwest packer, cereal from Nebraska, coffee from Colombia, and perhaps eggs and milk from a nearby community. Food purchased at a local supermarket may then be stored in a frost-free refrigerator-freezer and prepared on an instant-on gas or electric stove, or perhaps even in a microwave oven. All these appliances are heavy energy users.

The average consumer has little awareness of the implications of the energy costs for modern agriculture. In the following excerpt from their book *Plants, Agriculture, and Human Society,* Richardson and Stubbs describe the economic factors related to the mechanization of modern agriculture in the developed nations.

On the surface it might appear that intensive, mechanized agriculture has been an unmitigated benefit. Until quite recently, food production has been so high in the United States that the federal government yearly spent millions of dollars to subsidize farmers for *not* growing certain crops, such as wheat and corn. Fruits and vegetables tend to be larger and more attractive than those grown under less technological conditions, and the per-acre yield of grains has been increased. Mechanization has also reduced the number of people necessary for adequate agricultural output. In recent decades a greater number of individuals from farming families have pursued different life-styles.

Paradoxically, some of the short-term advantages of mechanized agriculture may be detrimental from a long-range economic and ecological standpoint. In the midst of our abundance, there are subtle factors that call into question the wisdom of continuous agribusiness expansion. Synergistic cycles have been set into motion which, unless these cycles are checked, threaten the future of our most important food crops.

Economic Considerations of Agribusiness

Let us first examine some of the economic aspects supporting the contention that highly technological agriculture is not all to the good. Consider the individual farmers who are attempting to maximize gains. They will be interested in producing the greatest quantity possible on the land available to them. If the crop is a grain, for example, it is unlikely to have any distinguishing qualities that confer an advantage over the crop of other individual producers. Cultivators of fruits and vegetables may focus some efforts on the appearance and size of their crops; but even so, the ultimate quantity remains important.

So a successful farmer will use whatever means are available to maximize the potential yield. It is worth noting that statistical estimates rate only about 25 percent of U.S. farmers as "successful"; the remainder are marginal producers. Nevertheless, agriculture in the United States more than supplies the needs of the country. Enough food is produced to provide for substantial annual exports as well.

Mechanization. The farmer who can afford to do so will purchase tractors, mechanical harvesters, trucks, and other labor- and time-saving devices, and will invest in chemical fertilizers. Many farmers are dependent on the industries that manufacture these materials; at the same time, the industries are dependent for their survival on agriculture's continuing need for their products. Thus, the modern farmer must compete to maximize production, and to maximize production must take advantage of technological innovations. As more machinery is bought, the greater is the financial investment; so that even if an agriculturist significantly increases the yield through mechanization and extensive applications of fertilizers and pesticides, the profit may be modest in terms of inflation. Yet the farmer must continue to make the most of the machinery if the investment is to pay for itself.

Monoculture. An especially disturbing facet of the dependence on high-yield, mechanized agriculture is that it emphasizes monoculture. The costliness of agricultural technology causes the farmer to grow large acreages of the same crop. The serious disadvantages inherent in mono-cultural practices are, naturally, of less interest to most farmers than the immediate financial necessity.

What are the problems with monoculture? Monoculture simpli-fies ecosystems. The more simplified an ecosystem becomes, the less stable it will be, and the more vulnerable it will be to disruptions, such as attacks by insects or fungi. . . . Economically, the farmer who practices monoculture must spend more on fertilizers to replace exhausted soil nutrients, because a single species removes the same elements from the soil year after year, whereas the rotation of several crops can replenish elements used by others. The farmer will have to apply more pesticides, also.

The effects of consumer attitudes. Consumer attitudes play a role in the nature of agribusiness. People usually equate the quality of fruits and vegetables with attractive appearance. Thus, a shopper browsing through the produce section of a supermarket is inclined to look for the largest and most appealingly colored fruits. To compete, a farmer uses all the technological means developed to produce the most attractive produce. No one knows the effects of the increasing residues of toxic materials which we consume in our foods because of the methods used to enhance appearance of produce.

The farmers are caught in a system for which they are not responsible and about which they can do little. Increased productivity per unit of land usually causes prices to drop, because a greater quantity is available. Then the farmer finds it necessary to produce *even more* to maintain the same profit. One cannot blame individuals who are merely attempting to make a living in the context of a complex economic dilemma. However, mechanized agriculture has expanded to the point that most successful farms operate on almost an industrial scale. Many smaller operations have been forced out of business because of an inability to compete adequately with large-scale agribusinesses.

Energy Use

The increased mechanization of agriculture is of particular concern in light of the contemporary scarcity of energy sources. "Modern, high-yield agriculture can reasonably be described as a system that turns calories of fossil fuel into calories of food."[1] Farm machinery cannot function without fossil fuels as an energy source. There are also less direct requirements: gasoline powers the trucks that distribute food nationwide; fuel is used in the manufacture of farming machinery. Fuels are consumed in the production of fertilizers and pesticides, both as energy sources and as raw materials.

During the past fifty years, the energy input into food production has increased impressively, not only in terms of energy used for farming but in terms of energy required in the preparation of commercial foods. Even aside from conserving energy, it is relevant that the complexities of food production in developed countries cause costs to be higher, and these expenses are passed on to the consumer. Food in the United States is relatively expensive when compared with most developing nations, but as Americans tend to have a high standard of living, the cost for an adequate diet is not yet prohibitive for the majority. In 1970, an average individual in the U.S. consumed $600 worth of food.[2] Considering that the per capita income is in many countries well below that figure, Americans clearly pay a higher absolute price for their food than do the citizens of the developing nations. Granted, Americans eat much better than do most people in those nations. But if an average East Indian were to pay for his or her food at American prices, it would cost $200, about twice the annual per capita income for that country.

For every calorie that is eaten by someone in the United States, approximately nine more were required for its production. The energy in the food eaten annually by Americans is about 250×10^{12} food calories (kilocalories) or 1.4 percent of the total of U.S. energy consumption. Accordingly, about 13 percent or 14 percent of all U.S. energy use is in some way involved in food production. The amount of energy devoted to producing food in the United States increased tenfold from 1920 to 1970, whereas the agricultural output was increased by only a factor of two. It is particularly striking that only one-fourth of the energy utilized in the food production system is expended on the farm; processing, distribution, and food preparation consume the remainder. Although the use of energy in food production has continued to grow, the increments of output have been smaller since about 1965.

These figures suggest that, in spite of projections by technological optimists who say that we need only implement mechanized agricultural techniques to allay or eliminate world food shortages, the problem is not that simple. For example, to raise the Indian calorie intake from its present level to 2000 to 3000 per day (the U.S. level) would require more energy if accomplished through mechanization than India currently expends in the total economy. To produce food for the entire world with a U.S. agricultural system would consume about eighty percent of the world's present estimated energy expenditure. Thus, it does not seem likely that the food crisis will be solved by transferring mechanized agriculture to the developing nations. There are not enough energy sources to do so, no matter how the equations are juggled.

An interesting perspective is that the apparently low number of individuals engaged in food production is misleading.[3] In the United States one farmer now feeds fifty or more people, and it is true that fewer farmers are providing more food than ever before. However, "yesterday's farmer is today's canner, tractor mechanic, and fast-food carhop." That is, the nature of food production has changed so radically in recent years that many indirect activities related to processing food have come into being. People who previously might have engaged in farming are now employed in food-related industries which previously had considerably fewer jobs.

Increased subsidies of agriculture correlate with the rise in energy use. From 1940 to 1970, total U.S. farm incomes ranged from $4.5 billion annually to $16.5 billion annually, while subsidies increased from 1.5 billion in 1940 to 7.3 billion in 1972. The increased use of machinery has interlocked the role of federal subsidy into our agricultural system. Increased production costs are not balanced by consumer prices, despite the sharp rise in food costs.

Can Energy Consumption Be Reduced?

There are reasonable possibilities for reducing the agricultural energy input in the United States, and such alternatives should be given serious consideration.[4] Better use of manure as fertilizer, instead of chemical synthetics, would reduce pollution from feedlot runoff. The use of manure could save as much as 10^6 kilocalories per acre. There would not be enough manure available to replace completely chemical fertilizers, but its use should reduce energy expenditures. Increased crop rotation and the planting of leguminous cover crops to provide nitrogen fertilizer would also reduce the quantity of commercial fertilizers needed.

The control of weeds and pests could be accomplished in ways more energetically and ecologically conservative. Use of a rotary hoe during cultivation, instead of the application of pesticides, would result in a 10 percent energy saving, and would reduce pollution as well. Biological pest controls could be more widely used. These techniques include the introduction of sterile males into the pest species' population, the introduction of natural predators, and other "natural" means. Such actions require a small fraction of the energy consumed in pesticide manufacture, distribution, and dissemination, and would lessen the serious environmental pollution that has occurred as a result of excessive and indiscriminate use of toxic chemicals. Also, a more discriminating policy of pesticide use is called for. When feasible, pesticides could be applied by hand instead of being sprayed from airplanes or ground machinery. Although the human labor would be increased, the energy expended in application would drop from 18 thousand to 300 kilocalories per acre.

Plant breeders might concentrate more on qualities of hardiness, resistance to diseases and pests, less moisture content (to reduce the natural gas needed to dry crops), reduced water requirements, and higher protein content—if yields were reduced somewhat by these emphases. Solar energy on the farm has scarcely been investigated. Wind-generated electricity provided by modern windmills is already in use in Australia. And methane gas can be produced from manure or garbage dumps. Such potentials have not been exploited to any degree, and need controlled experimentation and engineering. Hopefully such techniques could supply workable, nonpolluting alternatives to the more energy-consuming, environmentally hazardous methods now used in farming.

It has been proposed that chemical farming could be entirely eliminated without disastrous results. Reduced yield per acre would require most land in the soil bank to be put back into production. Some experts estimate that overall output would fall about 5 percent, and the price of farm products would increase by 10 percent. Farm income would rise by 25 percent, reducing or even eliminating the need for governmental subsidies. Consumers are not likely to react favorably to a 10 percent rise in the price of groceries. However, there would be long-term gains—a reduction in environmental pollution and less energy use, as well as a significant saving of tax dollars. These might, in the long run, outweigh the immediate displeasing effects. We believe that alternatives to the existing agricultural technology are going to be forced upon us sooner or later, unless new energy sources are developed to replace fossil fuels.

The role and attitude of government is important in changing the agricultural methodology. One aim of the U.S. Department of Agriculture has been to increase agricultural productivity through the development of more chemical agents. The department finances extensive research to improve and innovate chemical pesticides and fertilizers. It is no small undertaking to shift so broad and accepted an emphasis.

Agriculturists trained in the tradition that increased technology is unequivocally beneficial find it difficult to depart from that view. There is also an economic factor and the vested interests of the corporations that produce the fertilizers and pesticides. However, a change is imperative if we are to achieve a rational agricultural system not dependent on a high and ever-increasing energy expenditure. Surely long-range interests would be better served by research into some of the biologically conservative possibilities suggested in the preceding paragraphs.

Soil Conservation

A problem that is not unique to mechanized farming, but which may, in some cases, be aggravated by it is soil erosion. Repeated plowing during the growth of crops causes a continuous and cumulative loss of topsoil. It takes thousands of years to build up a single inch of topsoil, where *inches* may be lost in a single year. The practice of using the rotary hoe instead of herbicides and planting cover crops would alleviate soil loss to some degree, although the cover crops might have the disadvantage of competing for moisture and nutrients.

Topsoil conservation is important to future agricultural welfare. It is an issue that must be dealt with in any agricultural system, not just technological ones. The environmentalist Aldo Starker Leopold related a dismal tale of how quickly human beings can ruin the productivity of the soil.[5] Less than 200 years ago the foothills north of Mexico City were covered with forests of pine and oak. As the population of the Valley of Mexico grew, more land was cleared and planted in corn and wheat. Within a few years, the topsoil had been washed away and minerals had been leached out—leaving a barren subsoil that would no longer support corn and wheat crops. However, it was sufficient for the hardy *maguey* plants, from which fibers and tequila are obtained. Eventually, even the subsoil eroded. Under the subsoil there was a layer of hardpan on which not even maguey could be cultivated. Still, a few desert plants grew there, providing food for limited herds of goats and donkeys which soon eliminated even this sparse vegetation. Today, the area is totally a wasteland, productive of nothing.

The story is not an isolated one. As we have previously mentioned, the Sahara desert of Africa and the Thar desert of western India were lush only a few thousand years ago, and were altered drastically, largely due to deforestation and poor agricultural practices. To prevent the loss of topsoil, which is, for all practical purposes, irreplaceable, technological farming techniques should be balanced by practices that will minimize soil loss. Another "dust bowl" is not an impossibility, even in the United States.

It is clear that modern agriculture has given us more food per acre, but the effects of mechanization must also be measured in terms of energy consumption, environmental degradation, economic factors, and the biological hazard of monoculture. The current trend in agricultural energy input, to focus on continuous production increase, cannot continue unabated. For example, 10^3 kilocalories of fuel are required to cultivate a square meter of corn. At present, the yield from that land gives us 2×10^3 kilocalories of food. Presumably, more energy will be expended in the future, with little probability of further increases in yield. Clearly a more conservative, stable, and balanced system of agriculture must be developed—a more self-contained system less dependent on complex machinery and chemicals.

Notes

1. Paul R. Ehrlich, Anne H. Ehrlich, and John P. Holdren. *Human Ecology* (San Francisco: Freeman, 1973).

2. D. Pimentel et al., "Food Production and the Energy Crisis," *Science* 182 (1973):443–49.

3. John S. Steinhart and Carol E. Steinhart, "Energy Use in the U.S. Food System," *Science* 184 (1974):307–16.

4. D. Pimentel et. al., "Food Production."

5. Aldo Starker Leopold, *Wildlife of Mexico* (Berkeley: University of California Press, 1959).

Part IV

Consumer Perspective on Food

In previous sections of this text, following a discussion of nutrient cycles and nutrient needs, we dealt with a number of macroenvironmental issues related to nutrition. Selections emphasized the interdependent relationships of human beings, environment, and food supply. Throughout, an ecosystems framework has been stressed and ecological relationships emphasized.

Now we turn to matters of importance to the microenvironment of the home and family. Systems terms can be used to explain family functions and food selection and consumption behavior. The family, too, may be viewed as an ecosystem. As such, it is affected by economic, technical, social, psychological, and cultural factors that influence food choices. No matter what a family's socioeconomic level, it will be subject to cultural influences that make some available foods acceptable and others taboo. The cumulative consumer choices made by individuals and families have an impact on the larger environment—whether in India, as suggested by Marvin Harris in selection 25, or in the United States, as suggested by Harrison in selection 27.

Economic systems have been made possible by trade-offs in the amount and kind of energy used in food-getting and food-preparation technologies. In primitive societies firewood or cow dung may become an important energy resource. In our society, gas and electricity become important. Modern industrialized nations have come into being as a consequence of large agricultural surpluses. Today's urban dwellers exchange goods and services for money to pay for food rather than growing, preserving, and preparing all of it themselves. The fact that more and more families are becoming consuming rather than producing units is an important fact of modern economic life.

Food technology, responding to changing Canadian and American life-styles, provides a variety of foods with convenience features. It also provides various opportunities to eat or take home a great many meals prepared outside the home. An estimated one out of two meals will be eaten away from home by 1985. It now takes the average consumer more time to shop for food than to prepare it: Many foods can be purchased cleaned, trimmed, and ready for cooking. Such foods include oven-ready poultry, ground meat preshaped in patties or ready for meatloaf, salad greens grated and packaged, in addition to the vast array of dried, frozen, and canned foods that require only heating to serve.

Clearly, education is essential to an informed choice in the marketplace, whether meals are prepared at home or eaten out. Programs in nutrition education not only must emphasize the economic and health aspects of food selection and preparation, but also must take into account consumers' cultural and personal preferences as well as their budgets. Apart from the cultural influence on food choice, the family as consumers must also be aware of the impact of the mass media on how they eat. They must learn to filter through various appeals from advertisers and others to incorporate reliable information into their life-styles.

Selection 25 India's Sacred Cow

Marvin Harris

Editors' Introduction

The Western mind sometimes finds it hard to understand the seemingly irrational technology of less developed nations. When viewed in terms of energy costs, however, some practices regarded as unenlightened clearly have ecological benefit. One of the most widely misunderstood practices is the reverence for the cow practiced in India with its teeming millions bordering on starvation. A closer examination of that nation's food-production system shows that preservation of the cow has far-ranging value to the population at large. Westerners, who view meat eating as a basic right, can gain new perspective through understanding the basic efficiency of a food-production system that provides both food (milk protein) and fuel (cow dung) and assures a future supply of both through reverence for one form of life.

News photographs that came out of India during the famine of the late 1960s showed starving people stretching out bony hands to beg for

Source: Adapted from Marvin Harris, "India's Sacred Cow," *Human Nature*, February 1978, pp. 28–36. Reprinted with permission from *Human Nature* Magazine, Copyright © 1978, Human Nature, Inc. References appearing in this article are not included here; for further information consult the original version.

food while sacred cattle strolled behind them undisturbed. The Hindu, it seems, would rather starve to death than eat his cow or even deprive it of food. The cattle appear to browse unhindered through urban markets eating an orange here, a mango there, competing with people for meager supplies of food.

By Western standards, spiritual values seem more important to Indians than life itself. Specialists in food habits around the world like Fred Simoons at the University of California at Davis consider Hinduism an irrational ideology that compels people to overlook abundant, nutritious foods for scarcer, less healthful foods.

What seems to be an absurd devotion to the mother cow pervades Indian life. Indian wall calendars portray beautiful young women with bodies of fat white cows, often with milk jetting from their teats into sacred shrines.

Cow worship even carries over into politics. In 1966 a crowd of 120,000 people, led by holy men, demonstrated in front of the Indian House of Parliament in support of the All-Party Cow Protection Campaign Committee. In Nepal, the only contemporary Hindu kingdom, cow slaughter is severely punished. As one story goes, the car driven by an official of a U.S. agency struck and killed a cow. In order to avoid the international incident that would have occurred when the official was arrested for murder, the Nepalese magistrate concluded that the cow had committed suicide.

Many Indians agree with Western assessments of the Hindu reverence for their cattle, the zebu, or *Bos indicus*, a large-humped species prevalent in Asia and Africa. M.N. Srinivas, an Indian anthropologist states: "Orthodox Hindu opinion regards the killing of cattle with abhorrence, even though the refusal to kill the vast number of useless cattle which exists in India today is detrimental to the nation." Even the Indian Ministry of Information formerly maintained that "the large animal population is more a liability than an asset in view of our land resources." Accounts from many different sources point to the same conclusion: India, one of the world's great civilizations, is being strangled by its love for the cow.

The easy explanation for India's devotion to the cow, the one most Westerners and Indians would offer, is that cow worship is an integral part of Hinduism. Religion is somehow good for the soul, even if it sometimes fails the body. Religion orders the cosmos and explains our place in the universe. Religious beliefs, many would claim, have existed for thousands of years and have a life of their own. They are not understandable in scientific terms.

But all this ignores history. There is more to be said for cow worship than is immediately apparent. The earliest Vedas, the Hindu sacred texts from the second millennium B.C., do not prohibit the slaughter of cattle. Instead, they ordain it as a part of sacrificial rites. The early Hindus did not avoid the flesh of cows and bulls; they ate it at ceremonial feasts presided over by Brahman priests. Cow worship is a relatively recent development in India; it evolved as the Hindu religion developed and changed.

This evolution is recorded in royal edicts and religious texts written during the last 3,000 years of Indian history. The Vedas from the first millennium B.C. contain contradictory passages, some referring to ritual slaughter and others to a strict taboo on beef consumption. A.N. Bose, in *Social and Rural Economy of Northern India, 600 B.C.–200 A.D.*, concludes that many of the sacred-cow passages were incorporated into the texts by priests of a later period.

By A.D. 200 the status of Indian cattle had undergone a spiritual transformation. The Brahman priesthood exhorted the population to venerate the cow and forbade them to abuse it or to feed on it. Religious feasts involving the ritual slaughter and consumption of livestock were eliminated and meat eating was restricted to the nobility.

By A.D. 1000, all Hindus were forbidden to eat beef. Ahimsa, the Hindu belief in the unity of all life, was the spiritual justification for this restriction. But it is difficult to ascertain exactly when this change occurred. An important event that helped to shape the modern complex was the Islamic invasion, which took place in the eighth century A.D. Hindus may have found it politically expedient to set themselves off from the invaders, who were beefeaters, by emphasizing the need to prevent the slaughter of their sacred animals. Thereafter, the cow taboo assumed its modern form and began to function much as it does today.

The place of the cow in modern India is every place—on posters, in the movies, in brass figures, in stone and wood carvings, on the streets, in the fields. The cow is a symbol of health and abundance. It provides the milk that Indians consume in the form of yogurt and ghee (clarified butter), which contribute subtle flavors to much spicy Indian food.

This, perhaps, is the practical role of the cow, but cows provide less than half the milk produced in India. Most cows in India are not dairy breeds. In most regions, when an Indian farmer wants a steady, high-quality source of milk he usually invests in a female water buffalo. In India the water buffalo is the specialized dairy breed because its milk has a higher butterfat content than zebu milk. Although the farmer milks his zebu cows, the milk is merely a by-product.

More vital than zebu milk to South Asian farmers are zebu calves. Male calves are especially valued because from bulls come oxen, which are the mainstay of the Indian agricultural system.

Small, fast oxen drag wooden plows through late-spring fields when monsoons have dampened the dry, cracked earth. After harvest, the oxen break the grain from the stalk by stomping through mounds of cut wheat and rice. For rice cultivation in irrigated fields, the male water buffalo is preferred (it pulls better in deep mud), but for most other crops, including rainfall rice, wheat, sorghum, and millet, and for transporting goods and people to and from town, a team of oxen is preferred. The ox is the Indian peasant's tractor, thresher, and family car combined; the cow is the factory that produces the ox.

If draft animals instead of cows are counted, India appears to have too few domesticated ruminants, not too many. Since each of the 70 million farms in India requires a draft team, it follows that Indian peasants should use 140 million animals in the fields. But there are only 83 million oxen and male water buffalo on the subcontinent, a shortage of 30 million draft teams.

In other regions of the world, joint ownership of draft animals might overcome a shortage, but Indian agriculture is closely tied to the monsoon rains of late spring and summer. Field preparation and planting must coincide with the rain, and a farmer must have his animals ready to plow when the weather is right. When the farmer without a draft team needs bullocks most, his neighbors are all using theirs. Any delay in turning the soil drastically lowers production.

Because of this dependence on draft animals, loss of the family oxen is devastating. If a beast dies, the farmer must borrow money to buy or rent an ox at interest rates so high that he ultimately loses his land. Every year foreclosures force thousands of poverty-stricken peasants to abandon the countryside for the overcrowded cities.

If a family is fortunate enough to own a fertile cow, it will be able to rear replacements for a lost team and thus survive until life returns to normal. If, as sometimes happens, famine leads a family to sell its cow and ox team, all ties to agriculture are cut. Even if the family survives, it has no way to farm the land, no oxen to work the land, and no cows to produce oxen.

The prohibition against eating meat applies to the flesh of cows, bulls, and oxen, but the cow is the most sacred because it can produce the other two. The peasant whose cow dies is not only crying over a spiritual loss but over the loss of his farm as well.

Religious laws that forbid the slaughter of cattle promote the recovery of the agricultural system from the dry Indian winter and from periods of drought. The monsoon, on which all agriculture depends, is erratic. Sometimes it arrives early, sometimes late, sometimes not at all. Drought has struck large portions of India time and again in this century, and Indian farmers and the zebus are accustomed to these natural disasters. Zebus can pass weeks on end with little or no food and water. Like camels, they store both in their humps and recuperate quickly with only a little nourishment.

During droughts the cows often stop lactating and become barren.

In some cases the condition is permanent but often it is only temporary. If barren animals were summarily eliminated, as Western experts in animal husbandry have suggested, cows capable of recovery would be lost along with those entirely debilitated. By keeping alive the cows that can later produce oxen, religious laws against cow slaughter assure the recovery of the agricultural system from the greatest challenge it faces— the failure of the monsoon.

The local Indian governments aid the process of recovery by maintaining homes for barren cows. Farmers reclaim any animal that calves or begins to lactate. One police station in Madras collects strays and pastures them in a field adjacent to the station. After a small fine is paid, a cow is returned to its rightful owner when the owner thinks the cow shows signs of being able to reproduce.

During the hot, dry spring months most of India is like a desert. Indian farmers often complain they cannot feed their livestock during this period. They maintain the cattle by letting them scavenge on the sparse grass along the roads. In the cities cattle are encouraged to scavenge near food stalls to supplement their scant diet. These are the wandering cattle tourists report seeing throughout India.

Westerners expect shopkeepers to respond to these intrusions with the deference due a sacred animal; instead, their response is a string of curses and the crack of a long bamboo pole across the beast's back or a poke at its genitals. Mahatma Gandhi was well aware of the treatment sacred cows (and bulls and oxen) received in India. "How we bleed her to take the last drop of milk from her. How we starve her to emaciation, how we ill-treat the calves, how we deprive them of their portion of milk, how cruelly we treat the oxen, how we castrate them, how we beat them, how we overload them."

Oxen generally receive better treatment than cows. When food is in short supply, thrifty Indian peasants feed their working bullocks and ignore their cows, but rarely do they abandon the cows to die. When cows are sick, farmers worry over them as they would over members of the family and nurse them as if they were children. When the rains return and when the fields are harvested, the farmers again feed their cows regularly and reclaim their abandoned animals. The prohibition against beef consumption is a form of disaster insurance for all India.

Western agronomists and economists are quick to protest that all the functions of the zebu cattle can be improved with organized breeding programs, cultivated pastures, and silage. Because stronger oxen would pull the plow faster, they could work multiple plots of land, allowing farmers to share their animals. Fewer healthy, well-fed cows could provide Indians with more milk. But pastures and silage require arable land, land needed to produce wheat and rice.

A look at Western cattle farming makes plain the cost of adopting advanced technology in Indian agriculture. In a study of livestock production in the United States, David Pimentel of the College of Agriculture and Life Sciences at Cornell University found that 91 percent of the cereal, legume, and vegetable protein suitable for human consumption is consumed by livestock. Approximately three-quarters of the arable land in the United States is devoted to growing food for livestock. In the production of meat and milk, American ranchers use enough fossil fuel to equal more than 82 million barrels of oil annually.

Indian cattle do not drain the system in the same way. In a 1971 study of livestock in West Bengal, Stewart Odend'hal of the University of Missouri found that Bengalese cattle ate only the inedible remains of subsistence crops—rice straw, rice hulls, the tops of sugar cane, and mustard-oil cake. Cattle graze in the fields after harvest and eat the remains of crops left on the ground; they forage for grass and weeds on the roadsides. The food for zebu cattle costs the human population virtually nothing. "Basically," Odend'hal says, "the cattle convert items of little direct human value into products of immediate utility."

In addition to plowing the fields and producing milk, the zebus produce dung, which fires the hearths and fertilizes the fields of India. Much of the estimated 800 million tons of manure produced annually is collected by the farmers' children as they follow the family cows and bullocks from place to place. And when the children see the droppings of another farmer's cattle along the road, they pick those up also. Odend'hal reports that the system operates with such high efficiency that the children of West Bengal recover nearly 100 percent of the dung produced by their livestock.

From 40 to 70 percent of all manure produced by Indian cattle is used as fuel for cooking; the rest is returned to the fields as fertilizer. Dried dung burns slowly, cleanly, and with low heat—characteristics that satisfy the household needs of Indian women. Staples like curry and rice can simmer for hours. While the meal slowly cooks over an unattended fire, the women of the household can do other chores. Cow chips, unlike firewood, do not scorch as they burn.

It is estimated that the dung used for cooking fuel provides the energy equivalent of 43 million tons of coal. At current prices, it would cost India an extra $1.5 billion in foreign exchange to replace the dung with coal. And if the 350 million tons of manure that are being used as fertilizer were replaced with commercial fertilizers, the expense would be even greater. Roger Revelle of the University of California at San Diego has calculated that 89 percent of the energy used in Indian agriculture (the equivalent of about 140 million tons of coal) is provided by local sources. Even if foreign loans were to provide the money, the capital outlay necessary to replace the Indian cow with tractors and fertilizers for the fields, coal for the fires, and transportation for the family would probably warp international financial institutions for years.

Instead of asking the Indians to learn from the American model of industrial agriculture, American farmers might learn energy conservation from the Indians. Every step in an energy cycle results in a loss of energy to the system. Like a pendulum that slows a bit with each swing, each transfer of energy from sun to plants, plants to animals, and animals to human beings involves energy losses. Some systems are more efficient than others; they provide a higher percentage of the energy inputs in a final, useful form. Seventeen percent of all energy zebus consume is returned in the form of milk, traction, and dung. American cattle raised on western rangeland return only 4 percent of the energy they consume.

But the American system is improving. Based on techniques pioneered by Indian scientists, at least one commercial firm in the United States is reported to be building plants that will turn manure from cattle feedlots into combustible gas. When organic matter is broken down by anaerobic bacteria, methane gas and carbon dioxide are produced. After the methane is cleansed of the carbon dioxide, it is available for the same purposes as natural gas—cooking, heating, electricity generation. The company constructing the biogasification plant plans to sell its product to a gas-supply company, to be piped through the existing distribution system. Schemes similar to this one could make cattle ranches almost independent of utility and gasoline companies, for methane can be used to run trucks, tractors, and cars as well as to supply heat and electricity. The relative energy self-sufficiency that the Indian peasant has achieved is a goal American farmers and industry are now striving for.

Studies like Odend'hal's understate the efficiency of the Indian cow, because dead cows are used for purposes that Hindus prefer not to acknowledge. When a cow dies, an Untouchable, a member of one of the lowest ranking castes in India, is summoned to haul away the carcass. Higher castes consider the body of the dead cow polluting; if they do handle it, they must go through a rite of purification.

Untouchables first skin the dead animal and either tan the skin themselves or sell it to a leather factory. In the privacy of their homes, contrary to the teachings of Hinduism, untouchable castes cook the meat and eat it. Indians of all castes rarely acknowledge the existence of these practices to non-Hindus, but most are aware that beefeating takes place. The prohibition against beefeating restricts consumption by the higher castes and helps distribute animal protein to the poorest sectors of the population that otherwise would have no source of these vital nutrients.

Untouchables are not the only Indians who consume beef. Indian Muslims and Christians are under no restriction that forbids them beef, and its consumption is legal in many places. The Indian ban on cow slaughter is state, not national, law and not all states restrict it. In many cities, such as New Delhi, Calcutta, and Bombay, legal slaughterhouses sell beef to retail customers and to the restaurants that serve steak.

If the caloric value of beef and the energy costs involved in the manufacture of synthetic leather were included in the estimates of energy, the calculated efficiency of Indian livestock would rise considerably.

As well as the system works, experts often claim that its efficiency can be further improved. Alan Heston, an economist at the University of Pennsylvania, believes that Indians suffer from an overabundance of cows simply because they refuse to slaughter the excess cattle. India could produce at least the same number of oxen and the same quantities of milk and manure with 30 million fewer cows. Heston calculates that only 40 cows are necessary to maintain a population of 100 bulls and oxen. Since India averages 70 cows for every 100 bullocks, the difference, 30 million cows, is expendable.

What Heston fails to note is that sex ratios among cattle in different regions of India vary tremendously, indicating that adjustments in the cow population do take place. Along the Ganges River, one of the holiest shrines of Hinduism, the ratio drops to 47 cows for every 100 male animals. This ratio reflects the preference for dairy buffalo in the irrigated sectors of the Gangetic Plains. In nearby Pakistan, in contrast, where cow slaughter is permitted, the sex ratio is 60 cows to 100 oxen.

Since the sex ratios among cattle differ greatly from region to region and do not even approximate the balance that would be expected if no females were killed, we can assume that some culling of herds does take place; Indians do adjust their religious restrictions to accommodate ecological realities.

They cannot kill a cow but they can tether an old or unhealthy animal until it has starved to death. They cannot slaughter a calf but they can yoke it with a large wooden triangle so that when it nurses it irritates the mother's udder and gets kicked to death. They cannot ship their animals to the slaughterhouse but they can sell them to Muslims, closing their eyes to the fact that the Muslims will take the cattle to the slaughterhouse.

These violations of the prohibition against cattle slaughter strengthen the premise that cow worship is a vital part of Indian culture. The practice arose to prevent the population from consuming the animal on which Indian agriculture depends. During the first millennium B.C., the Ganges Valley became one of the most densely populated regions of the world.

Where previously there had been only scattered villages, many towns and cities arose and peasants farmed every available acre of land. Kingsley Davis, a population expert at the University of California at Berkeley, estimates that by 300 B.C. between 50 million and 100 million people were living in India. The forested Ganges Valley became a windswept semidesert and signs of ecological collapse appeared; droughts and floods became commonplace, erosion took away the rich topsoil, farms shrank as population increased, and domesticated animals became harder and harder to maintain.

It is probable that the elimination of meat eating came about in a slow, practical manner. The farmers who decided not to eat their cows, who saved them for procreation to produce oxen, were the ones who survived the natural disasters. Those who ate beef lost the tools with which to farm. Over a period of centuries, more and more farmers probably avoided beef until an unwritten taboo came into existence.

Only later was the practice codified by the priesthood. While Indian peasants were probably aware of the role of cattle in their society, strong sanctions were necessary to protect zebus from a population faced with starvation. To remove temptation, the flesh of cattle became taboo and the cow became sacred.

The sacredness of the cow is not just an ignorant belief that stands in the way of progress. Like all concepts of the sacred and the profane, this one affects the physical world; it defines the relationships that are important for the maintenance of Indian society.

Indians have the sacred cow; we have the "sacred" car and the "sacred" dog. It would not occur to us to propose the elimination of automobiles and dogs from our society without carefully considering the consequences, and we should not propose the elimination of zebu cattle without first understanding their place in the social order of India.

Human society is neither random nor capricious. The regularities of thought and behavior called culture are the principal mechanisms by which we human beings adapt to the world around us. Practices and beliefs can be rational or irrational, but a society that fails to adapt to its environment is doomed to extinction. Only those societies that draw the necessities of life from their surroundings without destroying those surroundings, inherit the earth. The West has much to learn from the great antiquity of Indian civilization, and the sacred cow is an important part of that lesson.

Selection 26 A Perspective on Food Patterns

Margaret Mead

Editors' Introduction

Anthropologists view human beings both as physical and products of a long line of human evolution and as embodiments of unique behavior patterns, or designs for living, called *culture*. Cultural patterns include all the ways of thinking and behaving practiced by a particular group of people. These ways of living result in distinctive sets of customs, including customs related to food. Food is an important cultural bond. At an individual level food choices may appear simple. They are in reality learned responses to a complex set of environmental and social conditions.

Psychologist Abraham Maslow has suggested that human needs can be ranked at five levels, creating what he has described as a hierarchy of human needs. In Maslow's hierarchy, needs are ranked from lowest to highest. At the baseline are physiological or tissue needs—essential for survival. At the apex of the hierarchy are self-actualization needs that meet the human being's potential for self-fulfillment. In between are safety or security needs, social needs, and self-esteem or ego needs. These needs are met within the context of a particular culture and set of environmental circumstances. They influence our behavior in both obvious and subtle ways. Simply stated, few people live just to eat or eat just to live. People meet a variety of other psychosocial needs in the way they select, prepare, present, and consume food. As Marvin Harris pointed out in selection 25, cultural factors can establish inhibitions on the free choice of available foods that can meet physiological needs. Clearly, eating is a complex form of human behavior, and each human group and subgroup accepts some ways of satisfying hunger while rejecting others.

Many people in Western culture are ambivalent about the

Source: Adapted from Margaret Mead, "Comments on the Division of Labor in Occupations Concerned with Food," *Journal of the American Dietetic Association* 68, April 1976, pp. 321, 325; Senate Select Committee on Nutrition and Human Needs: *Part I—Problems and Prospects*, statement of Margaret Mead before the 90th Congress, 2nd Session, December 1968; Margaret Mead, "The Problem of Changing Food Habits," *Bulletin of the National Research Council*, report of the Committee on Food Habits, National Research Council, Washington, D.C., 1943, in Margaret Mead, "A Perspective on Food Patterns," © J.C. Penny Company, Inc., *Forum* Fall/ Winter 1977, pp. 2, 3. Reprinted with permission of J.C. Penney Company, Inc.

decision to eat for health or enjoyment—or how to achieve both goals simultaneously. In an earlier article, "Comments on the Division of Labor in Occupations Concerned with Food," anthropologist Margaret Mead points out the negative impact on family health that occurs when control of food technology is disassociated from women's role.* This separation came about when agricultural and food technology, discussed in part III, became mechanized and industrialized. Dr. Mead suggests that the absence of women among the ranks of agricultural scientists and technologists has had serious consequences. This idea is worth examining and reexamining from time to time. In the following selection, Dr. Mead suggests many interlocking factors that influence family food choices.

As anthropologists looking at the world, one of our striking observations is that very few societies have relied on people's natural rhythms and hunger drives to determine the diets that they are expected to eat.

Traditionally, in all known societies including our own, we have eliminated many natural desires to eat, substituted for them cultural patterns, and enforced these cultural patterns with very heavy sanctions. "You eat this because you're a human being; if you ate that, you would be an animal," is one of the strongest. "These foods are foods that the next tribe eats," or "only pigs eat that," or "you, as an aristocrat instead of a peasant, eat steak."

In the past, this dependence on culturally imposed eating patterns kept homo sapiens alive. We must suppose that in any culture which had too deficient a diet, the people perished. Undoubtedly, many tribal groups disappeared because they did not have a good dietary pattern, or because one change was introduced into the pattern with which they did not know how to cope. For instance, the one source of their calcium or the one source where they obtained ascorbic acid may have become unfashionable in some way. Then the whole diet would have gone to pieces, and in a battle with the neighboring tribe, they would have gone down, and that would have been the end of that tribe. Thus, all the people we find today have a nutritionally viable eating pattern which they have somehow bullied, cajoled, threatened, and persuaded their children to eat. Each such pattern has been based on the empirical nutritional tenet: If it did not include all the absolutely essential nutri-

*Margaret Mead, "Comments on the Division of Labor in Occupations Concerned with Food," *Journal of American Dietetic Association* 68 (April 1976).

ents, the people would not have survived. Historically, people did not understand the physiological significance of the foods they ate. In addition, no one knew why they ate the things they ate, but gradually over a period of time, viable food patterns were established.

These patterns are important for a reason which I think is valuable to understand. In our prehuman history, if we can judge by what the primates do today, people did not have much time for anything except sleeping and eating. They ate all the time they were awake, and when they stopped eating, they went to sleep. Then they woke up and ate again.

In the course of evolution, people learned that it was appropriate to expect to be fed two or three or four times a day, with the rest of the time available for other activities—such as carving out a civilization. Talking in nutritional terms, in fact, we can almost say that civilization began with three innovations: persuading males to help feed the women and children; dividing up the labor of preparing food so that one person could cook for several, instead of each person picking his/her own grapes all day long; and establishing specified eating times, or mealtimes, so that you could persuade someone who would have been perfectly willing to eat almost continuously to eat only sometimes.

What are some of the dynamics of American dietary patterns that have developed during our contemporary mealtimes? Various investigations have highlighted a situation which is so commonplace to most of us, and especially to those who have specialized in questions involving attitudes toward food, that at first sight it will not seem to be a discovery at all: that resistances and acceptances of food are thought of in terms of morality. People feel that they ought to eat correctly, or, more concretely—"It's wrong to eat too much sweet stuff." Foods that are good for you are not good to eat, and foods that are good to eat are not good for you. So ingrained is this attitude that it may come as a surprise to learn that in many cultures there is no such contrast, that the foods which are thought to make people strong and well are also exclusively the foods which they like to eat, which they boast of eating, and without which they would be most unhappy.

The whole problem of food habits in the past has been variously discussed as a phenomenon of "habit formation" on the loose general basis that any habit once formed is hard to break, that Americans have learned bad food habits and that therefore it is difficult to teach them good ones. The assumption has been that food habits were just like any other kind of habit, and very little attention has been given to the particular way in which they were ingrained.

In order to be able to make a permanent impression on the dietary habits of Americans, it is necessary to know the plot of the life of the American child who is learning to eat, what attitudes are built up toward food, what part of the personality is most deeply involved. Here we find that an attitude far older than the science of nutrition is still holding sway in the home, in fact, an attitude which is inimical to all that we know about permanently establishing new patterns of behavior.

Each generation of children is taught that bad food habits are a possibility against which they must be continually on guard. That is, traditionally, we have tried to make the correct consumption of foods an act of repetitive personal choice, instead of a semiautomatic behavior. In many homes, the "right" food and the "wrong" food are both placed on the table; the child is rewarded for eating the "right" food and so taught that the "right" food is undesirable because, from the child's point of view, rewards are never given for doing things which are, in themselves, pleasurable or enjoyable. At the same time, children are punished by having the "wrong" food taken away from them. Here, again, the lesson is taught to the child that that which is delicious is an indulgence for which one is punished or with which one is rewarded. A dichotomy is set up in the child's mind between those foods which are approved and regarded by adults as undelicious and those foods which are disapproved but recognized as delightful. A permanent conflict situation is established which will remain with that child throughout life; each nutritionally desirable choice is made with a sigh, or rejected with a sense of guilt; each choice made in terms of sheer pleasure is either accepted with guilt or rejected with a sense of puritanical self-righteousness. Every meal, every food contact, becomes an experience in which one must decide between doing right and enjoying oneself. Furthermore, as doing right is closely associated with parental supervision, a secondary association is made linking autonomy, adulthood, and masculinity, with eating what one likes instead of what mother approves.

This situation is a perpetually self-defeating one, for as long as there is a plethora of nutritionally inferior, palate-pleasing, sugared, fatted, and salted foods pervading the media and marketplace, individuals will frequently be making the wrong choices about the foods they eat. As long as any given article of food is presented to children in an unfavorable context, the chances are high that they will reject this food for part or all of their lives. We may be able to make changes in diets, but unless we can disassociate eating habits from this type of training of children, we will never have a population which eats, happily and unquestioningly, the best foods which we have.

One of the consequences of our eating so much of those foods which have the least redeeming nutritional value is that we are becoming increasingly overweight and obese. And to remedy our corpulence, we spend huge sums of money on low-calorie drinks that are guaranteed to do absolutely nothing for us. In addition, we are increasingly the victims of heart disease, diabetes, and hypertension, all of which are almost certainly, or at least partially, attributable to our diets.

It is almost impossible for Americans, who see food as wrecking their figures and health, to understand what it means to be hungry, what it means for the majority of the world's people not to know where their food is going to come from a day or week in advance. Yet, the technology of television and Telstar has transformed us into a world community alerted to our common human heritage, irreversibly linked in intercommunication. We are in a period of great stress—a period of tremendous poverty for a very large number of people, aggravated by a totally disproportionate allocation of global resources. We are now in a period in which we are going to have to alter our food patterns both for our own personal health and for the maintenance of our interdependent world.

Selection 27 Cultures and Food Choices

Gail G. Harrison

Editors' Introduction

Food-consumption behavior is hard to change, especially since many food-consumption habits that have been established early in life and are reinforced daily over long periods of time are deeply engrained. Nevertheless, some factors do contribute to change— but not always change for the better. The author of the following selection, who co-authored a major nutrition textbook entitled *Nutrition, Behavior, and Change* (see bibliography) emphasizes the thesis that eating patterns are the product of a complex interplay of factors. Furthermore, a study of the eating patterns of individuals, families, and larger subcultural groups shows that new and

Source: Adapted from Helen H. Gifft, Marjorie B. Washbon, and Gail G. Harrison, *Nutrition, Behavior, and Change* (Englewood Cliffs, N.J.: Prentice-Hall, Inc., 1972) in *J.C. Penney Forum*, Fall/Winter 1977. Reprinted by permission of Prentice-Hall, Inc., and J.C. Penney. Diagram and complete notes and references appearing in this article are not included here; for further information consult the original version.

often surprising variations must be recognized and taken into account when making recommendations for improving food-consumption practices. Several interesting trends that indicate the impact of economic and social factors on changing food habits are seen in the Garbage Project examined in the next selection. Thus, food-behavior is affected by many variants.

We often think of food habits as particularly resistant to change. Indeed, studies of immigrant groups in various countries have shown that often the old food habits are retained long after language, clothing and other aspects of daily behavior have changed to blend into the new culture. Foods which are familiar to us are particular sources of comfort and security and often form a focal point for family traditions which endure for generations. The very term "food *habits*" implies a fixed, unchanging set of behaviors. But we are naive if we think of eating patterns as static. They do change. The eating habits we exhibit as a society reveal a great deal about our collective values and ideals, and the direction of change in eating habits reflects more general cultural change.

In order to examine some of the changes in U.S. eating patterns which have come about in the last few decades, we need first to consider the factors which influence food choices in any society. . . . The first consideration . . . is that the food must be *available* in the environment before any individual can make a decision to consume it. Many factors influence food availability; in the United States, the sophistication of systems of food processing, transportation, and marketing results in the availability of a great diversity of food items. Availability to the individual, however, is influenced strongly by economics, by the relative costs of different items, and by decisions made by others. The role of "others" who help determine what foods we will consume by deciding what foods will be made available is particularly noteworthy.

Kurt Lewin used the term *gatekeeper* to describe the person who makes the ultimate decisions about what food appears in the household; but there are gatekeepers at various points in the environment — parents, teachers, school administrators, food market managers and government regulatory agencies influence the availability of particular foods to individuals. Young children and those fed in institutional settings such as hospitals, nursing homes, and prisons are the most completely at the mercy of the decisions of others with regard to their food supply, but we are all affected to one degree or another by gatekeepers in the society.

The decisions made by gatekeepers, however, do not necessarily represent strictly a one-way flow of influence. The consumers or those affected by the decisions almost always exert some influence on the decisions made. For example, it has been shown in several studies that the requests of young children for particular food items influence the purchasing behavior of their mothers; this fact is well known by advertising agencies and the food industry, as can be observed by watching any Saturday morning's smorgasbord of television commercials directed toward children. Another example of the impact of consumers on gate keeping decisions is the resistance among consumers to proposed Food and Drug Administration bans on certain products in the U.S. food supply. When a food or an item which people perceive as important to them is threatened, there is usually a reaction. . . .

The second major classification of determinants of food choice [is] *acceptability*. After a food item becomes available, it will be accepted or rejected on the basis of the needs it fulfills for individuals. Acceptability is influenced by a complex network of factors, including taste, texture, appearance, familiarity, nutritive quality, and attitudes toward food developed from personal experiences and cultural norms. These factors determine which of the available foods will be consumed, and by whom.

Changes in eating patterns in a society come about through changes in either the availability or the acceptability of given food items. Since both contexts are constantly changing and impinging on a food supply which, in the United States, is highly diverse, changes in our eating patterns are neither simple nor easily explained. Some of the methods by which availability and acceptability are affected include (1) *changes in the physical environment* (for example, a hard freeze in Florida will affect the price, and perhaps the availability, of oranges and orange juice in much of the country), (2) *changes in the economic situation* (there is evidence that inflation generally over the last several years has had an impact on food consumption patterns), (3) *changes in the relative desirability or status value of food commodities* (for example, vegetarianism was regarded only a few years ago as an eccentricity; it has become more and more common, and some quite elegant vegetarian restaurants in many cities attest to its increasing cultural acceptability), and (4) *conscious attempts to bring about change* through policy decisions and educational efforts. The publication of *Dietary Goals for the United States* by the Select Committee on Nutrition and Human Needs of the U.S. Senate . . . is an example of this type of effort.

Dr. Norge Jerome, in an excellent article on U.S. culture and food habits, has listed seven basic cultural values or themes which are reflected in our eating patterns as a society. These are: individualism, democracy, capitalism, industrialism, leisure, pluralism, and youthfulness. It is worth considering how each of these themes is reflected in our food habits.

Individualism and democracy are tightly connected values which permeate our society. We tend to feel that people should be independent, resourceful, able to "pull themselves up by their own bootstraps," free to "do their own thing" as long as they don't interfere with the ability of others to do likewise. We feel that individuals should be responsible for their own welfare. Margaret Mead expressed this value eloquently in the choice of a title for her classic book on American culture, *And Keep Your Powder Dry*. In terms of eating behavior, we express these values by maximizing opportunities for individuals to express themselves through food. The modern supermarket offers thousands of products, many different from one another only in shape, size, color, or other minor characteristics. We use this tremendous diversity to let individuals express their own right to free choice. For example, this is reflected in the purchase of several different types of breakfast cereals, each because a different family member prefers it over all others, and the freedom of each child to select his or her own cereal in the morning. Imaginativeness and variety are valued over monotony in menus; cookbooks advertise hundreds of different ways to prepare basic staple items, such as ground meat. In many cultures, by contrast, the major underlying assumption in menu planning is to include the major staple in the same form in each meal. Instead, we strive for change and variety.

Capitalism and industrialism are also intertwined themes in American culture. We tend to accept readily the value of technology in producing bigger, better, and more specialized products. "New and improved" has become an advertising cliché in this country. We are always looking for a new improved product, even when we are basically satisfied with the old model. There seems to me to be a recent modification of these values, however, with increasing consumer activism and discontent with contrived demand and needs created by advertising. Vance Packard's book, *The Waste Makers*, may have been one of the initial indicators of this trend; certainly today many Americans are beginning to reexamine their need for always-increasing levels of technology.

Leisure as a cultural theme is related to the value we place on individual expression. Increasing availability of leisure time and our notions of how it ought to be used have resulted in definite changes in our food habits. The proportion of meals eaten away from home has increased dramatically over the last decade, reflecting not only the increasing proportion of women in the labor force but also the value that we place on leisure as a culture. The increasing use of convenience foods further reflects these trends.

Pluralism is a basic American value in spite of homogenizing influences of mobility and mass media. We are a society of many subcultures, and the food habits contributed by each are a source of richness and variety in the texture of our national eating patterns.

Youthfulness is a value which we express through food as well. Ours is a culture in which youth is equated with independence, productivity, and achievement as well as with freedom to express oneself. No wonder youthfulness is sought after and imitated, since it embodies so many of our other basic values! The popularity of foods and cosmetics which are thought to keep one young, the emphasis on low-calorie and diet foods, and a large "health food" industry all reflect the desire of many people to keep the attributes of youth as long as possible and to stave off the processes of aging.

Using Dr. Jerome's seven cultural themes, then, we can make better sense out of the trends in our own eating patterns over the last several decades. We have seen several major trends: a tremendous increase in the diversity of individual food products available, a large increase in food eaten away from home and packaged and convenience foods, an increase in the relatively high status of meat and other animal protein foods at the expense of grains and potatoes, an increased consumption of canned and frozen fruits and vegetables at the expense of fresh produce.

There is some evidence, however, that some of these trends are beginning to be modified or even reversed in the last few years. . . .

These [changing] trends, if they turn out to be representative of the larger society, indicate that changes in the direction of decreasing meat consumption and increasing fresh-produce consumption may already be underway. These changes, as we would expect, are related to cultural change in the society as a whole. There has been increasing concern in the United States with the possible health hazards of a highly processed food supply. The rise in consumer activism has provided a new public conscience to monitor the consequence of the operation of the profit motive of industry.

It has become clear that our major health problems are related now less to infectious diseases than to life-style, including sedentary living, smoking, and diet. Our basic cultural value of individuality makes us, as a society, responsive to the argument that we have to take responsibility for our own health. While we retain a strong commitment to each individual's right to make his or her own decisions, we are increasingly making it clear that such decisions have to be made on an informed basis.

Thus it seems to me highly appropriate that the publication and discussion of *Dietary Goals* should come at this time. It is a time of reexamination of our individual and societal decisions about our food supply and our use of it.

Selection 28 Food Waste Behavior in an Urban Population

Gail G. Harrison
William L. Rathje
Wilson W. Hughes

Editors' Introduction

In previous selections we have emphasized the importance of recognizing the finite limits of the world's natural resources and the futility of attempting to repeal the laws of thermodynamics. There is, indeed, no free lunch. This concept is illustrated in concrete terms in the following selection.

Food production in industrialized nations—especially in Canada and the United States—is energy- rather than labor-intensive. Economic theorists like to consider problems as though systems worked perfectly—that is, as though the production, distribution, and consumption of food operated in perfect harmony. However, not all the money spent by families on food is spent for food alone, since as much as 9 percent is spent on packaging. Furthermore, an important factor that is often overlooked is the amount of food that goes to waste because it is not available for consumption.

Food waste on the farm resulting from spoilage, damage, or contamination or food waste resulting from improper storage or transportation cause lowered food supplies at the marketplace. Such losses are passed on to the consumer by middlemen and retailers. What about food that reaches the consumer and is not utilized? These are household wastes. In a dramatic and important study, the "Garbage Project" of the University of Arizona, researchers have reached some important findings related to household refuse. The data developed by this research challenges our assumptions about supply and demand as they relate to food.

In the following selection the authors suggest new ways of monitoring food consumption and utilization trends at the community level. The suggestion is also made that we must raise our awareness of the serious problem created by extensive household waste while food prices at home are rising and hunger and starvation are all too real in other parts of the world.

Source: Adapted from Gail G. Harrison, William L. Rathje, and Wilson W. Hughes, "Food Waste Behavior in an Urban Population," *Journal of Nutrition Education* 7, no. 1 (January/March 1975):13–16. © Society for Nutrition Education. Reprinted with permission.

Growing awareness of the finite limits of natural resources under the pressure of an exploding population has made it necessary to look at human utilization of food resources in a new light. The concept of efficiency—ecological and economic—has assumed a new priority in nutrition policy and planning. At the household level, economic inflation has made efficient use of food resources more obviously important to more consumers than it has been in the past.

Recent analyses of the U.S. food-production system[1] have made it clear that food production in this country is extremely energy-intensive, and that the U.S. food system is reaching the point at which further investments of energy-intensive technology may produce only marginal increments in output. Notably absent from such analyses, however, is an evaluation of the extent, nature, and effects of food waste. No doubt some waste of food is inevitable in any system of production, distribution, and consumption, but little is known about how much waste of food takes place, why, or how much might be avoided.

Food waste in the field and in storage and transportation has been recognized as a significant factor in affecting the availability of food supplies.[2] It has been estimated that up to 40 percent of the total grain crop in some areas of the developing world may be lost through spoilage or other damage in the field, in storage, and in handling and processing. Opinion varies as to the potential for reducing such losses.[3]

Food waste at the household or consumer level has been studied even less. The fact that household food waste in industrialized countries is substantial has been often remarked upon but seldom documented. The U.S. Department of Agriculture, which conducts household food consumption surveys in the United States, has long recognized the need for reliable data on food waste. In the late 1950s, USDA undertook some studies of household food waste using records of weighed food waste kept by volunteer respondents.[4] These studies utilized small, nonrepresentative samples, and the authors noted that the behavior of the respondents was changed by participation in the study. Even so, caloric loss from waste of household food supplies in these studies ranged from 7 to 10 percent of total calories.[5]

A problem in studying food waste is that the concept of waste is fraught with moral implications in our culture. Few Americans like to admit that they unnecessarily waste food, and mere participation in a study of waste behavior is sure to bias results. What is needed, then, is a nonreactive measure—a means of estimating food waste which does not affect the behavior of the subjects.[6] We propose that the methods of archaeology may be useful in this context.

Household Refuse as a Nonreactive Measure of Behavior

The Garbage Project of the University of Arizona has been studying household refuse in Tucson, Arizona, for two years. The project is archaeological in background, theory, and method. Archaeologists have traditionally studied refuse and the remains of material culture in order to make inferences about ancient civilizations — their ways of life, social structures, and utilization of the environment. The Garbage Project is based on the assumption that the methods and theory of archaeology may offer useful perspectives for dealing with contemporary problems of resource utilization.[7]

The project is accumulating data on a wide variety of resource management behaviors including recycling behavior and purchase of food, drugs, household, and personal sanitation items, and other consumables. As a method for studying food utilization patterns and waste behavior, the study of household refuse offers two significant advantages.

First, it is a nonreactive measure of behavior. What goes into the trash can is evidence of behavior which has already occurred. It is the evidence of what people *did*, not what they *think* they did, what they think they should have done, or what they think the interviewer thinks they should have done. In this way, the study of household refuse differs from accepted methods of collecting data on household-level food-consumption patterns, all of which suffer from problems of reactivity — distortion of the behavior itself or the recall of the behavior.[8]

The study of household refuse has its own, but different, limitations as a measure of food-utilization patterns. In no way can the evidence of food input to the household, as reflected by packaging or other items in the garbage, be used as a measure of nutritional adequacy or of quantitative consumption of food by the individual household. Garbage disposals, meals eaten away from home, feeding of leftover food to household pets, fireplaces, compost piles, and recycling of containers all introduce biases into the data acquired from the trash can. However, these biases all operate in one direction — they decrease the amount of refuse. Thus garbage data can confidently be interpreted as representing *minimum* levels of household food utilization and waste. On this basis, population segments can be compared and changes over time observed.

A second major advantage to the study of household refuse is that it is inexpensive, relatively easy to do, and requires no time or active cooperation on the part of the subjects. The logistics of a study of household refuse should not be minimized (the Garbage Project requires the efforts of a full-time field supervisor, even at present sample size), but compared to other methods of monitoring food consumption and nutritional behavior, to which the study of refuse may offer a supplement, the study of household refuse is relatively simple. Data collection can be accomplished by workers with relatively little previous training; and there is little need for special equipment or facilities. This is a major departure from traditional epidemiological methods which usually demand a high level of subject input.[9] As a result, household refuse may be studied in a community on an ongoing basis or at frequent intervals in order to detect short-range changes in food-utilization behavior.

Methodology

The sample. The city of Tucson is an urban community of slightly under 450,000 inhabitants located in southern Arizona. It is characterized by rapid growth in population. The two major ethnic groups are Anglos (whites) and Mexican-Americans; with the latter comprising 27.1 percent of the population in 1973; the proportion of elderly individuals is relatively high with 12 percent of the population aged 65 or over.[10]

The sampling unit for the Garbage Project was the census tract. Tucson's 66 urban census tracts were grouped into seven clusters derived from 1970 federal census demographic and housing characteristics. Factor analysis was used to derive groups of significantly associated census variables, and cluster analysis was then used to order census tracts into clusters based on their association with these derived factors of census variables.[11] Data from thirteen census tracts in 1973 and nineteen in 1974, drawn to be representative of the seven census tract clusters identified by statistical analysis of the data, form the basis for this report.

Data collection. Refuse was collected for the project by Tucson Sanitation Department personnel from two randomly selected households within each sample census tract, biweekly in 1973 and weekly in 1974. Refuse was collected for a four-month period (February through May) in 1973 and again for the same period in 1974. Addresses were not recorded, in order to protect the privacy and anonymity of sampled households. Specific households were not followed over time—that is, a new random selection of households was done each time refuse was collected. Data from all collections in a given census tract were pooled; thus data analysis is based on the census tract as the unit sampled. Total refuse studied includes the equivalent of that from 222 households in 1973 and 350 in 1974. Households were not informed that their garbage was being studied, although there was local newspaper, radio, and television publicity on the project at frequent intervals with emphasis on procedures taken to protect the anonymity of sampled households.

Thus far community reaction to the project has been overwhelmingly supportive.

Fifty student volunteers sorted, coded, and recorded the items in the refuse working at tables provided in the Sanitation Department maintenance yard. After sorting and recording, all items in the refuse were returned to the Sanitation Department for deposit in the sanitary landfill. While the students were not paid for their participation in the project, they had the option of receiving academic credit for archaeological field experience, since they gained experience with the methods and theory of field archaeology while working on the project. Student workers were provided with lab coats, surgical masks, and gloves, and were given appropriate immunizations. In almost three years of the project's operation, there have been no illnesses attributable to garbage work.

Items found in the refuse were sorted into 133 categories of food, drugs, personal and household sanitation products, amusement and entertainment items, communications, and pet-related materials. For each item, the following information was recorded onto precoded forms: Item code; type (e.g., "ground chuck" as a type of "beef"); weight, as derived from labeling; cost, material composition of the container; brand; and weight of any waste. Fifty-two of the category codes referred to food items.

Waste was defined as any once-edible food item except for chunks of meat fat. Bone was not included, nor were eggshells, banana or citrus peel, or other plant parts not usually deemed edible. Food waste was further classified into two categories: *straight waste* of a significant quantity of an item (for example, a whole uncooked steak, half a loaf of bread, several tortillas), and *plate scrapings* which represent edible food but which occur in quantities of less than one ounce or are the unidentifiable remains of cooked dishes. Potato peels were classified separately, and are not included in "straight waste" for purposes of this paper. It is our guess (yet to be investigated) that "straight waste" may be more susceptible to directed change than is the type of waste we have classified as "plate scrapings."

For purposes of this report, the total weight of a given food item coming into sampled households, as derived from labeling on associated packaging materials which are discarded into the trash can, is termed "input" of that food item. It must be kept in mind that these "input" figures are minimal, and their deviation from actual household food utilization of a type of food item is variable depending on the characteristics of the given households sampled.

Results and Discussion

The following data summarize the evidence of food utilization and waste patterns for the entire sample for the time period specified....[12]

1. The refuse analyzed showed that sampled households waste a significant proportion of their food resources. In 1973, 9.7 percent of the total food input, by weight, was wasted; in 1974, 8.9 percent was wasted. (The downward trend was not statistically significant.) Actual waste, of course, was higher since 21.3 percent of the households in sampled census tracts have garbage disposals in good working order and probably grind up a great deal of their food waste.[13] We are currently undertaking a study which will allow us to estimate the effect of differential use of garbage disposals on the food waste found in garbage cans. These data on waste do not include milk or other beverages, since beverage waste usually goes down the drain; thus weight of beverages including milk was eliminated from the input figures for calculation of the above percentages.

2. In 1973, straight waste accounted for 55.3 percent of the food waste and in 1974 it totaled 60.6 percent. (The change is statistically significant at $p < .001$ using the difference-of-proportions test described by Blalock.[14] Thus, although the percentage of total food wasted remained stable from 1973 to 1974, the percentage of straight waste versus "plate scrapings" increased significantly.

3. There were some changes between 1973 and 1974 in evidence of utilization and waste of specific food groups (see tables 28.1 and 28.2). The total input of meat, poultry, and fish was significantly smaller in 1974 than in 1973 (normalized to the same sample size). The percentage of these animal protein foods which was wasted (total waste/total evidence of input, by weight) showed a sharp and statistically significant drop from 12 percent in 1973 to less than 4 percent in 1974, mainly due to a decline in the rate of waste of beef from 9 percent in 1973 to 3 percent in 1974. We find this interesting for two reasons. One is that the high 9

Table 28.1 Item Percentage of Total Household Input Evidence and Waste

Item	1973 Percent of Total Input Evidence	1973 Percent of Waste-Excluding Leftovers	1974 Percent of Total Input Evidence	1974 Percent of Waste-Excluding Leftovers
Selected protein foods*	19.56	21.74	18.50	11.84
Vegetables	24.40	34.77	19.85	38.62
Fruits	13.64	14.25	15.26	17.26
Grain products	11.23	14.68	14.80	15.80
Packaged goods	4.53	4.28	7.41	5.89
Sugar and sweets	10.10	5.74	9.72	6.55
Other	16.54	4.64	14.46	4.04

* Meat, fish, poultry, eggs, cheese, and nuts.

Table 28.2 Percent of Food Items Wasted

Item	Percent of Item Wasted	
	1973	1974
Selected protein foods, (meat, fish, poultry, eggs, cheese, and nuts)	12.09	3.44*
Vegetables	7.65	10.47*
Fruits	5.61	6.09
Grain products (excluding pies, cakes, and other sweet pastries)	7.02	5.73*
Packaged foods (TV dinners, takeout meals, packaged soups, stews, and sauces)	4.96	4.28
Baby foods	3.01	2.42
Fats and oils	1.39	1.08
Dairy (excluding liquid milk)	.92	.73
Spices	.77	4.49
Dips, whips	4.07	1.54
Sugar and sweets (including sweet pastries)	3.04	3.63

Note: Waste (weight) as percent of evidence of total input (weight).

* Significantly different from 1973 value at $p < .05$.

percent waste of beef occurred during the beef shortage in the spring of 1973. It is possible that during the shortage consumers were overbuying or purchasing unfamiliar cuts or quantities which could not be used efficiently. The change in beef waste is also interesting since there was front-page local newspaper coverage of the Garbage Project, reporting the high level of beef waste (and only beef was mentioned) just at the start of the 1974 data collection period. We don't know whether the publicity had any effect on waste behavior but believe that controlled investigations should be carried out to determine whether heightened awareness of waste behavior could have any effect on actual behavior.

Vegetable input decreased between 1973 and 1974 (again, normalized to the same sample size), but vegetable and fruit waste increased. Waste of fresh vegetables accounted for most of the increase. In both years, vegetable and fruit waste made up a larger percentage of straight waste than of the evidence of household input of food. Input of grain products increased from 1973 to 1974, but proportional waste of grain products decreased. In both years, grain products made up a larger percentage of straight waste . . . the waste being for the most part due to waste of bread.

Sweets and packaged foods in both years made up a smaller percentage of straight waste than of household input. Perhaps the most remarkable change in input occurred in packaged and convenience foods: TV dinners, takeout meals, canned stews, soups, and sauces. Evidence of household input of these items increased by over 30 percent between 1973 and 1974. The only explanation we can offer is to point out that the percentage of households in Arizona in which two persons held jobs increased sharply in the same period from 14 percent in November 1973 to 21 percent in March 1974.[15] With more households with two adults in the labor force, the consumption of convenience foods might be expected to rise.

4. The cost of the food waste we observed is high. Extrapolating average household waste (total food waste, divided by the number of household equivalents in the sample) over a full year and figuring at June 1974 prices, Tucson's annual food-waste bill may run between $9 and $11 million. For an average household over a year, the cost of waste was between $80 and $100 of edible food (see table 28.3). The biggest contributors to the cost of waste were beef and other meats (in spite of the decline in waste, beef waste is expensive), cheese, fresh vegetables and fruits, take-out meals, bread, and pastry.

Extrapolating from our data to the estimated 110,000 households in Tucson, we estimate that Tucson was likely to throw out 9,538 tons of edible food in 1974. It may be easier to grasp the significance of this waste if we focus on one item. The average sample household threw away 1.5 ounces of meat, fish, or poultry (straight waste) in each garbage collection. That comes to 5.1 tons each time the garbage is collected in Tucson,

Table 28.3 An Extrapolation of the Cost of Waste/Household/Year

Item	1973	1974
Beef	$20.80	$ 5.20
Other meat	4.58	5.10
Poultry	1.98	1.45
Cheese	3.11	3.86
Fresh vegetables	11.32	12.06
Canned vegetables	1.80	1.25
Frozen vegetables	1.29	.95
Fresh fruit	6.18	7.34
TV dinners	.82	1.01
Takeout meals	4.68	7.90
Soups, stews, etc.	.39	.31
Bread	5.12	4.21
Noodles	.24	1.58
Chips, crackers	1.54	1.28
Candy	1.36	.81
Pastry	5.93	6.83
Baby food	.50	.27
Potato peels	2.18	.92
Total	$73.82	$62.33
Total with plate scrapings:	99.14	82.91
Plate scrapings at 34¢/lb.	25.31	20.58

Note: Calculated by multiplying average quantities wasted per garbage pickup times the number of pickups a year (104) times current (7 June 1974) averaged Tucson prices.

which is twice a week. Using 1965 USDA data, we can estimate that a two-person urban household may consume about 9.4 pounds of meat, poultry, and fish each week.[16] Tucson's waste in one week would provide a week's worth of meat, poultry, or fish for over 2000 such households or a year's worth for 42 two-person households.

5. The quantitative estimates of food input to households derived from packaging materials in the garbage are similar to the quantitative estimates of food consumption for similar households achieved by the USDA household food-consumption surveys.[17] If we extrapolate for a year from the evidence of food input by weight in the average Garbage Project sample household, we estimate that the food input in our sample averaged 1.069 tons of food per household in 1973 and .9763 tons in 1974. The median household size in the census tracts in our sample is two persons.[18] If we add together the quantitative estimates for all food categories for the two-person urban household in the spring, 1965 USDA household food consumption survey, we get a total of .9752 tons of food—extremely close to the estimates obtained in our sample by observation of household refuse.[19]

Although the categories of food are not strictly comparable in all details, it is interesting to compare Garbage Project data for the two years with the percentage of total household food consumption obtained in the 1965 USDA survey for urban households (see table 28.4).[20] To the extent that the comparison can be made, it appears that people in Tucson in 1973 and 1974 were consuming somewhat less of some animal protein foods, less fruit, and more grain products, sweets, and fats and oils than the USDA sample was in 1965. The overall similarity of the food-input pattern shown in table 28.4 with the independent USDA household food consumption data is an encouraging indication of the validity of refuse data as an index of food-utilization patterns on the community level.

Table 28.4 Percentage of Total Household Food Input

	Food Groups as Percent of Household Food Consumption (by weight, USDA, urban households, spring 1965)	Food Groups as Percent Total Evidence for Food Input, by Weight, Garbage Project	
		1973	1974
Selected protein foods*	26.1	19.6	18.5
Vegetables	25.3	24.4	19.8
Fruits	18.3	13.6	15.3
Grain	11.6	11.2	14.8
Sugar and sweets	6.0	10.1	9.7

* Meat, fish, poultry, eggs, cheese, and nuts.

Conclusions

These preliminary data show that the study of household refuse offers a simple, inexpensive, and nonreactive means of monitoring food utilization and waste behavior on the community level. The data accumulated to date clearly indicate that food waste is a significant factor in food-resource utilization and should be seriously considered by nutrition planners and educators.

Notes

1. D. Pimentel et al., "Food Production and the Energy Crisis," *Science* 182 (1973):433; J.S. Steinhart and C.E. Steinhart, "Energy Use in the U.S. Food System," *Science* 184 (1974):307.

2. A.A. Woodham, "The World Protein Shortage: Prevention and Cure," *World Review of Nutrition & Dietetics* 13 (1971):1.

3. A. Berg, *The Nutrition Factor: Its Role in National Development* (Washington, D.C.: Brookings, 1973).

4. S.F. Adelson, E. Asp, and I. Noble, "Household Records of Food Used and Discarded," *Journal of the American Dietetic Association,* 39 (1961):578; S.F. Adelson et al. "Discard of Edible Food in Households," *Journal of Home Economics* 55 (1963):633.

5. S.F. Adelson et al., "Discard of Edible Food."

6. E.J. Webb et al., *Unobtrusive Measures: Nonreactive Research in the Social Sciences* (Chicago: Rand McNally, 1966).

7. W.L. Rathje, "The Garbage Project: A New Way of Looking at the Problems of Archaeology," *Archaeology* 27 (1974):236.

8. C.M. Young and M.F. Trulson, "Methodology for Dietary Studies in Epidemiological Surveys II. Strength and Weaknesses of Existing Methods," *American Journal of Public Health* 50 (1960):83; M. Pekkarinen, "Methodology in the Collection of Food Consumption Data," *World Review of Nutrition and Dietetics* 12 (1970):145.

9. J.W. Marr, "Individual Dietary Surveys: Purposes and Methods," *World Review of Nutrition & Dietetics* 13 (1971):105.

10. D.G. Bal et al., *Pima County ECHO Report* (Tucson, Ariz.: Pima County Health Department, 1973).

11. R.C. Tyron and D. Bailey, *Cluster Analysis* (New York: McGraw-Hill, 1970).

12. G.G. Harrison et al., "Socioeconomic Correlates of Food Consumption and Waste Behavior: The Garbage Project" (Paper delivered at the Annual Meeting of the American Public Health Association, New Orleans, La., October 21, 1974).

13. D.G. Bal et al., *Pima County ECHO Report.*

14. H.M. Blalock, *Social Statistics* (New York: McGraw-Hill, 1960).

15. *Arizona Daily Star,* June 6, 1974.

16. *Dietary Levels of Households in the United States, Spring, 1965: Household Food Consumption Survey, 1965–1966,* U.S., Department of Agriculture, USDA/ARS, 1969.

17. *Dietary Levels of Households Survey.*

18. D.G. Bal et al., *Pima County ECHO Report.*

19. *Dietary Levels of Households Survey.*

20. Ibid.

Selection 29 Cultural Food Patterns in the U.S.A.

American Dietetic Association

Editors' Introduction

Americans and Canadians enjoy the benefits of cultural pluralism which finds expression in a rich and diversified pattern of eating. Both countries also have extensive agricultural resources from which to draw for the production and distribution of a wide variety of foodstuffs. Many food patterns reflecting subcultural values coexist. This diversity reflects the many countries of origin, religious viewpoints, and regional preferences of these nations' populations. Some populations have maintained their distinctive food patterns since their ancestors immigrated to the New World from Europe. Others have retained their distinctive food patterns although other cultural traits are less evident. Each generation has welcomed new food traditions introduced by later waves of immigrants. Despite the influences of the mass media, universal public education, mass marketing of convenience and fast foods (which have tended to homogenize food tastes), a variety of subcultural differences in family eating patterns can still be identified.

In the following selection the American Dietetic Association has set forth some of the major food patterns followed in the United States. (Some of these are also evident among Canadian families.) Characteristic food preferences and ways to use traditional foods for improved nutrition are identified for menu planning that takes cultural preferences and food habits into account.

Chinese

In a large country, such as China, regional differences in eating habits exist. It is important to know the regional origin of Chinese families. Regional differences in food habits are indicated by N (for the northern and western regions), C (central region), and S (southern region). The styles of cooking vary and are known as Mandarin (north), Shanghai (central), and Cantonese (south).

Eating habits of the Chinese are influenced by belief in the importance of balancing the intake of "hot and cold" food—hot and cold

Source: Adapted from "ADA Cultural Patterns—Cultural Food Patterns in the U.S.A.," a pamphlet published by the American Dietetic Association © 1976 the American Dietetic Association. Reprinted by permission.

relating to the reaction a food has within the body, unrelated to temperature or seasoning.

In general, Chinese cooking involves much pre-preparation while the actual cooking time is brief. Methods of cooking used are steaming, boiling, or stir frying in small amount of hot fat. Ovens are not used.

Characteristics of Food Habits	For Better Nutrition and Economy
### Milk Group	### Milk Group
Restricted use of milk or milk products beyond infancy is due to traditional scarcity and expense. It is considered a luxury item. For some, milk is unacceptable and disliked.	Mix milk into cereals such as oatmeal. "Steamed eggs" using milk are well liked. (This product is like a pudding or custard, prepared the Chinese way in a covered dish on a rack over water).
Cheese is rarely used but a cheese-type product made from goat or cow's milk is eaten in northern China.	Encourage milk cheese which is usually acceptable, and ice cream which is popular. Bean curd is high in calcium and protein and usually well liked and economical.
### Meat Group	### Meat Group
The amount of meat used is very limited. In China, only the upper-middle class is likely to eat meat daily. In the United States, it is more common for all to have some daily, usually in mixed dishes. Pork, fish, and eggs are popular. Chicken and shellfish are less frequently used but are generally well liked.	Encourage increased use of meat, fish, poultry, and eggs. The thrifty buys in fish, poultry, and eggs may be the most acceptable.
Meat may be excluded from the diet of young children since it is considered difficult to chew.	For babies "baby food meat" may be introduced. Encourage use of minced and chopped meats for appropriate age group to become accustomed to taste and usage.
### Vegetable and Fruit Group	### Vegetable and Fruit Group
A wide variety of vegetables is used. Many farms are producing familiar and favorite Chinese vegetables. Widely used are spinach, broccoli, leeks, various greens (only recently grown in this country), bok toy (cabbage), carrot, pumpkin, sweet potato, mushrooms (as seasoning), soybeans, brussels sprouts, turnip, radish, watercress.	Continued use of a variety of vegetables and fruits for all members of family and at all times is desirable. Discussion of the cost comparison of fresh, frozen, and canned fruits and vegetables and seasonal fluctuations in price may be helpful.

Regional additions are: N—corn; C—kohlrabi, white eggplant; S—yautia, eggplant, bamboo shoots, and snowpeas (a delicacy).

Fruits considered to be a delicacy may be used as a snack food, not a dessert. (Some fruits are reserved for men).

Fruits in N—persimmon, peaches, plums, pears, and large dates. C—apples, figs, winter melon. S—abundant fruit, bananas, mango, red tangerines, papaya, pineapple, orange, litchi nuts, figs, small dates.

Encourage the use of some fruit or vegetable high in vitamin C daily, as a "snack" or as a dessert.

Bread and Cereal Group

Regional differences in consumption exist. N—mostly wheat products are eaten, including noodles, steamed bread. Millet and rice are also used. C—rice is the predominant food. S—rice, rice flour, and "sticky rice" are used extensively.

Bread and Cereal Group

Encourage use of enriched or brown rice. Affirm economy of this group in family meals.

Miscellaneous

Soybean oil, peanut oil, and lard are used.

Sweets used are sugar, molasses, brown sugar, and occasionally preserves. Seasonings most often used are salt, ginger, garlic, scallion, parsley, red and green peppers, sugar, and vinegar. More highly seasoned foods are eaten by northern Chinese families.

Miscellaneous

Affirm practice of limited use of fats but encourage liquid types.

Italian

Characteristics of Food Habits

For Better Nutrition and Economy

Milk Group

Most adults drink very little milk, except in coffee. Milk is considered an expensive beverage and seldom thought of as food. Children may or may not get recommended amounts of milk.

Milk Group

Encourage the use of milk for all the family. Stress that milk is a food and not expensive since it is rich in food value. Greater use of evaporated and dry skim milk can be encouraged.

Cheese is eaten frequently. It is also used in the preparation of many cooked foods. Imported varieties of cheese are preferred; however, American and Swiss cheeses, as well as domestic Italian types, are being used to greater extent.

Encourage wider use of cheeses in the traditional way (at the end of a meal with fruit) and in cooking. For economy suggest the use of domestic cheeses and the purchase of cheese by the piece to be grated at home.

Meat Group

Veal, beef, pork, and chicken are the most popular meats. Choice cuts are favored but all parts are eaten. Meat is often fried. . . . A small amount of meat or fowl may be used in many dishes.

Highly seasoned meats, such as sausages and salami, are frequently served.

Organ meats (liver, tripe, heart, lungs) are used, as well as the head of lamb.

All kinds of fish, including shellfish (shrimp, lobster), squid, snail, mussels are eaten. Fish may be fresh, canned (anchovies, tuna, sardines), or dried (cod). Fish is often fried in oil or used in stews or chowders.

Eggs are very well-liked, and are used in omelets and in preparing other dishes. The most expensive grades of eggs are preferred.

Many varieties of dried beans and peas are used in soups, stews, with pasta, and they are also served in salads.

Meat Group

Encourage cooking methods other than frying, when it is desirable to reduce the intake of fats and as a means of adding variety to the diet. Greater use of economical cuts of meat, especially in combination with other foods, can be suggested.

Discourage the use of highly seasoned fatty and fried meats. . . .

Continue to recommend the use of organ meats.

Fish, eggs, dried peas and beans, and ricotta cheese (like cottage cheese) make good low-cost meat substitutes. Inexpensive grades of eggs are satisfactory for cooking purposes.

Vegetable and Fruit Group

Large quantities of green vegetables, both cooked and raw, are used. Escarole, Swiss chard, mustard greens, dandelion greens, and broccoli are very popular. Salads are part of most meals.

Vegetables, especially green leafy ones, are often first boiled and then cooked in oil

Peppers and tomatoes are used in the preparation of many foods. Tomatoes are purchased fresh, canned (whole), and as tomato paste.

Vegetable and Fruit Group

The liberal choice of fruits and vegetables is a good one—encourage its continuation.

Discuss methods of cooking vegetables which require shorter cooking time and use less oil.

For economy encourage the purchase of canned tomatoes, especially when fresh tomatoes are out of season and expensive.

Potatoes are seldom eaten, probably because pasta is considered the "starchy" part of the meal.

Eggplant and zucchini are favorite vegetables. Artichoke, mushrooms, and fava beans are also well liked.

The use of eggplant and zucchini can be encouraged. Their nutritive value is enhanced by the tomatoes, peppers, and cheese used in their preparation.

All kinds of fruits are liked. Grapes, oranges, tangerines, and figs are among the most popular. Persimmons and pomegranates are holiday favorites. Raw fruit is often served for dessert.

Selection of fresh fruit in season should be recommended. Encourage the use of canned and frozen citrus fruit juices, when these are less expensive than fresh.

Bread and Cereal Group

Bread and Cereal Group

Pasta is a staple of the Italian diet. Cornmeal (polenta) is used in northern Italy. Rice is also used by Italian families.

Bread is eaten every day at each meal. Italian bread is preferred. Stale bread and day-old bread is used in preparing many main dishes.

Encourage the use of whole grain and enriched bread. Point out that Italian bread may not be made with milk and may not be enriched unless it is packaged and labeled as such.

Miscellaneous

Miscellaneous

Olive oil is the preferred cooking oil. Lard may also be used in cooking and salt pork for flavoring soups and tomato sauce.

Urge families to use some of the domestic oils and less expensive fats for cooking and seasoning foods, such as soybean, cottonseed, and corn oils. (Domestic oils with Italian labels or names are sold in cans by many stores).

Butter is preferred by many families for baking.

Olives are well liked.

Cakes, pastries, and frozen delicacies are used on festive occasions.

Italian food may be highly seasoned.

Japanese

Those of Japanese descent in the United States span four generations: a disappearing first generation; the aging second generation; the increasing third generation; and the beginning fourth generation. The practice of eating a typical Japanese meal, therefore, is infrequent, perhaps once a week to once a month or reserved for the dinner out.

Hence the eating habits described might apply to the still living first generation, or to a recent arrival from Japan.

Characteristics of Food Habits	For Better Nutrition and Economy

Milk Group

Milk and dairy foods are not easily available in Japan. Tea is the available and popular beverage.

Milk, fresh and canned, is used in small to moderate amounts. It is added to coffee and may be consumed in milk desserts, such as ice cream.

Cheese is used in only small amounts.

Milk Group

Encourage increased consumption of all forms of milk as a beverage and in cooking, such as in simple milk puddings, and greater use of cheese.

Meat Group

An excellent variety of saltwater and freshwater fish is eaten. These are broiled, baked, boiled, and used in soups. Raw fish is consumed on occasion, especially when available fresh from the sea. Smoked, dried, and canned fish are also consumed.

The main dish often is a combination of meat and vegetables, seasoned with soy sauce. Beef, pork, and poultry are preferred to lamb and veal. Variety meats are seldom used.

Eggs are frequently eaten raw, fried, boiled, scrambled, and in soups. The freshest eggs are preferred.

A limited number of dried beans and peas common to Japan is used in this country. They are hard-to-get items.

Meat Group

Continue to recommend (eating) a wide variety of fresh fish in season and frozen, canned, and dried fish the year around.

Encourage the use of highly nutritious variety meats and other meats. Hard and soft cheeses are easy-to-use protein substitutes. Cottage cheese can be tastefully combined with fruit.

Discourage the eating of raw eggs. Medium-size eggs may be a better buy than large eggs.

The use of easily available pea and bean dishes favored in the United States, as well as peanut butter, can be encouraged.

Vegetable and Fruit Group

A large variety of vegetables, both raw and cooked is eaten. Commonly used are: spinach, broccoli, carrots, green beans, peas, cauliflower, tomatoes, cucumbers, eggplant, peppers, and squash. These may be prepared with meat, fish, and chicken.

A large variety of fresh fruit is eaten, such as: oranges, tangerines, grapefruit, apples, pears, and melons.

Vegetable and Fruit Group

Encourage good cooking procedures to preserve nutrients. Discourage parcooking and draining of water.

Fruits and juices high in vitamin C should be emphasized, and the continued use of fresh fruits in season.

Bread and Cereal Group

Polished white rice is the staple. (The short grain, sticky variety, is preferred.)

Consumption of wheat products as in breads and cereals is a post-World War II practice in Japan.

Miscellaneous

Butter is used in small amount.

Deep-fat frying of fish, shellfish, and vegetables (tempura) is one of the few times when fat is used in food preparation.

Simple cakes and cookies made of sugar and rice flour, containing little or no fat, are eaten.

Soy sauce is used to season and flavor food whether main course, soup, or side dish and whether meat, fish, fowl, or vegetable. Miso sauce, a soybean product, is used as seasoning for these same dishes. The many varieties of pickles eaten accounts for the high salt content.

Bread and Cereal Group

Encourage the use of restored or enriched rice and discourage washing them prior to cooking. Suggest more frequent inclusion of potato cooked in the skin, in place of rice.

Urge the use of enriched and whole grain breads and cereals. Discourage sugar-coated cereals.

Miscellaneous

Seasonings and pickles should be used in moderation. Patients requiring sodium restriction should be advised of the high salt content of these products.

Jewish

Jewish Dietary Laws are observed in varying degrees by Orthodox, Conservative, or Reformed denominations. Orthodox families place great value on traditional and ceremonial rituals of their religion and observe the Dietary Laws under all conditions.

Characteristics of Food Habits

Milk Group

Dietary Laws prohibit using meat and milk at the same meal. (Six hours must elapse after a meat meal before dairy foods may be eaten; half an hour must elapse after eating a dairy food before meat may be eaten.)

Cheese, such as American, Muenster, and Swiss, is well liked and makes a good milk substitute. Cottage cheese and pot cheese are eaten plain or in blintzes and noodle puddings.

For Better Nutrition and Economy

Milk Group

The use of milk at breakfast and the dairy meal (many times lunch) needs to be encouraged to insure adequate milk intake.

Explain that cream cheese which is well liked is a fat, not a milk, substitute and suggest other cheeses high in protein and calcium.

Meat Group

Orthodox Jews use only the forequarters (rib section forward) of quadrupeds with a cloven hoof, which chew cud, i.e., cattle, sheep, goat, and deer. Animals and poultry must be slaughtered by a ritual slaughterer (shochet) according to specified regulations. Before cooking, meat is koshered by one of two methods: (1) Soaking it in cold water for half an hour; salting it with coarse salt (koshering salt); and draining it to let blood run off. It is then thoroughly washed under cold running water and drained again before cooking. (2) Quick searing. Liver, for example, cannot be koshered by soaking and salting because of its high blood content. It is, therefore, rinsed, drained well, and broiled on a grill. It may then be fried, chopped, or combined with other foods. This second method is preferred for patients on salt-restricted diets. Separate dishes and utensils must be used for preparing and serving meat and dairy products.

Meat of beef, lamb, goat, and deer, as well as chicken, turkey, goose, pheasant, and duck, is allowed. Liver and tongue are used liberally.

Discourage excessive use of delicatessen-type meats, such as corned beef, pastrami, and salami.

Meat is usually broiled, boiled, roasted, or stewed with vegetables added.

Encourage use of less expensive cuts of meat, since all kosher meat is expensive.

Fish that have fins and scales may be used, such as whitefish (fresh and as gefilte fish); smoked sable; carp; lox (salmon); and caviar.

Shellfish (oysters, crab, shrimp, and lobster) and scavenger fish such as sturgeon and catfish are not allowed.

Fish and eggs are considered "pareve" or neutral and may be eaten as dairy or meat.

Urge use of fish, cheese, and other sources of protein.

Eggs are eaten in abundance. An egg with a clot of blood must be discarded.

Dried beans, peas, lentils are eaten liberally, especially as soup.

Vegetable and Fruit Group

All fruits and vegetables may be used.

Some greens are popular. Spinach or sorrel leaves are used for Schav, a popular soup. Good use is made of broccoli, carrots, chicory, sweet potatoes, and yams. Green peppers are popular and are often served stuffed with meat or dairy mixture.

Vegetable and Fruit Group

Stress more variety in the use of dark green leafy and deep yellow vegetables. Emphasize the correct method of cooking vegetables: a small amount of boiling water, a covered pot, and short cooking time.

Fresh and canned tomatoes are extensively used. Green cabbage is cooked slightly and may be stuffed with a ground beef and raisin mixture with tomato sauce. Root vegetables and potatoes are liberally used. Potato pancakes (latkes) and potato pudding prepared with eggs are very popular. Noodles or noodle pudding, as a potato substitute, is preferred to rice. Beets are used in soup (borscht).

Orange or grapefruit or their juices are generally used for breakfast. Cooked dried fruits (prunes, raisins, apples, peaches, pears, apricots) are commonly served. Fresh or stewed fruits are often eaten as desserts with the meat meal.

Fruits are usually eaten in sufficient quantity as snacks and desserts. When prunes are served in the morning, orange juice is apt to accompany the meat meal. It may be necessary to point out the high caloric value of dried fruits when calories need to be limited.

Bread and Cereal Group

Water rolls (bagel), rye bread, and pumpernickel are often used, as these do not have milk or milk solids and, therefore, can be eaten with meat or dairy meals. They are considered "pareve" or neutral. Matzoth, also "pareve," is the only bread product allowed during Passover, but is commonly used throughout the year. Whole grains such as oatmeal, barley, brown rice, buckwheat groats (kasha) are used.

Bread and Cereal Group

Encourage the use of enriched white or whole wheat bread at dairy meals. Explain that matzoth, crackers, and saltines are not enriched and make little contribution to the diet, other than calories.

Miscellaneous

Sweet (unsalted) butter, usually whipped, is preferred to salted butter. Vegetable oils and shortenings are considered "pareve" or neutral. Chicken fat is often the choice for browning meats and frying potato pancakes.

Danish pastries, coffee cakes, homemade cakes and cookies may be eaten in large quantities. Honey cakes are served for various holidays.

There may be an overuse of relishes such as pickled cucumbers and tomatoes, horseradish, and condiments.

Miscellaneous

Certain margarines are permitted. The code "U" on a package indicates it is permissible; if in doubt check with local rabbinical authorities. Encourage greater use of vegetable oils.

Encourage desserts such as milk puddings, ice milk, ice cream for dairy meals and fruit with meat meals.

Soup may be used at every meal. Chicken noodle and chicken rice soup are commonly served.

Soft drinks are served with meat meals when milk beverages are forbidden.

Encourage soups that make good contributions to daily nutrient needs.

Discourage overuse of soft drinks.

Polish

Characteristics of Food Habits

For Better Nutrition and Economy

Milk Group

Children drink fresh (sweet) milk, while adults may prefer buttermilk. Sour cream is also popular and used in soup, salad dressings, with berries and raw vegetables.

Cheese is well liked.

Milk Group

Encourage recommended intake of milk or milk products for all members of the family.

Meat Group

Meat is commonly consumed. Beef and pork are the most popular meats. Pigs' knuckles, sausages, smoked and cured pork are very well liked as well as chicken, goose, duck, and variety meats (liver, tripe, tongue, brains).

A small amount of inexpensive meat may be made to go a long way in soups and stews.

Fish—fresh, smoked, dried, or pickled is used.

Eggs are well liked and are also used in the preparation of pancakes, noodles, dumplings, and soups.

Legumes are used in soups.

Cottage cheese is very well liked and may be served with sour cream.

Meat Group

For economy encourage greater use of meat substitutes, low-cost variety meats, and less expensive cuts of meat in the preparation of stews and soups.

Greater amounts of meat may be desirable to include in mixed dishes.

Vegetable and Fruit Group

Potatoes are a very important part of the Polish diet and are used in soups, stews, pancakes, and dumplings. Other popular vegetables include carrots, beets, turnips, cauliflower, kohlrabi, broccoli, sorrel, green pepper, peas, spinach, and green beans.

Vegetable and Fruit Group

The use of broccoli, kale, sorrel, green pepper, spinach, carrots, and the tops of beets and turnips may be encouraged for vitamin A.

Vitamin C–rich fruits are not traditionally popular in the Polish diet, but citrus fruits may be used more liberally today than in previous years.

The use of citrus fruits, green pepper, raw cabbage, fresh tomato in season, and canned and frozen citrus juices in off-season may be stressed for vitamin C.

Encourage proper cooking methods for retention of vitamin C values of cabbage, broccoli, green pepper, spinach, kale, sorrel, tomatoes, cauliflower, kohlrabi, potatoes (cook in the jackets).

Dried fruits are well liked.

For economy stress the use of root vegetables, and fruits and vegetables in season.

Bread and Cereal Group

Bread probably will be eaten at each meal. Pumpernickel, sour rye bread, and white bread are very well liked. Sweet buns are also commonly used.

Oatmeal, rice, noodles, dumplings, cornmeal, porridge, and kasha are also prominent in the Polish diet.

Bread and Cereal Group

Eating whole grain and enriched breads and cereals can be encouraged.

Miscellaneous

A wide variety of fats and oils is used.

Polish families are fond of candy, sweet cakes, and other sweets such as honey.

Coffee with cream and sugar is a favorite beverage. Tea is infrequently consumed.

Polish cooking may be highly salted and seasoned.

Miscellaneous

Suggest more frequent use of fruits as desserts.

Puerto Rican

Characteristics of Food Habits

For Better Nutrition and Economy

Milk Group

Milk may be used in insufficient quantities due to economic conditions rather than because it is not liked. Although milk may not be consumed as such, a cup of *cafe con leche* may contain two to five ounces of milk.

Milk Group

Use of milk as a beverage and in cooking may need to be encouraged, including evaporated milk, and nonfat dry milk may be used in cooking, in puddings, and on cereals.

The domestic American cheese is used in limited quantities. Native white cheese (resembling farmer cheese, but firmer and saltier) is used, but is expensive.

Greater emphasis can be placed on the use of cheese.

Meat Group

Chicken is eaten frequently; often in combination with other foods. Expensive cuts of pork and beef are selected more often than other meats and are usually fried.

Ham butts and sausage are used to flavor different dishes. The intestine of the pig is eaten either fried (cuchifritos) or stewed with native vegetables (salcocho) and chick peas.

Fish is used in limited amounts; salt codfish is a common choice.

Eggs are used more often in cooking than as a main dish; the highest priced eggs are often purchased. Fried and scrambled eggs are popular.

Beans are eaten almost every day, either cooked or served with rice. A sauce called "refrito" (green pepper, tomato, garlic, lard) is served with the beans and rice. Pigeon and chick peas are very popular.

Meat Group

Variety meats, especially liver, kidney, and heart may be used in increased amounts. Emphasize lean, less tender, and lower cost cuts of meat, and long, slow cooking methods for the less tender cuts.

Suggest that use of expensive cuchifritos be limited to the special holidays. If salcocho is used, encourage larger quantities of vegetables and meat as well as peas.

Suggest more frequent consumption of fish—fresh, frozen, and canned.

Greater use can be made of eggs as a main dish and as a meat substitute. Medium size rather than large eggs, often represent better value.

The use of larger amounts of beans than rice may be desirable. Some milk, meat, chicken, cheese, or fish should be eaten with the bean meal to provide complete protein. Pigeon peas are more expensive than chick peas. Use of chick peas should be encouraged since their protein is almost as good as that of the soybean.

Vegetable and Fruit Group

Expensive imported vegetables, such as yautia, apio, malanga, name, plantain are frequently used. In addition to being high in starch these viandas have fair amounts of B vitamins, iron, and vitamin C. Pumpkin, carrots, green pepper, tomatoes, and sweet potatoes are well liked. Pumpkin is used to thicken and flavor foods.

Head lettuce, cabbage, fresh tomatoes, and onions are often basic salad ingredients. Lettuce is believed to be very nourishing.

Vegetable and Fruit Group

Encourage the use of less expensive vegetables, such as carrots, beets, yellow squash, yellow or white turnips. Root vegetables may be prepared and served the same way as the Puerto Rican tubers (plantain, yautia, yucca, name).

Stress greater use of canned tomatoes except when fresh tomatoes are plentiful and less expensive. Urge the use of more cooked and raw, dark green leafy vegetables. Stress greater intake of other salad greens and green cabbage rather than the iceberg lettuce for salads.

Long cooking of vegetables, as in stews, is common.

Potatoes are eaten in small amounts and most often in stews, soups, or are fried.

Imported fruits are used often. Oranges are being used more than formerly. Bananas and fresh pineapple are quite popular and frequently eaten. Fruit cocktail, canned pears, and peaches are liked very much.

Peach, apricot, and pear nectar are commonly used.

Emphasize the correct method of cooking vegetables: a small amount of boiling water, a covered pot, and short cooking time.

Greater use of potatoes cooked in the skin can be suggested.

Oranges, grapefruit, and citrus juices—fresh, frozen, and canned, can be used in greater amounts. Encourage use of bananas and fresh pineapple in season, as well as apples and pears and other fruits in season. Recommend the use of fruits, canned in light rather than heavy syrup, as these are often better buys.

Point out that nectars are expensive and offer minimal food value.

Bread and Cereal Group

Bread may be used in only small amounts. Plantain is often eaten in place of bread. French bread, rolls, and crackers are the most frequent choices.

Breakfast cereals, especially for children, is increasing—oatmeal, farina, cornmeal, and cornflakes are the ones most commonly eaten. Cereals often are cooked in milk instead of water.

Bread and Cereal Group

Encourage use of whole grain and enriched breads; enriched or brown rice to replace white polished rice.

Use of breakfast cereals, especially whole grain and enriched ones, should be encouraged, as well as the practice of cooking cereal in milk. Use of sugar-coated cereals should be discouraged.

Miscellaneous

Butter is used in small amounts and only on bread. Lard and salt pork are used for flavoring many dishes, often in large amounts. Expensive oils are used on vegetables and salads. Olive oil is a favorite.

Sugar is very liberally used in sweetening beverages and prepared desserts. Cakes, pies, guava, orange and mango pastes, and boiled papaya preserves are favored often between meals.

Black malt beer is a favorite beverage. It is believed to be very nourishing and is combined with beaten egg for convalescents and pregnant women. In addition to being quite high in calories it contains a fair amount of iron and some of the B vitamins.

Miscellaneous

Suggest margarine in place of butter, and corn, cottonseed, or soybean oils in seasoning vegetables and other dishes, rather than lard and salt pork.

Encourage less frequent use of sugar and sugar-rich desserts. Guava and mango pastes retain some of the vitamin C even after boiling, but are expensive.

Recommend the use of other nourishing beverages, such as milk and fruit juices, rather than the expensive black beer.

Canned soups, such as chicken and vegetable, are often served as the main dish.

Stress meal planning around a main dish made of a protein food rather than soups of low protein value.

Southern United States

| Characteristics of Food Habits | For Better Nutrition and Economy |

Milk Group

Limited amounts of milk are consumed. Buttermilk is often preferred. Cheese may be used in sandwiches. Baked macaroni and cheese is well liked.

Encourage use of evaporated and nonfat dry milk for both cooking and drinking, and greater use of cheese, when milk intake is limited.

Meat Group

Chicken—especially as a "company" dish—is usually enjoyed. Pork and variety meats are very popular. Pigs' feet, hog jowls, ham hocks, cured ham, and heart are often eaten. These may be stewed, boiled with vegetables, or fried. Spareribs are baked or barbecued. Lungs, kidneys, and brains are floured and fried. Chitterlings (intestines) are cut, dredged with cornmeal or flour, and fried crisp. Beef is used in hash or stewed with vegetables. Cured tongue is also eaten. Game—rabbit, squirrel, opossum, and other small game are eaten, usually in a stew.

Fish and shellfish—fresh (as catfish and white buffalo) and canned fish are often eaten. Swannee River catfish dipped in cornmeal and fried is popular. Boiled shrimp, fried scallops, and fried, stewed, or raw oysters are popular in coastal regions.

Eggs—used frequently if the budget permits. They are usually fried.

Legumes and nuts—dried black-eyed peas and beans cooked with salt pork are popular and play a prominent part in meals. Peanuts and peanut butter are consumed.

Emphasize the lean, economical cuts of meat, and stress that salt pork and bacon are fats, not meats. Encourage stewing, baking, roasting, and boiling as methods of cookery.

Teach that white or brown eggs are equally nutritious. Stress grade B for cooking.

Urge that milk or cheese be served with the "bean meal."

Vegetable and Fruit Group

Vegetables generally are well liked. Few are eaten raw. Large amounts of leafy greens are consumed. Turnip greens, mustard greens, collards, cabbage, and green beans are cooked in water with bacon, ham hocks, or salt pork. The cooking liquid (pot liquor) may be eaten with cornbread. Tomatoes, fresh and canned, and white potatoes, are also favorite vegetables. Sweet potatoes, fried, baked, or candied with syrup or sugar, are popular.

Fruits are generally liked although little citrus fruit may be eaten. Fruits, especially those in season, may be eaten between meals rather than as part of a meal. Watermelon and lemonade are favorites in the summer.

Bread and Cereal Group

Few whole grain cereals are used. Hominy grits with gravy, hot biscuits with molasses, and cornbread are eaten extensively.

White or polished rice cooked and combined with ham fat, tomatoes, onion, and okra is especially popular. Dumplings, pancakes, and hoecakes (originally baked on a hoe) are favorite foods.

Miscellaneous

Fats—bacon and salt pork are liberally used in vegetable cookery. Lard is used for baking and frying. Butter is used for preparing desserts, and as seasoning in other types of foods. Gravies are used generously.

Sweets—cakes, cookies, pies, other pastries, and sweet breads are very popular. Molasses and cane syrup are employed as sweeteners. Ice cream, jams, and jellies are frequently eaten. Large quantities of soft drinks are consumed, especially by children.

Vegetable and Fruit Group

Discuss quick cooking of vegetables in very little water to save the vitamins. Note that the addition of baking soda to the water in which vegetables are cooked to make them stay green destroys the vitamins. Stress that a cooked or raw vegetable should be served in addition to potatoes or legumes.

Point out the value of fruits. For limited budgets encourage serving citrus fruit or juice as well as the cheaper grades of canned tomatoes, raw cabbage, "greens," and potatoes for vitamin C.

Bread and Cereal Group

Teach the use of whole grain or enriched breads and breakfast cereals. For economy, stress the use of cooked cereals such as oatmeal.

Emphasize the inclusion of a protein food such as meat or milk when this casserole is served.

Miscellaneous

Discourage the use of large amounts of bacon and salt pork as seasoning for vegetables where overweight or salt restrictions are factors. Suggest methods of cooking other than frying. Encourage the use of margarine and oil.

Since rich desserts may tend to displace the protective foods, especially in the low-income food budget, they should be used only in moderation. Excessive intake of sweets and beverages containing large amounts of sugar should be avoided, especially by small children.

Spanish-American–Mexican

The Southwestern part of the United States is a unique blending of several cultural backgrounds—the Anglo, the Indian, the Mexican, and the Spanish. A melding of food habits has resulted. The [following] food pattern . . . refers primarily to the Spanish or Mexican cultures although they are similar to the Indian.

Characteristics of Food Habits	For Better Nutrition and Economy
Milk Group	**Milk Group**
Milk may be limited due to availability and economy.	Utilizing various forms of milk in cookery and as a beverage would improve the overall nutrition pattern—dried milk, evaporated milk, or fresh milk.
Limited amounts of cheese are used.	Increased use of cheeses would improve the quality of protein in the diet.
Meat Group	**Meat Group**
Chicken, pork chops, weiners and cold cuts, and hamburgers are used predominantly but usually only once or twice a week.	Emphasis on variety of lower cost meats and cookery methods may provide more frequent use of meats, poultry, and fish.
Eggs are frequently used and are usually fried. In rural areas, many have their own chickens.	Eggs are a good meat substitute and daily consumption is encouraged.
Beans are usually eaten with every meal. Usually they are cooked, mashed, and refried with lard.	Beans and lentils provide a good source of protein and calcium. Their protein is enhanced when eaten with animal proteins such as milk, meat, eggs, or cheese.
Vegetable and Fruit Group	**Vegetable and Fruit Group**
Potatoes are a basic item—usually fried—and may be used three times a day.	Different cookery methods could be used.
Chilies from green and red peppers are popular at each meal. These items are good sources for vitamin A even when dried. Green peppers are usually called "mangoes."	Encourage the use of peppers but stress caution in home-canning methods.
Fresh tomatoes are purchased the year around and are a most popular vegetable. Occasionally canned tomatoes are used.	Stress increased use of canned tomatoes except when fresh tomatoes are in season.

Pumpkin, corn, field greens, onions, and carrots are used frequently.

Bananas, melons, peaches, and canned fruit cocktail are the more popular fruits. Oranges and apples are used occasionally as snacks.

Encourage wide variety of vegetables.

Recommend a variety of fruit canned in light syrup as a more economical purchase. Use of citrus fruits could be encouraged. Fruit drinks should not be substituted for fruit juices. Melons (cantaloupe in particular) are encouraged due to the high vitamin C content.

Bread and Cereal Group

Bread, purchased or homemade, is a popular item. Tortillas from enriched wheat flour are made daily. Sweet rolls are purchased. Purchased bread for sandwiches in sack lunches is a status symbol.

Breakfast cereals are usually the prepared type with emphasis on the sugar coated. Occasionally oatmeal is used.

Fried macaroni is prepared and served with beans and potatoes.

Bread and Cereal Group

Continue use of enriched flour. In some sections where corn tortillas are used, encourage use of dried skim milk.

Encourage whole grain cereals. Cooked cereals are usually more economical.

Encourage use of vegetables rather than excessive starch foods.

Miscellaneous

Lard, salt pork, and bacon fat are used liberally. Most foods are fried.

Soft drinks, popsicles, and sweets of all kinds are used liberally.

Miscellaneous

Encourage a variety of cookery procedures.

Purchased cookies, soft drinks, and sweets are expensive and do not contribute to nutritional needs. Utilizing more milk, ice cream, and juices would be helpful.

Selection 30 The Family: Nutrition and Consumer Problems

Effie O. Ellis

Editors' Introduction

As North American families have become more urbanized, their economic function has shifted from production to consumption. Food is an important emotional link among family members and is increasingly subject to such economic fluctuations as price of food, family income, and ways of supplying food to families with low incomes. In rural settings poor families have been able to maintain themselves by growing some food for themselves and exchanging services for food. They could often manage with little hard currency. Increasingly, as urbanized families are removed from opportunities to provide food for themselves, family income becomes an important factor in maintaining an adequate diet. Thus, government programs at every level are important in assisting disadvantaged families to supplement their food budgets. However, financial adequacy is not in itself a guarantee of good nutrition.

Certainly, at whatever income level a family exists, the choices available within their means are a critical factor in family well-being. Public policies are sometimes shortsighted. They appear to give with one hand what they take away with the other. Needy families, struggling to maintain themselves on the borderline of poverty, may actually be penalized for their attempts to supplement their incomes. Neglected groups, such as ethnic minorities (including native Americans), the elderly, and the handicapped, must also be provided for. The social consequences of fostering dependency on public assistance by making it more attractive than the deprivation associated with marginal independence are serious. All too often, those in power who make the policies have little understanding of the interlocking problems that confront disadvantaged families. When dealing with the problems of the poor, they often seek solutions that conform with their middle-class assumptions concerning family life-styles.

In the following selection Dr. Effie Ellis makes an impassioned plea for public policies and effective educational oppor-

Source: Adapted from Effie O. Ellis, "The Family: Nutrition and Consumer Problems," pp. 157–67. From *U.S. Nutrition Policies in the Seventies* edited by Jean Mayer. W.H. Freeman and Company. Copyright © 1973. Reprinted by permission.

tunities that will serve and strengthen families at every stage of development and at every income level.

The family is the basic unit of our society and a most important institution. It is the family that molds the early years of a child's life and establishes the life pattern of the individual. It is the family that determines the physical, mental, and spiritual growth and development of its members and establishes patterns of discipline, communication, and personal relationships.

Food and feeding have served from time immemorial to establish man's family relationships, to transmit tradition and cultural patterns from one generation to another, to fulfill family roles and to provide basic satisfactions in so doing.

Many experts in child growth and development have commented on the vital role of food and the act of feeding in establishing warm human relationships, first within the family, and later with others. After all, man's first experience with love and security is intimately related to food and the feeding process. The family meal can help to nurture and cement family life and enhance individual and group growth. It affords an occasion for parents and children to talk with each other and provides an opportunity for sharing and developing understanding. It can reinforce the role of parents as providers and givers of love and security.

Today, many traditional functions of the family are increasingly being assumed by other institutions—schools, restaurants, community agencies, and so forth. In all social strata fewer meals are being eaten at home. This development could weaken the stability of the family and threaten the uniquely important role it plays in shaping its members' destinies.

For these reasons, the recommendations of the White House Conference on Food, Nutrition and Health (1969) include suggested solutions to major nutrition and consumer problems at the family level. Full recognition was given by the conferees to the need for national policies that will enable the family to continue to function as a major food-delivery system.

Three Problem Areas

The policies that affect the family regarding food, nutrition, and consumer problems can be placed in three main categories: (1) problems associated with an inadequate income or inadequate assistance from federal, state, and local programs; (2) problems associated with budgeting, marketing, and food pricing; and (3) problems associated with a lack of education (in foods, nutrition, child care, home management, and consumerism).

The problems associated with budgeting are dependent upon an adequate income, since no person can obtain a nutritious diet unless he has the financial means to do so. The problems of marketing and food pricing, however, often stem from a consumer's lack of basic knowledge of food labeling, quality, and selection. Therefore, one must consider the total interplay of these three problem areas before one can determine the fate of the family and therefore of society itself.

Adequate Income

Adequate income is of major concern to millions of families in our country at the present time. (This is true, particularly, of the nonwhite minorities and the residents of Appalachia.) There is considerable variation in the amount of a family's income that can be allotted for food even among higher income groups; other essentials that the family needs—housing, clothing, transportation, and health care—compete for the dollar.

The high and constantly rising cost of food is considered to be the primary reason for the high cost of living. At least it seems safe to say that the food dollar buys very little. In order to make ends meet, it is common practice for families to cut the food budget, which provides some elasticity, to meet unexpected emergencies.

Although the existence of poverty and malnutrition is widely deplored, efforts to ameliorate these social conditions clash with the commonly held belief that a person's need for help is evidence that the person is not willing to work. There is an amazing amount of mixed feelings about the root causes of poverty and the remedial measures and methods that are needed for the prevention of poverty. This widespread ambivalence in public opinion is reflected in the provisions of the 1962 and 1967 amendments to the Social Security Act.

In general, welfare policies and practices present the needy family with many complex problems. Consider, for example, the almost unbelievable restrictions encountered in the provision of aid to dependent children of unemployed parents: the full-time earnings of an employed father may not be supplemented even if they fail to meet the family's needs. Also, assistance may not be given with federal matching funds until the father has been unemployed for thirty days—and then only if he has been previously employed for certain periods of time.

There are earned-income exemptions for adults and older children—the first $30 they earn per month plus one-third of the balance of their earnings are not counted as family income. But this applies only to families who are already receiving assistance. Families who apply for assistance are not allowed such exemptions and for this reason may be unable to get help.

Supporting social services are limited only to welfare clients in many states. As a consequence, potential and former welfare clients are denied preventive and maintenance social services. Thus, families who are near-poor or in need of special services are penalized for not being on welfare; because they are not on welfare, they cannot receive family-planning services, day-care services or family-counseling services.

Such policies yield a house divided, largely because the socio-economic realities of the life of the poor are not generally understood by those in power. In part, they are not understood because the problems of communications across socioeconomic lines are mammoth. Program-planning input from the families in need has been small, at best, since so many of the poor are unable to speak for themselves. Through a lack of understanding and ill-advised restrictions, the stated intent of the law does not prevail.

The ADC (Aid to Dependent Children) law, which was designed to keep families together, has failed to enhance the capability of the family to function and indeed leads to family decay. The law was based on the premise that the father in the home would be capable of working and supporting his wife and children. All too frequently this premise has proven to be false.

When a hard and honest look is taken of the situation, we recognize immediately that willingness to work is only a part of the picture. It is the actual earning power of the workers that is of highest importance. It is a well-established fact that opportunities for employ-ment are limited by race, ethnic background, place of residence, age, training, education, union regulations, state of the economy, etc.

For whatever reasons, when a father fails to earn enough money to support his family, he is in trouble. He is in danger of being alienated from society. In order to obtain aid for his family under the ADC law, he must abandon them. Should he seek help under the General Assistance Program, which is set up to cover family needs not provided for by ADC, he must be prepared to be treated as an unworthy person and willing to go through miles of red tape. As a rule, the funds for this program are insufficient, and the eligibility requirements and administrative policies exclude many needy families.

As a further handicap, recipients of these services, particularly those of very low incomes, are often subjected to much criticism by the general public. There is widespread belief that even when the poor are given sufficient resources, they are unable to improve their well-being. Examples of this belief are evident in statements as: "Those people are too lazy to learn," "Look at what they buy—the food carts are full of potato chips and soft drinks," "All these people want is money for alcohol and cigarettes," "They don't known how to buy," "How can these people be hungry when there are television sets and radios in every household?" In reality, most poor people would like to work, but are physically unable to work or cannot find a job. The reason their food baskets at the checkout counters emphasize quantity rather than quality is because the first object of eating is to avoid physical hunger. As for tobacco and alcohol consumption, they are far from being the monopoly of the poor.

An impoverished family that cannot provide all basic essentials, including nutritious food for its members, is without a doubt at high risk of falling apart. And, without a doubt, widespread disruption of family structure will weaken the nation.

The highest priority should be given to the development of policies that will enable every family to have an income that will allow for the purchase of a nutritionally adequate diet. Attainment of this goal would reduce the need for current government programs such as food stamps, food (commodity) distribution, and others. It would reduce the stigma and red tape associated with these programs as well. In addition, the responsibility for budgeting for the family food would be shifted from the government to the family.

A guaranteed adequate family income of necessity must be a long-range goal. Until such time as this goal can be accomplished, strong effort must be directed toward improvement of current food programs.

Food stamp program. Since the White House Conference, the food stamp program has been strengthened substantially as a money-equivalent resource. However, there is still much room for expansion and extension of the program. The purpose of the program administered by the Department of Agriculture is to improve the diet of low-income consumers by supplementing their food-purchasing power. Presently, the maximum purchase price of stamps cannot exceed 33.5 percent of a family's total income. A family of four with a monthly income of $100 would spend $25 for food stamps in order to receive $106 worth of food. Although this amount may seem to be adequate at first glance, the consensus is that this allowance falls slightly below the standardized USDA low-cost food plan. (This is a menu plan that meets the minimal nutrient needs of a family without any provision for the family's cultural food likes and dislikes.) In addition, no provision is made for nonfood items necessary for personal hygiene, cleanliness, and home sanitation.

Eligibility for stamps varies within and between states because of the differences in the standard of living. Problems of welfare impose an additional hardship in providing for the needs of the family. For example, a father or mother who gets a job loses food stamp allowances. Usually the decrease is not compensated for by the increase in family income, because the latter is taxable.

A method of self-certification would help to alleviate the humiliation of applying for stamps, which today strips away a person's right of privacy. Since no one knows his needs better than himself, criteria for eligibility should be established by the government only after consultation with the poor person. Presently the food allowance is determined by USDA, which defines an average meal cost at 35 cents per person. The free–food stamp plan, for which the poorest of the poor are eligible, is still in an experimental stage and is not available nationwide. Under this plan, a family of four with an income less than $100 per month will be able to receive $125 worth of groceries. Presently that family pays a maximum of $22 per month.

Eligibility requirements arbitrarily define the meaning of the word "household" to include family members under sixty years of age. As a result, a large percentage of elderly people who are living alone or with families are deprived of food stamp benefits. The elderly are perhaps the most neglected group in the United States nutritionally, socially, and culturally. That more efforts are not made to meet their needs is a fault of all programs.

Food stamp procedures should be flexible enough to benefit recipients with special needs. This would include a provision for increased benefits for those with a special nutritional requirement for additional foods or special dietary foods. In times of emergency, such as a loss of a home due to fire, stamps should be provided free or at a greatly reduced price. In addition, ways should be developed to strengthen the use of stamps for people in nursing homes, communal groups, or other similar groups. Special consideration should be given to those families who have no cooking facilities and depend on higher priced prepared foods.

The present method of distributing stamps from a central office directly to the recipient is humiliating for those who pride themselves on their independence. This could be remedied by establishing the policy of issuing stamps by mail. Such a plan would be most beneficial to people who are unable to pay the round-trip bus fare and to those who are disabled.

For people who receive a daily or weekly paycheck instead of pay on a monthly basis, the policies should be flexible enough to permit weekly stamp distribution. Likewise, clients should be allowed to determine the amount of stamps they need to buy at a given time; minimum purchase requirements should be eliminated.

School lunch. For many children the school lunch is the primary source of nutritious food. Many others who need additional food are prevented from participating in the school-lunch program because of restrictive administrative policies. New policies should be designed to utilize food stamps as payment for the school lunch.

In the light of the poor food habits of large numbers of children and youths, efforts should be directed toward providing a free school lunch for all regardless of income. . . .

Budgeting, Marketing, and Food Pricing

There are many interrelated factors involved in the development of a meaningful, workable budget. Often problems of budgeting are easily traced to lack of consumer education and unfamiliarity with public services available to consumers in the community. The nutritional needs of the family must be viewed within the family context in relation to other basic family needs—housing, clothing, health care, etc.

Services should not be limited to a specific family member or age group. Witness the feelings of frustration and inferiority which are generated when a pregnant mother is given supplemental food for her personal use and her young children are hungry. Imagine what happens in terms of sibling relationships when the young children in a poor family are given food at school and the older children are hungry during the school day. Careful coordination of community education, public health, social service, and other agency programs can go a long way in reducing problems for many families.

In this connection, people with small sums of money sometimes cannot spend money for adequate food because of health problems that need immediate attention. On the other hand, a mother may decide to forego needed prenatal care because she cannot afford the high cost of baby sitting or day-care services. A working father may postpone needed medical attention because he cannot take time from his job without losing pay. Nutritious foods, which are furnished by the Commodity Distribution Program, may not be utilized because they fail to meet the family's ethnic needs. It is difficult to overstress the fact that food must be consumed in order to nourish. To make food available is not sufficient. It is of little value to suggest that the family can obtain sufficient calcium to meet nutritional needs from nonfat dry milk if families refuse to drink this milk.

Knowledge of food labeling is helpful, if not essential, in planning budgetwise meals. The consumer relies upon labels attached to packaged foods as a prime source of information about the contents, nutritional value, and safety of those foods. Policies that will improve food labeling are essential.

Three actions that would provide needed consumer information are:

1. Improvement in labeling all packaged and processed food products by listing the name and amount of each ingredient, including the nutritive value of each major ingredient per serving. Food

ingredients should be declared in terms of these sources, such as: "wheat-protein hydrolysate" rather than "protein hydrolysate"; "potato starch" rather than just "starch"; and "peanut oil" rather than "vegetable oil."

2. Strict enforcement of existing standards of actual nutritive values to which food manufacturers must conform if they promote, advertise, or label a given product as nutritive.

3. Informative labels on all foods and food products including those that have an established standard. These standards of identity are not defined for laymen. Certain food items are exempt from listing ingredients because the contents follow a recipe that is consistent for all brand names. U.S. standards have been set for a large number of foods such as ice cream, peanut butter, catsup, hamburger, etc. Consumers cannot be expected to remember all of these standards when making purchases.

Every shopper knows the burden of comparing food items, particularly canned goods, when the content varies between brand names. Weights should be standardized in order that "unit pricing" can be a facilitating factor in budgeting for family needs.

There are many problems of budgeting and food purchasing simply because food-distribution facilities are not conveniently located. In small, inner-city neighborhoods, the conveniently located, privately owned store is known for higher priced items. Often the produce is of lower quality, and display cases are not maintained in accordance with public health regulations.

It follows that the larger chain economy stores are located away from ghetto areas and also from rural residents. Three actions that would improve distribution of foods to these areas include: development of new facilities in needed areas or improvement of existing facilities; provision of mobile food stores, particularly in rural areas; transportation of residents to nearest food-distribution centers.

Nutrition Education

Nutrition education is a necessary component of any program. The head of the family can set an example for its members that will give them a foundation in good nutrition. For the basic concepts of good nutritional habits and health to be learned at an early age, it is essential that the parents have sound information in these areas. Some people have emphasized that attempts at parent education have been directed to the middle class and that the parents who need it the most don't get it. However, recent programs conducted by various voluntary and service organizations have shown that parent education for low-income people is succeeding. This is evidenced by the fact that low-income mothers are eager to take advantage of the opportunity to learn and to have their children increase their living skills. Evaluation of the success of these programs cannot be made objectively, but many mothers have expressed their appreciation for this type of assistance.

While it has been more common for women to be involved in nutrition education, it is equally important for the father to be involved. A mother who has accepted a new idea and prepares a new recipe for a meal will be depressed to find that the father won't accept the new dish.

Nutrition education is particularly important for adolescent girls. Current statistics indicate that one out of every four babies is born to an adolescent and that many are born prematurely following a lack of total prenatal care. Childbearing is an example of a situation in which appropriate care can prevent untimely death or lifelong disability, and may simultaneously serve to move an entire family forward to new levels of healthier living. However, in producing normal, healthy infants, nutrition begins at (or before) the moment of conception and depends on the health of the mother. Of prime concern is the fact that many adolescents are malnourished and suffer from anemia. Often, the adolescent's only nutrition advice is provided by sources that may not be reliable, and the adolescent's dietary habits are conditioned by peer group approval. For this reason, a great effort should be made in schools, clinics, community health centers, privately owned centers, and more importantly, at home, to see that accurate information is relayed. It is of extreme importance that adolescents are motivated enough to seek these services when in need. The same is also true for nonadolescent housewives. If nutrition education programs are to succeed, they must give much attention to the women that produce the next generation.

There are various considerations to be made for any nutrition education program. Persons living in poverty are those who have the least—and yet are expected to know the most. They lack such basic necessities as stoves and refrigerators, yet they need ways to prepare nutritious meals. Because of these drawbacks, the woman resigns herself to preparing the same monotonous meals. Many do not have the confidence to try something new. Acceptance of new ideas must begin with demonstrations using familiar recipes, showing ways in which the recipe can gradually be improved.

Eating fulfills a psychological need. In order for education to be effective, the family's food preferences in meeting this psychological need should be known. In this way, the family culture is maintained. The satisfaction derived from a family eating together or a mother nursing her baby can hardly be overemphasized.

The important contributions of the family members in determining the quality of family life also need to be recognized. Business, industry, and communications media can do much to emphasize the importance of the homemaker's role. Even in financial terms, the services provided by a mother for her family—and society—are hard to overestimate. Too often, we disparage the homemaker's role, as in the phrase "only a housewife."

Efforts to provide family-life education should be supported. The subjects studied should include the importance of good nutrition in relation to family relationships; home management; cognitive and intellectual development of the children; the stages of life and their relation to nutrition. Materials can be developed to illustrate "The Family Life Cycle" and explained by trained paraprofessionals. This education can be made a part of the elementary and high school curriculum.

Much can be done to illustrate the role of the father or father-substitute as family provider. It is estimated that it costs between $15,000 and $19,000 for a family to raise one child to age eighteen if they live on the low-cost food plan. If one multiplies this factor by the number of children and includes additional family expenses, it is not hard to see the importance of the father as family provider. Anything that denies this family member's right to provide for his family is threatening to fragment the family unit. In our strongly work-oriented, money-based society, profitable productivity is vastly more popular than idleness in poverty.

Recognizing the need for education in the areas of foods, nutrition, child care, consumer education, and home management, there are various ways in which this need can be implemented. A comprehensive program should be provided to the public by a trained home-service corps of paraprofessionals. Community-sponsored programs can be carried out in neighborhood centers, supermarkets, by public instruction in schools for children and adults, as well as in churches and other community meeting places. Nutrition associations are planning on sponsoring consumer-education programs in large chain supermarkets nationwide. One is currently in progress in Chicago in which free nutritional advice is given on topics of current interest such as weight control.

Nutrition education based on past experience, current knowledge, and research can make a difference in the quality of life for many Americans. Nutrition alone can play an important role in the growth and development of all people, and be a major influence on the way a person performs on the job, at home, and in society as a whole. What we need is the best way to educate the public with the resources at hand in order for families to attain a new status in life. Factual information presented in an understandable way at the time of decision is needed in solving some of the nutrition and consumer problems at the family level.

Selection 31 Feeding America's Poor

Joan Higgins

Editors' Introduction

In the previous selection Dr. Effie Ellis makes a plea for reconsidering some underlying assumptions concerning domestic food policies. The Scots poet Robert Burns once remarked how marvelous it would be to have the gift of seeing ourselves "as others see us." Certainly, nutritionists, home economists, and public officials the world over have had their eye on American food policy. On the one hand they are concerned with the disposition of American and Canadian food surpluses in the face of world food shortages. On the other hand they are quick to note how American domestic food programs contrast with American notions of democracy and equality when faced with the problem of alleviating domestic hunger in the midst of affluence. Certainly, no social, economic, or political system has yet worked out perfect solutions to the problems of modern living. But perhaps we have something to learn from constructive criticism.

In the following selection Joan Higgins, a lecturer in Social Administration at the University of Southampton, gives us an opportunity to see our policies as others see them.

When Jimmy Carter signed the . . . [1977] Food Stamp Act on 29 September, it marked a significant change in policy towards America's hungry poor. The most important feature is that food stamps will be provided free of charge to many of those eligible for the program. It is extremely surprising that this proposal, which has caused so much controversy and debate in the past, should now slip so easily into the legislative package. To understand the real significance of the new act it is necessary to go back some years to the origins of food programs.

They began in 1935 as part of Roosevelt's New Deal and combined subsidies to farmers with the distribution of surplus commodities to the poor. The main aim, at that time, was to dispose of surplus foods and provide price support for farmers. Feeding the poor was a secondary consideration.

It was the beginning of a long controversy about whether food programs were really intended to benefit farmers, rather than the hun-

Source: Adapted from Joan Higgins, "Feeding America's Poor," which first appeared in *New Society*, London, the weekly review of the social sciences, January 5, 1978, pp. 14–15. © New Science Publications, London. Reprinted by permission.

gry. The fact that the administration of the program was handled, then as now, by the Department of Agriculture (and not the Department of Health, Education and Welfare or its predecessors) led many critics to believe that this was so. There were times, of course, during the depression when many farmers themselves were hungry; but, in recent years, the picture has changed considerably. It was estimated in 1967, for example, that less than a million farmers grew most of America's food and, of these, the richest 25 percent got 75 percent of the federal subsidies.

The first food stamp program began in 1939. It was an administratively complex scheme whereby eligible families could purchase orange stamps with a minimum value of $1.00 per week, and a maximum of $1.50, for every family member. For every dollar's worth of orange stamps purchased, the family was entitled to 50 cents worth of blue stamps free of charge. Orange stamps could be used for a variety of foods and household goods (excluding tobacco and alcohol) and could be spent at those local grocery stores in the program. Blue stamps, on the other hand, could only be used for those commodities which the Department of Agriculture ruled were in surplus at that time.

The program was excessively complicated and had only limited benefits for the farmers, whose surplus products were guaranteed a market, and for the poor, whose diets were regulated more by the availability and nonavailability of certain foods than by their needs and desires. The program was abandoned in 1943 when World War II created an increased demand for agricultural products.

The current food stamp program began in 1961 with a series of pilot projects to test its feasibility. It became a nationwide program in 1964, with the signing of the Food Stamp Act. Its immediate effect was to reduce, dramatically, the numbers of people receiving federal food aid. As counties and states switched from the commodity distribution program to food stamps, these numbers fell by between 18 percent and 85 percent. These percentages represented literally thousands of poor people. The Department of Agriculture attributed this enormous reduction to the fact that people had been receiving commodities which were actually surplus to their requirements and concluded that most of them did not really need food aid.

A more likely explanation is that the purchase requirement, in the new program, deterred many who either had no income or who had too little to be able to afford the minimum outlay for food stamps. In order to participate in the program, families had to pay a minimum of $2.00 a person, a month. It was to be paid in a lump sum and had to be paid in advance. For this they received $2.00 worth of stamps, plus a number of free, bonus stamps, which could be exchanged for a wide variety of foodstuffs, not simply surplus foods. The actual requirements were determined according to a sliding income scale and on the basis of an estimated "normal expenditure for food." It was this purchase requirement which caused so much conflict. Bob Choate, a well-known lobbyist for the hungry, complained that the Food Stamp Act, 1964, "amounts to criminal extortion of the poor." . . . [The 1977] Food Stamp Act has helped remedy the situation.

The real effects of this minimum-purchase requirement were uncovered when the Citizens' Board of Inquiry (ad hoc group of doctors, academics, and businessmen) published their findings on hunger and malnutrition in America. Their report, *Hunger USA*, became available in 1968, four years after the introduction of the food stamp program. The first case they quoted was of a woman, in Birmingham, Alabama, who had twenty children (nine of which were her own and the rest she had taken in to give them a home). Her total monthly income was $104 and, out of this, her contribution was assessed as being $74—in order to receive $108 worth of stamps. This left her $30 with which to house, clothe, and cater for all the other needs of her family.

There was also the case of Annie White of Cleveland, Mississippi and her six children. She registered for the food stamp program, but was unable to receive stamps because she had no income with which to make the initial payment. Another mother qualified for $99 worth of stamps, but couldn't afford [them because her] income was only $27.

They were not isolated cases. The findings of the Citizens' Board of Inquiry corroborated those of the six doctors sponsored by the Field Foundation to investigate hunger in Mississippi and those of the Senate Subcommittee on Poverty, whose most prominent member was Robert Kennedy. Abolishing the purchase requirement for food stamps was one of the main demands of the Citizens' Crusade against Poverty. It had the support of Martin Luther King and his successor, Ralph Abernathy, and was one of the reasons for the Poor People's March on Washington in 1968.

There was, and is, no agreement on the number of hungry people in America and estimates vary between 20 million and 40 million. Even taking the lower figure of 20 million, this still leaves a massive problem of hunger and malnutrition which is not being adequately dealt with. Attempts to relieve the problem, in recent years, have met with considerable opposition and the food stamp program, in particular, has been the subject of a great deal of criticism. There is a widely held belief that the poor misspend their stamps on Coca-Cola and potato chips and that there are many people (especially students and strikers) illicitly receiving stamps.

Many Americans categorically refuse to believe that hunger, malnutrition, and even starvation exist in their country. They are aided in their belief by the fact that many hungry Americans do not actually *look* malnourished. In fact, large numbers of them, through eating starchy foods (including surplus foods provided by the federal government), are extremely overweight. Governor Johnson of Mississippi was only one of many southern politicians to deny that hunger existed in their area when he remarked, in 1967, that "all the Negroes I've seen round here are so fat they shine!"

Even at their most generous, food stamp allocations do not allow for nutritionally adequate diets and it is not so much ignorance of what to buy which prevents the poor from securing the right food, as lack of money. Examples of poor families living off "junk food" and TV dinners can certainly be found, but studies have shown that the poor make relatively better use of their money than people on higher incomes. A Department of Agriculture survey in 1965 showed that poor families get more nutrition for their food dollar than the nonpoor and that most food stamp recipients spend their money on nutritious food and not "luxuries."

Some of these issues will be unaffected by the recent legislation, but other ambiguities and administrative anomalies, have been given some attention. The main provision of the Food Stamp Act, 1977, is the elimination of the purchase requirement. This means, in principle, that people who were excluded from participation, through lack of income, should now be able to receive assistance. When the legislation takes effect, participants will receive bonus stamps, as they did before, but will not be required to make any financial contribution. If a family had been paying $100, say, to receive $150 worth of food stamps they would now receive just $50 worth of bonus stamps.

The federal government also seems preoccupied with the British "cars outside council houses" problem. It has ruled that the value of any car worth more than $4,500 will be taken into account in calculating assets. This is some concession to the critics who claim that food stamp recipients eat better, have bigger color televisions and more expensive cars than they could ever afford.

Although some rules have been relaxed, like that excluding applicants without cooking facilities (perhaps a group most needing help), the new act has introduced a number of other restrictions. These include the requirement to register for, and actively seek, work—a central feature of all Carter's welfare reforms. On the other hand, one important advance is the issuing of a national food stamp application form, where previously each administrative unit (and there are hundreds of them) had its own. At the same time, states will have to provide "appropriate bilingual personnel and printed material" where there are substantial numbers of non-English-speaking people. However, these welcome changes are unlikely to standardize the administration of the food stamp program to any great degree.

In Phoenix, in 1974, for example, it was discovered that people were queuing up at midnight in order to apply for food stamps the next morning. Those who arrived at 4 AM were usually too far back in the queue to get seen and had to wait a further day. Some areas had appointment systems, but applicants might be given a date several weeks away. One writer alleged that "waits of two months for an appointment are not infrequent" and claimed that, in Hawaii, sixteen weeks was the normal period. In many areas food stamp offices are open only for a few hours a day, making it impossible for the working poor to attend. In Vermont, food stamp recipients are required to report monthly for recertification, while in parts of Indiana, assistance has been denied to people who own dogs.

These regional variations are unlikely to be eliminated under the new legislation and, as long as responsibility for administering the program rests at the local level, practices will vary widely from area to area. To some extent, regional differences are necessary and desirable. This is underlined by a reference in the act to the fact that, in "remote areas of Alaska" food stamps may be exchanged for hunting and fishing equipment! Nevertheless many of the variations are unjustified.

Finally, the question remains of whether the food stamp program—even in its new form—is the right program for solving the problem of hunger in America. It has been argued that it would be better dealt with through policies which would guarantee a minimum income for the poor. Programs of this type are being tried, on a very limited scale, in Massachusetts and California.

To British observers, this might seem the obvious solution. But in America, support for such a program remains small. To many Americans it smacks of "creeping socialism" and undermines the traditional ethic of self-help. While the poor in America await a more effective solution to their problems, the Food Stamp Act, 1977, should rescue a few more of them from hunger and malnutrition.*

---

* *Editors' Note:* The food Stamp Program (FSP) has changed considerably since this article was written. As of 1980, food stamps are issued at no cost, a major change that helps make it much easier to use them. The application process is a little easier and also quicker for those who need immediate help. Some households that were in the old program had their benefits reduced or eliminated completely under the new program. Others found the amount of their benefits increased. Therefore, before including food stamp purchases in family food budgeting, the latest program regulations must be consulted.

Selection 32 Space Program Technology
Applied to Meals for Elderly

Johnson Space Center

Editors' Introduction

The needs of astronauts in space have proved a challenging research frontier for nutritionists and food technologists. On manned space flights the provision of a self-contained environment where wastes are recycled and converted to food will become necessary, if flights continue for long periods. Research on space menus has had some beneficial secondary effects. For example, food technology and packaging techniques developed by NASA's Johnson Space Center in Houston to feed Apollo and Skylab crews have been adapted to a pilot program to provide balanced meals to elderly persons who live alone. In the future these technologies may also have applications in solving the world food crisis.

The following short excerpt describes some of the important ways in which space technology has been used to assist the elderly.

While three square meals a day are taken for granted by most Americans, getting even one balanced meal each day is a problem for some of the nation's elderly.

Food technology and packaging techniques, developed by NASA's Johnson Space Center (Houston, Texas) to feed Apollo and Skylab crews during space flight, are being applied in a pilot program to help provide balanced meals to elderly persons who live alone. Physicians, nutritionists, and biomedical engineers at the center are working together to design and develop a meal system to supplement the existing National Nutrition Programs for the Elderly.

The effort is part of the agency's Technology Utilization program, in which space-developed technology is applied in the solution of Earthbound problems.

Project engineer Gary R. Primeaux reported that surveys have shown that many elderly Americans do not receive adequate nutrition.

Source: Abridged with permission of publisher from "Space Program Technology Applied to Meals for Elderly," *Astronomy*, February 1978. Copyright © 1978 by AstroMedia Corp., all rights reserved. Reprinted by permission.

He cites as contributing factors lack of single serving products, limited mobility, loss of skills needed to prepare balanced meals, limited finances, and often a sense of loneliness or rejection that reduces the incentive to cook and eat nutritious meals alone.

Primeaux says the goal of Meal Systems for the Elderly "is to develop nutritious, shelf-stable, convenient, and easily deliverable meals for the elderly."

While several programs for home-delivered hot lunches for the elderly are being tried in some cities, there is usually no weekend service and spoilage risk is high. The NASA team developing the meal system is striving to come up with a shelf-stable, multimeal package that can be distributed by several methods—even parcel post—to senior citizens who live beyond the range of hot-meal delivery, or to those in cities where weekend meals are not provided. The team is working toward a meal system that can be opened, cooked, eaten, and cleaned up by elderly people living alone.

The basic meal will consist of an entrée, two side dishes, dessert, and beverage, with a twenty-one-day menu cycle to provide variety from a list of ten entrées, twenty side dishes, ten desserts, and five beverages. Each meal will provide at least one-third the daily dietary allowance for elderly persons.

In addition to the Johnson Space Center team developing the meal system technology, the University of Texas Lyndon B. Johnson School of Public Affairs in Austin will assist in demonstrations and distribution of meals. The Texas Research Institute of Mental Sciences in Houston has surveyed attitudes and food preferences, and has run taste tests among potential users.

The program is expected to cost $240,000 of which NASA will fund $125,000; Johnson School of Public Affairs, $90,000; Texas Research Institute of Mental Sciences, $8,000; and United Action for the Elderly, Inc. $17,000. Technology, Inc. and Martin Marietta Corp. are contractors in the development program.

Selection 33 The Family as an Ecosystem

Nancy C. Hook
Beatrice Paolucci

Editors' Introduction

In earlier selections we discussed the planetary ecosystem and its relation to the food supply essential for human survival. We noted that a fragile balance is maintained on the man-food continuum. As a species we realize that our life-support system depends upon maintaining biogeochemical cycles, food chains, and food webs. Every species—except the human species—survives in its own ecological niche. Only the human species can survive in the widest possible variety of environments. In each environment, cooperative effort is basic to survival. The family in every society provides a basis for such cooperative endeavors. The family, as a human institution, may also be viewed as a life-support system for its members. Families take on a variety of types and forms and differ in composition and cultural orientation. Despite such differences, the family is the fundamental unit of all human societies. Continued cooperative effort at the microenvironmental (family) level is essential for human survival.

The profession of home economics, since its founding in 1902, has emphasized the family as its focus of study and service. Spurred by its founder, scientist Ellen H. Richards, the field has maintained a focus on the processes that take place through the interaction of the near environment of the family and the larger environment of neighborhood, community, and world. This ecological emphasis is especially meaningful today. It has provided a common perspective for home economists, nutritionists, dietitians, human ecologists, and others concerned with improving the family's utilization of resources, both human and material.

In the following selection Hook and Paolucci reiterate the historical ecological focus of home economics. Furthermore, they describe the unique relationships and transactions that take place in families in systems terms. They describe these interlocking activities as constituting the family's life-support system. Basic to

Source: Adapted from Nancy C. Hook and Beatrice Paolucci, "The Family as an Ecosystem," *Journal of Home Economics* 62, no. 7 (May 1970):315–18. Reprinted by permission of the American Home Economics Association. Complete notes and references appearing in this article have been omitted here; for further information consult the original version.

their concept is the link between the family system and other systems—including the physical environment with its energy dependency. They note that the family operates, as open systems do, to process energy in various forms to sustain individual and family functions; the family also processes information in the interests of well-being. When we consider the family in terms of energy-information transformations, this new paradigm, or model, of the family provides a unique frame of reference for understanding the family as a consumer of material resources and a producer of human resources.

The quality of man's life and the prospects for his continued survival within a limited environmental setting are today receiving national and international attention. Over time home economists, along with other professionals, have been concerned with developing and promoting social, economic, and technological innovations which at one level have enhanced man's quality of life but which at another level may have unwittingly limited the potential for life. The rapid depletion of essential resources and the necessity to maintain man's humanness have forced us to reconsider the interdependence of man and his environment.

Home economics was defined by the participants of the Lake Placid conferences as the study

> of the laws, conditions, principles and ideals which are concerned on the one hand with man's immediate physical environment and on the other hand with his nature as a social being, and is the study specially of the relation between those two factors.[1]

As viewed today, these pioneers were defining an ecological framework. They considered and discarded the term *ecology* based on the fact that "botanists had already appropriated this word and established its use in their science." Historically, Ernest Haeckel in an effort to formulate a logical scheme in the zoological sciences coined the word "ecology" (oecology) around the 1870s to emphasize "the fact that the structure and behavior of organisms are significantly affected by their living together with other organisms of the same and other species and by their habitat." Ecology is derived from the Greek word *oikos*—a house or place in which to live. From this same root word come the terms *economy* and *economics*. In the early twenties Robert E. Park and Ernest W. Burgess adopted the use of "human ecology" within the field of sociology. Generally ecology is the study of the relation of organisms or groups of organisms to their environment.

In retrospect, ecology might have been a suitable choice of name for the area of study now known as home economics, for the term forces one to emphasize the interdependent relationship between man and his environment. In the field of home economics, this interdependent relationship basically focuses on the home as a life-support system for family members; that is, provision of both physical and social nurturance.

This approach of viewing the home and/or family as an ecosystem provides a framework to assist home economists in meeting the challenge of man's survival. What constitutes the study of the home as an ecosystem?

> Ecologists use the term ecosystem to refer to a community together with its habitat. An ecosystem, then, is an aggregation of associated species of plants and animals, together with the physical features of their habitat. Ecosystems . . . can be of any size or ecologic rank. Thus, a drop of pond water together with the organisms that live therein constitutes a small ecosystem. At the extreme, the whole earth and all its plant and animal inhabitants together constitute a world ecosystem. The concept of ecosystem emphasizes the interrelations between the group of organisms that form a community, and . . . its environment.[2]

At the 1908 Lake Placid conference, home was defined as "the place of shelter and nurture for the children and for those personal qualities of self-sacrifice for others for the gaining of strength to meet the world. . . ." Interpretation of this definition has sometimes become a limiting stereotype of one-family dwellings with an overemphasis on the material aspects. Home economists have tended to take a unifocal view of both the environment (that is, food, clothing, and shelter) and the family (its relationships and development of individuals). They have neglected to look at the family as an interdependent life-support system.

The family as a life-support system is dependent upon the natural environment for physical sustenance and upon the social organizations which are related to man's humanness and give quality and meaning to life. Home economists for some time have emphasized the social-emotional environment. It is necessary for the field (as it focuses on the family) to link both the natural environment and the social environment. Therein lie its uniqueness and strength.

Understanding and accepting the consequences of this interdependence is critical to man's survival. A noted ecologist, John Cantlon, recently stated:

> The Congress should undertake to expedite eliminating the serious lack of environmental understanding in the public-educated citizenry of the country. . . .
> One example of a place to start would be to encourage the home economics curricula in the United States to adopt as a curricular focal point "the home as an ecosystem." Learning to think of each household as a system of inputs and losses of energy and materials would provide a means of relating to the larger urban and rural ecosystems. It would be rather simple to quantify the coupling of each individual in a systems

way to his requirements from air, water, and food sheds, from fuel and other resources; as well as coupling his waste outputs to these regional sheds and man's larger ecosystems. Learning how these systems operate and where he fits in the picture may help alleviate some feelings of alienation between the individual and various components of his environment. Learning what affects the health of the ecosystems that sustain and inspire him may make him a better informed voting citizen.[3]

The primary question is: What constitutes the study of the family as an ecosystem?

We define family as a corporate unit of interacting and interdependent personalities who have a common theme and goals, have a commitment over time, and share resources and living space. Hawley defined the family as:

> A relatively small association of individuals, differing in age and sex, who, as a result of their close physical association in a common residence and their mutually sustaining activities, form a distinguishable entity or unit within a larger aggregate.[4]

These definitions are seen as mutually compatible.

The writers of this paper recommend the blending of perspectives of human ecology as traditionally developed by sociologists and biologists. The approach is ecological: a search for *understanding* and *controlling* the mutually sustaining relationships that couple man with his environment.

An Approach for Home Economics

A single profession can bring knowledge to bear on only a limited part of the environment; hence, home economists generally define their sphere of concern as the *family* and that part of the near environment that impinges directly upon the family and is subject to manipulation by the family. Home economists attend to the *interaction* of man as a total being and his near environment, *especially as this interaction is managed by the family.*

The approach using concepts developed by sociology is that of Duncan's ecological complex or POET model—population, organization, environment, and technology. How does this complex relate to the way home economists can view the family as an ecosystem?

Population

According to Duncan, population refers to a concrete population of human organisms more or less circumscribed territorially. This population aggregate has unit character and significant properties which differ from the properties of its component elements. A family may be viewed as the population. The family is a corporate unit with symbiotic relationships. The position of this paper views the family as a population aggregate or system*—that is, a corporate unit which is circumscribed territorially within a household and which has some unit character differing from the characteristics of its individual members such as its theme or value system and cyclic development.

Organization

Organization arises from sustenance-producing activities. It is a property of the population aggregate, is indispensable to the maintenance of collective life, and must be adapted to the conditions confronting a population. Organization is a communication and control system which functions to maintain unity and to accomplish work. This is a major concept of family managerial behavior. The assumptions of organization made by Duncan come close to those of the family management specialist. Examination of information flows in the ecosystem is as pertinent as examination of energy flows. According to Duncan ". . . information serves to control" is one function of management. This is related to the decision-making function of the family and is fundamental to the ecological approach. In addition to the traditional food, clothing, and shelter arenas of family decision-making to which home economists have attended, attention must now be focused on value considerations which include controlling population and technology for the ultimate benefit of mankind.

Environment

In a very general sense, environment can be defined as whatever is external to and potentially or actually influential on a phenomenon (a system, an organism, an object). The environment is seen as providing resources potentially useful for the maintenance of life. The population acts upon the environment and the environment acts upon the population. This adjustment is a continuing dynamic process.

*A system can be defined as a set of parts (units or components) together with the relationships between the parts and the properties of the parts. A system has interrelationships with other systems. In addition, it is characterized by interdependence of its parts; they are reciprocally dependent upon each other. This definition was adapted from A.D. Hall and R.E. Fagen, "Definition of System," in W. Buckley, ed., *Modern Systems Research for the Behavioral Scientist* (Chicago: Aldine, 1968, pp. 81–92 by the Committee on Undergraduate Program Development, College of Home Economics, Michigan State University, Progress Report, East Lansing, 1968, pp. 12–13 (mimeographed).

Components of the environment with which the family interacts and with which it is interdependent may be considered as: the physical and biological environment, which includes land, water, air, space, the solar system, plants and animals, sources of food, and energy. The social environment includes the social institutions of society: the kinship, religious, political, economic, productive, recreative; and the symbolic and ideological systems. Within this total environment can be superimposed three human systems: (1) the biophysical—physiological and metabolic processes, the organic life cycle; (2) the psychosocial—interpersonal relationships expressed by individual and collective patterns of behavior; and (3) the technological—materials, tools, and techniques.

The technological subsystem includes parts of both the physical and the social environments; for example, a dishwasher utilizes water from the physical environment, which is controlled through the social environment. The availability of a pure water supply depends upon elaborate social organizations which provide service to homes in this country, in addition to the technological developments which have led to the construction of dams, purification systems, and the like.

Man, being both biophysical and psychosocial, serves as a connecting and controlling link between these systems. The family is seen as both an environment for the individual and as existing in a larger physical and biological environment and social environment. The family exists within only part of the total environment; there are spatial and temporal dimensions which need to be considered. This is especially true in a postindustrial society.

Technology

This has been included within the environment in the preceding discussion. Technology refers to a set of techniques employed by a population to gain sustenance from its environment and to facilitate the organization of sustenance-producing activity. In effect, technology has the potential for redefining the environment.

A simple approach to viewing the family as an ecosystem is to consider energy flows. Adams has listed two major ways in which energy relates to human organizations: (1) an organization is an ordering of energy and (2) human organizations are converters of energy.[5] Examination of this aspect requires knowledge of biological ecology and an understanding of caloric intake, coupled with the energy requirements necessary for carrying out social and economic functions of household and family activity and work patterns.

One consideration might be the material inputs that come into the family, such as purchases from the grocery. Computations could be determined of the energy inputs from food, paper, detergents, plastics, cloth, cosmetics, drugs, and other commodities, in addition to energy sources such as electricity, heat, and labor, which are essential in converting matter for consumption. Balancing against these energy inputs would be computations of family activity and work-pattern outputs. It also is important to realize the essentiality of overall balance, recognizing that costs ensue from energy and material losses. For example, the material inputs from the grocery result in human and nonhuman waste which contributes to the pollution problem. Waste that is recycled is not a problem; that which is not recycled mars the landscapes and pollutes the environment. Much of this recycling is now left to chance. In the future, families will need to recognize their role in maintaining an energy balance and living in harmony with nature.

These approaches do not have mutually exclusive variables; it is readily observable that there is overlap. The approaches may be useful in helping students understand interdependencies of man with man and with his environment. Interdependencies of man with man could be seen as the reciprocal effects of individuals within a family and reciprocal effects of families with other families, and the effects of both on the environment.

Rapid scientific and technological developments have pushed scientists to consider the alternatives of present action in terms of their long-range consequences. Since the industrial revolution, the ecosystem has included the machines devised by man, their products, and their incalculable capacity to alter the natural balances.

> There is no longer an "away." One person's trash basket is another's living space . . . there are no *consumers*—only users. The user employs the product, sometimes changes it in form, but does not consume it—he just discards it. Discard creates residues that pollute at an increasing cost to the consumer and to his community.[6]

A solution to these problems requires welding together the physical, biological, and social sciences to help define and achieve an environment of a quality satisfactory to human well-being and aspiration. As Cain stated, "The only true synthesis would be that which recognizes the real nature of human ecosystems, a recognition of all the significant relationships between man and environment."[7] The centrality of this approach to man's survival and the role for home economics [were] . . . pointed out. . . . The charge and challenge are clear.

Notes

1. *Lake Placid Conference on Home Economics, Proceedings of Conferences 1 to 10, 1899–1908* (Washington, D.C.: American Home Economics Association. Proceedings of the Fourth Annual Conference, 1902), pp. 70–71.

2. L.R. Dice, *Man's Nature and Nature's Man* (Ann Arbor: University of Michigan Press, 1955), p. 2.

3. J. Cantlon, in *Colloquium to Discuss a National Policy for the Environment.* Joint hearing before U.S., Congress, Senate, Committee on Interior and Insular Affairs and, House, Committee on Science and Astronautics, 90th Cong., 2d sess., 1968, pp. 153–54.

4. A.H. Hawley, *Human Ecology,* (New York: Ronald Press, 1950), p. 211.

5. R.N. Adams, "Energy Analysis of Social Organization" (Unpublished paper, Michigan State University, November, 1959).

6. *Waste Management and Control,* National Academy of Sciences. National Research Council Publication 1400, 1966, pp. 3, 5.

7. S.A. Cain, "Can Ecology Provide the Basis for Synthesis Among the Social Sciences?" in M.E. Garnsey and J.R. Hibbs, Eds., *Social Sciences and the Environment* (Boulder: University of Colorado Press, 1967), p. 40.

Selection 34 Know How to Read the Food Labels

Changing Times

Editors' Introduction

Few consumers have at their fingertips the nutritional knowledge necessary to make on-the-spot food choices without some kind of easily understood guidelines. Food labels provide important point-of-purchase information for consumers. However, informed consumers also need to know what labels mean and where to look for information of importance in identifying and selecting nutritious foods for well-balanced meals.

In the United States, since the passage of the Pure Food, Drug and Cosmetics Act in 1938, the Food and Drug Administration has been charged with the responsibility of monitoring the safety of foods offered to the public. Product-labeling regulations issued in 1973 provided for greater emphasis on nutritional information printed on food labels. Nutritional information is important in planning balanced diets. The presence of detailed data enables consumers to evaluate comparable products on a cost-nutrition basis. Labeling also assists the consumer in learning how unfamiliar conventional foods, as well as new foods, can be combined to provide balanced meals.

Nutritional labels require the cooperation of the food in-

Source: From "Know How to Read the Food Labels," *Changing Times,* The Kiplinger Magazine, February 1978, pp. 36–38. Reprinted with permission from *Changing Times* Magazine, © Kiplinger Washington Editors, Inc.

dustry, except where a nutrient is added to a food or a nutritional claim is made. In such cases full disclosure becomes mandatory. For example, foods that are normally sold as "enriched," "fortified," or for "special dietary use" require nutritional labeling. The term *enriched* applies to flours, breads, and cereals that are nutritionally improved by replacing the thiamin, riboflavin, niacin, and iron removed in processing. *Fortified* refers to the addition of specific nutrients in amounts beyond the level normally found in the food, for example, when vitamin D is added to milk or vitamin C is added to nonfruit beverages. Nutrients not considered appropriate for the general public may be added to certain foods known as diet foods. This category also includes foods that should be used under a physician's directions for weight reduction or treatment of disease.

Whenever a food is labeled, information must be presented in standard form and include the following:

On the front panel
1. The complete name of the product, for example, "Blend of Cane and Maple Syrup." This product may not be labeled "Maple Syrup."
2. The name of the company that manufactures or distributes the product must appear.
3. The net weight or quantity of the product must be identified. Drained weight is given only when the manufacturer desires to provide this information. Net weight means everything in the can, jar, or package and thus might mislead the consumer.

On the right-side panel
1. Ingredients of the food must be listed in descending order by weight. This means that the predominant ingredient is listed first. An exception is a food that conforms to a *standard of identity.* (The 1938 Pure Food Act established standards for seventeen groups of food items. Standards were published stating the basic "recipes"—that is, the ingredients and proportions that must be in such standard products as chocolate and cocoa products, cereal flours and related products, macaroni and noodles, cheeses and cheese products, catsup, salad dressing and mayonnaise. The terms *artificial color, artificial flavor,* and *chemical preservatives* must be declared on the labels of all foods containing them except butter, cheese, and ice cream.
2. The name and address of the manufacturer or distributor must be identified.

3. Nutritional information per serving includes:
   a. serving size;
   b. number of servings per container;
   c. caloric content;
   d. number of grams of protein;
   e. number of grams of carbohydrate;
   f. number of grams of fat;
   g. fatty-food and/or cholesterol-composition information (when declared) must immediately follow the statement on fat content and, in the case of cholesterol, the fat content or the fatty-acid content (if stated);
   h. percentage of the U.S. Recommended Daily Allowance of protein and seven important vitamins and minerals.

Although nutritional labeling has not yet been perfected, and many still do not undertand the meaning of such detailed labels, the program represents an important step toward consumer protection. One major drawback in nutritional-labeling regulations is the failure to define "serving." The manufacturer designates serving size. The tendency is to make the serving size as large as possible to allow for higher percentages of U.S. RDAs. The nature of nutritional labeling is such that fabricated foods fortified with a certain nutrient may look better to consumers than conventional foods exhibiting a greater nutrient profile but with lesser nutrient content. The following selection presents explanations that may be useful in interpreting this important information.

If you know how to read a food label, you're in for some marvelous moments of discovery. Liquid in a bottle may look like orange juice, but if you read the label, you see it's "orange drink" and contains only 10 percent orange juice. The "bran" bread is a luscious dark color, but the label shows "enriched white flour" as the first and primary ingredient. Also present is "caramel color," which means the bread gets much of its dark hue artificially. Look on a jar of real mayonnaise and you'll see a calorie count of 100 per tablespoon; the same amount of "imitation" mayonnaise has forty calories per tablespoon and less fat and more water. You can even find out whether your potato chips were fried in cottonseed, peanut or corn oil, or lard.

Unquestionably, you want more information on food labels, and you are getting it as a result of federal government pressure and the voluntary actions of food companies. Still, some authorities and consumer groups believe food labels do not tell nearly enough.

Here's what you can find out now by reading food labels and what you can expect to see on them in the future.

What's in a Name?

Every food label must carry the name of the product, the net contents or net weight, and the name and place of business of the manufacturer, packer, or distributor.

Even the product name can be revealing. For example, "Quaker Oats" says in those two words what it is. When a brand name is not self-explanatory, the label must carry a definition of the type of food it is; for example, the brand name of a cereal might be followed by "a sweetened rice cereal." Cheese is another food that need be identified by name only. But when you see the words "processed cheese food," you know the cheese has been diluted somewhat with water, whey, and skimmed milk, as the label will note. Likewise, the word "spread" is often used to denote a dilution of an ordinary food. "Strawberry spread," "margarine spread," and "peanut spread" have less of the major ingredient—fruit, oil, peanuts—and perhaps fewer calories.

And what about all those foods concocted or manipulated in the laboratory? The Food and Drug Administration has laid down rules: If a food is nutritionally inferior to the real thing, it must be called "imitation," as in "imitation margarine," or "imitation mayonnaise." However, simply lowering the fat and calorie content does not, in the FDA's view, make a food inferior. In fact, for people trying to lose weight it may be a definite plus.

On the other hand, a new food that's judged nutritionally equal to the food it is patterned after must be called a "substitute" and can be given a descriptive name. Such products as Eggbeaters and Scramblers are considered egg substitutes. Consumer advocates have widely attacked the government's policy of allowing fabricated foods to be called substitutes because they believe the government cannot guarantee that they are nutritionally equivalent and buyers are thus misled.

The net weight on canned and frozen fruits and vegetables tells the weight of the product exclusive of packaging and is a guide for comparing prices. But you may want to know the weight of the solids. The FDA gave the canning industry reasonable time to come up with a solution. Most major companies are already putting the solid-content weight on the labels of their canned fruits and vegetables.

Inside the Package

Ingredients must be listed on most packaged foods and are an excellent source of information about the general quality of the food. The ingredients must be listed in descending order by weight—the main one first, the least last. If a presweetened cereal lists sugar as the first ingredient, there's more sugar in the food than anything else.

The ingredient panel usually also reveals whether a food is artificially colored or flavored, but not specifically which chemical or color was used. Many people think all artificial ingredients—Red No. 40, Yellow No. 5, etc.—should be specifically named so that anyone allergic to certain colorings can avoid them. The FDA has, as an exception, agreed to ask companies to list Yellow No. 5 because of its capacity to induce allergic reactions.

Some fabricated foods, such as nondairy whipped creams, instant breakfasts, and meat substitutes made of soybeans, have ingredient lists that read like chemical dictionaries. Many of these chemicals are nutritious; some are functional and cosmetic additives. You can almost always spot the preservatives (BHA, BHT), flavor enhancers (monosodium glutamate), and thickeners (modified starches) on the ingredient label. Sometimes, however, the formidable-sounding names are merely vitamins and minerals with which the product has been fortified—for example, ferrous sulfate is iron, pyridoxine hydrochloride is vitamin B_6. On many products you'll now find both the common and the chemical names of the ingredient.

Ingredients do not have to be listed when a government "standard of identity" has been set for a food. The food must contain all basic ingredients set forth in the standard. For example, all colas must contain caffeine, so caffeine doesn't have to be declared on the label. Food companies, however, must now list all optional ingredients they use in addition to those required by the standard. As a result you'll be seeing longer lists of ingredients. Some companies give the basic ingredients as well.

Merely listing ingredients often does not give you a true picture of the food's contents. One brand of frozen meat patty might have 70 percent meat and another 90 percent, but there's no way for you to tell the difference. There's also no way to determine how much of a jar of baby food is fruit or vegetable or meat and how much is water and fillers. Particularly offensive to consumer advocates is the failure of many manufacturers to list the percentage of sugar in processed foods. Some cereals, for example, are over 50 percent sugar, yet buyers generally don't know it.

Is It Good for You?

Many foods carry a nutritional panel listing protein, fat, calories, carbohydrates, and seven or more vitamins and minerals. The protein, fat, and carbohydrates are listed in grams per serving. The protein, vitamins, and minerals are given in percentages of the U.S. Recommended Daily Allowances. This means that if the label says a serving of food supplies 25 percent of the U.S. RDA for protein, you need to find foods to make up an additional 75 percent of the U.S. RDA to get your quota of protein for that day. The same is true for vitamins and minerals.

Though only seven main nutrients in addition to protein must be listed—vitamin A, vitamin C, thiamine (vitamin B_1), riboflavin (vitamin B_2), niacin, calcium, and iron—companies may list twelve other nutrients, such as magnesium, zinc, pantothenic acid. They can also include figures on cholesterol, sodium, type of fat (saturated or polyunsaturated) and fiber. This information is sometimes valuable, sometimes misleading. The labels on some cereals, for example, state that they contain no cholesterol. It's true, but one would not expect to find cholesterol in grain or vegetable products, only in animal products, such as meat, fish, poultry, eggs, and butter.

It's not likely the government will soon require cholesterol labeling because the relationship between cholesterol level and health is a matter of considerable controversy. However, it may in the near future move to require the labeling of sodium, or salt, believed to aggravate high blood pressure. Those who want to avoid a high-salt diet often can't find the necessary information on labels.

Why do some foods have nutritional labels while others don't? Nutritional labeling is not mandatory across the board; foods are required to carry a nutritional panel only if they make a nutritional claim or have added nutrients. Almost all cereals bear nutritional labels because they are fortified with vitamins and minerals, but such foods as frozen entrées, potato chips, and canned foods are not fortified and usually do not have nutritional information. Some companies provide a nutritional rundown on their labels even if they're not required to. Several bills have been introduced in Congress to make nutritional and ingredient labeling mandatory.

Fancy, Prime, and AA

Only a few foods have grades on their labels, mainly milk, butter, eggs, meat, and poultry. Since most supermarkets carry only top grades, you don't have to worry much about deciding among them. However, the grading system is confusing and often reflects cosmetic features (taste, flavor, appearance) rather than nutritional qualities.

Prime beef, for example, has more marbling than lesser grades of beef, making it more tender but also higher in fat content and slightly lower in protein. Eggs are graded on how well their yolks stand up after they come out of the shell. Fresh vegetables and fruits are graded for wholesalers as Fancy, A, B, and C, according to their appearance, but shoppers rarely see such grades. Grades do not usually appear on processed fruits and vegetables. Some people believe the whole food-grading system should be completely overhauled if it is to be useful to consumers.

What Labels Shouldn't Say

Federal regulations prohibit food companies from making health claims on labels. Manufacturers of the new high-fiber breads made with cellulose claimed they are beneficial for a number of diseases. The FDA is making them delete such statements from labels, although some occasionally crop up. The FDA does not have prior approval of labels and can take action only after it finds violations.

Nevertheless, you'll see numerous food labels that say "low calorie," "dietetic," "low fat," or "sugar-free." FDA officials admit these are often confusing and misleading. To partially correct the problem, the FDA has proposed a new rule about calorie claims. Some companies are following it now. According to the proposal, a food cannot be called low calorie unless it contains 40 or fewer calories per serving. This puts such foods as celery and green beans in the low-calorie category. A food cannot be labeled as "reduced" in calories unless it has one-third fewer calories per serving and at least twenty-five fewer calories. Also, the food must show a "before" and "after" comparison of calories on the label. For example: "diet snack food, sixty calories per serving; ordinary snack food, 100 calories per serving." When buying foods with such words as "dietetic," be sure you're getting what you think. "Dietetic," for example, can mean low in sodium.

Other Kinds of Labels

Most perishable foods now carry stamps or tags saying the food should not be sold after a specific date. The date labeling is the result of state, not federal, action and voluntary labeling by food companies.

Canned goods carry mysterious code numbers embossed on the can. These tell when and where the food was processed, sometimes even the batch and hour. The code is a precaution in case the food spoils and must be recalled. Nearly all labels these days also carry a code panel that enables the product to be put through automatic checkout computers.

Food labels are changing and will continue to change. Food companies say that extensive labeling adds a certain cost to the product, but consumer groups doubt that the extra cost is as great as the industry says and argue that shoppers should have nothing short of total disclosure about something as important as food. Of course, as critics point out, all that information is valuable only if you use it.

Selection 35 How to Eat without Meat

Citibank

Editors' Introduction

Inflationary pressures on the food budget are evident in the high
cost of meat. However, consumers cannot shop for food by referring only to cost. They must consider the nutritional value of their
purchases. They must calculate the per portion cost of food in
terms of nutrient density. The cost of protein, rather than the cost
of meat, is a critical consideration in menu planning. Sometimes
the most expensive meats are high in saturated fat. Therefore, a
less expensive cut such as chuck or a meat substitute such as
cottage cheese may represent wiser choices from the viewpoint of
health. One can eat like a gourmet for less by stretching meats in
combination with grains and vegetables and by using less expensive protein sources. The following selection explains how to
protect protein intake—for the sake of both budget and health.

That big "beef" over runaway meat prices . . . [recently] resulted
in the first sizable decline in beef eating in the United States in many
years. But the average American may still eat thirty-four pounds more
beef this year than twenty years ago. And at a high price!

The fact is that meat won't ever be cheap again. World demands
for protein foods have been rising and will continue to rise. This will
keep meat prices high and supplies tight.

As a source of protein, the beef animal is actually a very inefficient
machine as a converter of protein from feed into meat. For instance,
twenty-one pounds of grain protein must be fed to a steer to get a single
pound of protein in meat back to us. Turkey or other poultry is a more
efficient converter of feed into protein than are large beef animals; pork
is more efficient than poultry.

With meat prices grooved in at a high level, experts are now
advocating the consumer use of plant proteins such as beans, peas, and
grains more directly. By combining plant foods (which have *incomplete*
proteins) meals can be built up to provide complete protein-food values,
and can also have satisfying flavors and the textures that make them
interesting to eat.

Such meals save dramatically on the cost of food. The most careful

Source: Adapted from Citibank, "How to Eat without Meat," *Consumer Views*, vol.
4. no. 11 (First National City Bank, New York), pp. 1–4. Reprinted with permission of Citibank's *Consumer Views*.

shopping to find a cheaper cut of meat that costs, say, [$1.79] a pound instead of [$2.29] will give four servings at [45 cents] each. Add another [15 cents] to [20 cents] to each for the vegetables.

That cannot compare with the savings from shopping that skips the beef. A complete main dish could cost only [32 cents] per total serving, for example, if it is half an acorn squash stuffed with wheat cereal, egg, soy granules, cheese, and seasonings.

The protein? It is equal in value to the beef, or better.

Of course, you don't always want to eat without meat. But even when meat is in good supply it's more economical to s-t-r-e-t-c-h meat values. The thrifty hamburger, for example, is a better investment and, many families think, better eating if you extend the meat by adding the new soy granules now available to consumers.

This "protein extender" is now sometimes added by the store, or you may be able to buy it separately in the nonmeat department. If you add about a cup to a pound of hamburger the meat will make six servings, not four. Or half again as much.

Don't Skip Protein

Your body's need for protein cannot be overestimated. Proteins are essential for life; they make up our skin, hair, nails, muscles. Proteins are necessary to adults for tissue repair and maintenance; to children for growth; to all of us for vitality and body regulation, to fight infections, and to restore damaged tissues. Proteins are used up every day and need to be replaced every day.

But your body couldn't care less how much you pay for its proteins. Given the right materials, your own body will convert protein from cottage cheese just as effectively as from sirloin steak—or more effectively.

If that last statement is startling, the experts explain that despite its gilt-edged price, the edible flesh of animals, while a source of complete protein, is actually not our best source in terms of *protein use by the body.*

Dairy products (eggs, milk, and cheese) and fish actually rate ahead of meat in what experts call efficiency of protein use. Legumes (dried beans, peas), soybeans, and rice are close behind.

And the "marbling," or white fat, that you find in the top-grade, most expensive meat is not only the villain that helps run up costs, but also the source of the saturated fats many experts hold responsible for major current health problems.

So there are plenty of reasons to get to know our entire protein market—including the low-cost incomplete protein sources.

To choose and use those incomplete proteins properly you need to learn just a few facts about proteins and how our bodies "build" them.

The protein in our bodies is made up of some twenty-two amino acids. Most of these can be made by our bodies. However, eight are called *essential* amino acids because our bodies cannot make them and yet they must be available to the body at the same time and in the right proportions.

If this does not occur, however much incomplete protein you eat, it works only partially, which is roughly like trying to run your car with some of the cylinders blocked.

Many vegetable proteins are incomplete in some amino acids. So they must be balanced with other protein sources at the same meal in order to permit your body to absorb their protein fully. Nutrition experts measure this by what they call the net protein utilization (NPU).

At this point, you may be thinking that maybe the expensive meat animal—which combines incomplete proteins for us—has earned its keep! But you can easily learn to combine proteins. Let's start with the foods you may be less familiar with as proteins.

1. Good cereals and grains. A large part of the world uses grain as a protein source. The protein content and quality both vary, particularly in wheats, depending on the type and the processing.

Whole wheat has more protein (and vitamins and minerals) than even enriched white flour. Gluten flour is still higher in protein. (But remember that if your family prefers white bread, the whole wheat they don't eat will do them no good.) Firm chewy breads—such as French breads—are generally made with "hard," higher protein flour. Many soft American breads more than make up for the difference with added milk solids. Check the label.

You can make grains most efficient when you eat them together with milk or cheese or *small amounts* of meat, fish or poultry—even sesame seeds.

Rice and whole wheat eaten together, or other grains and nuts eaten together, balance each other's amino acid pattern and make for a very efficient protein utilization by the body.

The grain proteins are, nevertheless, lower in quantity and efficiency than those in meat, fish, or cheese, so you need more of them to satisfy body needs.

2. Dried beans, peas, lentils, soybeans. Americans are rediscovering the biblical bean—in baked bean dinners, chili meals, newly popular soybean dishes, and in the soybean curd (tofu) now selling in Chinese markets.

But while beans have a very high proportion of protein, they don't have certain amino acids—such as *tryptophan*. You can make up for this tongue-twister basic element by adding rice, wheat, milk, peanuts, or sesame seeds. (Cooks can serve Boston baked beans with nutted brown bread; chili meals with rice or cheese.

3. Nuts and seeds. These can take on new importance if you have a life-style that includes lots of snacks. Use nuts and seeds in place of sweets.

In meals, a peanut butter sandwich *is* a sound nutritional substitute for a meat sandwich, especially if served with a glass of milk. Or combine nuts with beans or grains in a main dish. The cook can chop them into a "do-your-own-thing" burger, using chopped vegetables and an egg to bind the mixture.

Just remember that the nuts also carry a good proportion of calories! The new soy "nuts" (made of soybeans) have more protein and fewer calories.

4. Fruits and vegetables. These also give you some proteins, small "penny-bank" proportions and not complete, but helpful. To get the most from them, combine them with cheeses, nuts, rice, chopped hard-cooked egg, or small amounts of fish, poultry, or meat. Add flavor with soy sauce or tomato sauce.

5. Dairy products and eggs. The protein of eggs is almost fully utilized by the body. In fact, as we've noted, both eggs and milk (and all the cheeses) are better utilized than beef. Dairy products have a complete amino acid profile and are particularly strong in specific amino acids that make them especially good with cereals and bread.

6. Fish and seafood. These, of course, rate tops as a protein source, and are especially recommended for our overall well-being. They offer the best protein value at the lowest calorie cost.

Fish has a high content of *lysine*, one of the eight essential amino acids. Even small amounts of fish or seafood, either in or with rice, can provide up to half the day's protein needs.

How much protein do you need daily? The current specified allowances are considered high by some researchers, but the National Academy of Sciences recommends about . . . [44] grams for a woman of average weight (120) lbs.) and about . . . [56] grams for a man (154 lbs.). Your individual needs may vary, and your doctor may have his own standards.

Here are some foods that supply . . . [more than] one-third of a day's proteins: There are about 20 grams of protein in a three-ounce portion of boneless meat, poultry, or fish; one pint of milk; ½ cup of peanuts; about ⅓ cup of soy "nuts"; one cup of cooked bean casserole; or a little over ½ cup cottage cheese. There are 14 grams of protein in two large eggs.

Those proteins vary in cost from about [16] cents per portion for the beans to "you name it" for meat. . . . [These costs are subject to inflationary pressures and must be calculated according to current market prices. (See Selection 36 "A Ready Reckoner of Protein Costs.")]

A New Image

"Nutritionists hail meat shortage as bona fide bonanza," says a recent newspaper headline. The point was health: Many nutritionists believe that vegetables and fruits should be substituted often for the high-cholesterol animal meats. They also advise more frequent use of fish and poultry.

Meats supply vitamins and other food values along with proteins, but that is even more true of vegetables, which now supply more than half of many key vitamins and minerals we need.

It all adds up to our need to reshape our image of the ideal meal. The status-symbol steak—too big, too fat, too expensive—is losing rank. The experts are looking with new respect, *nutritional* as well as economic, at some international traditions of good eating. Consumers are rediscovering the creative pleasure of combining the good things of the earth, available in our supermarkets, to make unusual meals. . . .

Without Meat—
Delicious Main Dishes to Try

Stuffed Acorn Squash

Grams of Protein per Serving: 23

2 acorn squash (about ¾ lb. each)	3 eggs, medium
Oil, salt, pepper	½ cup finely chopped onion
½ cup soy granules	1 cup (4 oz.) grated cheddar cheese
½ cup water	1 rounded tablespoon prepared
½ cup wheat germ	mustard

Scrub squash well, split in half, discard seeds and fibrous matter. Place in a baking pan, cut-side up, in 1 inch boiling water. Cover the pan and bake in a hot oven (400° F) about 30 to 40 minutes, until squash is almost tender. Brush cut surfaces with oil, sprinkle with salt and pepper. Soak soy granules in water 5 minutes. Add remaining ingredients, salt and pepper to taste. Mound filling in the hollows of squash halves. Bake uncovered in a hot oven (400° F) in a baking pan with 1 inch boiling water, until stuffing and squash are lightly browned, about 20 minutes. Makes 4 servings.

Bean Loaf

Grams of Protein per Serving: 21

3 cups pureéd cooked or canned
  kidney beans
4 oz. seasoned, textured soy protein
  meat extender
1 cup water to moisten soy, or as
  directed

1 onion, chopped
½ cup slivered celery and leaves
1 cup whole wheat bread crumbs
2 eggs
1 tablespoon ketchup

Use canned beans (2 cans about 1 lb. each, drained) or cook 1–1½ cups dried beans, as directed on package. Drain well, mash or whirl in blender to pureé. Soak soy protein in water for 5 minutes. Combine with beans and remaining ingredients. Adjust seasoning, if necessary, with salt and pepper. Bake in an oiled 9×5-inch loaf pan in a moderately hot oven (375° F) about 40 minutes, until the loaf is crusty and browned. Makes 6 servings.

Seafood Paella

Grams of Protein per Serving: 31

2 tablespoons oil
1⅓ cups converted rice
3 cups boiling water
1 teaspoon salt
1 can (1 lb.) seasoned stewed
  tomatoes

1 lb. shrimp, shelled and deveined
  or 1 lb. fish fillets, fresh or frozen
1 quart clams, fresh or canned

Heat oil in a saucepan, add rice and stir over moderate heat until rice is golden. Add boiling water and salt, cover the pan, cook until rice is tender, about 20 minutes. Add the tomatoes, heat. Add shrimp or fish fillets, cut into 1-inch strips, and clams. Cover, cook 5 minutes, until seafood is cooked through and has lost its translucency. Makes 6 servings.
Note: If canned clams are used in this recipe, use the clam broth instead of part of the water in cooking the rice.

Selection 36 A Ready Reckoner of Protein Costs

Flora L. Williams
Catherine L. Justice

Editors' Introduction

Protein-rich foods, especially those of animal origin, are the most expensive items in the average family's food budget. It, therefore, pays to learn more about the amount of protein you and members of your family really need each day and the variety of food sources that can be used to get the most protein value for your money.

Americans tend to overestimate their protein requirements. The average adult in the United States may consume about 100 grams of protein per day within a range of 80 to 150 grams. Of these, it has been calculated that 73 grams come from animal products, primarily meat rather than dairy sources. In selections 14, "Eating in the Dark," and 15, "Changing Public Diet," we considered some of the health problems associated with eating too much meat and other animal protein. Americans have been urged to cut down on the consumption of animal products to avoid excessive intakes of saturated fat and cholesterol, contributing factors in the development of coronary heart disease.

The Food and Nutrition Board recommends a daily intake for the healthy adult of 0.8 grams of protein per kilogram of body weight. Hence the RDA for a 70–kilogram reference man over 18 years of age is 56 grams of protein per day; for a 55-kilogram reference woman over 18 years of age the RDA of protein is 44 grams. If you are over 18 years of age, you can calculate your own protein allowance by dividing your weight in pounds by 2.2 (the result is your weight in kilograms) and then multiplying your weight in kilograms by 0.8. Because children and adolescents are growing and their bodies are developing, they have proportionately higher needs in relation to body weight. For example, teenagers, 11 through 14 years of age, should receive 1 gram of protein per kilogram of body weight. As they mature, teenagers

Source: Adapted from Flora L. Williams and Catherine L. Justice, "A Ready Reckoner of Protein Costs," *Journal of Home Economics* 67, no. 2 (March 1975):20–21, as adapted from Journal Paper No. 5446, Purdue University, Agricultural Experiment Station. Reprinted by permission of the American Home Economics Association and Purdue University. Notes and references appearing in this article have been omitted here; for further information consult original version.

require less protein in relation to body weight. Thus, the male, 15–19 years of age, requires 0.85 grams of protein per kilogram of body weight, and the female, 15–19 years of age, requires 0.84 grams of protein per kilogram of body weight. Thus the RDA for an 18-year-old male who weighs 66 kilograms is 56 grams. However, the RDA for a 20-year-old male who weighs 70 kilograms would also be 56 grams because of the decrease in protein per kilogram of weight. Similarly, for an 18-year-old female who weighs 55 kilograms, the RDA is 46 grams, while for a 20-year-old female of the same weight, the RDA is 44 grams.

Table 36.1 Recommended Dietary Allowance for Protein [1980]

Family Member	Age	Weight (lbs)	Weight (kgs)	Protein RDA (gms)
Father	44	154	70	56
Mother	40	120	55	44
Male child	12	99	45	45
Female student	18	120	55	46
Male student	20	154	70	56

As discussed in selection 8, "The Requirements of Human Nutrition," the RDAs for protein are not minimums. They represent a margin of safety over the requirements. You and your family can improve your health and save money if you reduce your consumption of animal protein products—particularly meat—to an amount no more than the RDA level each day.

Furthermore, the RDA for protein was established on the assumption that protein food would be chosen from a wide variety of sources of both vegetable and animal origin. These sources include meat, fish, poultry, milk and cheese, legumes and nuts, and bread and cereals, as well as starchy vegetables such as potatoes. These foods differ in the quantity of protein they yield per serving. For example,

— 1 cup of milk yields 8 grams of protein;
— 1 medium egg yields 6 grams of protein;
— 1 ounce of cooked lean meat yields 7 grams of protein;
— ½ cup cooked kidney beans yields 8 grams of protein;
— 2 tablespoons of peanut butter yields 8 grams of protein;
— 1 slice of enriched bread yields 2 grams of protein;
— 1 medium potato yields 2 grams of protein.

From this list it can be seen that animal protein foods and legumes and nuts are the most concentrated sources of protein. Protein-yielding foods also differ in their amino acid composition.

The term *protein quality* refers to whether or not the protein is complete and supplies all the eight or nine essential amino acids in the relative amounts and proportions needed by the body for protein synthesis. Animal sources such as eggs, meat, fish, poultry, milk, and cheese supply high-quality protein. Proteins from plant sources are generally of low quality. When legumes and nuts are appropriately used, they are nutritionally equivalent to animal protein foods.

The general recommendation is that 40 to 50 percent of the RDA of protein should be high-quality protein and that a high-quality protein should be included in each meal. Two that more than meet this recommendation are (1) 2 cups of milk plus 2 ounces of cooked lean meat, fish, or poultry and (2) 2 cups of milk plus 1 egg and ¼ cup of cottage cheese. The rest of the protein allowance can be provided by such common foods as legumes, breads and cereals, potatoes, and other starchy vegetables that are not usually thought of as protein sources.

Meeting protein requirements from a wide variety of food in a 50:50 ratio of animal and vegetable protein sources means that most Americans would cut down on the consumption of high-cost animal proteins. Hopefully, this reduction would produce long-term benefits by decreasing the incidence of cardiovascular disease.

Williams and Justice provide a means of computing the best protein buys in a marketplace where food costs change from week to week. Serving sizes on the worksheet are expressed in units of 14 grams of protein—equivalent to 2 ounces of cooked lean meat. Each of the units presented in the worksheet supplies between one-third and one-fourth of the 1980 RDA. Protein-yielding foods other than the foods usually thought of as protein sources may be added and their cost compared to other conventional sources by following the methodology explained in the selection.

At a time when food costs are rising rapidly, some home economists have to recalculate protein costs among a number of foods about as rapidly as the prices change.

Other home economists in teaching are faced with the need to have *current* price information on protein-yielding foods available to use in teaching wise consumer choices: 1970 or 1972 food price information just will not do.

For home economists in a number of professional situations dealing with informed choice in food buying, an easy way to select protein "best buys" is shown in the buyers' worksheet . . . "A Ready Reckoner of Protein Costs" [shown in table 36.2].

Table 36.2 A Ready Reckoner of Protein Costs

Item	Serving Size to Provide 14 Grams Protein	Multiplication Factor		Current Retail Price per Pound		Cost of 14 Grams Protein
Dry beans	1 cup cooked	.128	×	_____	=	_____
Peanut butter	3½ tablespoons	.123	×	_____	=	_____
Eggs	2 eggs	.269	×	_____	=	_____
Bologna	4–5 slices (if 18 slices/pound)	.255	×	_____	=	_____
Beef liver	(6–7 servings/pound)	.155	×	_____	=	_____
Milk	1¾ cup	.881	×	_____	=	_____
Dry milk	9 tablespoons dry	.086	×	_____	=	_____
Cottage cheese	(4–5 servings/pound)	.227	×	_____	=	_____
Hamburger	(5–6 servings/pound)	.172	×	_____	=	_____
Ocean perch, fillet, frozen	(6 servings/pound)	.160	×	_____	=	_____
Tuna fish	(3 servings to a 6-ounce can)	.128	×	_____	=	_____
American process cheese	2½ slices (if 16–18 slices/pound)	.133	×	_____	=	_____
Chicken, whole	(4 servings/pound)	.244	×	_____	=	_____
Ham, whole	(4–5 servings/pound)	.228	×	_____	=	_____
Pork sausage links	6 links (if 16 links/pound)	.329	×	_____	=	_____
Frankfurters	About 2½ (if 10/pound)	.247	×	_____	=	_____
Pork chops with bone	(4 servings/pound)	.239	×	_____	=	_____
Bacon, sliced	5½ slices (if 20 slices/pound)	.403	×	_____	=	_____
Sirloin steak, choice grade	(4⅓ servings/pound)	.229	×	_____	=	_____
Rib roast of beef	(4–5 servings/pound)	.227	×	_____	=	_____
Round pot roast	(6–7 servings/pound)	.158	×	_____	=	_____

Note: To figure the cost per pound for large eggs, multiply ⅔ times the price per dozen; for milk, divide the cost per gallon by 8.6; for dry milk, calculate the cost of 5 quarts of reconstituted milk; and for tuna, multiply ⅔ times the cost of a 6-ounce can.

The worksheet can be used on a daily, weekly, or monthly basis. To figure comparative protein costs, the buyer records the current retail price per pound of the meats or meat alternates listed, multiplies those prices by the factor given, then makes the assessment of the wisest choice among a number of protein foods, based on comparative price.

Serving sizes on the worksheet are expressed in units of 14 grams of protein. Each of these units supplies between a third and a fourth of the . . . Recommended Dietary Allowance (RDA) of daily protein (protein RDA is . . . [44] grams per day for the reference woman and 56 grams for the reference man). Students should be reminded that 2 cups of milk will provide slightly more than one-fourth of the protein RDA.

Serving sizes to provide 14 grams of protein were determined from information in U.S. Department of Agriculture publications. It will probably be necessary to point out . . . that the serving size required to provide 14 grams of protein is not necessarily the serving size generally considered acceptable or "adequate" in our culture. However, 14 grams of protein in addition to milk at each meal is all that is required in the type A school lunch; that same amount of protein is all that is required for a main dish at either lunch or dinner with a well-balanced menu.

How to Add Foods to the Worksheet

Protein-yielding foods not listed on the worksheet can be added and their costs compared. To find the multiplication factor (M) for a food—

— determine the grams of protein yielded from the edible portion of 1 pound of the food as purchased (example: there are 90.3 grams of protein in 1 pound of beef liver);
— divide 14 by the grams of protein (g) in 1 pound of the food (example: 14 grams ÷ 90.3 grams = 0.155, the multiplication factor (M) for beef liver).

In summary, then, the formula for finding the multiplication factor for a food not given on the worksheet is $M = 14 \div g$.

To find the number of servings of a food, each containing 14 grams of protein—

— divide the grams of protein per pound by 14 (example: 90.3 ÷ 14 grams = 6.45 servings per pound).

Selection 37   What Price Nutrition?

Citibank

Editors' Introduction

Although food prices have steadily risen in recent years, the total of disposable income spent on food has declined. Also, about 25 cents of every food dollar is now spent on eating out. Although low-income families spend a larger proportion of their money on food than families with higher incomes do, malnutrition is often common among the poor. Lack of knowledge concerning principles of nutrition may be more important than lack of money in providing an adequate diet. Too often junk foods or empty-calorie foods are selected in preference to foods of equivalent cost that could provide sound nutrition. Low-cost, high-quality choices require information, thoughtful advance planning, and the willingness and desire to make sound nutrition a priority. Money is often spent on high-priced meat and convenience foods, and not enough attention is paid to inexpensive sources of proteins, vitamins, and minerals. Many families could improve their diets by purchasing and preparing more fruits and vegetables, and milk and milk products rather than giving preference to highly advertised convenience foods.

Food selection can be made easier by reference to the Basic 4 discussed in selection 7. The following case studies illustrate the importance to a family of planning economic and nutritious meals.

American families now spend more for food than ever before—and many are buying less in nutrition for their money. . . .

Another fact of today: Diet-conscious Americans are using high-priced meats more often in place of less expensive foods for their protein and vitamins.

But studies show that families could actually improve their diets if they put greater emphasis on fruits and vegetables and on milk and milk products—and less emphasis, in at least some cases, on meat proteins.

The U.S. Department of Agriculture studied two groups of families spending a weekly average of . . . [approximately] $12 per person

Source: Adapted from Citibank, "What Price Nutrition," *Consumer Views*, vol. 3, no. 12 (First National City Bank, New York), pp. 1–4. Reprinted with permission of Citibank's *Consumer Views*. Charts appearing in this article are not included here; for further information consult the original version.

on food. One group had "good" diets according to the daily Recommended Dietary Allowances for each of the seven major nutrients — protein, calcium, iron, vitamin A, thiamine, riboflavin, and vitamin C (ascorbic acid). The other group had "poor" diets.

The study found that the households with good diets spent, on the average, 11 cents more of their food dollar on two food groups — fruits and vegetables, and milk and milk products — than did the households with poor diets.

Both groups spent about the same percent on flour, cereal, and bakery products.

But the homes with good diets used 7 cents *less* of each food dollar for the fourth food group — meat, poultry, fish, eggs, dry legumes (beans), and nuts — than the poor-diet group used.

In the diets rated poor the low nutrient levels were most frequent for calcium, vitamin A, and vitamin C. Iron intake may also be a problem, especially for women and girls after adolescence, in the light of current RDA standards for iron.

Today we are all more aware of nutrition needs. More vitamin supplements are being sold than ever before, health food stores are opening from coast to coast, and special diets seem to travel the consumer grapevine like electronic communications.

But the typical eating patterns of most Americans still ignore the basics of good nutrition.

Fat and Undernourished

Case 1. Commuter Jones, who makes the early train each day, gulps orange juice at home, a roll and coffee at the station and has another cup of coffee and a Danish pastry at his morning office meeting. No real meal yet, and he's downed 555 calories.

Jones' lunch (often a business meeting) begins with a cocktail. He skips hors d'oeuvre but takes the garlic bread (a fat-trap: 125 calories a slice). His steak is a half-pound whopper of well-"marbled" (that means saturated fat) beef. Salad and only half a baked potato — *he's watching his figure.* But he has Roquefort dressing on the salad and sour cream on the potato. No dessert, tea. This lunch: 1,330 calories.

Jones joins his wife for a cocktail before dinner and nibbles at a cheese tray and a new dip. Mrs. Jones sets out pot roast, potatoes, buttered peas, salad with the Roquefort dressing he likes, ice cream. Calories? 1,715.

By 7:30 P.M. he's had a total of 3,600 calories, or 1,000 more than he needs for the day — before his evening beer. That is enough to account for a gain of about a pound a week (or the 10 pounds he put on since his last diet bout). The meals were too high in saturated fats, expensive in dollars, and poor in nutrition.

Case 2. Mr. Brown calls his truck-driving job hard with long hours, lots of tension. He wants meals that "stay with him." Breakfast—western omelette, side of potatoes, coffee, doughnut. Lunch—meat loaf sandwich, side order of fried onion rings, apple pie with cheese wedge, two coffees. Dinner—spaghetti with sausage and peppers, Italian pastry, coffee twice. The calories on that food road: 3,345, not calculating the candies he nibbles on the road to "wake up." He's had too little vitamin C. And those meals take a big bite from his pay.

Cases 3 and 4. Mrs. Jones and Mrs. Brown live differently but have similar meals. Neither husband is home for breakfast and each wife has coffee after the children go to school. Mrs. Jones stops to snack about 11 A.M. (she feels "pooped"); Mrs. Brown has a break on her job at 10:30 A.M.—each takes a sweet muffin and coffee. Neither has a real lunch.

Mrs. Jones has dinner with her husband, but no potato; Mrs. Brown eats with the kids and they have spaghetti—a quick prepared version. Neither woman gets adequate vitamin C or calcium during the day; Mrs. Brown is chronically low in B vitamins, also; and Mrs. Jones' doctor tells her she is somewhat anemic.

From breakfast skipping to obesity, parents' nutritional hang-ups are often passed on to children. The Jones and Brown children, like six out of ten teenaged American girls, and four out of ten boys, according to studies, have poor diets in terms of RDAs, and could develop health problems. A disturbing number of high school students studied at the University of Iowa, for example, had surprisingly high cholesterol levels and intakes of fat above those recommended by the American Heart Association.

What Price Protein?

Protein foods are the costliest and most essential of the food values needed every day for body maintenance, repair, and growth. Daily recommended allowances: for an adult man, . . . [56] grams of protein; for a woman, about . . . [44]; for a teenage boy, . . . [over 14 years of age, 56].

A small serving of lean meat, poultry or fish (about 3 ounces) averages 20 grams of protein. Milk has 9 grams a cup; a 1-ounce slice of cheddar cheese, about 8; an egg, 6; bread, about 1.9 a slice.

Food experts note that there is incomplete protein in grain foods and in some vegetables which is better utilized by the body when eaten together with a complete protein. So the generations of international cooks who combine small bits of meats, poultry, fish, cheese, or eggs with beans, pastas, and rice are right in terms of nutrition as well as flavor. Sandwiches, pastas with cheese or meat sauces, and cereal with milk are also efficient nutritionally, and budgetwise. (But be careful of fat-traps in rich sauces.)

More about protein costs: The protein quality is the same in mackerel . . . as in lobster . . . and there is more fish on the fork in a pound of mackerel than in lobster. Turkey leg and thigh . . . offer as good protein as turkey breast . . . beef liver . . . rates as high as calves liver. . . .

The vitamins we most often miss are A and C, the experts say. A is found in green and yellow fruits and vegetables, and in butter and margarine. Calorie counters who skip butter and margarine might use thrift carrots often for A.

Vitamin C can't be stored in the body and must be replenished daily. . . . a day's recommended allowance: 60 milligrams for adult males, about 60 for adult women generally.

The prime source for calcium is dairy products. The daily recommendations (with some exceptions) are one quart of milk (or cheese equivalents) for children, one pint for adults. An ounce of cheddar or Swiss cheese equals about a cup of milk.

Milk you make from dry nonfat milk solids, . . . has slightly more calcium than fresh whole milk. . . . Cottage cheese holds its own in nutrition with expensive imported Brie. So pamper your taste if you can, but calcium is yours on a budget, too.

If you need more iron: Meats, particularly liver, and eggs, are good sources. Dried fruit snacks such as raisins or prunes, in place of empty-calorie sweets, are a mineral mine.

Don't overlook our most essential food need for survival and maintenance of body balance—water. We get water in many foods, and in soft drinks at 20 to 60 cents a quart. These earn their way in entertainment. But if you need to cut calories and costs, rediscover water!

And "Health Foods"?

Happily, those whole grain cereal mixtures that are "in" this year for breads and breakfast have needed vitamin B values. But they sometimes cost quite a bit more than homemade mixtures, and more than an old-fashioned dish of cereal to which you add fruit and milk at the table. Also, many of the traditional prepared cereals in supermarkets have been fortified nutritionally in the past year.

The currently popular health foods offer good nutrition, fun, good taste, and convenience at no more than the cost of many empty-calorie snacks. Comparison shop for them.

Natural brown rice, for example, costs . . . [more] in health food stores . . . [than] in supermarkets in the same metropolitan area. But remember that prices do not measure differences in taste, texture, and other qualities that provide enjoyment.

The food experts are pleased that because of today's interest in the nutritious foods, more of the natural grains, wider varieties of dried beans and nuts, and high-quality flours are becoming more available at practical prices in the supermarkets.

However, they warn that no *one* of the many new nutrition-conscious products is a panacea. It is costly and self-deluding to expect any single food to be an instant cure-all.

Nutrition information now appears on food cans and labels. They will tell the contents in terms of protein, iron, calcium, essential vitamins, and other basic foods, and may give calorie counts.

But whether this labeling actually helps or not, families should begin *now* to shop harder for good nutrition—at the lowest possible price. . . .

Whenever you are in the supermarket, check your cart for these four basic foods: vegetables and fruits; milk foods; meats, fish, poultry, and eggs, dried beans, nuts, and peanut butter; and breads and cereals. You can add some oil or fat, and sweets, *within* your calorie allowance. But are the basic foods—which you and your family need *every day*—in the cart?

Selection 38 Accounting for Taste

James C. Boudreau

Editors' Introduction

When Senator Gaylord Nelson introduced the Food Protection Act of 1972, he said, "I believe that it is time to find out which of the chemicals we are ingesting daily are safe from toxicity and long-range harmful effects, and how they react with other chemicals affecting the human body. I believe that food can be colored, doctored, flavored, fattened, preserved, stabilized, and spiced with

Source: Adapted from James C. Boudreau, "Accounting for Taste," *The Sciences* (March 1980):14–15, 30. Reprinted with permission from *The Sciences*, March 1980. Copyright © 1980 by the New York Academy of Sciences.

fewer chemicals that are currently in use." In selection 38, food chemist James C. Boudreau voices yet another concern over food produced in today's complex food system—the loss of taste. He gives us insight into how food manufacturers can reconstruct flavors and fragrances to provide the consumer with "natural" taste—artificially!

Our modern system of food production, with its revolutionary technologies and miraculous yields, has brought us greater and greater quantities of goods, but less and less that is truly tasty. As anyone with a palate and a memory knows, many of our staple foods just aren't what they used to be: turkey and tomatoes, for example, or chicken and eggs, or fruits and vegetables. We are witnessing—and on many fronts at once—the virtual destruction of flavor.

Just what is going wrong? The answers are complex; to understand why so many of our foods have become less tasty, we must examine the nature of nutrition and of taste itself.

Choice after Choice

The plant and animal substances we consume promote complex and essential physiological activities. We need compounds for structural repairs and replacements, and other compounds for the metabolic energy systems, and still others for the combat of pathological organisms and the regulation of temperature (the thermal function of food is well known to peoples of the Orient, who separate foods into those that cool the body and those that warm it). So our food selection must be selective in the extreme, designed to be receptive to that which we highly require, and repulsed by that which we might find an irrelevance or an interference. Almost without exception, natural foods that taste good are good for us, and foods with compounds that are needed taste good even though the stomach is full. Toxic compounds almost invariably have noxious tastes; the one exception for land foods is the *Amanita phaloides*, a mushroom with a delicious taste that leaves you dead.

Taste and smell are the manipulators of appetite. Although these days taste is much maligned in its capabilities, and usually assigned a role subordinate to that of smell, there is evidence that the taste systems are much more complex than traditionally assumed, and play the primary role in the perception of flavor. Smell seems to serve mainly as an initial screening system for food selection, since foods with bad smells will rarely be tasted. Many foods, however, have only feeble or uninteresting odors—oysters and beer, for instance—but complex and delicious tastes. Furthermore, even some foods with objectionable odors will be consumed for their pleasant tastes: Roquefort cheese, blue cheese, and the durian fruit, which is a large, oval, delicious but foul-smelling fruit with a prickly rind. In fact, many of the compounds functioning in food odor are nutritionally inconsequential, whereas taste-active substances comprise a cornucopia of nutritionally important compounds.

Recent investigations of the physiology and psychophysics of taste show the taste systems to be eminently qualified for their role in the analysis of complex flavor. Studies of peripheral taste systems have revealed a wide variety of distinct chemoresponsive systems sensitive to many of the basic constituents of foods. Many of the compounds which had once been assumed to function as odors have been shown to be taste active. These neurological studies have been complemented by human psychophysical studies on the chemistry of food flavor—studies, mostly conducted by either industrial or agricultural investigators, which have demonstrated that many more tastes than the traditional "front four" of sweet, bitter, sour, and salty are required to reconstruct food flavors.

A recent study of seafood flavor, for instance, used twenty-nine terms to describe the flavor of oysters: five of these terms referred to texture, eight to odor, and sixteen to taste, including such sensations as "typical oyster," "earthy" and "boiled-potato-like." Reconstructing Swiss cheese flavor required taste sensations such as "nutty," "burned," and "buttery." Although some of these novel sensations are still inadequately described, a recent list of the taste sensations with a certain degree of experimental validation (i.e., distinct oral locus of elicitation and unique chemistry) encompasses twelve distinct sensations. With intensive experimental investigation the list could readily be extended to over twenty taste sensations.

Indeed, a hard look at the chemistry of taste may uncover hundreds of chemical surprises and new sensations. As we now know, there are at least two distinct sweet sensations and two distinct bitter sensations. Certain amino acids maximally evoke sweet and bitter from the front of the tongue, but the sweet sensation elicited by the dihydrochalcone sweeteners and the bitter sensation of certain salts originate from receptors on the back of the tongue. Prominent in the perception of apples, tea, and wine is the astringent sensation, which is elicited by many polyphenols. The pungent sensation is elicited by certain compounds found in chili peppers (capsaicin), black pepper (piperine), mustard (sinigrin), and ginger (gingerone). A metallic sensation from the back of the tongue may be perceived when eating oysters or mushrooms.

Umami

One of the most elaborately studied of these new taste sensations is the "umami," arising from the back of the tongue and mouth. This exotic taste is entirely the discovery of Japanese researchers, particularly

S. Yamiguchi and others at the Central Research Laboratory of the Ajinomoto Company. "Umami," often described as delicious or brothy, is elicited by certain amino acids and monophosphate nucleosides, notably monosodium glutamate (MSG). The sensation (or possibly *sensations*, since the monophosphate nucleosides stimulate an oral locus distinct from that stimulated by the amino acids) is one of the primary psychophysical components of meat and fish flavors, tomatoes, soy sauce, cheese, and a host of other common foods. The "umami" and all the other diverse oral sensations newly identified are an index of the complexity of the underlying chemical inputs; and though the chemistry of most of these taste sensations has not yet been elucidated in any detail, their study promises a complete revision of our conception of taste chemistry, and the interaction of the eaters and the eaten.

Though the study of taste-active compounds in food still lags behind the study of odorous food compounds, we now know that in meat and fish flavor, the prominent substances are inorganic ions, amino acids, peptides, amines, thiamine, and nucleotides. Japanese scientists have demonstrated that the taste of crab can be largely reconstructed with a mixture of compounds, which they identified in crab extract. Lovers of crabmeat may be enlightened to learn that the nucleus of the crab taste is produced by glycine, glutamate, arginine, AMP, CMP, sodium ions, and chloride ions. Similarly, the tastes of other shellfish, fish, and meat can be shown to be primarily determined by the inorganic ions, free amino acids, peptides, and nucleotides naturally present. These compounds, of course, are fundamental constituents of living matter.

Enter the Chef

Humankind has made some basic alterations in this natural nutritional ecosystem. Two of these changes, fermentation and cooking, increase the number and diversity of taste-active compounds in our foods. Fermentation, a transformation of food compounds by microorganisms, is more or less natural, in that most of the new flavor compounds created are commonly found in nature. Fermentation plays a role in an extraordinary variety of foods: not only in sauerkraut, kim chi, and pickles, but also cheese, bread, soy sauce, anchovies; tea and chocolate; and, of course, all alcoholic drinks. Fermented food tastes are strong and complex, and lists of the flavor compounds present in fermented foods like wine, beer, chocolate, and tea fill many pages of text.

Cooking is the most common method of modifying food compounds; but whereas the flavor compounds of fermentation are seminatural, many heat-produced compounds are not found in nature in any quantity. The variety of flavor compounds produced by cooking is vast, especially when—as is common—foods of different chemical compositions are heated together. But this is not entirely a good thing. Though cooking does sometimes increase food value by making certain starches and proteins more available to us, most foods could be eaten raw with little or no loss in food value; and cooking, in fact, destroys or transforms many useful vitamins and amino acids and can produce compounds known to be detrimental to health. Toxic compounds, some carcinogenic, have been demonstrated to be produced by grilling or by deep frying. The third major change which humans have effected in their nutritional ecosystem is more recent, and unlike fermentation and cooking, is definitely detrimental to good taste. The development of modern industrial agriculture has brought about a profound decrease in food·flavors. Traditional agricultural systems, existing since the neolithic period, approximated a natural nutritional ecosystem in that human beings were part of an integrated system, and food was produced by small, diversified farms. In the past 100 years or so (and accelerating since 1940) major changes have occurred in the methods of food production and distribution, and agriculture has become geared toward quantity production and various distribution needs, and not at all toward the production of good taste. We have eliminated most naturally occurring species of crops and intensively farmed only a few of the most successful. We raise foods for yield, appearance, and ease of transportation.

There are several agricultural practices which contribute to the general inedibility of American agricultural produce.

Fruits are picked green and then artificially ripened—a technique that in no way approximates normal ripening and has been shown to result in a decrease in the quantity of flavor compounds. Typically, the fruit is picked unripe and stored in a cool, airtight place, in which it can remain fresh, or semifresh, for a long period of time. Then, just before the fruit is shipped, it is exposed to ethylene gas, which brings about several changes, primarily in color, but cannot replace the flavor compounds which would have been present had the fruit ripened naturally on the tree or vine.

Animals usually undergo forced growth and are slaughtered earlier than they used to be. Until recently, steroids were widely used to promote the growth of cattle. We have selected our breeds of chicken for rapid growth, and achieve it partly with the help of massive administrations of medications.

The reliance on a few fertilizers with high nitrogen content and a few simple compounds in no way approximates the chemical complexity found in a natural nutritional ecosystem or in a traditional farm: Many vital nutrients may not be available to plants. Sulfur deficiency in soil for instance, has been linked with a decrease in flavor of onions and garlic. Since sulfur deficiency is becoming more and more common (sulfur compounds are usually not supplied in commerical fertilizers), the flavors of other vegetables with sulfur flavor compounds such as cabbage, watercress, broccoli, and asparagus are also affected. A sulfur deficiency in plants may also be implicated in the decline of some meat flavors. In England, the shift from traditional agriculture to high intensive chemical farming has been linked to a flavor loss in cider—and also to cider's shorter shelf life.

Novel Flavors

The chemical composition of our foods is being radically altered. The chemical used to loosen oranges for mechanical picking, for example, has been found to introduce novel chemicals—with off-tastes—into the oranges. Nematicides have been reported to produce large changes in the chemical composition of tomatoes. The use of various chemical compounds for herbicides, fungicides, insecticides, and medications has introduced various new compounds into our foods, often in high concentrations: DDT, toxaphine, aldrin and dieldrin, heptachlor, diazinon, parathion, chlorobenzilate, dithiocarbimate, dalapon, dimethoate. And besides the novel food compounds directly added to our food by agriculture, many industrial compounds such as polychlorinated biphenols have found their way indirectly into our food supply. [See selection 21, "Tragedy of a Michigan Farm Family," which recounts the effects of PCBs (polychlorinated biphenols) accidentally entering the food chain.]

No studies have been undertaken yet to determine what possible novel flavor compounds might be produced when DDT, dieldrin, or parathion are fried in olive oil with garlic and onions. But it can be predicted that the chemical composition of the product bears little resemblance to the foods eaten in our primeval natural nutritional ecosystem—the system within which our tastes evolved. In the course of only twenty years or so, foods selected over the millenia for flavor and nutrition have become bland or objectionable, and possibly detrimental to good health. Ironically, the foods which have incorporated the most agricultural chemicals are fresh fruits and vegetables, the very foods most commonly advocated for good health by nutritionists.

The impact of industry upon foodstuffs and taste is staggering, and since we live within a closed ecosystem, almost everything produced by industry sooner or later and in one form or another ends up on the dinner plate.

Selection 39 Let Them Eat Junk

William Serrin

Editors' Introduction

Selection 39 takes the consumer behind the scenes of the food-processing industry. Waiting in the wings for consumer approval are an amazing array of "plastic" foods—that is, foods that are the products of modern technology rather than conventional agriculture. Food technology has come out of the closet: it is no longer merely a means to preserve foods but has now embarked on producing foods that never saw a farm, feeding lot, or fishery. Many highly processed foods are promoted to consumers through nutritional claims. Fortunately, nutritional claims can be analyzed by informed consumers, and manufacturers are, ultimately, held accountable for misleading claims. In one case a bread manufacturer was forced to provide several months' worth of "corrective advertising" for a product about which the public had been misinformed.

The food-processing industry is highly energy-intensive. Although economies of scale—for example, baking bread in mass production rather than home baking—may be energy-conserving, other food-processing technologies such as freeze-drying may not. Perhaps economics rather than informed choice will return nature's bounty to our dining tables in place of technology's triumphs. In 1980, for example, Donald Wiggans a professor of chemistry at the University of Texas Health Science Center in Dallas noted that soy flour, although a good source of protein, could run as high as $14 per pound. In comparison ground chuck costs less than $2 per pound and better cuts of beef cost about $4 per pound.

In the following selection William Serrin, a national correspondent for the *New York Times*, reports on the technological feats of food processors. How attractive consumers will find this chemical cuisine remains to be seen.

Hundreds of men and women laden with plastic shopping bags wander a vast midway of booths. Some wear straw hats, party favors from a turn-of-the-century gala the night before. All around them, on placards hanging from the roof of the Cervantes Convention Exhibition

Center in St. Louis, are signs hawking their companies' products.

— Prefabricated pork chops triumph with H&R natural and artificial flavors;
— VD has the scoop on True-to-Life flavors;
— Nutrifox VDD sodium tripolyphosphate is the one for meat-curing applications;
— Now Amazio adds more eye and mouth appeal to processed foods faster than you can say "pregelatinized starches."

These men and women are food scientists. More than farmers, ranchers, or nutritionists, they determine what Americans eat. At a recent convention of the Institute of Food Technologists (IFT), they bustled up and down the corridors between display booths, nibbling on the products that the large food companies hope to place on the nation's dining tables: low-calorie watermelon punch, imitation vanilla cookies, fudge made from artificial chocolate, imitation cream cheese, imitation mozzarella cheese, imitation provolone cheese, sausages made with artificial meat flavor, popcorn flavored with imitation butter, freeze-dried raspberry yogurt chunks, peppermint-flavored mints.

Until the past generation, food scientists concerned themselves largely with techniques of preservation—canning, refrigeration, cellophane wrapping. The technology explosion that occurred during World War II and the decades afterward helped to create an industry more concerned with producing new foods in new forms than with preserving and transporting the existing ones economically and conveniently. Two new practices that had enjoyed immense growth in the twenty years before the war, market research and national advertising, were of great assistance in the birth of what amounted to a whole new enterprise—the modern food industry.

Today Americans spend $260 billion annually on food, almost half of which goes toward the purchase of highly processed items, including convenience and snack foods. We also eat about 40 percent of our meals away from home, spending an additional $105 billion on what is known as the food-service business. Food science is the backbone of this industry as well.

Not long ago the food business, as well as the food-service business, consisted of local entrepreneurs with their own factories, or warehouses, or shops. Today not only the frozen, wrapped, uniform food at the grocery store but also the fast-food restaurants, many of the farms, the food research groups, and even the seeds are controlled by a handful of huge conglomerates with names like General Foods, General Mills, Procter and Gamble, Kelloggs, along with such nonfood companies as ITT and General Electric. Many of these firms sell literally hundreds of products and spend vast amounts of money on marketing and advertising to convince the public that the new items are somehow different from their predecessors. The lack of competition among these firms has led to charges that food prices are artificially high, as well as, in one case, an FTC antitrust suit. Companies have also been charged with manipulative and deceptive advertising. Critics of the food business are also distressed that the industry has managed almost to saturate the American market and is now looking abroad, especially to the developing nations of the Third World, for new consumers. This internationalization has raised the fear that America will soon be blanketing the world with frozen french fries. But all of these criticisms pale before the essential one: that food-processing companies have succeeded in debasing the American diet.

Just what have technologists done to our food? The answers can be found not only in the foods they put on American plates but in the ideas they put into the minds of American consumers by means of marketing and sales promotion.

"Today's consumers really don't need anything in the way of new products," the research director for Libby, McNeill & Libby, the large Chicago-based food company, told the IFT a few years ago. Nonetheless, he contended, "they are constantly searching for something just a little better or different. . . ." An aggressive company, he pointed out, must capitalize on this. Though one firm might look at a proposed orange-juice product and ask, "Who needs it?" a go-getter, the marketing man suggested, would know better. "A company could come along with an orange-juice product to which an additional color or sweetness . . . or . . . an important nutritional component has been added, and do well in the marketplace."

Enter the food technologist. He can add ingredients that extend the shelf life or keep processed foods stable so that, for example, chocolate pudding doesn't turn into a mess of separated layers of goo, all different colors. He can add substances that produce what the industry calls "fine surface gloss." He can simplify production, saving labor and its costs. Raw foods—milk, meat, eggs, grains, fruits, vegetables—are not important. They exist only to be simulated in the laboratory, with the manufactured copies transformed into new foods, those known in the trade as "fun foods" or "consumer hot buttons." Companies can capitalize on almost any characteristic of these products—the novelty, the taste, the cooking time, a new or unusual container—whatever might pique the fancy of the consumer thumbing through the newspaper food section or strolling the aisles of the supermarket.

"The technology is skewed toward anything that can make a buck and away from anything that improves quality," says James S. Turner, a Washington, D.C. attorney and author of *The Chemical Feast*, a study of the regulatory policies of the Food and Drug Administration. "Nothing is heard from the scientific community about quality. . . . The scientists say to the companies, 'We can improve your sales,' and then they come up with the flavors, colors, and extenders that are added to food substances to make them appear to be food. But it's not food. We don't even know what food is in our society."

The overwhelming dominance of manufactured foods in the American diet belies the idea that we are experiencing a revolution in taste and cooking, a notion largely advanced by food editors and writers. A casual inspection of big-city newspapers and magazines suggests that everyone is puttering around a brick-lined kitchen, a gourmet cookbook in hand, the food processor purring, turning out some delicate, exotic dish. But the reality is that consumers have accepted food technology, and our ever-more homogenized diet is destroying the nation's rich culinary traditions.

Regional and ethnic distinctions are disappearing from American cooking. Food in one neighborhood, city, or state looks and tastes pretty much like food anywhere else. Americans are sitting down to meals largely composed of such items as instant macaroni and cheese, soft white bread, oleomargarine, frozen doughnuts, and Jell-O. "Today it is possible to travel from coast to coast, at any time of year, without feeling any need to change your eating habits," according to a brochure printed by the IFT. "Sophisticated processing and storage techniques, fast transport, and a creative variety of formulated convenience-food products have made it possible to ignore regional and seasonal differences in food production. . . ."

The success of food scientists can be charted by the radical transformation of the American diet in recent years. Consumption of fluid milk, for instance, has slipped more than 30 percent since 1960; soft drinks are now the nation's number-one beverage. Potato products, largely frozen french fries, became 464 percent more popular between 1910 and 1976, a year in which more fries, in tons, were sold than any other frozen vegetable. In 1940, homemakers bought 50 percent of the flour sold in the United States; today they buy 11 percent. Most flour now goes into processed breads, cakes, pies, and buns sold at grocery stores and fast-food restaurants (40 percent of the beef consumed here is hamburger).

One of the great recent triumphs of food science is Procter and Gamble's potato-chip-like product, Pringles. The baby of several years of research, Pringles are made not from potato slices, like traditional chips, but from a potato paste. They have a salt taste on only one side: Why put taste on both sides, the manufacturer reasoned, when only one will touch the tongue? Without food science, all milk shakes would still contain milk. Many are now made instead from vegetable oils such as coconut or palm, milk-food solids, emulsifiers, flavors, and sugars.

Fast-food restaurants, a booming sector of the economy, depend upon the miracles of modern food science no less than do the drinks and snacks you buy in the grocery store. A firm like Denny's, for example, has some 700 outlets in 41 states, and others scattered across Great Britain and Japan. With labor turnover in the industry running at about 350 percent a year, Denny's must serve foods that can be prepared by almost anyone. Their cooks are not likely to have high culinary skills. Even though Denny's puts pictures on its food containers to make sure employees with limited reading ability can manage the cooking, the chain still relies on food science to make preparation even easier. The foods Denny's chooses are ready for eating when heated to 90 degrees, and are palatable at temperatures between 75 and 105. Though the chain used frozen foods heavily at first, the ballooning costs of refrigeration are dictating a switch to dehydrated foods. In the future, Denny's plans to use foods packaged in retort pouches—flexible aluminum cans whose contents can be quickly warmed under the kitchen faucet. The firm is looking for preportioned servings that will keep for the longest possible time. . . .

A change in public taste has led to a rash of "natural" items, products with some crucial vitamins restored. But food scientists and the companies that they represent do not feel that the diet they have created is deficient in any fundamental way. They do not take well to criticism of it—as one scene at the IFT convention demonstrated. In one part of the program, 400 scientists gathered to watch movies about the health aspects of their business.

Murmurs of approval ran through the audience during the screening of *Chemicals: A Fact of Life*, filmed through the courtesy of the Monsanto Company. *Adventures in Packaging*, by the Package Research Laboratory, enjoyed a similar reception. But the background commentary changed tone with the appearance of the "controversial" films. . . . No discussion followed the films. The movies were uniformly ridiculed from the beginning.

Why show them, then? I.D. Wolf, the program's moderator, and a professor of food science from the University of Minnesota, said that the controversial movies were full of "inaccuracies and exaggerations," but that they were representative of the sort of information about processed food now reaching the public. Since laymen might take such charges seriously, she continued, it was up to food scientists to familiarize themselves with them and rebut them.

They have a great deal of rebutting to do. As Americans have become more concerned about their health, and somewhat more circumspect about what they put into their mouths, allegations like those in the "controversial" films have become common coin. Dr. Michael Jacobson, a well-known food activist and author, claims that the American diet "promotes high blood pressure, strokes, heart disease, obesity, tooth decay, diabetes, and probably certain forms of cancer—surely bowel cancer and breast cancer. Diet is not the only cause of these afflictions, but it is significant. . . . And if you add them all up, they cause half the deaths Americans succumb to annually."

More bad news comes from the Senate Select Committee on Nutrition and Human Needs, which points out that processed food is exceptionally high in sugar and salts. The committee reported that six out of the ten leading causes of death are linked to overconsumption of fats, cholesterol, sugar, salts, and alcohol.

Food executives often don't take the comments about overweight Americans too seriously. They like to joke that their industry has been so successful at providing wholesome, good-tasting food that the nation's major nutrition problem is obesity. And they are attacking even that condition, the executives say, through edibles that are low in calories.

But food executives do not usually joke when confronted with the allegations about the hazards of their products. Dr. Jack Francis, president-elect of the IFT, concedes that sugar contributes to tooth decay and that high consumption of fats "probably" leads to obesity; but he testily labels other charges "a lot of speculation." Francis calls for more research. And what if further investigation confirms the dangerous consequences of eating processed food? "What is the alternative?" he asks. "Go back to the diet we had 100 years ago? . . . People aren't going to go back to the salt pork, cabbage, carrots, and potatoes that they ate in New England a century back. We have to feed people, and we have to transport food, and we have to make food delivery as efficient as we possibly can. . . . That means more processing, not less."

The bewildering diversity of canned, frozen, and dehydrated foods on the grocer's shelves gives the mistaken impression that the food business is teeming with small, competitive firms as it was in Francis's "old days," when food meant fresh produce. . . . The number of food companies, according to Carol Tucker Foreman, assistant secretary for Food and Consumer Services for the Department of Agriculture, has declined from 44,000 in 1947 to 22,000 in 1972 and is still dropping. Researchers J.M. Connor and Russell C. Parker say that 200 corporations control 63.5 percent of food- and tobacco-processing sales. They have estimated that monopoly overcharges in the food manufacturing industries totaled $10 billion, or about 6 percent of food sales, in 1975.

Indeed, concentration has become the rule throughout the food business. Farms, the equipment that they use, as well as the crops that they produce, have come more and more under the domination of a shrinking number of conglomerates. Regional supermarket chains have all but eliminated substantial local competition in many cities. The processed-food market is no less concentrated. Campbell's makes 90 percent of our soup. And only four other firms sell us a large majority of many canned fruit and vegetable products.

The billion-dollar food-processing companies not only manufacture hundreds of consumer goods but they have extended their grasp throughout the food business. For example, General Mills sells a long list of cereals, including Wheaties and Cheerios, Betty Crocker cake mixes, Saluto pizza—and owns Red Lobster inns. General Foods has Burger Chef restaurants and markets Maxwell House coffee, Post cereals, Kool-Aid, Jell-O, and Tang. Ralston Purina sells Chicken of the Sea tuna, Chex cereals, and a long list of pet food, and owns the Jack-in-the-Box restaurant chain. Del Monte, which is itself part of the R.J. Reynolds tobacco company, has seed farms and engages in food and agricultural research, agricultural production, transportation, storage and distribution, as well as food processing and service. . . .

Since many of their products are essentially alike, an advertised image may provide the critical difference in the mind of the consumer. Lay's potato chips, for example, may not differ intrinsically from Wise potato chips; but who could fail to be moved by the sight of Bert Lahr gazing rapturously at Lay's finest? With this kind of clout in mind, food companies have turned heavily to television advertising.

Here, too, government regulatory agencies have stepped in to halt what they consider systematic abuses. Spurred by a series of petitions from public-interest groups, the Federal Communications Commission tried to persuade manufacturers of presweetened cereal, candy, and toys to reduce the numbers of their television commercials to children and to include messages that might mitigate some of the ill effects of their products. Broadcasters and advertisers agreed to decrease slightly the hourly time allotted for advertising on children's TV but have otherwise proved intransigent. The cereal industry has lobbied intensely on the issue, reportedly spending $30 million (peanuts compared to the $600 million spent on children's TV advertising), and has so far staved off further reform.

Action for Children's Television (ACT), a Boston-based group, continues to pressure the FCC. Peggy Charren, the president, argues that children should "be protected from deception in the marketplace the same way adults are. . . . Nobody's ever told a child that Milky Way causes cavities; the message is 'Milky Way at work, rest, or play.' After 10 years of this argument they could at least say, 'at work, rest, or play, and if you don't brush your teeth you're going to get a cavity'." ACT would prefer, however, that commercials for sweets be removed from children's TV entirely.

Whatever the marketing strategies and advertising finesse, the food industry faces one apparently intractable problem: America can eat just so many Pringles. The food-processing business has already responded to the problem of satiation by inventing new packages, new slogans, and yet more exotic products. But the national population is stabilizing and the food companies must look for growth opportunities elsewhere—to pets, for example: Americans now feed 40 million dogs and 30 million cats, whose taste buds remain more or less unexplored territory. Grocery shelf space devoted to pet food has expanded dramatically in the last few years, and dogs now enjoy a variety of comestibles not much less impressive than their masters'.

The biggest growth area of the future is neither new products nor new species, but new countries. General Foods now sells coffee and powdered drinks in Europe, ice cream in Brazil, candy and gum in Mexico, and Tang, that venerable pick-me-up of astronauts, to Japan. Borden's foreign sales account for 20 percent of its total volume. The cerealmakers, with no new mouths to conquer at home, have turned increasingly to the Third World nations of South America and the Middle East. Indeed, the upper crust of the Third World, a vast market full of people who have never so much as seen a frozen apple pie, represents the next great market for many food-processing companies. "The most compelling job," said Kellogg International's Vice-President Charles Tornabene in a *Business Week* interview, "is to change people's food habits." Converting the entire world to the processed-food gospel may prove a daunting task.

In his closing speech to the IFT delegates, William Beers, retired chairman of Kraft, Inc., proposed that underdeveloped nations be encouraged to revamp their food systems into miniature versions of our own. Third World nations, said Beers, "must acquire modern infrastructures—industrial, technological, and marketing." Farmers, said Beers to the cheering scientists, "must be motivated to adopt and use modern agricultural technology." And finally, developing nations must pattern their food marketing systems after our own. Then, he concluded, "there will be demands for new types of processed foods, packaging, transportation, and distribution."

The consequences of selling and aggressively advertising sophisticated food products to Third World consumers have been painfully illustrated in the case of infant formula milk. Most manufacturers of infant formula—Nestlé, Borden, Carnation, and Bristol-Myers, among others—market their product to mothers in developing nations. The companies sent "milk nurses"—employees dressed up as nurses—into maternity wards, where they handed out free samples of the formula. Then the companies launched highly effective advertising campaigns. Mothers in the Ivory Coast were found feeding their children Nescafé after a radio message proclaimed that "Nescafé makes men stronger, women more joyful, and children more intelligent."

Besides taking the message too literally, mothers often do not understand how or simply are not able to use the formula: Once back in the village, clean water may not be available to mix with the formula powder. The instructions may be written in the wrong language, or the mother may be illiterate. Money runs out, they can no longer afford the formula, and they have lost their own ability to nurse. For these reasons, according to INFACT, an antiformula group, as many as 10 million infants die annually from diseases related to bottle-feeding. But the milk companies have done little to counteract the damage they may have caused.

If the past is any indication, however, the companies will survive these complaints and controversies. The food-processing industry has shown itself to be extraordinarily adaptive. When the American consumer began clamoring for "natural foods," the industry stuck "natural" on its labels. While its very success depends on its ability to abolish the past, the industry suggests that its goods have the taste and quality of old-fashioned foods. Running out of Americans to feed, the food business has moved into the Third World, proclaiming itself a force of economic liberation rather than a purveyor of dubious goods.

Of course, the industry is not wholly responsible for the decay of the American diet. After all, no one is forced to choose the laboratory's products over the farm's; no one has to buy orange drink instead of oranges. The industry has found willing customers in the American public.

Yet the questions remain: How do we deal with the technology we have spawned? What kind of food system should we move toward in the future, not only for ourselves but for the rest of the world? Are world hunger and malnutrition to be combated with massive doses of instant junk foods? Unless we choose to confront these questions, we can be assured a steady diet of frozen pizza and cupcakes.

Selection 40 Safe at the Plate

Richard L. Hall

Editors' Introduction

In recent years public attention has focused on the presence of additives in food. What is an additive? An *additive* may be defined as a substance or mixture of substances intentionally or unintentionally added to food and consumed with the food. Many such substances perform useful functions and some, such as smoking and salting, have been used for centuries to preserve foods. *Intentional*, or direct, *additives* are those that

1. preserve and prevent spoilage;
2. add or enhance flavor or appearance;
3. maintain or improve nutritional value;
4. produce an acceptable consistency.

The legal definition of an additive set forth by the Food and Drug Administration (FDA) includes only intentional additives. It does not include *incidental*, or indirect, *additives* that are not deliberately added. These are the substances that have become part of food as a result of some phase in the production, processing, storage, or packaging of food. Some substances such as pesticide residues when found in foods are usually found in trace quantities. Other substances migrate or transfer from the package or processing to the food itself.

We cannot assume that every processed or new food that makes its appearance on the market shelf is good for us. Neither can we assume that all processed foods with additives are bad simply because they contain chemicals. All foods are chemicals. Many traditional ingredients in foods—such as salt, pepper, sugar, clove, garlic, dill, ginger, and mustard—are technically additives, just as those nutrients deliberately added to enrich and fortify foods with minerals and vitamins are. Consumers should not become alarmed just because additives and unfamiliar chemical names appear on food labels. Moreover, consumers should resist scare tactics and alarmist headlines and announcements concerning, for example, the dangers of mercury in fish or pesticides on cranberries. This is not to say that adulteration of our food supply

Source: Adapted from Richard L. Hall, Ph.D., "Safe at the Plate," *Nutrition Today* Magazine (November/December 1977):6–9, 29–31. Reproduced with permission of *Nutrition Today* Magazine, 101 Ridgely Avenue, Annapolis, Maryland 21404. © November/December, 1977.

can go unchallenged. However, we now have little scientific evidence about the extent to which the human body can ingest these materials and store them in toxic amounts. We do not know whether human beings possess a capacity not shared with test animals to excrete or break down these substances, nor do we even know the extent to which biochemical individuality can make certain substances safe for some people but dangerous for others.

An estimated 1,300 intentional additives are currently approved for use by the FDA. The exact amount of these additives consumed is not known. However, a study prepared by the FDA in 1976 estimated that the average daily consumption of just artificial colors among children one to five years of age may be 60 milligrams, and the average consumption by children age six to twelve may be about 75 milligrams. The study found that the largest category contributing to artificial-coloring consumption among children consists of beverages.

Food additives now in use are considered safe by the FDA based on varying degrees of testing, review of scientific findings, expert opinions, and long-time use. In accordance with the 1958 Food Additives Amendment to the Food and Drug Act of 1938, the major responsibility for proving the safety and efficacy of an additive was given to the food companies. After careful review of material concerning an additive, the FDA authorizes its use under specific conditions. The Delaney Clause, a rider to the amendment, prohibits the use of additives in any quantity if the additive is found to induce cancer when ingested by humans or animals. This clause has created a great deal of controversy among members of the food industry, FDA officials, nutritionists, and consumerists. Some feel that the clause should be strictly enforced; others criticize it for not allowing for the difference in effects of varying dose levels on the body.

When the 1958 Food Additive Amendment and the Delaney Clause were passed, many substances were exempted from complying with procedures to establish their safety because they had been in use for some time without any known harmful effects. These substances were put on what has become known as the GRAS (Generally Recognized As Safe) list. In 1969 the White House Conference on Nutrition recommended the gradual review of the GRAS list, particularly for artificial flavors and colors. Testing of substances on the GRAS list by the FDA is now in progress. The U.S. Senate Select Committee on Nutrition and Human Needs: Dietary Goals for the United States (1976) stated that although food additives as a category may not justifiably be considered harmful, the varying degrees of testing and quality of testing and the continuing discoveries of apparent connections between certain additives and cancer, and possibly hyperactivity, give justifiable cause to seek to reduce additive consumption to the greatest possible degree.

Among the additives that many authorities classify as possibly hazardous to health are nitrates and nitrites. Nitrates are being phased out as food additives. Nitrites, however, are still used extensively to cure ham, frankfurters, bacon, and luncheon meats. Nitrites are added to check the growth of botulinum, a bacteria that produces a deadly toxin, to impart a typical pink color to these meats, and to prevent a warmed-over flavor. Nitrates and nitrites are not in themselves harmful, but they may combine with other chemicals in the intestines to form nitrosamines that are known to cause cancer. Therefore, authorities feel that the FDA should limit the addition of nitrites to the amounts no more than needed to check the growth of botulinum bacteria.

What can consumers do? The best idea is to eat a variety of foods. Try to cut down on high-fat processed meats, candies, sweet baked goods, and soft drinks. Do not eat excessive quantities of any one food. You do not have to go to the unnecessary inconvenience or expense of buying "natural" or "organically grown" fruits and vegetables. Nutritionally, their vitamin and mineral content is no more or less than those grown commercially. As for pesticides, washing fresh fruits and vegetables before using will assure a measure of safety.

We face a real problem in the United States and Canada due to the way many people, indeed too many people, regard food ingredients and the way modern food is processed as it moves from the farm to the table. Unless some way can be found for physicians, dietitians, home economists, food technologists, and nutritionists to respond convincingly to the questions being raised by the average person, the nutritional health of the entire public will be adversely affected.

One response, a vivid portrayal of some unreasonable concerns about the safety of the foods we eat, is presented here.

But first let us look at the reason why the purity and virtue of our food supply is suspect by so many people. The reason is wrapped up with many other popular dissatisfactions and disenchantments. First, food supply is business, an enormous business, and we all know that the business community is mistrusted by many people. It always has been, only today, perhaps, it is more so. In a different but parallel vein, we all know—indeed we all share—a distaste for the anonymity and complexity of an urbanized, industrialized, increasingly regulated society.

Both attitudes affect our views of food, particularly industrially processed food.

Food, moreover, occupies a special place in our lives. It is not only a biological necessity, it is a social activity, an aesthetic experience, and a cultural expression. All of these impose a heavy load of emotional involvement, beginning in infancy.

The Mystery of Food

Several generations ago, most of our food was prepared at home, "from scratch," largely from ingredients that were themselves home-made or locally grown. This intimacy bred the confidence that comes from familiarity.

For another thing, in that day the germ theory of disease was new, and very few people other than scientists knew about it or were concerned with its implications. Vitamins were unheard of. People knew what they meant when they spoke of "wholesome food." Analyses for insect contamination, microbiological quality, or pesticide residues were certainly not done on home-grown produce and rarely on foods sold in the "grocery store." The safety of food ingredients was seldom questioned and virtually never tested. We all enjoyed the confidence that comes from innocence.

Today, of course, our food is often grown hundreds or thousands of miles away. In order to assure a continuing supply of wholesome food of uniform quality to 250 million people spread from the Rio Grande to the Arctic Ocean, most foodstuffs travel thousands of miles and are stored for long periods. How this is possible is a mystery to many. Also most food is "processed" by people and equipment we never see. The fact that today's food is cleaner, safer, more varied, and proportionately cheaper than ever before still doesn't inspire the confidence in our food supply that at one time came from personal involvement.

Ironically, the same science and technology that have made our present food supply possible, nutritious, and safe is, at the same time, based on a body of knowledge so large and complex that only a few dedicated people comprehend it. To most, food science and technology are mysteries. In this light, the current worries and misconceptions about the safety and nutritional value of our food supply become more understandable—not more correct—just more understandable. The time has come for those of us in food technology and the health professions and enlightened laymen to allay the fears of the public and to assuage their emotional reactions to this circumstance.

For one thing, we must have production in the most suitable growing areas. The economies of volume and sophistication from industrialized food processing, fertilizers, pesticides, additives, and packaging are necessary merely to feed ourselves properly and economically. Without the wise use of them, we have no hope of feeding the world.

Food Hazards

We should point out that there are risks associated with food, as there are with everything else in our lives. Food does pose problems of disease, poor nutrition, and potentially hazardous components. But we had better appraise these risks clearly and accurately, or we will, in that appropriate phrase from the Gospel of Matthew, "strain off a gnat, yet swallow a camel."

In virtually everything we see or do, we need a sense of perspective. This need is particularly true in coping with food hazards. Without perspective we will concentrate on the trivial and miss the significant.

What are the sources of food hazards? Foremost are the microbiological hazards—those which result in food-borne disease which affects perhaps 10 million persons a year. We do not even have a good grip on numbers, because our reporting practices are so poor. Second are the nutritional hazards—from overconsumption, poor food choices, and less than optimal intakes of many essential nutrients through ignorance, indifference, or poverty. While vastly more serious in the developing countries, nutritional hazards in some degree affect millions in the United States and Canada. Perhaps one-thousandth as significant as these in terms of known human effects are the hazards in food due to environmental contaminants—the mercury in lakes and rivers, the PCBs and similar careless or inadvertent pollutants. While we must work to minimize or eliminate them, as food hazards they are remote and improbable, although rare cases of human injury and even death have occurred.

The natural toxicants in food are unfamiliar to many of us, but have been an important source of human illness and death in other times and places. And it still happens. Mushroom hunters whose enthusiasm exceeds their skill, uncritical imitators of Euell Gibbons, food faddists, and those who eat bizarre diets are by no means uncommon.

Finally, a hundred or more times less significant than these are hazards from pesticide residues on food and from food additives, the intentionally added minor ingredients in food. There is no known case of human injury or death from a pesticide residue on food. Those rare instances of harm from food additives are not only curiosities widely reported in the scientific literature and general news media, but are invariably associated with extremely distorted food intakes, themselves a source of harm. In part, the pesticide residue and food additive risks are extremely low because a great deal of scientific and regulatory effort has gone into their evaluation, prevention, and control. In part also, they are low because the substances involved are in virtually all cases used by people with some knowledge, or even expertness, in their use. The microbiological and nutritional hazards are large because they are affected by the way the 238 million people in the United States and Canada handle and choose food, and few are experts.

This ranking of hazards is supported by an enormous body of evidence. It is thus paradoxical and frustrating that many people persist in viewing these hazards virtually in inverse and perverse order of importance. It is quite obvious that many people fear what they see as chemical, and are uncritically admiring of what they consider to be natural. Beyond that, many others fear what is new and pay undue respect to the old. We are in the simultaneous grip of two phobias, chemophobia and novophobia, the fear of chemicals and the fear of anything new. They are, like all phobias, irrational. Chemophobia is irrational because chemicals are not a thing apart. Our whole world is chemical. We are each a bundle of chemicals. Nor is the new necessarily hazardous and the old safe. We may be, and in fact often are, simply unaware of the near misses from hazards that we do not recognize.

Toxicologists carefully judge the safety of chemicals in our environment by animal testing, human experience, and informed scientific judgment. . . . (See table 40.1.) Even if animal tests tend to indicate

Table 40.1 Food Testing

Toxicologists derive the information by which they judge the safety of the chemicals in our environment using two principal sources of information. By testing the effect of a substance fed to animals, we may reach some tentative conclusions on how the same substance may affect man. These results are *always* tentative. Rats, mice, or even monkeys are not simply small humans. Each species may react differently, and these differences must be studied. Within each species, individuals may differ. It is customary to allow for these differences by applying a safety factor of a hundredfold, more or less, as we derive safe levels for human use from such animal experiments. Stated more precisely, the highest level fed to animals which causes no apparent adverse effect is normally divided by 100 in order to determine the total amount to which a human may be exposed. If the test data are not extensive, or the effects are serious, then a larger safety factor may be required. If the background of information is very broad and the adverse effects are not serious, then a somewhat smaller safety factor may be tolerated. Our Food and Drug Act, however, stipulates one major exception to this scheme. It provides that a substance that is found to cause cancer when ingested by man or animal shall not be permitted as a food additive in any amount. This is the so-called "Delaney Clause."

The second source of information about food safety is human experience. This may be experience with the substance in nature, from accidental or industrial exposures, or as a result of drug or other use. Human experience has the great advantage that it involves the species with which we are most concerned — man himself. But it has a correspond-

Table 40.1 (continued)

ingly great disadvantage. It is experience, not an experiment. It is almost never controlled. Other things are happening, other influences are at work, which may alter or cloud the results. Thus, it is seldom that we are able to associate a particular cause with a particular effect. We can speak of correlations, but not of a clear connection unless it is supported by other kinds of information.

In summary, animal tests are difficult, subject to a variety of major uncertainties, and often hard to reproduce. With all their weaknesses and with the need for wide safety factors, they still remain a valuable source of insight into the extent of risk or safety associated with a particular substance. Yet human experience remains the final determinant. No matter how many animal tests tend to indicate safety, if a substance harms humans, we will be reluctant to use it. Conversely, we continue to eat, drink, and do many things which are hazardous, because we attach other values to them, or because the hazards appear to be small.

Other types of tests may supplement or replace these two kinds of information. A critical third factor is informed scientific judgment. This is usually based on knowledge of the chemical structure and the physiological effects of substances that are chemically or pharmacologically related. Such judgment tells the toxicologists what adverse effects to look for, what kinds of tests to run, what special conditions to apply, how much to trust the results, and when further testing is likely to be profitless.

---

safety, if a substance is found to have adverse effects on humans, we will be reluctant to use it. In fact, the "Delaney Clause" of the Food and Drug Act stipulates that a substance that is found to cause cancer when ingested by man or animal shall not be permitted as a food additive in any amount. Therefore, by statute, intentional additives that are carcinogens are not allowed in any amount. However, naturally occurring carcinogens are not restricted in any way.

Sometimes we gain a better perspective by looking at objects from a fresh angle. We shall go through that exercise now, employing on the known, natural components of ordinary foods the same criteria of safety we would apply if those components had *not* been put there by nature, but had instead been added by man. We will look at what adverse effects of these substances are known from animal testing or human experience.

We will apply the hundredfold or other appropriate safety factor and the professional judgments customarily employed. And we will apply the Delaney Clause with its prohibition of added carcinogens as relentlessly as the most ardent advocate could wish. We will do this to the things nature put there, or at least to those we know about. Obviously, we can't do a complete job because our knowledge of the composition and safety of food is now and always will be incomplete. For this exercise, we will take the menu we might be served at a fine restaurant. Imagine yourself there as we serve you a tasty luncheon with delicious foods and wine, coffee, tea, or milk.

Appetizers

Now let's pass the relish tray with carrots, radishes, onions, and olives.

Everybody from Bugs Bunny to night fighter pilots knows that carrots are good for you. What is less well known is that carrots contain carotatoxin, a fairly potent nerve poison, with a chemical structure which would excite suspicion in any toxicologist's mind. Chronic feeding studies have not been done, but the acute toxicity and structure are sufficiently alarming so that we could not possibly consider carotatoxin an acceptable food ingredient. Carrots also contain myristicin. This substance is a hallucinogen and is thus wholly inappropriate for food use. Carrots also contain some unknown substances, probably isoflavones, that show an estrogenic effect; i.e., they mimic one of the female sex hormones. Obviously, by these criteria we should not eat carrots.

Have a radish? Radishes raise a different problem. They contain two substances which are goitrogens; i.e., they promote goiter by interfering with our use of iodine. About fifty grams of radishes, a little less than two ounces, could be expected to have a clinically noticeable effect on iodine metabolism. So, no radishes.

Don't those spring onions look good? Onions contain some fascinating sulfur compounds, including those that make us cry. But the ones we are crying about here are found in a complex, messy, smelly mixture of disulfides and trisulfides, which also exhibit antithyroid or goitrogenic acitivity. Your friends may not tell you, as they say about halitosis, but we will. Scratch the onions.

Like olives? Yes, but consider this: olives, of course, are processed—soaked in dilute lye to remove a bitter flavor, then washed and brined. They contain far too much sodium to be acceptable within the safety factors we must apply here. In addition, they have tannins, which we shall discuss later. But we really need not debate processed or natural, sodium or tannins. Olive oil, obtained from olives, usually contains low levels of benzo(a)pyrene, a potent carcinogen, or cancer-causing agent.

Under the Delaney Clause, no level of carcinogen is permitted. Olives, too, must go. They're illegal! Melons wrapped in thin slices of ham are tasty appetizers. You can enjoy them if you ignore the fact that ham is smoked, and most smoked ham contains traces of polynuclear aromatic compounds, including, again, our old friend benzo(a)pyrene. Goodbye ham. For the moment, however, we are left with the melon crescents.

Main Course

Well, we have avoided acute food intoxication so far, but we're still hungry. Don't those shrimps look delicious? Sorry. Shrimps are a rich source of several minerals, and among them, pride of place must go to arsenic. Arsenic enjoys a popular reputation largely unjustified in fact. Probably most of the people allegedly done in by arsenic actually succumbed to something else. Nevertheless, shrimps contain some 40 to 170 or more parts per million of arsenic, vastly more than we can tolerate or the Food and Drug Law would allow with our hundredfold safety factor. Not only that. Shrimps are out on any one of several other counts. They can also contain iodine at very high levels and are one of the richest known sources of copper. Two hundred parts per million of copper in the diet is probably the maximum no-effect level in man, and shrimps may contain twice that. We could not possibly eat shrimps with an acceptable margin of safety for at least these three reasons, and that leaves us the Newburg sauce.

Our chef's Newburg sauce consists of lobster butter, brandy, flour, and fish stock. An important constituent of butter is vitamin A. Vitamin A presents us with a significant and curious dilemma. In test animals, both deficiency and excess are teratogenic; that is, it produces deformities in the unborn. Pregnant women beware. Our safety factor for vitamin A does not approach 100; therefore, no butter.

Brandy, of course, contains alcohol, and we do not need to go to animal experiments to study the adverse physiological effects of alcohol. Beyond that, brandy also contains fusel oils which, with alcohol, are responsible for hangovers. Without lobster, butter and brandy, the Newburg sauce is pretty unattractive, so let's forget that.

Ah well, you'll say, "I'll just make a meal of potatoes." Let's see whether you'll be safe. One thing is sure: if you don't want to eat foods that contain additives, then you shouldn't want to eat foods containing similar chemicals added by nature.

Potatoes, like all members of the nightshade family, contain glycoalkaloids. The alkaloid in potatoes is solanine. It is a cholinesterase inhibitor; that is, it interferes with the transmission of nerve impulses in much the same way as nerve gases. The solanine is near the skin, along with the vitamin C. Therefore, the solanine content is particularly high in potatoes that have a high skin to volume ratio; that is, in new potatoes. The safety factor may only be ten or less. If you find yourself feeling drowsy or paralyzed or having difficulty breathing after your next bite of potatoes, it might have been the solanine at work. Potato poisoning is no joke. It was common years ago when potatoes were a major item of the diet and in times of food shortages.

What about the parsley and butter. Sorry, relief is not yet in sight. Butter we have discussed. Parsley contains psoralen, a photosensitizer. Rubbed on the skin or consumed by mouth in sufficient quantity, it produces an unusual sensitivity to sunlight, resulting in severe sunburn or tanning. Furthermore, parsley contains the hallucinogen, myristicin, same as carrots. No parsley for you.

Broccoli contains not one, but *five* goitrogens, two of them in large quantity. These different promoters of goiter, and the chemicals our bodies produce from them after we eat the broccoli, act at five different points in our metabolism—our use—of iodine. It is somewhat like kinking your garden hose in five different places. Skip the broccoli.

Hollandaise sauce without anything to eat it on is not very attractive, but our food is getting scarce, and we will not discard it on that account. Let's see now. Our hollandaise sauce was made with egg yolk, butter, and lemon juice. We'll skip the cholesterol in egg yolk, and in this toxicology exercise consider only its vitamin A and vitamin D content. We know about vitamin A. Vitamin D, another of the fat-soluble vitamins, is tolerable only with an even narrower margin of safety. For adults, the safety margin with vitamin D is about tenfold; for infants, it is probably less than five. Lemon juice contains a host of very questionable substances. Citral, for example. Given orally to animals, citral damages the lining of the circulatory system, and the optic nerve, and is a vitamin A antagonist; that is, it counteracts the good effects of vitamin A. Synephrine is a pressor amine, which we shall discuss shortly, and isopimpinellin is a photosensitizer, similar to the psoralen in parsley. Nix the hollandaise.

A nice white wine is just the thing for such a tasty meal. Well, it might have been but you don't have to be a teetotaler to ask the waiter to take it away. The principal ingredient of toxicological interest in wine is, of course, the alcohol. It may also contain pressor amines, and a number of other substances not acceptable under these criteria. Carry Nation would feel vindicated.

Salad

In our salad, watercress, like the radishes and broccoli already discussed, contains a goitrogen. That would be enough to eliminate watercress. But in addition to that, weight for weight, watercress contains twice as much dangerous vitamin A as butter, and also an un-known something, an "antivitamin," that ties up and renders vitamin B_1 ineffective.

A moment ago when discussing lemons we mentioned synephrine, a pressor amine. Such chemicals tend to raise the blood pressure. Avocados contain a number of pressor amines. For most of us, the consumption of a normal diet containing pressor amines has little effect because our bodies contain an enzyme system, monoamine oxidase, which rapidly and effectively chews these amines up into fragments we can utilize or excrete. But some people have reduced monoamine oxidase capacity, particularly if they have been taking antidepressant drugs, such as Parnate. Moreover, the potential adverse effects of the pressor amines are not restricted to those on antidepressants. We will take this point up later on. However, we have good reason to pass up the avocado.

Lemon-herb dressing is a "no-no" by our far-fetched application of the federal standards for added toxicants to those naturally occurring in our food. We have already discussed the hazards of lemon juice. Among the herbs, the pepper contains myristicin, the parsley has myristicin and psoralen, and the onions have the disulfide goitrogens. Egg white contains avidin, a biotin antagonist which ties up that vitamin in an unusable form. The red pimento contains vitamin A. The dill contains more myristicin; the vinegar, acetic acid; and the vegetable oil, like most samples of vegetable oil, contains the now familiar benzo(a)pyrene, a carcinogen, apparently as a result of biosynthesis in the plant. That leaves just the hearts of palm and we don't know what all they contain.

Butter

We have already eliminated butter as an ingredient, so we cannot tolerate it as a separate, visible item. "Waiter, remove the butter, please."

Cheese

Cheese would be nice to have after our meal—if we'd had a meal to have something after. But cheese, like avocados, is a rich source of pressor amines, particularly tyramine. So, goodbye cheese.

Fruit

But we are not done with the pressor amines. Bananas are a major source of pressor amines, particularly serotonin. We've seen that hazards from pressor amines are not restricted to those persons taking antidepressants. Here we can draw again from human experience. Those

African tribes that eat a large amount of bananas and plantains show an unusual incidence of a peculiar type of heart diease, right-sided valvular lesions. Furthermore, individuals in our own population who suffer from a tumor called "carcinoid syndrome," which causes them to produce a large amount of serotonin, suffer from the same heart lesions. This is fairly persuasive evidence that our margin of safety with bananas is not all that great. These hazards are from the *dietary* consumption of bananas. The pressor amines are most effective when injected. In fact, one gram, $\frac{1}{28}$ of an ounce, $\frac{1}{6}$ of a teaspoonful, of banana pulp is equivalent to about 50,000 bee stings, which certainly makes one grateful that bananas do not have sharp points.

An apple a day keeps the doctor away? Well, let's apply our regulatory yardstick of toxic chemicals to its content. Apples' most interesting component is phlorizin, which interferes in a number of enzyme systems in our cells and produces glucosuria; that is, glucose in the urine. Several dozen apples a day will not keep the doctor away, but they would scare off your life insurance agent.

A day without oranges is like a day without sunshine? But oranges contain the flavone, tangeretin, which is embryotoxic. It is found not in the pulp juice, but in the peel juice, some of which gets into ordinary orange juice. Here the safety factor is fairly wide, probably more than 100, although one ordinarily regards embryotoxic effects as more serious than some other categories of toxicity. Oranges also contain tyramine, synephrine, and citral. So our tray of fruit is bare.

Beverages

Of our nonalcoholic beverages, the most studied of all, because of its popularity and cost, is coffee. To date, nearly 500 different chemical substances have been isolated and identified in coffee aroma. Informed estimates suggest that if and when tireless chemists ever tease out all of the chemicals in coffee aroma, the total number will amount to 15,000 different substances. Most have never been tested or evaluated for safety, and some we could not possibly consider for intentional addition to food. Coffee is also a rich source of tannins. Free tannins cause growth depression, intestinal damage, and are implicated, not necessarily firmly, in human esophageal cancer. Drinking moderate amounts of coffee and tea may contribute about one gram of tannin a day to our diet, and we consume these with a safety factor of thirty or less. They also contain the stimulant caffeine, for which the safety factor is only about twenty or thirty. Coffee, being a roasted product, also contains traces of three, four-benzo(a)pyrene. Tea not only contains the tannins and the caffeine, but is our richest dietary source of fluorine and manganese. Fluorine can be regarded as an essential nutrient. Certainly it is essential in proper bone formulation. But eight to ten parts per million of fluorine in the diet can lead to skeletal fluorosis, with pain, stiffness, and excessive calcification. The safety factor is less than ten. Manganese is consumed in our diet with about a tenfold safety factor.

Milk, of course, contains milk sugar, or lactose, and vitamin D. Galactose, a component of lactose, causes cataracts in test animals when given at only fairly low multiples of normal intake. It may be the cause of an unusually high incidence of cataracts in India where yogurt is a large part of the diet. We have already discussed vitamin D.

So, What's Left?

We are then left with the melon crescents, hearts of palm, pastry shell, roll, and mineral water. Not a terribly attractive menu, but the end is not yet.

Melons have relatively little in them, except water, which should make them safe. Right? Wrong. It is widely assumed that water is safe, and nothing could be further from the truth. We are not discussing drowning, but dilution. There is a considerable literature on the toxicity of water in animal-feeding studies. A recent human death and at least two cases of coma induced by excessive voluntary drinking of water indicate a safety factor for water between ten and twenty. This excludes both the melon and the mineral water from our meal. The hearts of palm we leave here, even though the water content may be a bit high. There are no significant other toxicants yet known in hearts of palm, but that is undoubtedly because we have not yet studied them with sufficient attention. For, in fact, we possess today the means to indict any substance to which we care to devote sufficient, or sufficiently uninterpreted, testing. We can indict; we cannot necessarily convict or declare innocent.

— Melon crescents — Water
— Mineral water — Water
— Hearts of palm — ?
— Wheat and other grains — Phytic acid
— Rolls — Phytic acid

We still have the rolls and pastry shell. These are not really natural foods, but a blend of ingredients themselves fairly highly processed. They therefore fall outside the frame of reference we have employed here. But they are not wholly irrelevant. They do not contain any of the kinds of toxicants we have discussed because, in the process of refining their ingredients, the toxicants have been refined out. We hear occasional criticism of such items in our food supply because of the loss of nutrients consequent upon the refining process, even though the important nutrients are restored by fortification. But in the same refining of wheat and other grains, we have also lost phytic acid. Phytic acid has a strong affinity for iron, zinc, and other minerals in the diet. In many areas of the world, such as Iran, where unleavened whole grain bread is a major item of the diet, one finds iron and zinc deficiencies with their attendant symptoms such as anemia and hypogonadism, failure to develop sexually.

We are obviously at the end of our meal, our time, and our rope.

If you wonder "What is really safe?" or "Why is he bad-mouthing all food?" then we will have failed grievously in trying to convey an essential message about the safety of our food supply.

Misplaced Concern

The message is that a lot of people—and to a considerable extent, our own government—do too much worrying about the wrong things. We must not neglect any aspect of food safety. But we should pay the most attention to the greatest risks.

Through popular, misplaced, and overzealous concern we have devoted disproportionate effort and placed stringent requirements on certain minor food ingredients and exaggerated their risks. To them we apply safety standards we dare not apply to major or natural ingredients, or we would have virtually nothing to eat, as you can see from what's been said.

Behind the irony of these absurd but true examples there's a serious point. Let us have no misunderstanding. The goods in our menu are *not* dangerous when consumed as a normal part of a balanced and varied diet. They are nutritious and they are safe. Nothing else is implied. Nor does this suggest that we should go to the other extreme and say that because too much of anything will hurt you, we should throw caution to the winds and abandon completely any effort to weigh risks and to choose wisely. The whole point of this exercise is that there is a middle course and it is the only sensible course. Safety lies not in avoiding all risk, because we *never* avoid all risk. We simply choose among risks. Safety is, in fact, a path between risks, sometimes broad, sometimes narrow, sometimes clearly marked, sometimes indistinct. We cannot follow that path if we look at only part of it, if we preoccupy ourselves with only one type of risk, or the most remote risks. In total reality, pesticide residues and additives are far "safer"—used with wider safety factors and more careful appraisal—than many natural components. Their risks are tiny compared with the risks we run every day, through carelessness and ignorance, from food insanitation and poor nutrition. We can only make progress safely if we see the whole scene and deal with risks in the priority of their importance. We owe it to ourselves to concentrate most of our efforts on the greatest risks in our food supply and on those which can most easily be reduced. The key to food safety is three simple words: sanitation, variety, and moderation. All of us connected with the food industry, as I am, have a substantial responsibility to help people achieve understanding of this perspective—in seeing the whole picture.

Selection 41 Diet for Two: But Dinner for Five

Jean Mayer

Editors' Introduction

In the typical family nutritional needs differ on the basis of age, sex, occupation, state of health (including pregnancy), and specific biochemical uniqueness such as allergies to foods. Meal management that provides each person with the greatest benefit from family meals requires advance planning and imagination and resourcefulness in the selection and preparation of foods that can satisfy a number of different family needs and tastes.

In the following selection the problem of a typical three-generation family is analyzed. A three-day sample menu plan designed to meet all of the family members' individual needs is suggested. Although the plan assumes that the husband is the family's wage earner, the approach to menu planning is the same, whatever the makeup of the family. From single-parent households to "empty-nest" retired couples, the food needs of family groups are rarely identical.

Happily, people still come in two sexes. They are separate and in many ways not the least equal. A weight-control diet for one person might be an overabundance for the other. And the very same diet might not answer the special needs of both.

Source: Adapted from Dr. Jean Mayer, "How a Husband and Wife Can Go on a Diet Together," *Family Health* Magazine, January 1972, pp. 26–30, 35, and 46. Reprinted with permission of the author and *Family Health* Magazine, January 1972 ©. All rights reserved.

But since both sexes—and all ages—do share a great number of similar characteristics and bodily needs, a basic meal plan can be adapted for all, so long as it meets their common nutritional needs. And a wife can contemplate dieting together with her husband without sacrificing the nutrition of her children or resident grandparent.

For example, we all need sufficient but not excessive calories, enough proteins, carbohydrates, fats (or at least certain types of fats), water-soluble and fat-soluble vitamins and minerals, and an abundant supply of water (in whatever form it comes). But the amounts needed vary considerably from one person to another.

. . . [In this report] we're presenting . . . a new three-day sample meal plan showing how basic menus can be adapted for all members of a family, without cheating anybody of food they need or overwhelming anybody with food they don't. [See table 41.1.]

These examples were planned for a family of five—father, mother, preschool child, teenager, and elderly grandparent—by my colleague at Harvard, nutritionist Johanna Dwyer, and myself. They offer a means of meeting the different food needs within the family while keeping a husband's weight and a wife's weight in line.

Specific Problems

Let's take a look at the specific problems of the basic family members, beginning with the heart of the family, husband and wife.

The husband in many ways is the most vulnerable member of the family. Everyone depends on his earning capacity, as well as his leadership and his example. Yet from a medical viewpoint, there he is—usually overfed, underexercised, on a diet high in saturated fats and salt, with too much stress and too little rest, a prime candidate for heart-and-artery diseases (which cause over half the deaths in the 40–60 male age group). We know some of the main contributing factors and how the husband endangers himself.

First, there's undiagnosed high blood pressure. He not only claims he is too busy for a checkup, but he keeps eating peanuts with his beer and oversalting his meat, french fries, and onion rings.

Second is the danger of overweight. That flabby waist on what used to be your favorite athlete is visible to all except him. He formed his body image as a high-scoring halfback or Marine second lieutenant and has not taken a real look at himself since then. He downs cheeseburgers and malted milks with the children, martinis and steaks with his customers, and a prebedtime glass of milk plus a slice of banana-cream pie with the girl he married. Then he wonders why his favorite golf slacks are splitting (poor workmanship, no doubt). . . .

Third is the matter of high saturated-fat diets. That's the added hazard of eating the cheeseburgers, steaks, french fries, fried clams, milk, cream pie, and so on.

Fourth and fifth are heavy cigarette smoking and lack of physical exercise. He usually thinks of himself not as sedentary, which he most probably is, but as moderately active, because he thinks he will be able to play golf next weekend. If he has actually played golf once on each of the preceding two or three weekends, he thinks of himself as very active. But walk an hour or at least a solid half hour a day? "Who has the time to do that?"

Finally, there is lack of sleep. How many cups of coffee does he take? Does he wait up for the 11 o'clock news and then take in one of those late shows—for which he usually expresses nothing but scorn anyway?

The fact is that Father, living as he does, needs to cut down his caloric intake drastically—from over 3,000 calories to no more than 2,500—and he shouldn't reach 2,500 until after he has submitted himself for the next year to no more than 2,000 calories a day, to get rid of those extra dozen pounds.

A calorie is a calorie is a calorie, which means that if he has a couple of drinks one night, he better cut off 300 calories at dinner or at least during the course of the twenty-four hours following the drinks. He also needs to cut down on fat, salt, and cholesterol. Starting with breakfast, if there is one dish he does not need it is high-fat, high-cholesterol, high-calorie fried eggs and bacon. If he is very careful the rest of the week, he can have two poached eggs on Sunday. That's it! The rest of the week, breakfast should consist of a glass of orange juice, a muffin with some marmalade, or some cereal with low-fat milk and coffee or tea. Nothing else—unless he can convince the rest of the family that he is going to spend the morning chopping down trees or plowing a rocky field behind a brace of insubordinate oxen. . . .

For lunch, a single sandwich and one cup of soup—or a limited amount of grilled meat or fish, with a boiled or baked potato, a salad with low-calorie dressing, and or fruit—should enable him to last until a light, low-fat dinner, emphasizing low-fat fish and poultry.

If he likes a just-before-bed bite, make it even lighter. Cottage cheese makes a fine snack. Fresh, frozen, or canned fruit is the ideal dessert, but go easy on the syrup in canned and frozen fruits. If there is one source of calories that the dieter can cut down without any real loss of useful nutrients, it is sugar.

The wife actually eats more sensibly than other members of her family. She watches her figure. She does not eat large meals but spreads her intake over the day. The main nutritional problem is often anemia, particularly if she menstruates fairly heavily each month. She should seek sources of iron.

Less vulnerable to cardiovascular diseases than her husband (at least until the menopause), she can afford to eat an egg every morning and is, in fact, well advised to do so. She should still avoid bacon. Enriched bread, toast, or a muffin with some margarine go nicely with the egg. And, of course, she needs orange juice, or another good source of vitamin C, as much as anybody. A light lunch or a couple of nutritious snacks stand her in fine stead until dinner. Cottage cheese is a high-protein, high-calcium, low-calorie dish. A dish of chicken livers and a slice of calf liver, each once a week, are excellent sources of the iron she needs. Her dinner (and after-dinner snack) can be the same as the one she serves the other members of her family.

But while she is being kind to herself, she should try not to keep on feeding her sedentary (executive, professional, or bureaucratic) husband as if he were a high school sophomore going out for wrestling. She should try not to chide her teenage daughter for eating less than Father (and twice as much as Mother) and try not to complain that her teenage son (who is on the cross-country track team) is nibbling all the time and not honoring the massive amounts of meat, french fries, pie, and ice cream that she periodically places before him.

General Rules

She should keep in mind certain general rules that apply not only to her husband and herself, but to all those in her dietary care: young or old, active or sedentary.

For example, everybody in the family needs plenty of fluids, particularly in the summer and particularly as far as water requirements are concerned, it matters little whether it is provided by whole or skim milk, fruit juices, tea, coffee or beer, soft drinks high or low in calories, fizzy water or aqua pura. Obviously, these beverages do differ in calories and in their effect on the teeth and arteries.

Although everyone in the family needs enough calories, no one should eat too much. All foods contribute calories—not just carbohydrates or "fattening food" or solid foods, but all foods: avocados or apples, beans or beer, cabbages or cucumbers, and so on down the alphabet. Carbohydrates and proteins contribute 120 calories per ounce, fats 270 calories per ounce, and 100-proof alcohol 105 calories per fluid ounce. Again, while the form of the calories makes little or no difference as far as how "fattening" they are, it makes a lot of difference in terms of how healthy one is.

Everybody in the family needs enough protein. This does not mean the enormous amounts of protein most American males think necessary. A little over two ounces a day is plenty for each member of the family, except perhaps a rapidly growing teenager or a pregnant woman. Even in their cases, the recommended three ounces is meant to give them a very large margin of safety. You could get your two ounces of protein daily by eating merely four ounces of chicken, one cup of beans, one egg, two slices of bread, and two cups of milk. Half the protein requirement can be adequately covered by animal products—such as milk and cheese, eggs, meat and fish—and half by vegetable products, bread, and cereal products (beans, peas, nuts, rice, corn, breakfast cereals, macaronis).

Everybody in the family needs some polyunsaturated fatty acids (corn, cottonseed, soybean, peanut or safflower oil, polyunsaturated margarines, fish) and a generous supply of vitamins and minerals. . . .

These are found in animal products and in whole grain or enriched cereals; but the best sources come from a generous intake of fruits and vegetables. Certainly, if we look at the diet of Americans of all ages, the most serious fault is an insufficient intake of fruits and vegetables.

Let us look now at the ways in which the other members of a family differ.

Teenagers, especially athletic ones, have higher requirements for protein and nutrients than adults of the same sex. It is very important that their diet be varied and that they avoid fad diets that might cut out whole classes of food, such as bread or animal products. On the other hand, this is an age group often particularly addicted to sugar in every form—soft drinks, candy bars, gooey desserts, and so on.

Teenagers should certainly not be exposed to temptation at home. Remember that active boys and girls need and want a lot of fluid, particularly in the summer, and that a six-pack of sweet soft drink will vanish very fast. So if you stock up on soft drinks, buy the low-calorie or calorie-free variety. And keep alternative sources of fluid in the icebox.

The skeleton in adolescents is still developing; therefore, make sure that there are good sources of calcium in the refrigerator: cheese, cottage cheese, yogurt, as well as milk. And remember, too, that anemia is a common risk during young womanhood. Give your teenage girl a couple of poached eggs every day; encourage her to eat enriched bread and chicken or calf liver. The teenage boy should taper off some of those high-cholesterol eggs as he reaches manhood.

The child, oddly enough, is the only member of the whole family who can appropriately consume the typical American diet. Those fried eggs and bacon, so deadly for the father (who usually eats them), are a fine breakfast for children (who usually don't). Breakfast cereals and milk are all right for them if they go easy on the sugar. (Aside from the empty-calories problem, how many children do brush their teeth after breakfast?)

Enriched bread and a glass of milk are a good substitute for the cereals—or a good addition to the lot. And don't forget the orange juice. There is a long morning ahead for the schoolchild; school lunch may not be served until 1 P.M., and you'll never know if your child even ate it.

Regarding soft drinks, candy, and similar items, don't make a fetish of forbidding sweets (any strict, emphasized prohibition is likely to be as effective as the Volstead Act), but don't use sweets as rewards or have them around as temptations. Above all, don't fall into a rut and feed children very few types of foods. Get them accustomed to a variety of foods, particularly those such as liver and fish, that will be healthful to them as adults, even though they can well tolerate the omelets, fried eggs, butter, and ice cream which Daddy should eat sparingly.

In the Boston area, we find that close to 20 percent of youngsters are obese by the time they graduate from high school, half of them having entered first grade too fat. Which leads me to an important point. Milk is a great food for children, but even they can overconsume it. No child needs more than a quart a day. We see a number of small children who are fat and anemic because they have had too much milk and too little iron-containing vegetables, enriched cereals, or liver.

The elderly don't get around as much as they once did, so they require less food than a middle-aged adult. This makes it all the more important that Grandfather's and Grandmother's diet be varied. Lack of teeth, fatigue, and loneliness (even when they don't live alone) too often militate in favor of a monotonous diet. And, of couse, a restriction of choices can spell danger. Anemia is common in older men as well as older women.

It is important for the heart and blood vessels of older people, as well as for the enjoyment of continued ease of motion, that their weight not go up. The bones of the elderly are already likely to lose calcium, without adding the risk of a low-calcium diet. A breakfast of enriched cereals, skim milk and fruit; a lunch with liver at regular intervals; and a lighter version of the adult dinner, with some fish, lean meat, or cheese, salads for bulk and nutrients, fruit, and skim milk for a beverage, will do splendidly.

Remember, a wise planner and good cook will serve food that everybody enjoys and will continue to enjoy in good health and good shape for a long time.

Table 41.1 Three-Day Family Meal Plan

	Day 1	Day 2	Day 3
Breakfast			
Mother	1 boiled egg, 1 English muffin and margarine, ½ cup orange juice, coffee	1 cup oatmeal with tablespoons raisins and milk, ½ cup orange juice, 1 slice cinnamon toast, 1 cup skim milk, coffee	½ cup 100 percent bran cereal with skim milk, ½ cup prune juice, 1 slice toast with margarine, coffee
Father (dieting)	Dry cereal and skim milk instead of egg; otherwise, same as mother	Same as mother	Same as mother, but 1 cup cereal, 2 pieces toast
Grandmother	Same as mother	Same as mother but no toast	Same as mother
Teenage boy	Same as mother but *also* bowl of cereal; no coffee	Same as mother but twice as much toast and orange juice	Peanut butter sandwich, 1 glass milk, 8-ounce glass orange juice
Preschool girl	Same as mother but only half a muffin and skim milk, no coffee	Same as mother, but half portions	Same as mother although she may choose a different cereal
Morning snack			
Mother	Coffee, ½ cup water-packed peaches	Coffee, 1 slice toast and jelly	Coffee, 1 English muffin, and 1 teaspoon marmalade.
Father	Coffee only	Coffee only	Coffee only
Grandmother	No snack	Coffee only	No snack
Teenage boy	No snack—in school	No snack	No snack
Preschool girl	Same as mother but skim milk instead of coffee	Milk instead of coffee plus apple later in the morning	Same as mother but milk instead of coffee
Lunch			
Mother	1 tuna salad sandwich, dark bread; 1 cup skim milk; ½ cup applesauce; 3 carrot sticks	1 cup tomato soup, 1 cup raw spinach, 1 hard-boiled egg, 1 ounce sardines, low-calorie salad dressing, fruit gelatin, skim milk	¾ cup chili-beef soup, ½ cup cottage cheese on 2 peach halves and lettuce, skim milk
Father	Same as mother	Eats at work: 1 cup skim milk, lean steak sandwich, green beans, coffee, fruit cup	Carries lunch: 1 sliced-chicken sandwich, (lettuce but no mayonnaise), coffee, skim milk, pear
Grandmother	Same as mother	Same as mother	Same as mother
Teenage boy	Eat hot lunch at school (600–700 calories)	School lunch (600–700 calories)	Same as mother School lunch (600–700 calories)

Preschool girl	Same as mother but half portions	Same as mother except for salad; she has American cheese sandwich instead.	Soup, peanut butter and jelly sandwich, milk, peach half for dessert
Afternoon snack			
Mother	Tea, 1 English muffin and diet jelly, skim milk	Tea, 2 molasses cookies	Tea, 1 cup strawberry yogurt
Father	Coffee only	Coffee only	Coffee only
Grandmother	Same as mother but no milk	Same as mother	Tea, English muffin and marmalade
Teenage boy	2 glasses skim milk, 2 English muffins and jelly	1 cup skim milk, 4 cookies	1 glass milk, English muffin and marmalade, 1 cup strawberry yogurt
Preschool girl	Same as mother but half portions	Same as mother, plus ½ glass milk mixed with tea	½ cup strawberry yogurt
Dinner			
Mother	4 ounces liver and onions, ½ cup broccoli, 1 small boiled potato, cucumber and tomato salad with low-calorie dressing, skim milk, ice cream	½ cup clear chicken consommé (from cubes), 4 ounces broiled chicken, ⅔ stalks broccoli, tossed salad with vinegar and oil, ½ cup rice pilaf, ½ cup fruit	½ cup 3-bean salad, 4 ounces fish sticks (with tomato sauce), ½ cup mashed potatoes, ½ cup peas, ½ cup fruit gelatin, skim milk, coffee.
Father	Same as mother except 6 ounces meat, and 2 potatoes	1 cup soup, ¾ cup rice, 6 ounces chicken, 2–3 stalks broccoli, salad with lemon juice, 1 cup fruit	Same as mother but 6-ounce serving fish sticks, ¾ cup potatoes, and ¾ cup gelatin
Grandmother	Same as mother	Same as mother	Same as mother but no coffee
Teenage boy	Same as father but no coffee	Same as father plus milk and nuts	Same as father but no coffee
Preschool girl	Same as mother	Same as mother plus milk and nuts	Same as mother but smaller servings
Evening snack			
Mother	3-ounce glass sauterne, 2 Swedish crisp crackers	8-ounce glass beer, 5 wheat thins	1 cup cider, 1 apple
Father	2 (8-ounce) glasses beer, 4 Swedish crisp crackers	2 (8-ounce) glasses beer, 10 wheat thins	1 glass beer, 2 apples
Grandmother	Tea, ½ cup water-packed fruit	No snack	Cider
Teenage boy	Milk shake of 1 glass skim milk whipped with ice cream	1 cup skim milk, ½ cup sherbet, apple, 10 wheat thins	Twice as much as mother plus leftover gelatin (about ½ cup)
Preschool girl	Same as brother	½ cup sherbert, 1 apple	Same as mother

Selection 42 Updating the Basic 4

Patricia Hausman

Editors' Introduction

Selection 14, "Eating in the Dark," alerts us to the fact that overconsumption of fats generally—and saturated fats in particular—as well as excessive intake of cholesterol, sugar, and salt have been related to the development of diseases currently cited as the leading causes of death: coronary heart disease, hypertension, diabetes mellitus, and atherosclerosis. In an effort to reduce the incidence of these chronic diseases, the U.S. Senate in its January 1978 report suggests the following changes in food selection and preparation:

1. Increase consumption of fruits and vegetables and whole grains;
2. Decrease consumption of meat and increase consumption of poultry and fish;
3. Decrease consumption of foods high in fat and partially substitute polyunsaturated fat for saturated fat;
4. Substitute nonfat for whole milk;
5. Decrease consumption of butterfat, eggs, and other high-cholesterol sources;
6. Decrease consumption of sugar and foods high in sugar content;
7. Decrease consumption of salt and foods high in salt content.

Most nutritionists accept these goals as a pattern that we should strive for, but also point out that decisions lie with the individual consumer who must be educated to make wise choices. The updated version of the Basic 4 incorporates these dietary goals and suggests ways they may be implemented. Caloric intake also must be adjusted to achieve and maintain desirable, or ideal, weight and thus further aid in preventing these chronic diseases. To avoid overweight, consume only as much energy (calories) as expended; if overweight, decrease energy intake (number of calories) and increase energy expenditure through exercise.

For almost twenty-five years, the last word in nutrition has been USDA's Basic 4 food guide. The four food groups—milk, meat, fruit-

Source: Adapted from Patricia Hausman, "Updating the Basic Four," *Nutrition Action* (January 1979): 8–9. Copyright © 1979, Center for Science in the Public Interest, 1755 S St., NW, Washington, D.C. 20009. Reprinted by permission.

vegetable, and grain—grace virtually all nutrition education materials, and are the basis for countless nutrition programs.

Nutritionists devised the Basic 4 in the mid-fifties to translate a myriad of nutrient recommendations into simple food choices that most people could understand. Much planning and thought went into the food guides, and what emerged was a food classification system that placed foods rich in protein, vitamin A, vitamin D, riboflavin, and calcium in the milk group; products high in protein, B vitamins, and iron in the meat group; foods especially rich in vitamins A and C and certain minerals in the fruit-vegetable group; and grain foods providing B vitamins, iron, carbohydrates, and protein in group four. Sweets, fats, and oils fall into the miscellaneous group.

But the Basic 4 has become a paradox: It was designed for good nutrition, but today it condones the major problems in our food supply. Half of all adult Americans have blood cholesterol levels above the value suggested in the National Heart, Lung, and Blood Institute's (NHLBI) handbook for physicians, yet the Basic 4 says nothing about the diet high in saturated fat and cholesterol that is so closely linked to this problem. NHLBI also estimates that 60 million Americans have definite or border-line high blood pressure, yet the Basic 4 does not address the sodium content of the American diet, which experts say contributes to this startling rate of high blood pressure. At the same time, though few Americans have nutrient deficiencies, the Basic 4 focuses on the vitamin, mineral, and protein content of the diet.

Still, the Basic 4 does provide a simple approach to nutrient adequacy, and the importance of nutrients should not be dismissed. Modifying the Basic 4's message is really all that is needed to turn its unfortunate acceptance of foods rich in salt, fat, and cholesterol into a health-promoting food guide designed to keep intake of these trouble-makers at reasonable levels. . . . [See table 42.1.]

Table 42.1 New American Eating Guide

	Anytime	In Moderation	Now and Then
Group 1: beans, grains, and nuts (Four or more servings/day)	bread and rolls (whole grain) bulgur dried beans and peas (legumes) lentils oatmeal pasta, whole wheat rice, brown rye bread sprouts whole grain hot and cold cereals whole wheat matzoh	cornbread[8] flour tortilla[8] granola cereals[1 or 2] hominy grits[8] macaroni and cheese[1, (6), 8] matzoh[8] nuts[3] pasta, except whole wheat[8] peanut butter[3] pizza[6, 8] refined, unsweetened cereals[8] refried beans, commercial,[1] or homemade in oil[2] seeds[3] soybeans[2] tofu[2] waffles or pancakes with syrup[5, (6), 8] white bread and rolls[8] white rice[8]	croissant[4, 8] doughnut (yeast leavened)[3 or 4, 5, 8] presweetened breakfast cereals[5, 8] sticky buns[1 or 2, 5, 8] stuffing (made with butter)[4, (6), 8]
Group 2: fruits and vegetables (Four or more servings/day)	all fruits and vegetables except those listed at right applesauce (unsweetened) unsweetened fruit juices unsalted vegetable juices potatoes, white or sweet	avocado[3] cole slaw[3] cranberry sauce (canned)[5] dried fruit french fries, homemade in vegetable oil,[2] commercial[1] fried eggplant (vegetable oil)[2]	coconut[4] pickles[6]

Group 3: milk products
(Children: 3 to 4 servings/day; adults: 2 servings/day)

buttermilk made from skim milk
lassi (low-fat yogurt and fruit juice drink)
low-fat cottage cheese
low-fat milk, 1 percent milkfat
low-fat yogurt
non-fat dry milk
skim milk cheeses
skim milk
skim milk and banana shake

fruits canned in syrup[5]
gazpacho[2,(6)]
glazed carrots[5,(6)]
guacamole[3]
potatoes au gratin[1,(6)]
salted vegetable juices[6]
sweetened fruit juices[5]
vegetables canned with salt[6]

cocoa made with skim milk[5]
cottage cheese, regular, 4 percent milk fat[1]
frozen low-fat yogurt[5]
ice milk[5]
low-fat milk, 2 percent milk fat[1]
low-fat yogurt, sweetened[5]
mozzarella cheese, part skim-type only[1,(6)]

cheesecake[4,5]
cheese fondue[4,(6)]
cheese soufflé[4,(6),7]
eggnog[1,5,7]
hard cheeses: bleu, brick, Camembert, cheddar, Muenster, Swiss[4,(6)]
ice cream[4,5]
processed cheeses[4,6]
whole milk[4]
whole milk yogurt[4]

Group 4: poultry, fish, meat, and eggs
(Two servings/day)[9]

fish
cod
flounder
gefilte fish[6]
haddock
halibut
perch
pollock
rockfish
shellfish, except shrimp
sole
tuna, water packed[6]
egg products
egg whites only

fish (drained well, if canned)
fried fish[1 or 2]
herring[3,6]
mackerel, canned[2,(6)]
salmon, pink, canned[2,(6)]
sardines[2,(6)]
shrimp[7]
tuna, oil packed[2,(6)]
poultry
chicken liver, baked or broiled[7] (just one)
fried chicken, home-

poultry
fried chicken, commercially prepared[4]
egg
cheese omelet[4,7]
egg yolk or whole egg (about 3/week)[3,7]
red meats
bacon[4,(6)]
beef liver, fried[1,7]
bologna[4,6]
corned beef[4,6]
ground beef[4]
ham, trimmed well[1,6]

Table 42.1 (continued)

Anytime	In Moderation	Now and Then
poultry chicken or turkey—boiled, baked or roasted (no skin)	made in vegetable oil[3] chicken or turkey, boiled, baked, or roasted (with skin)[2] red meats (trimmed of all outside fat) flank steak[1] leg or loin of lamb[1] pork shoulder or loin, lean[1] round steak or ground round[1] rump roast[1] sirloin steak, lean[1] veal[1]	hot dogs[4,6] liverwurst[4,6] pig's feet[4] salami[4,6] sausage[4,6] spareribs[4] untrimmed red meats[4]

[1]Moderate fat, saturated.

[2]Moderate fat, unsaturated.

[3]High fat, unsaturated.

[4]High fat, saturated.

[5]High in added sugar.

[6]High in salt or sodium.

(6)May be high in salt or sodium.

[7]High in cholesterol.

[8]Refined grains.

[9]Vegetarians: Nutrients in these foods can be obtained by eating more foods in groups 1, 2, and 3.

"Anytime" foods contain less than 30 percent of calories from fat and are usually low in salt and sugar. Most of the "now and then" foods contain at least 50 percent of calories from fat—and a large amount of saturated fat. Foods to eat "in moderation" have medium amounts of total fat and low to moderate amounts of saturated fat or large amounts of total fat that is mostly unsaturated. Foods meeting the standards for fat, but containing large amounts of salt or sugar, are usually moved into a more restricted category, as are refined cereal products. For example, pickles have little fat, but are so high in sodium that they fall in the "now and then" category.

Important: To cut down on salt intake, choose varieties of the foods listed here that do not have added salt, such as no-salt cottage cheese, rather than the regular varieties.
This guide is not appropriate for individuals needing very low-salt diets.

Part V

Alternatives for the Future

The first four parts of this text deal with various aspects of the food problem. This part deals with the avenues open for the future in three important areas: (1) alternative dietary patterns, (2) alternative food sources, and (3) programs, policies, and priorities for the future. Alternatives exist for individuals when making choices concerning both personal and family nutrition. Alternatives also exist for governments and public and private agencies when supporting proposed and formulated food policies.

At the microlevel the consumer should carefully weigh alternatives to the affluent diet. Eating can no longer be considered automatic behavior or a simple response to a physical need. We must ask ourselves what foods can be combined to provide substitutes for the protein customarily consumed in meat. What novel foods might be explored as possible protein sources? How can habitual eating patterns and those spawned by technology be modified in the future? Each of us must become aware that food is no longer a resource that can be taken for granted, but rather one that should be prized and utilized wisely.

Genetic engineering allows human intervention in plant breeding and makes possible the creation of new varieties of grains with improved amino acid patterns and the development of varieties that are higher in total protein content. Today, thousands of varieties of grains are being bred, collected, and analyzed in an attempt to identify those with desirable nutritional traits that genetic manipulation could then transfer to other strains. While some success has been achieved with new varieties of maize (corn), barley, and sorghum, scientists have made little progress in changing the amino acid pattern of wheat and rice. Often, however, even with those varieties developed such engineered strains are rejected in the marketplace because their texture, taste, or color differs from familiar products acceptable in a given culture.

The selections in this part begin with a look back to the early research on protein and close with a look forward to an ethically and ecologically responsible future. In considering alternatives, each of us shares responsibility not only for our own personal well-being but for the rest of the world's population in the struggle for survival. Where do *you* stand on these important ecological issues? Perhaps the following pages will help to clarify your options and suggest ways in which you, personally, can take a stand consistent with today's ecological realities.

Selection 43 Protein Requirement of Maintenance in Man

H.C. Sherman

Editors' Introduction

The historical work of Sherman and other researchers during the first half of the twentieth century provided the foundation and methodology for establishing current protein requirements and protein allowances. The critical examinations by Sherman in 1919 and 1920 of 109 experiments in 25 independent investigations, including work done in several countries, gave an average of 44 grams of protein per 70 kilograms of body weight or 0.6 grams of protein per kilogram of body weight as the minimum requirement. Later, in 1946, Stare and his co-workers reported on experiments in which 26 healthy adults were placed on a low-protein diet that was adjusted to the energy needs of the subjects, and the protein requirement was found to be between 30 and 40 grams for a 70-kilogram adult.

From the results of these classical studies, as well as more current data based on nitrogen determinations, the National Research Council RDA Committee now estimates the average minimum requirement to be 0.47 grams of protein per kilogram of body weight. The term *nitrogen balance* refers to the relationship between the nitrogen content of all the food eaten and the amount of nitrogen excreted in the feces and urine. The rationale for using the nitrogen-balance technique as a means of determining protein requirements is based on the fact that, on the average, protein contains 16 percent nitrogen, so that every gram of nitrogen going

Source: Adapted from H.C. Sherman, "Protein Requirement of Maintenance in Man and the Nutritive Efficiency of Bread Protein," *Nutrition Reviews* 35 no. 7 (July 1977); originally appeared in *Journal of Biological Chemistry* 41 (1920):97–109. Reprinted with permission of the Nutrition Foundation. Notes and references appearing in the article have been omitted here; for further information consult the original version.

in or out of the body can be assumed to be equivalent to 6.25 grams of protein. To check nitrogen balance, the subject's output is subtracted from the intake. If the nitrogen or protein in the diet is equal to or more than necessary to replace losses, nitrogen balance or equilibrium exists. Such a state is normal for the adult and indicates that there is a status quo between concurrently occurring processes in which tissues are constantly being broken down (catabolism) and tissues are constantly being synthesized (anabolism). If the intake is greater than the output, positive nitrogen balance exists. It means that new tissues are being synthesized as normally occurs during growth in childhood and during pregnancy and lactation. If the intake is less than the output, the subject is said to be in negative nitrogen balance and net decrease in body protein occurs. This undesirable state occurs in an otherwise healthy individual when the quantity or quality of the protein in the diet is inadequate for tissue replacement or when the diet does not contain adequate amounts of carbohydrate and fat, and protein is used as a source of energy.

The following selection, a nutrition classic, is an abstract of an article that appeared in the *Journal of Biological Chemistry* in 1920. Sherman reports on protein requirements and points out that cereal proteins supplemented with small amounts of milk are as efficient as high-quality protein in an ordinary mixed diet in maintaining nitrogen equilibrium. His work is of particular significance today when we are concerned about the ability to meet quantitative and qualitative protein requirements throughout the world.

In connection with our studies of nutritive requirements and of the efficiency of the proteins of the cereal grains in the maintenance metabolism of man we have taken occasion to bring together the results of such of the earlier experiments upon the protein requirement of maintenance as seem to lend themselves to direct quantitative comparison. The purpose of the present paper is to present as concisely as possible the net result of this study of the literature together with the data of our own experiments upon a dietary in which nearly all the nitrogen was taken in the form of wheat bread.

Probably the best present indication of the normal protein or nitrogen requirement is to be obtained by averaging the observed nitrogen output in all available experiments in which the intake appears to have been barely sufficient or not quite sufficient to result in equilibrium of intake and output.

Since the protein minimum thus determined is influenced by the protein-sparing action of carbohydrates and fats, the results will be comparable, and will bear directly upon the practical problems of protein requirement in food economics, only in those cases in which the energy value of the experimental ration is at least approximately adjusted to the energy requirement of the subject.

In order to minimize the personal equation in our interpretation of the work of others, we have uniformly excluded from table 43.1 all experiments showing a loss of body nitrogen greater than 1 gram per day even though in some cases this necessitated the omission of data of undoubted value.

There remained 109 experiments belonging to 25 different investigations and including 67 experiments upon 29 men and 42 experiments upon 8 women subjects. For convenience of comparison the total nitrogen output per day (urine and feces) is computed to a basis of 70 kilograms of body weight and multiplied by 6.25 to express the corresponding amount of protein which is tabulated as the "indicated protein requirement" in each of the 109 experiments as shown in table 43.1.

The general average of the 109 experiments shows an indicated requirement of 0.635 gram of protein per kilogram of body weight, or 44.4 grams per "average man" or 70 kilograms, per day. Two considerations, one favorable the other unfavorable, should be kept in mind in attempting to judge the scientific value of this average. On the one hand, it represents a very large amount of work in several different laboratories and on many subjects, both men and women, so that errors due to individual peculiarities of subjects, diets, or conditions, or the personal equation of the investigator are minimized. On the other hand, the data of individual experiments are rather divergent, ranging from a minimum of 21 grams to a maximum of 65 grams per 70 kilograms. It should perhaps be noted that the very large majority of these experiments (94 in 109) yield values within the limits of 29 to 56 grams per 70 kilograms, and that these more concordant data taken separately show an indicated protein requirement averaging 42.8 grams per 70 kilograms based on 94 experiments covering 34 subjects (26 men and 8 women) studied in 23 different investigations. If we go a step further in rejecting the extremes, we find within the limits of 30 to 50 grams per 70 kilograms per day, 76 experiments belonging to 19 different investigations, including 24 subjects (20 men and 4 women) and averaging 40.6 grams per man of 70 kilograms, or 0.58 grams per kilogram of body weight per day.

The efficiencies actually found in our typical experiments in which the protein consumed was almost entirely in the form of ordinary wheat bread, or of hard bread made from cornmeal or oatmeal.

The proteins of wheat, corn, and oats appear to be about equally efficient in adult human nutrition and need only be supplemented with small amounts of milk in order to be fully as efficient as the proteins of ordinary mixed diets have been found to be in earlier investigations. Our

Table 43.1 Indicated Protein Requirements per 70 Kilograms of Body Weight

Experiment Number	Indicated Protein Requirement (grams)	Experiment Number	Indicated Protein Requirement (grams)	Experiment Number	Indicated Protein Requirement (grams)	Experiment Number	Indicated Protein Requirement (grams)	Experiment Number	Indicated Protein Requirement (grams)
1	39	23	45	45	31	67	56	89	37
2	38	24	49	46	37	68	57	90	38
3	45	25	56	47	45	69	60	91	39
4	33	26	47	48	50	70	57	92	39
5	30	27	62	49	39	71	54	93	39
6	65	28	61	50	52	72	51	94	43
7	61	29	55	51	52	73	52	95	40
8	41	30	53	52	42	74	54	96	39
9	50	31	53	53	42	75	54	97	43
10	43	32	61	54	24	76	53	98	38
11	37	33	40	55	21	77	53	99	37
12	29	34	56	56	33	78	44	100	33
13	59	35	43	57	32	79	45	101	37
14	57	36	42	58	32	80	46	102	41
15	49	37	41	59	39	81	46	103	51
16	42	38	39	60	50	82	42	104	44
17	50	39	48	61	58	83	41	105	42
18	48	40	46	62	37	84	36	106	32
19	49	41	38	63	41	85	38	107	35
20	54	42	47	64	44	86	39	108	34
21	36	43	36	65	59	87	39	109	32
22	47	44	37	66	60	88	38		
Average	44.4								

findings for these cereal proteins are therefore similar to that of Hindhede for wheat bread and show their efficiency to be much higher than was reported by Karl Thomas for either wheat or maize.

Thus from the more recent and more carefully controlled experiments it appears that, even when the protein of the food is almost entirely derived from bread or other grain products, with a diet adequate in energy value a daily intake of about 0.5 grams of protein per kilogram of body weight is sufficient to meet the actual requirements of maintenance in healthy men and women. While if numerous older experiments having a tendency to high results are included the average is somewhat less than ⅔ gram of protein per kilogram of body weight. A standard allowance of 1 gram of protein per kilogram of body weight per day appears, therefore, to provide a margin of safety of 50 to 100 percent as far as the requirements of adult maintenance are concerned.

Selection 44 World Food Patterns and Protein Economy

Marion McGill
Orrea F. Pye

Editors' Introduction

Health, economic, and ecological advantages result from curbing excessive consumption of (1) meat and other animal protein products, (2) food in general (a lower caloric intake will allow us to achieve and maintain normal weight), and (3) convenience foods. Let us review some basic facts in order to better understand why our present eating patterns result in the uneconomical use of food and energy resources.

A pound of animal protein requires seven times as much energy on the average to produce as a pound of plant protein. Using USDA data, Frances Moore Lappé, author of *Diet for a Small Planet,* has shown that the production of one pound of beef, pork, turkey, chicken, and eggs requires 16, 6, 4, 3, and 3 pounds of grain and soy, respectively. The RDA for protein per day for a woman

Source: Adapted from Marion McGill and Orrea F. Pye, "World Food Patterns and Protein Economy," pp. 3–4. © 1975 UNA, N.J. Division (P.O. Box 4068 Ampere Station, E. Orange, N.J. 07019). Reprinted by permission.

over 19 years is 44 grams and for a man over 22 years is 56 grams. These protein recommendations are not minimum requirements; they include a generous safety margin above the average requirements. The average American consumes 101 grams of protein per day. Over 69 percent of the protein comes from animal products. This consumption pattern reflects our nation's overconcentration on meat, poultry, and fish as a source of protein.

Liberal nutritionists recommend a dietary pattern in which the protein content is reduced to the RDA and in which 40 to 50 percent of the protein comes from animal sources. The excessive use of protein foods, and particularly the excessive consumption characteristic of the affluent American diet in the Satisfied World, represents a tremendous waste of grain and soy products that could be used to feed people in the Hungry World. Convenience or prepared foods often require more energy to produce than do individual items cooked from basic ingredients.

In part II we note that fuel energy is scarce and that developing nations need this energy to manufacture and produce machinery and nitrogen fertilizers as well as to develop irrigation systems necessary to increase agricultural productivity.

If some countries turn to grain for the production of fuel (gasohol) this conversion must be recognized as a potential diminution of food stores. This conversion would have serious consequences in areas of the world where food is already in short supply.

In the following selection Marion McGill, a well-known nutritionist and magazine food editor, and Professor Orrea F. Pye, a distinguished nutrition educator, explore a number of alternatives for those who would like to move toward greater conservation of protein and food energy resources. Among the suggested alternatives for meal planning is the use of smaller, rather than larger, portions of meat, fish, and poultry in combination with grains and vegetables. Those who wish to achieve even greater levels of conservation may decide to exclude animal flesh from their diets and meet their protein requirements by using milk and eggs in combination with grains and vegetables or by using vegetable protein combinations for meatless meals.

Recipes for all levels of conservation are given in the following selection. In the spirit of food adventure, you may find it rewarding to experiment with these dishes that are representative of cuisines from all over the world.

Many Americans may wish to cut down on their consumption of meat, especially prime beef, for humanitarian reasons, to help over the long term in making more calories and protein available for starving and malnourished children, as world food supplies become increasingly scarce. Meanwhile we can develop worldwide plans for wiser policies of food distribution to supply surplus food to starving areas.

Other Americans may feel no moral responsibility for food crisis conditions of death, starvation, and malnutrition in underdeveloped, overpopulated lands. But for these other Americans there are other compelling reasons to curb excessive consumption of meat and other animal protein foods, an uneconomical use of food energy. . . .

Health authorities for some time have been telling us that Americans have been consuming too much meat containing saturated fat, increasing one risk factor related to the highest incidence of coronary heart disease in the world. The American Heart Association has advised that meat consumption be reduced at least by one-third. Recent studies stress the importance of fiber in diets, another reason eating more whole grain and vegetables and less meat is indicated for health. So Americans would help themselves by curbing meat consumption.

Very persuasive reasons for cutting down on meat consumption (especially for the future) are the ecological and economic ones. Excessive meat production uses more of the scarce basic energy resources of the United States and runs up the price of grain and other food for Americans as well as those in other nations.

Americans have been profligate with their abundant resources but continued waste of food and basic energy reserves cannot continue unchecked in the future without dire consequences for generations to come. A fundamental question . . . is: Will we continue on our current extravagant course or will we start to plan and to conserve resources for future Americans?

The pages of explanation that follow and the recipes are for those citizens who would like to move toward greater conservation of food energy resources. There are suggested recipes for all levels of conservation:

1. including smaller amounts of meat combined with grains and vegetables rather than larger servings of meat;
2. using more fish, poultry, and especially milk and eggs combined with grains and vegetables;
3. using vegetable protein combinations for meatless meals. . . .

Wheat

Wheat is the major grain of the Western world because of its pleasing flavor and versatility. It is still eaten in the Mediterranean countries similar to the way the men who built the pyramids ate it. Steamed plain or spiced, with or without meats and vegetables, pilaf or couscous are the main dishes of the diet. Wheat was used for the unleavened bread of that area, as it is today. But one of the proteins in wheat, gluten, makes it possible for wheat to become a workable and stretchable dough. As such it makes the pasta of Italy; and as other cuisines developed, wheat became noodles, dumplings, all sorts of breads or cakes cooked on a griddle and leavened bread. Leavened bread was termed the *the staff of life*, which it has been for many people for many centuries. In the light of present day science we know wheat protein is low in the essential amino acid, lysine; in other words, it is not a complete protein. However, . . . all essential amino acids do not need to come from one food protein. Again, one complete protein, or one complete and one incomplete protein, or two or more incomplete or partially complete food proteins (if they are truly complementary in essential amino acid composition) can supply all needed amino acids when eaten together. The age-old custom of having a bit of broiled meat with pilaf or in the couscous, including yogurt in a meal, sprinkling cheese on pasta, adding dumplings to a meat dish, and serving a bite of cheese with crackers or bread, completed the wheat protein pattern, and even lentils supply complementary protein to wheat. Thus a large amount of meat is unnecessary, and wheat protein is fully utilized.

One point to be kept in mind is that the best quality protein of the grain is in the germ. Therefore, whole wheat and in general whole grain contains a slightly better quality of protein than the milled grain. Thus, for example, whole wheat flour is superior to white flour, including enriched flour, in terms of protein quality and certain other nutrients.

Baked Macaroni *(Switzerland)*

Total protein 87.5 grams
Protein per serving 14.6 grams

1 package (8 ounces) elbow macaroni
3 tablespoons butter or margarine
1 cup grated process Swiss cheese
    (4 ounces)
1 cup fresh bread crumbs
2 eggs

2 cups milk
½ teaspoon dry mustard
¼ teaspoon salt
¼ teaspoon pepper

Preheat oven to 350° F. Cook macaroni in boiling salted water, according to package directions; drain; pour into a 2-quart baking dish. Melt butter in a small saucepan; drizzle 2 tablespoons over hot macaroni; stir in cheese until melted. Toss bread crumbs with remaining butter in saucepan. In small bowl beat eggs slightly with milk, mustard, salt, and pepper; pour over macaroni mixture; sprinkle with buttered crumbs. Bake 45 minutes or until set. Serves 6.

Bread Pudding *(England)*

Total protein 85.6 grams
Protein per serving 11 grams

12 to 15 day-old slices small French
    bread, ½-inch thick
4 cups milk
4 tablespoons butter or margarine
4 eggs

½ cup sugar
¼ teaspoon salt
¼ teaspoon nutmeg
1 teaspoon vanilla extract

Preheat oven to 325° F. Arrange about ⅓ of the bread in single layer in a buttered, shallow, 6-cup baking dish. Place remaining slices overlapping on top. Heat milk and butter until butter is melted. Beat eggs until blended; beat in sugar, salt, nutmeg, vanilla extract, and the hot milk. Strain over bread, moistening pieces evenly. Set baking dish in a pan on oven rack. Pour boiling water into pan to 1-inch depth. Bake 45 minutes or until knife inserted in custard comes out clean. Remove baking dish to wire rack. Serve warm or chilled. Serves 8.

Tamales *(Panama)*

Total protein 153.3 grams
Protein per serving 25.5 grams

2 cups white or yellow cornmeal
1 cup sifted all-purpose flour
2 teaspoons baking powder
2 teaspoons salt

1½ cups water
½ cup shortening, softened
    meat filling for tamales
    [see following recipe]

In top of double boiler mix cornmeal, flour, baking powder, and salt. Stir in water until dry ingredients are moistened, then blend in shortening. Cook over low heat, stirring constantly, until mixture bubbles at edge. Place over boiling water. Cook, stirring once or twice, 20 minutes. Mixture will be very thick. Remove from heat. Cut 12 pieces cooking parchment 12 × 8 inches. Spread warm cornmeal dough about ¼ inch thick over parchment, spreading to one 12-inch edge and leaving 1 inch uncovered on opposite side, and leaving 2 inches uncovered on each end. Spoon 2 tablespoons filling lengthwise down center of cornmeal dough. Fold dough-covered edge a little more than half way over filling, then fold opposite side over so dough just overlaps. Fold over ends of parchment to meet in center. Place tamales, folded side down, in a large colander. Place colander in deep kettle and pour water into kettle to within 1 inch of colander. Bring to boiling, reduce heat, but water must continue to boil, cover, and steam tamales for 1 hour. Add more boiling water as needed. Remove tamales with tongs, to heated serving platter. Serves 6.

Meat Filling for Tamales

2 tablespoons olive or vegetable oil
1 pound boneless pork, cubed
2 onions, sliced
1 clove garlic, crushed
1 can (8 ounces) tomato sauce
2 teaspoons salt
½ teaspoon pepper

¼ teaspoon dried oregano leaves
1 tablespoon vinegar
1 whole chicken breast, boned
1 apple, peeled, cored, and diced
12 stuffed green olives or pitted ripe
    olives, halved
2 tablespoons dark raisins

In Dutch oven in hot olive oil brown the pork cubes on all sides. Reduce heat and sauté onion and garlic until golden. Stir in tomato sauce, salt, pepper, oregano, and vinegar. Add chicken breast. Cover, cook over low heat, stirring frequently, 1 hour or until meat is soft. (Add small amounts of water or tomato juice if mixture becomes dry.) Remove chicken breast and dice finely. Return diced chicken; add apple, olives and raisins. Cook 5 to 6 minutes. Remove from heat. Let cool. Makes enough for 12 tamales.

Succotash   (United States)

Total protein 30.5 grams
Protein per serving 5 grams

1 package (10 ounces) frozen baby
    lima beans
1 package (10 ounces) frozen kernel
    corn

¼ cup milk
salt
pepper

Cook lima beans according to package directions; drain. Cook corn according to package direction; drain. Add milk to beans, mashing a few to thicken liquid. Add corn and season with salt and pepper. Cook, stirring gently until not quite boiling. Serves 6.

Tacos   (Mexico)

Total protein 76.8 grams
Protein per serving 6.4 grams

⅓ cup olive or vegetable oil
1 package (9 ounces) frozen tortillas
1½ cups refried beans (Frijoles
    Refritos) . . . [see
    following recipe]

¾ cup grated cheddar cheese
chopped green onions
shredded lettuce

Heat oil in small skillet. With tongs drop each tortilla in oil and fry 3 or 4 minutes. Remove to paper towel and fold in half. Fill each with 2 tablespoons refried beans, then a tablespoon grated cheese, a sprinkling of onion and then shredded lettuce. These are eaten like a sandwich. Makes 12.

Frijoles Refritos   *(Mexico)*

Total protein 91.6 grams
Protein per serving 11.5 grams

2 cups red or pinto beans
6 cups water

2 teaspoons salt
½ cup lard or bacon fat

Soak and cook washed beans according to directions . . . cooking beans at least 2 hours or until very tender and liquid is like gravy. Drain beans, reserving liquid. Melt half the lard in a heavy skillet. Add some of the beans, and mash them with a fork into the fat. Continue adding beans and lard until all are used, at the same time adding some of the bean liquid until mixture is smooth and the fat absorbed. Serve with grated cheese. (This may also be served with meats.) Serves 8.

Note: A quick version of Frijoles Refritos can be made with canned kidney beans. Use 1 can (16 ounces) red kidney beans and 4 tablespoons lard or bacon fat. Drain beans. Heat lard. Add beans and mash as above. Add bean liquid, a small amount at a time until all fat has been absorbed. Serves 4.

Egg Pasta   *(Italy)*

Total protein 57 grams
Protein per serving 9.5 grams

3 cups all-purpose flour
1 teaspoon salt

3 eggs
3 tablespoons water

Sift flour and salt into a bowl. Make a well in center. Add eggs and water. Work liquid into flour to make a stiff dough. Turn out dough on a lightly floured board and knead until smooth and elastic, about 10 minutes. Cover with a bowl and let rest 1 hour. Divide into quarters. Keep pieces covered until ready to roll out. Roll out one-quarter at a time into a rectangle about 14×10 inches and almost paper thin. Cut into ⅛ to ¼-inch wide strips for noodles, or cut in squares for ravioli or manicotti. Serves 6. Serve with meat or tomato sauce and cheese. 1 tablespoon grated Parmesan cheese contains 2.2 grams protein.

Meat Sauce for Pasta   *(Italy)*

Total protein 88 grams
Protein per serving 11 grams

1 cup chopped onion
1 clove garlic, crushed
1 tablespoon olive or vegetable oil
½ pound ground beef
½ pound ground pork
1 can (39 ounces) peeled
    tomatoes with basil leaf
1 can (6 ounces) tomato paste

½ cup water or wine
1 tablespoon chopped parsley
1 tablespoon sugar
2 teaspoons salt
1 teaspoon dried basil leaves
½ teaspoon dried oregano leaves
dash pepper

In large skillet sauté onion and garlic in oil until transparent. Add beef and pork and sauté, stirring frequently, until red color disappears. Stir in tomatoes, tomato paste, water, parsley, sugar, salt, basil leaves, oregano leaves, and pepper. Bring to boiling, cover. Reduce heat and simmer, stirring occasionally, 1 hour, adding water if needed. Serves 6 or 8, or enough for 1 pound of pasta.

Spaghetti with Clam Sauce   *(Italy)*

Total protein 91.6 grams
Protein per serving 15 grams

1 package (16 ounces) spaghetti
2 cloves garlic, crushed
3 tablespoons butter or margarine
1 tablespoon olive or vegetable oil

1 can (3 ounces) sliced mushrooms
2 cans (about 7 ounces each) minced
    clams
¼ cup chopped parsley
¼ teaspoon pepper

Cook spaghetti in boiling salted water according to package directions; drain. While spaghetti cooks, sauté garlic in butter and oil until transparent. Stir in mushrooms and liquid, clams and liquid, parsley, and pepper. Simmer 5 minutes. Place drained spaghetti in large bowl; pour sauce over; toss to mix well. Serves 6.

Stuffed Fish Fillets   *(Scandinavia)*

Total protein 143 grams
Protein per serving 22 grams

1 egg
2 cups fresh bread crumbs (4 slices)
1 tablespoon chopped parsley
½ teaspoon dried dill weed

½ teaspoon salt
6 fresh fillets of sole or flounder
2 tablespoons butter or margarine
1 tablespoon lemon juice

Preheat open to 350° F. Beat egg. Add bread crumbs, parsley, dill weed, and salt. Mix well. Lay fillets flat, spread with stuffing, dividing evenly. Roll up lengthwise; fasten with wooden picks. Place seam side down in shallow baking dish. Dot with butter, and drizzle with lemon juice. Cover dish with foil. Bake for 30 to 35 minutes or until fish flakes when tried with a fork. Serve with lemon butter or parsely sauce. Serves 6.

Wheat Pilavi   *(Turkey)*

Total protein 14.3 grams
Protein per serving 3.6 grams

1 small onion, chopped
2 tablespoons vegetable oil
½ cup bulgur or cracked wheat

2 cups beef broth or 2 beef bouillon
    cubes and 2 cups water

Preheat oven to 350° F. Sauté onion in oil until golden. Add wheat and stir until oil is absorbed. Cook 1 or 2 minutes, stirring constantly, then add beef broth. Pour into a baking dish. Cover and bake 1 hour or until wheat is tender. Serves 4.

Pasta e Fagioli *(Italy)*
(Pasta and Beans)

Total protein 93.3 grams
Protein per serving 12 grams

1 cup chopped onion
1 clove garlic, crushed
2 tablespoons olive or vegetable oil
2 chicken bouillon cubes
4 cups water
1 package (8 ounces) macaroni shells
1 can (16 ounces) tomatoes

2 cans (16 ounces each) red kidney
    beans
1 bay leaf
1 teaspoon salt
½ teaspoon dried oregano leaves
¼ teaspoon pepper
½ cup grated Parmesan cheese
chopped parsley

Sauté onion and garlic in oil in Dutch oven until golden. Add bouillon cubes and water and bring to boiling. Add macaroni shells; cook 10 to 12 minutes or until almost tender. Add tomatoes, kidney beans, bay leaf, salt, oregano, and pepper. Cook 15 minutes or until flavors are well blended and macaroni is tender. Serve in soup bowls sprinkled with Parmesan cheese and parsley. Serves 8.

Minestrone *(Italy)*

Total protein 151 grams
Protein per serving 19 grams

1 cup dried large white beans
5 cups water
2 pounds beef shank, crosscut
2 tablespoons vegetable oil
1 cup chopped onion
1 clove garlic, crushed
4 cups shredded cabbage

2 cups sliced carrots
1 can (16 ounces) stewed tomatoes
2 teaspoons salt
1 teaspoon dried basil leaves
¼ teaspoon pepper
1 cup elbow macaroni

Wash beans and drain. Combine with water in large kettle or Dutch oven; bring to boiling. Remove from heat, let stand 1 hour. Brown beef shanks in oil; remove and add to beans. Sauté onion and garlic in drippings until golden; add to beans. Cover, bring to boiling, reduce heat and simmer 1½ hours or until meat is tender. Remove shanks and cut meat from bones; cut meat in small cubes and return to beans. Add cabbage, carrots, tomatoes, salt, basil, pepper, and a little water if needed. Cook 30 minutes or until vegetables are tender. Add macaroni and cook 15 minutes longer or until macaroni is tender. Serve in large soup bowls sprinkled with Parmesan cheese. Serves 8.

Parathas *(India)*
(Filled Whole Wheat Turnovers)

Total protein 97.3 grams
Protein per turnover 5.4 grams

4½ cups whole wheat flour
2 teaspoons salt
1¾ cups water
¼ cup milk

6 tablespoons melted butter or
    margarine
Spicy green pea filling [see following
    recipe]
2 tablespoons vegetable oil

Combine flour and salt in large mixing bowl. Beat in water and milk. (Mixture will be very thin.) Let stand 1½ hours. Meanwhile make the spicy green pea filling. When ready, beat the batter 15 to 20 times or until it becomes an elastic dough. Turn half of dough onto a lightly floured board. Roll out as thinly as possible into a square. Brush with 1½ tablespoons of the melted butter. Fold in half. Brush with another 1½ tablespoons butter and fold in half in opposite direction, to make a square. Roll out to ⅛-inch thickness (about 9 × 9 inches). Cut into 3-inch squares. Measure out half of filling. Place a mound of filling in center of each square, dividing evenly. Moisten squares around edges and fold diagonally to make triangles. Press edges together well to seal. Repeat with remaining dough, butter, and filling. Heat oil in large heavy skillet. Sauté triangles, 3 or 4 at a time, until crisp and golden on each side, adding oil if needed. Keep warm until all are sautéed. Makes 18.

Spicy Green Pea Filling   *(India)*

Total protein 15.3 grams

1 package (10 ounces) frozen green
    peas
2 tablespoons butter or margarine
1 tablespoon finely chopped mint
1 tablespoon finely chopped parsley

1 teaspoon onion salt
¼ teaspoon cayenne pepper
2 tablespoons water
2 teaspoons lemon juice

Thaw frozen peas. Heat butter in a heavy saucepan and add mint, parsley, onion salt and pepper. Sauté 1 minute. Add peas and water; stir to mix. Cover, and cook over very low heat until peas are tender. Remove from heat. Puree peas in a blender or press through a sieve. Stir in lemon juice. Let cool.

Rice

The rice bowl is the symbol of the Orient, as rice has been the mainstay of the peoples of that vast region. Rice does not have the versatility of wheat, because it does not have a protein like gluten, which enables it to be used in many forms. Rice is eaten as rice. But it is combined in myriad ways and accompanies many spiced and flavorful meats and vegetables and combinations of both as the fried rices and curries of the Orient. As rice became known in the Mediterranean lands it was used the same way as wheat in pilafs and such dishes. When it moved to northern Europe, its bland flavor made it popular to use with cheese and milk in croquettes and puddings.

Rice has a reasonably good assortment of amino acids although rice proteins are not complete. Hence to obtain sufficient quantities of the essential amino acids, rice proteins must be eaten with complete food proteins or food proteins complementary to rice proteins. The rice combinations that follow represent such complementary mixtures. The rice and bean dishes used by Puerto Ricans and others represent naturally selected complementary combinations. Nuts also supplement rice in protein quality. The foods containing complete animal protein used in relatively small amounts (milk, cheese, eggs, poultry, fish, and meat) with rice can supply an excellent essential amino acid pattern.

Rice Custard Pudding   *(England)*

Total protein 53.4 grams
Protein per serving 9 grams

2 cups milk
3 eggs
⅓ cup sugar
¼ teaspoon salt

1 teaspoon vanilla extract
1 cup cooked white rice
¼ cup light raisins

Preheat oven to 325° F. Heat milk in heavy saucepan just until steaming. In large bowl beat eggs, sugar, salt and vanilla extract until well blended. Beat in milk; stir in rice and raisins. Pour into a 6-cup baking dish. Place baking dish in a pan on oven rack. Pour boiling water into pan to depth of 1 inch. Bake 45 minutes to 1 hour or until knife inserted in center of pudding comes out clean. Remove baking dish to wire rack to cool. Serve warm or chilled. Serves 6.

Chicken Curry   *(India)*

Total protein 245.4 grams
Protein per serving 40.9 grams

1½ cups chopped onion
1 clove garlic, crushed
5 tablespoons vegetable or peanut oil
2 tablespoons curry powder
½ teaspoon ground ginger
1½ cups diced apple or peach
2 tablespoons flour
1 fresh tomato or ½ cup tomato
    juice

2 cups chicken broth
Cooked chicken from a 3½ to 4 pound
    chicken [see following recipe]
¼ cup seedless raisins
6 cups hot cooked rice (1½ cups
    raw)
Mango chutney

In large skillet with cover sauté onion and garlic in 4 tablespoons of the oil until golden. Stir in curry powder and ginger and cook 2 minutes or until curry powder darkens. Stir in apple and remaining tablespoon oil; cover and cook until soft. Push vegetable mixture to one side; stir flour into oil and cook 1 or 2 minutes. Stir into vegetable mixture, then stir in tomato or juice, and broth. Cook, stirring constantly, until mixture comes to boiling. Add chicken and raisins. Cover, reduce heat to low; simmer 30 to 35 minutes to blend flavors. Serve with hot cooked rice and mango chutney. Serves 6.

Cooked Chicken and Broth
(For Chicken Curry)

3½ to 4 pound chicken, cut up
1½ cups water
1 small onion, sliced
1 carrot, sliced

1 chicken bouillon cube
1 teaspoon salt
¼ teaspoon pepper

Plate National   *(Haiti)*
(Rice and Red Beans)

Total protein 60 grams
Protein per serving 7.5 grams

1 cup dried pinto or red kidney beans
3 cups water
½ cup chopped onion
1 clove garlic, crushed
1 tablespoon chopped parsley

6 tablespoons bacon fat
2 teaspoons salt
½ teaspoon pepper
¼ teaspoon ground cloves
1 cup raw regular white rice

Wash and drain beans. In heavy Dutch oven or kettle bring water to boiling. Add beans, cover, and cook 5 minutes. Remove from heat; let stand 1 hour. When beans have soaked 1 hour, sauté onion, garlic, and parsley in bacon fat until onion is golden. Add salt, pepper, and cloves. Drain the beans, saving the liquid. Sauté the beans in the onion mixture for 5 minutes, then return all to Dutch oven. Measure the bean water and add enough water to make 5½ cups. Add water to beans and cook, covered, 1 to 1½ hours or until beans begin to soften. Stir in rice, and cook, stirring once or twice until rice is tender. (Add water if needed.) Pour mixture into a well-greased 8-cup casserole. Bake at 250° F for 30 minutes. Serves 8 to 10.

Rice with Chick Peas   *(Italy)*

Total protein 56.8 grams
Protein per serving 9.5 grams

1 clove garlic, crushed
½ cup olive oil
1 cup raw long-grain white rice
2 tablespoons minced onion

1 can (10½ ounces) condensed chicken
    broth
1 cup water
¼ cup tomato sauce
1 can (20 ounces) chick peas

In large heavy skillet sauté garlic in oil until golden. Remove and discard. Add rice and sauté, stirring constantly until lightly toasted. Stir in onion, then broth and bring to boiling. Stir in tomato sauce and chick peas. Reduce heat, cover and cook 25 to 30 minutes or until rice is tender and liquid absorbed. Serves 6. (In place of chick peas, you may use 1 package (10 ounces) frozen peas.)

Corn and Potato Chowder   *(United States)*

Total protein 32.1 grams
Protein per serving 5.3 grams

1 small onion, thinly sliced
3 tablespoons butter or margarine
2 cups diced, pared potatoes
1 cup water

1 can (17 ounces) cream-style corn
1½ cups milk
1 teaspoon salt
½ teaspoon sugar

In medium-size saucepan sauté onion in butter until golden. Add potato and water; bring to boiling. Cover, cook about 10 minutes or until potato is tender.

Stir in corn, milk, salt, and sugar. Cover and simmer 5 minutes or until hot. Season with fresh ground pepper, if you wish. Serves 6.

Corn Pudding *(United States)*

Total protein 36 grams
Protein per serving 4.5 grams

2 eggs
1½ cups hot milk
2 cups corn kernels, fresh, canned,
   or frozen
2 tablespoons butter or margarine

1 tablespoon grated onion
1 tablespoon sugar
1 teaspoon salt
¼ teaspoon pepper

Preheat oven to 350° F. Beat eggs well. Stir in hot milk, corn, butter, onion, sugar, salt, and pepper. Pour into a lightly greased 1½-quart baking dish. Set dish in a pan on oven rack; pour hot water into pan to 1-inch depth. Bake, uncovered, 50 to 60 minutes or until knife inserted in center comes out clean. Serve hot. Serves 8.

Cornmeal Soufflé *(Canada)*

Total protein 51.5 grams
Protein per serving 13 grams

2 cups milk
½ cup yellow cornmeal
¼ cup grated cheddar cheese
1 tablespoon butter or margarine

1 teaspoon salt
¼ teaspoon paprika
few drops hot pepper seasoning
3 eggs, separated

Preheat oven to 350° F. In heavy saucepan heat milk to boiling. Slowly stir in cornmeal. Cook, stirring constantly, until mixture thickens. Reduce heat, stir in cheese, butter, salt, paprika, and pepper seasoning. Beat egg yolks with a fork. Beat in about 1 cup hot cornmeal mixture, then return all to saucepan. Cook, stirring, 1 minute longer. Let cool. Beat egg whites and fold into cornmeal mixture. Pour into a 5-cup soufflé dish. Bake for 25 to 30 minutes or until puffed and golden. Serves 4.

Oats, Barley, Rye

Oats, barley, and rye are grains of Europe and northern Asia and have never attained the popularity of wheat. Oats in the form of oatmeal and rolled oats are the ways in which this grain, which has a high protein value, is mostly used. Eaten as a cereal with milk, or as oatcakes and oatmeal bread with cheese, the amino acid pattern is complete.

Barley is a popular addition to the soups of many lands, adding a good amount of protein as well as texture, flavor, and interest. And in some lands it is the grain favored above rice for pilafs and stuffings for meats and poultry.

Rye is most commonly used as a half-and-half mixture with

wheat to make bread. An all-rye bread is extremely heavy and dark. In Scandinavia, Poland, Germany, and Russia the people enjoy great breads of many combinations of grains with as many kinds of cheese or slivers of smoked fish which complete the amino acid patterns.

Barley Custard Pudding *(Scotland)*

Total protein 62 grams
Protein per serving 7.7 grams

1¼ cups quick-cooking barley
1 cup water
2 cups milk
1 teaspoon salt
⅔ cup sugar

1 teaspoon ground cinnamon
½ teaspoon ground nutmeg
2 tablespoons butter or margarine
3 eggs

Preheat oven to 350° F. Combine barley, water, 1 cup of the milk, salt, sugar, cinnamon, and nutmeg in medium-size saucepan. Bring to boiling, reduce heat; cook, stirring occasionally 10 to 12 minutes. Remove from heat, stir in butter. Beat eggs with remaining 1 cup milk, and stir into barley mixture. Pour into 8 buttered custard cups, dividing evenly. Bake for 20 to 25 minutes or until knife inserted in centers comes out clean. Serves 8.

Cream of Barley Vegetable Soup *(Russia)*

Total protein 60.5 grams
Protein per serving 10 grams

3 cups water
⅓ cup pearl barley
2 cups diced, pared potatoes
1 cup chopped onion
2 carrots, peeled and diced

1 cup shredded cabbage
4 cups milk
1 tablespoon butter or margarine
1 teaspoon salt
⅛ teaspoon pepper

In large saucepan heat water to boiling. Add barley; cook, covered, 30 minutes. Add potato, onion, carrot, and cabbage; cook, over low heat, 30 to 35 minutes longer or until barley and vegetables are tender, stirring occasionally and adding water if needed. Heat milk until steaming. Remove barley mixture from heat; stir in hot milk, butter, salt and pepper. Return to low heat 5 minutes to blend flavors. Serves 6.

Limpa *(Sweden)*

Total protein 50.6 grams
Protein per slice 2 grams

2 packages active dry yeast
1½ cups lukewarm water
⅓ cup sugar
¼ cup molasses
2 tablespoons melted butter or
   margarine

2 tablespoons finely shredded
   orange rind
1 tablespoon salt
2½ cups sifted rye flour
2½ cups sifted all-purpose flour

World Food Patterns and Protein Economy 367

Sprinkle yeast into warm water in small bowl. Stir until yeast dissolves. Let stand 15 minutes. In large bowl combine sugar, molasses, melted butter, orange rind, and salt. Stir in yeast mixture. Stir in 1 cup of the rye flour, then 1 cup of the all-purpose flour. Beat until smooth. Beat in remaining rye flour, a half cup at a time, then remaining all-purpose flour to make a soft dough. Turn out dough on to lightly floured board; cover with bowl. Let stand 10 minutes, then knead dough until smooth and elastic. Place in greased bowl; turn dough to grease entire surface. Cover and let rise in warm place (85° F) free from drafts, 2 hours or until double in bulk. Punch down dough. Turn out on lightly floured board; knead 5 minutes, then let rise again about 45 minutes. Punch down and divide in half. Shape into 2 round loaves. Place on lightly greased cookie sheet. Cover with damp tea towel. Let rise in warm place about 1 hour, or until double in bulk. Preheat oven to 375° F. Bake loaves 35 to 40 minutes or until well browned and loaves sound hollow when rapped with knuckles. Remove to wire rack. Cover with towel; let cool. Makes 2 loaves.

Oatcakes *(Scotland)*

Total protein 38.4 grams
Protein per oatcake 1.6 grams

1½ cups old-fashioned rolled oats
1½ cups sifted all-purpose flour
¼ cup light brown sugar, firmly
     packed
1 teaspoon salt

½ teaspoon baking soda
⅔ cup shortening
⅓ cup milk

In large bowl combine rolled oats, flour, brown sugar, salt, and baking soda. Mix well. Add shortening and cut in with a pastry blender until fine. Add milk, a tablespoon at a time, mixing with a fork until dough holds together. Divide dough in thirds. Chill. Preheat oven to 375° F. On lightly floured board roll out one-third at a time to ⅛-inch thickness. Cut in 4 × 2-inch strips. Place on ungreased cookie sheets. Bake for 8 to 10 minutes or until lightly browned. Makes 2 dozen oatcakes.

Barley Pilaf *(Bulgaria)*

Total protein 37.3 grams
Protein per serving 6 grams

1½ cups quick-cooking pearl barley
4½ cups water
2½ teaspoons salt
¼ pound sliced fresh mushrooms
½ cup chopped celery

½ cup chopped onion
¼ cup slivered blanched almonds
4 tablespoons butter or margarine
½ teaspoon dried thyme leaves
¼ teaspoon dried sage.

Preheat oven to 350° F. Heat barley in a shallow pan in oven for 30 to 35 minutes or until toasted. In medium saucepan bring water to boiling. Add toasted barley and salt. Reduce heat, cover, simmer, stirring occasionally, 10 to 12 minutes or until tender. Drain. In large skillet sauté mushrooms, celery, onion, and almonds in butter until golden. Stir in barley, thyme leaves, and sage. Cover, cook over low heat, stirring once or twice, 10 to 12 minutes or until hot. Serve with broiled meats. Serves 6.

Potatoes

Potatoes are a staple food also originally American, but having once been introduced to Europe have become great favorites. The Mexicans like them topped with a hot chili pepper cheese sauce, a custom that probably came down from the ancient Maya. And we like them in the many, many potato products in our supermarkets today. We all know a baked potato is good eating but we don't think of it as containing a small amount of good quality protein, which it does. The fish cake made of potatoes and dried or salt fish is a use of these foods as old as the early crossings of the Atlantic, and is a sound combination in terms of amino acid patterns.

Chile con Queso   *(Mexico)*

Total protein 30.7 grams
Protein per serving 5 grams
Protein in 1 (5 ounce) baking potato 4 grams

1 can (16 ounces) whole peeled
    tomatoes
¼ cup chopped onion
2 tablespoons butter or margarine
1 can (4 ounces) green chilies, drained
    and chopped

1 teaspoon salt
dash of pepper
½ pound Monterey cream cheese
    or Muenster cheese, cubed
1 cup light cream

Drain tomatoes well, saving juice; cut in quarters. In a saucepan sauté onion in butter until translucent. Add tomato, chilies, salt, pepper and ¼ cup of the tomato juice. (Use remaining for another purpose.) Bring to boiling; reduce heat and simmer 3 to 5 minutes. Stir in cheese until melted, then cream. Heat just until hot. Serve over hot boiled potatoes or other vegetables. Serves 6.

Leek and Potato Soup   *(France)*

Total protein 31 grams
Protein per serving 5 grams

3 leeks
4 tablespoons butter or margarine
4 medium-size potatoes
4 cups chicken broth or water with
    bouillon cubes

2 cups milk
salt
¼ teaspoon pepper

Wash leeks well. Trim to about 6-inch lengths, then slice thinly. In large saucepan sauté leeks in butter until soft. Peel and thinly slice potatoes. Add to leeks with chicken broth. Bring to boiling; cover, reduce heat and cook about 1 hour or until vegetables are very soft. Put mixture through a coarse sieve, pressing vegetables through. Return to saucepan; add milk and season with salt and pepper. Heat just to boiling. Serves 6.

Hochepot *(Belgium)*

Total protein 151.7 grams
Protein per serving 19 grams

2 pounds boneless lamb shoulder
¼ cup flour
1 teaspoon salt
1 large Bermuda onion, sliced
4 medium-size potatoes, peeled and
    sliced
½ teaspoon dried rosemary

½ teaspoon dried thyme leaves
¼ teaspoon pepper
1 cup chicken broth (or 1 cup water
    and 1 bouillon cube)
1 tablespoon butter or margarine

Preheat oven to 350° F. Trim fat from lamb and discard. Cut meat into 1-inch cubes. Toss cubes in flour and salt until evenly coated. In a 12-cup baking dish make layers of half the lamb, onion, and potato. Sprinkle with half the rosemary, thyme, and pepper. Repeat. Pour broth over; dot top with butter. Cover with lid or foil. Bake 2 to 2½ hours or until lamb is tender. Uncover and bake ½ hour longer or until top is browned. Serves 8.

Salad Nicoise *(France)*

Total protein 79.5 grams
Protein per serving 13.2 grams

2 cups diced raw potatoes
6 tablespoons oil and vinegar dressing
2 cups fresh green beans in 2-inch
    lengths
2 tomatoes

2 hard-cooked eggs
1 can (7 ounces) solid white tuna
12 ripe olives
6 anchovy fillets

Cook potatoes in boiling salted water just until tender. Drain. Place in a bowl; pour 2 tablespoons dressing over; mix gently. Chill. Cook green beans in boiling salted water just until tender. Drain. Place in a bowl; pour 2 tablespoons dressing over. Chill. When ready to serve: In salad bowl combine potatoes and green beans and remaining 2 tablespoons dressing. Toss to mix. Cut tomatoes and eggs in wedges. Flake tuna. Arrange over potatoes and green beans. Garnish with olives and anchovy fillets. Serves 6.

Legumes

The high-protein vegetables, the legumes, require little or no supplementation to make them as complete a protein food as animal protein sources.

The soybean contains the best of the vegetable protein and has an amino acid pattern that meets human needs completely. The garbanzo or chick pea, another good protein source, is found the world around as different varieties and under different names. The soybean, long a food of the Orient, is now a major American crop.

Lentils have been a food of the Old World since Babylonian times and are probably what were used to make Esau's pottage, whereas, most of the beans popular here and in Europe are from the New World. Lentils and beans have the same advantage as grain in that they can be dried and stored until the next crop, providing a year round, high-protein staple, for both nomadic and settled peoples.

We think of lentils, dried beans and peas in hearty soups and bean pots but in the hot countries these foods are popular cold with a dressing of lemon juice and olive oil. Either way they require little additional source of amino acids, for example, the egg in the lentil salad.

How to Prepare Dry Beans for Cooking

All need soaking. First wash the beans. Place beans in a colander and wash in cold water; drain well. Then soak the beans before cooking so they will take up part of the water lost in drying. To retain the fine natural flavor and to save valuable minerals and vitamins, always use the soaking water for cooking.

Quick method. Bring the required amount of water for the beans to boiling; add washed beans. Boil 2 minutes only. Cover. Remove from heat. Allow to stand 1 hour. That is the equivalent of soaking in cold water for 12 to 15 hours.

Overnight method. Pour the required amount of cold water for the beans over the washed beans. Cover and let stand overnight. To prevent souring place in a cool place, or boil the beans for 2 minutes as in the quick method.

Hard-water method. Hard water slows down the cooking. It helps to add 1/8 teaspoon baking soda to 1 cup dry beans, if tap water is hard. Too much soda is harmful to flavor and nutritive value.

For cooking beans use a large heavy kettle or Dutch oven that will hold two or three times the amount of dry beans with water to cover.

Great Northern Beans

— Soaking: For each 1 cup dry beans use 2½ cups water.
— Cooking: Cook in unsalted soaking water for 1½ to 2 hours.
— Yield: 2½ cups beans plus liquid.

Pinto Beans and Red Beans

— Soaking: For each 1 cup dry beans use 3 cups water.
— Cooking: Cook in unsalted soaking water for 2 hours.
— Yield: 2½ cups beans plus liquid.

Pea Beans and Navy Beans

— Soaking: For each 1 cup dry beans use 2½ cups water.
— Cooking: Cook in unsalted soaking water for 1 hour.
— Yield: 2½ cups beans plus liquid.

Cream of Pea Soup *(France)*

Total protein 59.1 grams
Protein per serving 7.4 grams

1 can (10¾ ounces) condensed chicken
   broth
3½ cups fresh green peas or 2 packages
   (10 ounces each) frozen peas
½ cup chopped onion
½ teaspoon salt
¼ teaspoon pepper
2 tablespoons cornstarch
1 cup milk
1 cup light cream
1 tablespoon chopped fresh dill

Add enough water to the condensed chicken broth to make 2½ cups. In medium-size saucepan combine 2 cups of the broth with peas, onion, salt, and pepper; bring to boiling and cook over low heat until peas are tender. Stir cornstarch into remaining broth until smooth, then stir into the peas. Cook, stirring constantly, until broth is thickened, 3 to 5 minutes. Cool; then puree in an electric blender until smooth. Stir in milk and cream and sprinkle with dill. Chill. Serves 8.

Ensalada de Garbanzo *(Mexico)*

Total protein 66.4 grams
Protein per serving 16.6 grams

1 can (20 ounces) garbanzos or
   Mexican chick peas
3 green onions, thinly sliced
1 jar (2 ounces) chopped pimiento
1 tablespoon chopped parsley
3 tablespoons olive oil
3 tablespoons wine vinegar
¼ teaspoon hot pepper seasoning
1 cup grated sharp cheddar cheese

Drain garbanzos and rinse under cold water. Drain well. Place in a bowl, add green onion, pimiento, parsley, oil, vinegar, and hot pepper seasoning. Toss to mix well. Chill several hours to marinate. Serve sprinkled with grated cheese. Serves 4.

Lentil Salad *(Ethiopia)*

Total protein 111 grams
Protein per serving 14 grams

½ cup olive oil
⅓ cup red wine vinegar
1 clove garlic, crushed
1 teaspoon black pepper
2½ teaspoons salt
2 cups quick-cooking lentils
6 cups water
1 onion stuck with 3 cloves

3 bay leaves
1 medium-size green pepper
½ cup thinly sliced green onions
¼ cup chopped pimiento
1 hot green chili, finely chopped
crisp lettuce leaves
2 hard-cooked eggs, quartered

Combine olive oil, vinegar, garlic, pepper, and ½ teaspoon of the salt in jar with tight-fitting cover. Shake well. Set aside. Rinse lentils under cold water; drain. Combine with water, onion, bay leaves, and remaining 2 teaspoons salt. Bring to boiling; reduce heat; simmer, uncovered, about 15 minutes or until just tender. Drain well. Cut green pepper in thin strips. Add pepper strips, green onions, pimiento, and chopped chili to lentils. Pour dressing over. Toss. Chill several hours or overnight. To serve: Arrange in lettuce-lined bowl. Garnish with egg quarters. Serves 8. (Note: This may be served as a hot lentil dish. Place in casserole and heat in a preheated moderate oven (350° F) 15 to 20 minutes or until hot.)

Pea Soup *(France)*

Total protein 123 grams
Protein per serving 15.3 grams

1 pound dried green peas
12 cups water
½ pound salt pork or 1 ham bone
1½ cups chopped onion
2 carrots, finely diced
1 stalk celery, diced

¼ cup chopped parsley
3 bay leaves
3 whole cloves
½ teaspoon dried thyme leaves
2 or 3 teaspoons salt
½ teaspoon black pepper

Wash and drain peas. In large kettle or Dutch oven combine with water; bring to boiling. Remove from heat; cover; let stand 1 hour. Add salt pork, onion, carrots, celery, parsley, bay leaves, cloves, and thyme. Bring to boiling; reduce heat; cover and simmer 1½ to 2 hours or until peas are soft. Remove salt pork, bay leaves, and cloves. Puree pea mixture in a blender or press through a coarse sieve, if you wish. (If using ham bone, remove meat, dice, and return meat to soup.) Add salt and pepper to taste. Reheat soup on low heat. Serves 8.

Red Bean Soup *(Colombia)*

Total protein 75.6 grams
Protein per serving 19 grams

1 cup red beans
7 cups water
1 ham bone (½ cup diced meat)
1 medium-size onion, cut in quarters
1 carrot, sliced
1 stalk celery, sliced

2 whole cloves
1 bay leaf
2 teaspoons Worcestershire sauce
½ teaspoon dry mustard
dash of nutmeg
1 hard-cooked egg

Wash and drain beans. In large kettle or Dutch oven, soak in 3 cups of the water, using quick or overnight method. . . . Add ham bone, onion, carrot, celery, cloves, bay leaf, and remaining 4 cups water. Bring to boiling, reduce heat, cover and simmer (bubbles should just break surface) 3½ to 4 hours, or until beans are soft. Remove ham bone. Cut meat from bone; dice and set aside. Skim fat from beans. Puree beans in a blender or press through a coarse sieve; return to kettle. Mixture should be as thick as heavy cream; add water and salt if needed. Add Worcestershire sauce, mustard, nutmeg, and diced ham. Reheat soup on low heat. Serve topped with hard-cooked egg slices. Serves 4. (Note: If you wish, 2 or 3 tablespoons sherry or Madeira may be added just before serving.)

Lentil Soup *(Saudi Arabia)*

Total protein 34.2 grams
Protein per serving 4.3 grams

½ cup lentils
2 cups chopped onion
2 teaspoons salt
2 quarts (8 cups) water

1 cup chopped spinach
2 tablespoons olive oil
1 tablespoon lemon juice

Wash lentils. In large saucepan combine lentils, onion, salt, and water. Bring to boiling; cook over low heat 1 hour or until lentils are tender. Add spinach, olive oil, and lemon juice. Cook 10 minutes longer or until spinach is tender. Serves 8.

Baked Beans *(America)*

Total protein 193.4 grams
Protein per serving 16 grams

4 cups pea beans
2½ cups cold water
½ pound salt pork
¾ cup molasses

1 tablespoon salt
2 teaspoons dry mustard
1 large onion, peeled

Wash and drain beans. In large kettle or Dutch oven, soak in the water using quick or overnight method. . . . Bring to boiling, reduce heat, cover and simmer 30 minutes. Drain beans, saving liquid. Preheat oven to 300° F. Slice salt pork ¼ inch thick; lay half the slices in bottom of bean pot. Stir molasses, salt, and mustard together, then stir into beans; pour into bean pot. Bury onion in middle of beans; lay remaining pork over top. Add bean liquid until it just covers pork; add water if needed. Cover bean pot. Bake 6 hours. Stir beans every hour and add a little water if beans seem dry. One hour before end of cooking, uncover pot to let beans brown. Serves 12.

Chili   *(Mexico)*

Total protein 66 grams
Protein per serving 11 grams

1½ cups chopped onion
3 tablespoons olive or vegetable oil
1 tablespoon chili powder
2 cans (16 ounces each) red kidney
    beans

2 cans (16 ounces each) stewed
    tomatoes
2 teaspoons sugar
1 teaspoon oregano
¼ teaspoon hot pepper seasoning

In large frying pan sauté onion in olive oil until golden. Push to one side. Add chili powder and heat in oil 1 minute. Add undrained beans, tomatoes, sugar, oregano, and pepper seasoning. Heat to boiling, reduce heat, cover, simmer 45 minutes, stirring occasionally. Uncover and simmer 25 minutes or until slightly thickened. Serves 6.

Chili con Carne

Total protein 106.7 grams
Protein per serving 17.8 grams

Add ½ pound ground beef or pork to . . . [chili] recipe. Sauté with onion in oil until lightly browned.

Lemon Pepper Lentils   *(Algeria)*

Total protein 99.7 grams
Protein per serving 16.6 grams

2 cups lentils
4 cups water
½ cup chopped onion
2 tablespoons butter or margarine
2 chicken bouillon cubes
3 whole allspice

½ teaspoon ground coriander
¾ teaspoon salt
1 tablespoon flour
1 tablespoon water
1 tablespoon lemon juice
½ teaspoon pepper

Soak lentils in the water overnight. Sauté the onion in butter until golden, then add the soaked lentils and water, bouillon cubes, allspice, coriander, salt. Bring to boiling; cover; reduce heat; simmer for 45 minutes, stirring occasionally. Uncover and cook until lentils are tender and all but ½ cup liquid has evaporated. Remove allspice. Mix flour and water to make a smooth paste. Stir into lentils with lemon juice and pepper; cook 3 minutes longer. Serves 6.

Lima Beans and Squash *(Peru)*

Total protein 32.4 grams
Protein per serving 5.4 grams

1½ cups fresh lima beans or 1 package
    (10 ounces) Fordhook lima beans
2 medium-size yellow summer squash
¼ cup chopped onion
¼ cup chopped green pepper
1 tablespoon butter or margarine

1 teaspoon salt
⅛ teaspoon dried thyme leaves
⅛ teaspoon pepper
¾ cup milk
1 tablespoon chopped parsley

Preheat oven to 350° F. Cook fresh lima beans in small amount of boiling water until tender, about 20 minutes. Or cook frozen beans a little less than time in package directions. Wash squash and cut into ⅛-inch slices. In medium-size skillet sauté onion and green pepper in butter about 5 minutes or until tender. Add squash and sauté 10 minutes longer. Stir in salt, thyme, and pepper. In 6-cup casserole layer half the lima beans, add half the squash mixture; repeat. Pour milk over all. Sprinkle top with parsley. Cover and bake 25 minutes. Serves 6.

Peanut Kiufta *(Russia)*

Total protein 95.9 grams
Protein per serving 24 grams

1 cup boiling water
1 cup coarse cracked wheat
6 tablespoons flour
1 tablespoon chopped parsley
½ teaspoon salt
¼ cup chopped onion
1 clove garlic, crushed
1 tablespoon butter or margarine
¼ cup peanut butter

¾ cup chopped unsalted peanuts
1 teaspoon ground coriander
1 teaspoon ground cumin
¼ teaspoon cayenne pepper
6 cups water
3 tablespoons instant chicken bouillon
1 egg, beaten
¼ cup fresh lemon juice

Pour boiling water over cracked wheat in saucepan and let stand 10 to 15 minutes, or until water is absorbed. Stir in flour, parsley, and salt; set aside. In small skillet sauté onion and garlic in butter until golden. Remove from heat. Blend in peanut butter; add peanuts, coriander, cumin, and pepper. Divide wheat mixture into 8 portions. Shape each portion into 2 flat patties; spoon about 1 tablespoon of peanut mixture on one and cover with other; press around edge to seal. When all are filled, moisten hands and shape into balls. In a large saucepan over medium heat, bring water and chicken bouillon to boiling. Add wheat-peanut balls and simmer 10 to 15 minutes. Place 2 in each of 4 serving bowls. Stir lemon juice into chicken broth and with a wire whisk slowly beat in egg. Pour broth over wheat-peanut balls. Serves 4.

Peanut Patties *(United States)*

Total protein 208.9 grams
Protein per serving 34.8 grams

5 cups soft whole wheat bread crumbs
2 cups cocktail peanuts, finely
    chopped
2 cups shredded process cheese
½ cup chopped onion
2 tablespoons chopped parsley

1 teaspoon paprika
1 teaspoon ground coriander .
2 eggs
½ cup milk
2 tablespoons butter or vegetable oil

In a bowl toss together 4 cups bread crumbs, peanuts, cheese, onion, parsley, paprika, and coriander. Beat eggs with milk and stir into bread mixture. Divide mixture into 6 portions and shape into patties. Dip patties in remaining 1 cup bread crumbs to coat. In skillet over medium-low heat sauté patties in butter or cooking oil until lightly browned on both sides. Serve with peanut sauce. Serves 6.

Selection 45 The Revered Legume

Aaron M. Altschul

Editors' Introduction

Legumes, like grains, are among humankind's oldest cultivated crops. Legumes are gaining increased attention as alternative sources of protein. The soybean, a legume, is an especially good source of vegetable protein. Although it has long been a staple of Oriental cuisine, the soybean has only recently been gaining popularity with Western consumers. It can be used in its natural form in many ways. As demand grows, modern industrial techniques will provide soy protein in forms acceptable to an affluent society that previously obtained most of its protein from meat. Extrusion and spinning of soy concentrates can produce vegetable products with textures that approximate those of many meat

Source: Adapted from Aaron M. Altschul, Ph.D., "The Revered Legume," *Nutrition Today* Magazine (March/April 1973):22–29. Reproduced with permission of *Nutrition Today* Magazine, 101 Ridgely Avenue, Annapolis, Maryland 21404. © March/April, 1973.

products. It must be noted that textured vegetable protein (TVP) requires energy-intensive technology.

In the following selection Dr. Aaron M. Altschul, professor of Community Medicine and International Health and head of the nutrition program at the School of Medicine, Georgetown University, suggests some reasons for the new popularity of this ancient food.

Soybeans may now be coming into their own as a staple source of food for Western man. If so, it is because of the achievements of food technologists. Only they, it seems, have been able to accomplish what native Chinese have done for centuries: make the soybean appetizing for Western palates.

Time was, as for example during World War II, when necessity made soy protein widely used as a replacement for meat, that the end product was so unappetizing that even the word "soy" or "soya" (either is acceptable) was something of a nutritional epithet. In fact, in one battle the legume that the Chinese revere was even the code word for "disaster." The occasion was the Allied invasion of Burma when British Empire Troops and American Air Commandos launched an airborne attack which was the greatest in history at that time. The operation took place at night when American transports towed gliders, crowded with Empire troops and equipment from India, over the Lushai Mountains and set them down in Central Burma, 160 miles behind the Japanese lines. To protect the element of surprise, the invaders observed absolute radio silence until they were on the ground and had established a stronghold in the enemy's backyard. Then they were to wireless back to Allied headquarters one of two messages: "pork sausage" if everything was going according to plan, or "soya link" if disaster impended. And that night, military as well as nutritional history was made for soya link, it was . . . everything went wrong.

Long Way

But we have come a long way in food technology since nutritive but altogether awful wartime soya links were used in making of edible foodstuffs from soy protein. Today, at long last, it is possible to enjoy the many rich nutritive benefits of the great soybean without paying any price in taste.

Even now in the United Kingdom, not many people have forgotten the peculiarly bitter taste of soya flour. It was added to countless numbers of foods. The present products bear little resemblance to their earlier mealy counterparts. They have been seasoned and colored, and by an ingenious process of making the soy into long fibers, the end products are very hard to distinguish from the meats they are designed to replace. Certainly no one would every use present day, textured soy protein as a code word for disaster.

There's nothing new about man eating soybean foods. He's been doing it as long as anyone knows. That is, the Orientals, especially the Chinese, have been living off the products of soy for centuries. They call it *shi-yu* and that sounds like soya to us. They are the only people with the patience and skill to make the soybean palatable.

The soybean itself may take pride in being the first legume of which a written record was made. This occurred in 2800 B.C. when the Emperor Shen Nung described the five principal and sacred crops of China: rice, wheat, barley, millet, and soybeans. The deification is deserved for to the soybean, the Chinese owe much.

The beans are raised more extensively in the north than in south China. Now it is cultivated throughout Asia. It is no wonder that, while Asia (India excepted) has certainly not been spared the burden of extensive malnutrition, that part of the world is not the home of kwashiorkor, the hunger of protein-calorie deficiency which is endemic in Africa and some regions of the Americas. The reason seems to be that the Asiatics, for all their deprivations, always had the mighty soybean as the backbone of their diet.

This point has not escaped the attention of nutritionists who have been enthusiastic about introducing soybeans in other areas of the world, where it would seem to be the ideal crop. It is rich in protein, fat, and other nutrients. Under not-too-careful cultivation the crops yield a great many "calories per acre". Hence, soybeans would seem to be the perfect solution for world malnutrition but for one thing, when boiled, fried, or cooked in the ordinary way that legumes are prepared everywhere else but Asia, soybeans are almost inedible. It has to be rather elaborately processed by methods which the Orientals have learned over the ages and which are not easily adopted in other cultures. As W.R. Aykroyd and J. Doughty have pointed out in their altogether enjoyable book, "Legumes in Human Nutrition," published by the FAO in Rome in 1966, "The soybean needs rather special treatment to make it an acceptable human food."

The Chinese go to great lengths in their use of soybeans. They make curds, cheeses, sauces, and pastes with which they enrich their staple diet of cereals. The traditional methods used today are the same as those described in Chinese writings of the time of Julius Caesar. They don't boil the beans whole, or fry them, or simply grind them up and mix them with cereals the way one ordinarily prepares other legumes. Instead, the Chinese subject the bean to germination and long, elaborate, and in a sense very Chinese processes of fermentation urged on by various fungi, bacteria, and yeasts. In addition, many kinds of sauces, cheeses, and the like are prepared with different flavors being imparted by aromatic leaves, ginger, citronella, onions, or somewhat decomposed fish and chicken. For example, one of their favorite cheeses, an Oriental staple for centuries, is made by encouraging a mold of the penicillium species to permeate the cheese. The end result is highly nutritious and reminds one of the best Gorgonzola. It is not easy to envision natives of other lands, lacking the Asiatic's temperament, accomplishing such feats.

For the affluent Oriental, soybeans are a principal raw material out of which Chinese gourmet cooks create their works of art. Beans have been looked upon as menial foods since biblical times. Yet anyone who would scorn soybeans or would use the word to signify ill fortune might reflect on the superiority of Chinese cuisine and the contributions this legume has made to the practicality and pleasures of life.

Perhaps another, if not the principal, reason that people in the developed nations of the West have never fully utilized soybeans in their daily diet is that they had no need to. The Slavs, Europeans, with the notable exception of Great Britain during World War II when soy meal was used in a variety of foods, and North Americans have always had enough animal protein to satisfy their needs. We did not need meat substitutes and we may not even need them today. Thus we have never had to develop a taste for *tofu,* the soybean curd popular in China and Japan; or *miso,* the soybean paste, a soybean-rice innoculate of *Aspergillus oryzae;* or *tempeh,* a dish made by treating soybeans with the fungus *Rhizopus oryzae* that Indonesians like; or *natto,* a Japanese dish made by fermenting whole soybeans through the action of *Bacillus subtilis.* Of all the great products having soybean as the primary ingredient, only soy sauce *(shoyu)* has achieved any popularity in the West and of that we use only the primary component, monosodium glutamate, characteristically extracted by American chemists.

Commodore Perry's Present

The soybean did not arrive in the Western world until the German botanist, Egelbert Kalmpfer, returned from Japan with many sprouts. These and other specimens were grown in several botanical gardens as a curiosity. The first mention of the plants in North America was by James Mease in 1804 who noted that they did well in a private garden in Pennsylvania. They really came into prominence when Commodore Matthew C. Perry brought back two varieties of the "soja bean" as gifts from the mikado. For years after that, soybean was referred to as the "Japan pea."

For decades soybean was used as a forage crop and for "green manure." Then uses of the pressed oil were found and these were and still are employed in such edible products as shortening, margarine, and salad oils. Today more than 69 percent of the oil in margarine, 47 percent of that in shortening, and 35 percent of that in other edible products, including cooking and salad oils, is derived from soybean. Soybean flour, grits, and flakes are used in bread, doughnuts, cakes, and cookies. It is a splendid emulsifier and binder in sausages and related meat products, in breakfast foods, low-starch health foods, macaroni, noodles, confections, ice cream, and as whip toppings. Food manufacturers use about 85 percent of the soybean oil produced in the United States. None of these data includes the soybean used in textured meat analogs.

Enlarged Dimensions

The day may not be far off when foods fabricated from soybeans may become an important part of the U.S. diet. The foods won't resemble Oriental delicacies. They will be fibers of soybean disguised as Western beef, bacon, and the like. In recent years technological scientists of the American food industry have been able to make soy protein into delectable food products that can make this ancient source of rich protein available to millions for the first time. In this sense, their achievement assumes a greatly enlarged dimension. By fabricating soybeans into analogs that can imitate almost any meat, the food technologists have surmounted a barrier that has denied this remarkable foodstuff to much of the world that is starving for protein. One may hope that having scaled one barrier, they have not erected another: costliness. It would be a sad paradox, if having made soybeans acceptable to the hungry of the world we find people still starving because our invention is too expensive.

In the United States, soy products are being more widely used each year. The popularity of the new soya "meats" ("imitation" is not a popular adjective in this context) is amply revealed by the USDA estimates that in the United States alone we consumed more than 700 million pounds of soybean products last year. This replaced only a trivial amount of meat. In fact, in protein value it represents but 1 percent of the meat eaten. However, the amount we are consuming is increasing proportionately. At our present per capita rate it is expected that we will each consume about 205 pounds of meat by 1980. But the agriculture economists forecast we will each be eating from ten to twenty times as much soybean as we do today.

The new soybean protein fills a growing need. Certainly within ten to twenty years, if we are to provide enough protein for everyone, we must continue fabricating high-quality protein that looks and tastes like meat but which actually is made from oil seeds such as soybeans. The U.S. Department of Agriculture announced in 1971 their approval of textured vegetable protein products for use as a protein alternate in order to meet part of the minimum requirements specified for type A school lunch, plus meeting the requirements for the special food service meal program for children. The allowable proportion of vegetable protein products is 30 percent hydrated vegetable protein to 70 percent animal protein.

It is, therefore, important to understand the properties of these textured soy products, of which each of us is going to eat more, and the role they are surely going to play in the diet of the average North American. While it is true that the relatively abrupt arrival of this new food on the American menu has aroused some apprehension among knowledgeable men, there seems to be little question but that soybean products can meet all protein requirements safely.*

First, a look at the soybean itself. Being a legume, it has the properties of that species, which means that its amino acid profile reveals an abundance of lysine and little methionine. It contains tri- and tetra-saccharides, e.g. stachyose, trypsin inhibitors, and hemagglutinins. It is . . . [the] protein content that distinguishes soybean. It contains more protein than any other legume, 40 percent as compared to 20 to 25 percent usually found in other legumes.

In developing the nutritional role for the soybean, Western nutritionists have done so much research that one might say that soybean is probably the best understood of all vegetables.

Three derivatives make up the products forming the basis of soy foods in general use. These are 50 percent soy flour, 70 percent protein concentrate, and the 95 to 100 percent protein isolate.

The first, soy flour, becomes immediately available when the lipids and seed coat are removed from the bean. About half is protein. The flour then yields soy concentrate when the soluble carbohydrates are removed. The protein content increases to 70 percent. Furthermore, in the concentrating process unwanted flavors and other components are removed. The final product, isolate, is obtained by extracting protein with water and then precipitating it in a manner similar to that used in the production of casein from milk. The end product is nearly pure protein. The cost of each product increases the further it is removed from the raw bean.

All three of the above-mentioned soy products, flour, concentrate, and isolate, can be converted into textured products by a combination of procedures. The first meat analogs were made by spinning pure soybean isolate in a spinnerette in the same way synthetic fabrics are made. This produced a structure analogous to muscle fiber. Hence, a powder (the form in which the isolate is usually available) is converted into a material

---

*"Some Things You Might Not Know about Foods Served to Children," *Nutrition Today* (September–October 1972).

that has some of the properties of a linear polymer. Because the starting material is the isolate, this is a very costly way of producing texture.

In recent years other methods have been developed for producing texture. These use soy flour or concentrate, thus saving one processing step. These methods involve a range of procedures from merely allowing soy grits to be extracted and dried, to thermoplastic extrusion. These result in textures of quite satisfactory protein content.

There is a wide variety of ways to create texture and a number of mixtures of textures that can be formulated into one product. Thus it is not surprising that we are now offered many different products ranging from the simplest to the most sophisticated kind of texture, with obvious variations in cost of production. The complex textures are the basis for meat analogs in which meat is imitated by textured soy and other protein products. It is the less sophisticated and less expensive textures that one finds in "helpers" to be mixed with real meat.

The soybean can be the sole source of protein for humans or animals. This of course is the best test of a protein. The soybean protein has more lysine than is necessary for the usual balance of amino acids and, because of this, it can effectively supplement the proteins of cereals which are deficient in lysine. It is deficient, as are all beans, in methionine, but this is usually added to cereals in order to achieve a better nutritional balance. Since cereals have more methionine than is needed, they complement the soybean making diets with soybeans and cereals complete and adequate for human protein nutrition.

When the soybean is supplemented with methionine, it becomes equivalent in protein value to casein. Such supplementation is necessary when the soybean is the sole source of protein, but it is not required when the soybean is mixed with other highly nutritional materials such as casein or meat or is mixed with cereals in adequate proportions.

Like many other foodstuffs, and certainly like all other legumes, soybeans contain certain antinutritional factors identified as trypsin inhibitors and others. Therefore, raw soybean has never been a source of protein for man or animals. This is equally true of many peas and beans. The soybean is always cooked or toasted. The right amount of heat (a subject in which considerable research has been done) when applied to soybean, effectively destroys the antinutritional factors and renders the remaining protein completely suitable for consumption. Moreover, such treatment improves the flavor of the final product. In this respect soybean is not different in principle from raw egg white which, if ingested in large quantities, can cause biotin deficiency because of the presence of avidin, which combines with biotin. When cooked, avidin is denatured.

Soybeans have an advantage over many other protein sources in that there is no evidence of it having allergenic properties. Therefore, it is recommended in cases of infants who are allergic to cow's milk.

The various soybean products mentioned earlier have slightly different nutritive properties but they all have in common the inherent soybean quality. Soy flour contains all of the components of the bean except oil and the seed coat. It has all of the protein and retains all of the flavor components and all of the carbohydrates. Its advantage is low cost. The concentrate is more refined. It has much less antinutritional activity and, therefore, requires less heat treatment. Most of the soluble sugars are removed as well as a good bit of the flavor component. The isolate is free from all components other than protein and, therefore, does not seem to require heat treatment. While it has little flavor, there is enough remaining after processing that it still has to be masqued.

The nutritional value of the soy products in meat analogs follows closely that of the raw materials involved in their preparation. The nutritive value of extruded soy products made from soy flour or concentrate is very close to that of the original materials. The value of the spun fiber will vary depending on how the fiber is incorporated in the final product. The fibers, just as the isolate, have a lower protein value since considerable methionine is fractionated out in the process of extraction of the protein. However, in all applications of spun products, the fibers are mixed with other sources of protein, wheat gluten, egg protein, etc., and hence, the nutritional value is the resultant of a mixture of protein sources. In all instances the nutritive value, as measured in rat tests, is improved by the addition of methionine.

Great Strides

When describing a new food or a new food application one usually tends to be somewhat on the defensive and to try to prove that what is being done is no worse than what has been done before. But, the advent of new textured soy foods adds a new dimension to the American food supply and totally unexpected benefits. One of the problems for which the new soy products may be beneficial is in dealing with "affluent malnutrition."

We have made great strides in nutrition in the United States. We are probably among the best fed people in the world; probably a greater proportion of Americans are better fed than any group of people in history but we continue to want to do better and we wonder about the incidence of certain diseases that come along with affluence: obesity, hypertension, coronary heart disease, diabetes, and gout.

Is diet an important component of the etiology of these diseases? Is it possible to enjoy food and still make needed corrections in the diet that might be helpful? In the last century sugar intake has reached the level of 25 percent of our calories; we have increased fat intake to 45 percent of the calories; and we have reduced cereal intake. Our animal protein intake has increased from one-third of the total protein to close to two-thirds of the total protein in our diet. And, at a level of 15 to 16 percent of the total calories. This is a high intake indeed. These are rather profound changes. Some would argue that these changes, together with other environmental changes that affect amount of exercise, tension, and smoking must be altered or better controlled if we are to limit or delay some of these diseases of affluence.

It is very difficult to change food patterns and yet maintain a high sensory quality in the diet. The introduction of the soybean analogs makes it possible to eat foods that satisfy the desire for meat-type patterns and yet have no cholesterol. With soy products in the food we can control fat intake. We can control total fat in the food and change the fat composition. Other changes, such as reduced or modified salt intake, can be made if desired. The soybean foods and the fabricated foods made with them offer an opportunity to affect changes in the American diet in a practical way in the direction of reducing excesses of certain nutrients.

The maintenance of a safe and healthful food supply in a complex society requires constant vigilance. It requires regulation of food ingredients and it requires accurate labeling. A new class of foods, particularly one that is likely to become a major component of the American diet, provides a challenge and an opportunity to the regulating agencies as well as to the food manufacturers. The school lunch authorities were rather careful about defining the properties of textured soy so it can be used to supplement meat. The general philosophy was that anything purported to be eaten like meat should offer the same nutritional properties of meat insofar as these are known.

A "standard of identity" for textured vegetable proteins is being developed by the Food and Drug Administration. Regulations are being developed to allow for orderly supplementation with amino acids when considered desirable to improve protein value. Vitamin and mineral addition is being regulated to bring these levels equal to those found in meat. As a result of the efforts made to define accurately the properties of the textured soy products, it is likely that such products will be better defined than many natural products which vary markedly in nutritional value.

The ability to produce texture out of soy flour will probably rank with the invention of bread as one of the truly great inventions of food. It now becomes possible to separate protein and fat in products that are modeled after meats and it is possible to allow people the enjoyment that they expect from meat-like compounds and yet avoid the excesses in calories, fat, and a high proportion of saturated fat that ordinarily come from such consumption.

Surely one cannot say that we know all about nutrition, whether we are talking about new products or continue to look at age-old products in a modern setting. Some foods looked upon with opprobrium by millions even today and considered appropriate as code words for misfortune only yesterday are taking on a new respectability as our understanding of food chemistry and technology improves. And so society will be continuing to refine its knowledge of nutrition and make proper adjustments as necessary in both old and new foods. The beauty of the concept of engineering, both for nutrition and sensory quality in foods, is that new nutritional problems that might develop in a society can be met. This goal will be attained more easily through use of fabricated foods, something the Chinese have been doing for centuries.

Selection 46 An Alternate Diet

U.S. Senate Select Committee

Editors' Introduction

Many Americans are seeking ways to conveniently, economically, and pleasantly modify their diets in order to reduce the risk of developing atherosclerotic heart disease. The new way of eating that has been proposed will not only offer hope of a healthier, longer life for many Americans but will also favor protein and energy conservation. People tend to cling to established food patterns and to resist abrupt changes in their customary eating habits. However, habits can be changed through a reeducation program that provides the individual with the opportunity to experiment gradually with new foods and meal patterns and develop a taste for recommended foods and food combinations that will nourish the body and also decrease the amount of cholesterol and fat consumed. Dietary modification (rather than an abrupt change in the affluent diet) will be a key to success. It takes from two to ten years or longer to make radical changes in your manner of eating. The U.S. Senate Subcommittee on Nutrition and Human Needs outlined a program for individuals interested in altering the affluent diet described in the following selection. Three or more phases are included in the program so that

Source: From U.S. Senate, Select Committee on Nutrition and Human Needs, report to 94th Congress, 1st Session, Appendix C, Washington, D.C., December 1975, pp. 87–89.

you can gradually move toward the desired alternative dietary pattern.

The Thompson and Tobias model, The Survival Seven, presented in table 46.2 serves as a guide in selecting an adequate diet and includes the food groups presented in table 46.1. You may compare this model with the Basic 4 described in selection 7.

The macronutrients for the sample of foods from the Survival Seven are listed in table 46.3. The sample pattern for the Survival Seven plan meets National Research Council protein allowances (56 grams per day for an adult male and 44 grams for an adult female) providing at least 1210 calories per day. Addition of grains, legumes, or fruits as well as some nuts will increase the calories to meet individual allowances. The sample pattern has been planned for the initial phase of the alternate diet, and approximately 63 percent of the protein in the plan comes from animal sources. In later phases people will be encouraged to increase their consumption of legumes to at least two servings a day and to reduce the amount of lean fish, poultry, or meat from

Table 46.1 The Survival Seven Food Groups and Their Nutritive Values

Food Group	Nutrition Contribution
Grains (particularly whole grain breads and cereals); also enriched breads and cereals	Important source of complex carbohydrates, thiamine, niacin, riboflavin, vitamin E, phosphorus, magnesium, zinc, and other trace minerals
Legumes	Important source of protein, complex carbohydrates, iron, potassium, and other trace minerals
	Good source of B-complex vitamins (thiamine, niacin, pyridoxine, and folacin) except for riboflavin, vitamin E, and zinc
Fruits	Important source of vitamin C and vitamin A
Vegetables	Important source of vitamin A, folacin, riboflavin, vitamin C, and calcium
Skim milk and skim milk products	Important source of protein, vitamin B_{12}, riboflavin, calcium, and vitamin D (in fortified milk), and carbohydrates.
Low–fat animal products other than skim milk	Important source of protein, thiamine, niacin, pyridoxine, folacin, vitamin B_{12}, iron, phosphorus, magnesium, and other trace minerals
Oils	Important source of polyunsaturated fats, vitamin A, and vitamin E

Note: Developed by the authors, Alice L. Tobias and Patricia J. Thompson.

Table 46.2 The Survival Seven Plan

Food Group	Sample Foods	Rec. No. of Servings	Approx.[1] Grs. Protein (total for group)	Approx.[1] Cal. (total for group)
Grains Whole grain or enriched breads, cereals, rice, and pasta	Oatmeal, ½ cup cooked; whole grain bread, rather than enriched preferred, 3 slices	4	10	270
Legumes Dried beans and peas and soy textured protein products	Navy beans, ½ cup cooked, dried	1	8	115
Fruits A wide variety including 1 citrus fruit	Orange juice, ½ cup; apple, 1 medium	2	1	130
Vegetables A wide variety, including 1 leafy, dark green or deep yellow vegetable; also may include potatoes and other tubers	Carrots, ½ cup cooked; potato, 1 medium	2	4	115
Skim Milk and skim milk products Skim milk or skim milk yogurt	Skim milk, 2 cups	2	17	175
Low-fat animal products other than skim milk Includes such foods as fish, poultry, lean meat, low-fat (or filled) cheese, eggs, and egg whites	Fish, poultry, or meat, 3 ounces cooked; or 1 egg (no more than three times per week) plus ½ cup cottage cheese, uncreamed	1	23	185
Oils Liquid vegetable oils, soft stick margarine, vegetable shortening, nuts, and seed products	Oil for cooking or in salad, 3 teaspoons; margarine as a spread, 3 teaspoons	2	–	225
Total			63	1215

Note: Developed by the authors, Alice L. Tobias and Patricia J. Thompson.

[1] Typical figures can vary somewhat depending on the choices within each group.

[2] Two tablespoons or the equivalent.

Table 46.3 Macronutrients in a Sample of Foods from the Survival Seven Plan

Food Group	Carbohydrates (grams)	Fat (grams)	Protein (grams)	Calories
Grains				
2 slices of enriched, white bread	26	2	4	140
1 slice whole wheat bread	14	1	3	65
Oatmeal, ½ cup cooked	11.5	1	2.5	65
Group total	51.5	4	9.5	270
Legumes				
Navy beans, ½ cup cooked	20	.5	7.5	112.5
Fruits				
Orange juice, ½ cup	15	—	1	60
Apple, 1 medium	18	—	—	70
Group total	33		1	130
Vegetables				
Carrots, ½ cup cooked	10	—	.5	22.5
Potato, 1 medium	21	—	3	90
Group total	31		3.5	112.5
Skim Milk and skim milk products				
Skim milk, 2 cups	24	—	17	175
Low-fat animal products other than skim milk				
Cooked hamburger, 3 ounces		10	23	185
Oils				
Oil, 1 tablespoon	—	14	—	125
Margarine, soft, 1 tablespoon	—	11	—	100
Group total		25		225
Total	159.5	39.5	63	1210

Note: Developed by the authors, Alice L. Tobias and Patricia J. Thompson.

three ounces of cooked weight to two ounces of cooked weight per day. Thus, approximately 50 percent of the protein allowance comes from animal sources.

However, some nutritionists question whether such a reduction is desirable because of difficulties in meeting the RDA for zinc. Although most nutritionists agree that Americans have to reduce their consumption of fat, especially saturated fat, a good deal of controversy and debate regarding the appropriate level of intake still exists. Do not be alarmed if you regularly consume four to six ounces of cooked meat per day. A consistent intake of eight- to 12-ounce portions of steak or prime ribs is another matter. You probably do not need that much fat or calories. Much of the protein in that superlarge serving of meat will probably be used as a source of energy. Once your immediate need for amino acids for protein synthesis is met, the extra amino acids are not stored for future use. They are converted into carbohydrates or fat and used as a source of energy or stored as body fat—a potential source of energy.

The Survival Seven plan includes one whole egg that is permitted three times per week in an effort to limit cholesterol. This rate represents a substantial reduction in egg consumption for many Americans. The first phase of the dietary pattern outlined by the Senate Subcommittee calls for the substitution of egg whites for whole eggs. This recommendation may be too drastic a change for many people who are accustomed to eating eggs. Furthermore, disagreement over the level of cholesterol in the diet of a healthy person with a normal cholesterol level is evident. Some nutritionists believe that Americans should consume no more than 300 milligrams of cholesterol per day in an effort to prevent atherosclerosis. Others believe that the normal, healthy adult does not need to restrict the intake to below 412 milligrams daily, the current level of consumption.

We propose to approach the alteration of food habits in a gradual manner with each phase introducing more changes toward the alternative dietary pattern desired. The major objective of these changes is to lower the blood cholesterol level.

Phase I

The first phase will be to advise people to decrease gradually the amounts of meat, egg yolks, and certain dairy products eaten in order to avoid food items extremely high in cholesterol, saturated fat, and total fat and to use substitute products, i.e., margarine for butter, vegetable oils, and shortening for lard, skim milk cheeses for whole milk and cream cheeses, and egg whites for whole eggs.

Following is an example of how phase I may be approached.

Eat a Balanced Diet

1. Increase use of legumes, grains, grain products, fruits, and vegetables;
2. Use low-fat animal products—skim milk, egg whites, and rinsed cottage cheese;
3. Be sparing in the use of table salt and "salty" foods.

Control Cholesterol Intake

1. Decrease the amount of meat and shellfish per day.
2. Use skim milk and water ices or sherbets made from skim milk; avoid egg yolks, whole milk, cream, and ice cream; egg whites, dried egg whites or products simulating eggs which are made from egg whites are cholesterol-free and perfectly acceptable.
3. Use margarine, vegetable shortenings, and oils instead of butter and lard.
4. Use rinsed or dry cottage cheese in preference to other cheeses.

Regulate Saturated Fat Intake

1. Eat small amounts of lean meat, fish, or poultry per day rather than fatty meats;
2. Use low-fat animal products—skim milk and rinsed cottage cheese—instead of whole milk, cream, and cheese;
3. Use margarine, vegetable shortenings, and oils instead of butter and lard;
4. Limit saturated vegetable fat-cocoa butter and coconut oil—and the products made from them (chocolate, many simulated dairy products, and certain shortenings).

Consider the Total Amount of Fat in Your Diet

1. Eat small amounts of lean meat, fish, and poultry per day;
2. Use moderate quantities of those foods which are by nature predominantly fat—margarines, shortenings, oils, nuts, peanut butter, olives, and avocado;

3. Use sparingly those foods which are comparatively high in fat by reason of their manufacture—regular salad dressings, potato chips, and similar snack foods, fried foods, "fancy breads," rich desserts.

Restrict calories if you are overweight.

Phase II

In phase II people will be encouraged to change their habitual diet further by the incorporation of the recipes developed in "alternative diet product development laboratories" for:

1. *Meatless entrées* with emphasis on legumes to ensure adequate protein;
2. *Baked products* which are cholesterol free and low in fat;
3. *Appetizers and party snacks* which are cholesterol free and low in fat;
4. *Meatless sandwiches* and other products used in snack lunches.
5. Acceptable substitutes for currently popular high-fat, high-cholesterol products.

Those recipes will contain little or no salt (sodium chloride and other sodium-containing condiment).

As more and more recipes are developed people will be encouraged to incorporate these into their own repertoire of recipes. At the same time they will be encouraged to use less meat and fat.

Phase III

Phase III will be to develop directly the philosophy of the alternative diet. It is planned to take a historical approach to the consumption of meat. Man has always eaten meat. What he hasn't done is to eat meat every day, let alone several times day. Even today daily meat consumption is only possible for the affluent minority of the world's population. It is neither healthy nor economical to consume large amounts of meat every day. Therefore, we plan to suggest ultimately that people adopt the pattern of eating meat occasionally.

Editors' Note: In view of existing uncertainty concerning the role of dietary cholesterol in elevating serum cholesterol levels, the discard of egg yolks (a valuable source of nutrients) may be viewed as ecologically unsound.

Selection 47 The Vegetarian Diet

U.D. Register
L.M. Sonnenberg

Editors' Introduction

In recent years the popularity of vegetarianism has increased, particularly among young people. For health, ecological, philosophical, or religious reasons, a growing number of people are choosing an eating pattern that differs from the customary Western model by excluding meat, poultry, and fish. Although vegetarian diets differ in the kinds of foods that they contain, the diets usually include vegetables, fruits, whole grain or enriched breads and cereals, dry beans and peas, lentils, nuts, peanut butter, and seeds. Some diets are more liberal than others.

A *lacto ovo diet*, the most popular type, includes eggs and dairy products as a supplement to vegetable foods. The *lacto vegetarian diet* includes only dairy products, but not eggs, as a supplement to plant foods. *Vegans*, or *strict, total vegetarians* avoid all foods of animal origin including eggs and dairy products. Vegetarian diets may include meat analogs that are made from various proportions of legumes, nuts, and cereals flavored to resemble beef, ham, chicken, and fish. These analogs provide nutrients comparable to those of the animal products that they are intended to replace. Unusual types of foods, such as miso, a fermented paste made of soybeans, salt, wheat, or barley and water; tofu, a curd or "cheese" made from fresh soybeans, also known as bean curd; seaweed; brewer's yeast or nutritional yeast, a source of high-quality protein that does not have the rising properties of baking yeast, are also included in the diets of some vegetarians.

U.D. Register and L.M. Sonnenberg are noted authorities on the vegetarian diet. For many years they have investigated the nutritional status of groups practicing the different forms of vegetarianism. In a number of excellent articles, they review their findings and present practical guides for planning an adequate vegetarian diet. Perhaps you are now following a meatless diet or

Source: U.D. Register and L.M. Sonnenberg, "The Vegetarian Diet," *Journal of the American Dietetic Association* 72, no. 3 (March 1973):253–61. First presented at the Fifty-fifth Annual Meeting of the American Dietetic Association in New Orleans on October 11, 1972. Copyright The American Dietetic Association. Reprinted by permission from *Journal of the American Dietetic Association* 72:253, 1973. Complete notes and references and selected tables appearing in this article have been omitted here; for further information consult the original version.

are considering changing to a vegetarian diet. In order to help you evaluate the pros and cons of lacto ovo vegetarianism, lacto vegetarianism, and veganism, we will summarize some of the basic characteristics and principles of these food patterns as outlined in their reports.

The complete vegetarian diet. Both the lacto ovo vegetarian diet and the lacto vegetarian diet are regarded as complete diets, because they can provide all the essential nutrients in amounts that meet or surpass the NRC Recommended Dietary Allowances. A carefully selected meatless diet chosen from a wide variety of plant foods plus fair amounts of milk, with or without eggs, can be superior to diets in which the meat intake is high. The "affluent diet" consumed by many Americans is often poorly balanced because of the large intake of meats, sweets, pastries, and fats and the limited use of whole grains, fruits and vegetables, vegetable oils, milk, and such dairy products as yogurt and cheese. In the vegetarian diet, protein and other nutrients ordinarily obtained from meat are provided by milk and dairy products, eggs, and legumes. The vegetarian diet may or may not include eggs. The milk group requires special attention. Two glasses of milk can be relied on to furnish 75 percent of the calcium, 43 percent of the riboflavin, 22 percent of the protein, and 100 percent of the vitamin B_{12} in the typical lacto ovo vegetarian diet.

The pure vegetarian diet. There are a number of hazards in adhering to a pure vegetarian diet. Plant foods do not contain vitamin B_{12}. Milk and eggs are satisfactory sources of this nutrient, but an all-vegetable diet does not include these foods. This nutrient must be obtained through the use of vitamin B_{12}–fortified soy milk or by taking vitamin B_{12} supplements. Calcium and riboflavin tend to be in short supply in a pure vegetarian diet, because it precludes the use of milk. Although a calcium supplement may be necessary, particularly for infants, children, adolescents, and pregnant women, the adult male and nonpregnant adult female may meet calcium requirements through the use of dark green vegetables such as broccoli, brussels sprouts, collards, dandelion greens, and nuts such as almonds, Brazil nuts, and peanuts. Adequate amounts of riboflavin may also be obtained from the above greens as well as from okra and winter squash if these foods are consumed frequently and in large amounts. Many plant foods are low in calories and when food selections are not well balanced, the energy value of the diet will not meet the individual's needs. The amount of food to be eaten to meet requirements for calcium, riboflavin, and calories may be difficult for an individual—especially a child—to handle. When caloric intake is inadequate, the body will preferentially use protein to meet energy needs. However, when the caloric intake is adequate and plant proteins are carefully selected and judiciously combined, it is possible to obtain protein in adequate quantity and of high quality.

Planning a vegetarian diet. According to Register and Sonnenberg, the most important considerations in planning an adequate vegetarian diet are:

1. To select from a wide variety of plant foods;
2. To minimize the use of empty calorie or junk foods, including soft drinks, candy bars, and other concentrated sweets as well as alcohol that are high in caloric value but carry only insignificant amounts of vitamins, minerals, and protein;
3. To use the Four–Food Group Pattern shown in table 47.1 in selecting foods and in planning menus;
4. To maintain caloric intake at the appropriate level to maintain normal weight; to increase amounts of all the four food groups and include some vegetable oil, margarine, and nuts to supply adequate calories;
5. To replace meat with such protein-rich foods as legumes, nuts, and meat analogs; (Low-fat cheeses such as cottage cheese and small amounts of hard cheese and eggs in moderation may be used. Eggs are optional but in some diets can be used as a meat substitute. Individuals with high serum cholesterol levels should include no more than three to four eggs per week in their diet.)
6. To include at least two cups of milk in your diet each day; (Milk is an important source of calcium, riboflavin, protein, and vitamin B_{12} in a complete vegetarian diet.)
7. To increase the intake of bread and cereals, especially whole grain products; (They supply complex carbohydrate protein, thiamine, iron, and trace minerals.)
8. To include a variety of fruits and vegetables in your diet; (Be sure to include a raw source of vitamin C such as citrus fruits, strawberries, or cantaloupe and at least one serving of a dark leafy green vegetable such as romaine lettuce, kale, broccoli, or chard in the diet each day.)

The total vegetarian, one who follows the vegan diet, excludes eggs and dairy products. To satisfactorily replace the

Table 47.1 The Four-Food Group Plan for Vegetarian Diets

Food Group	Sample Food	Recom. No. of Servings	Approx. Grms. Protein (total for group)	Approx. Cals. (total for group)
Fruits and Vegetables	orange, 1 banana, 1 small broccoli, ⅔ cups cooked potato, 1 medium	4 or more	8	275
Breads and cereals	oatmeal, ¾ cup, cooked whole wheat bread, 3 slices	4 or more	10	200
Milk Nonfat milk **Protein-rich foods**	2 cups cottage cheese, ½ cup legumes, ½ cup cooked	2 cups 2 cups 2 or more	17 17 22	330 175 225
Total			57	1,100

* Nonfat milk calories are not added in computation of total-calorie figure.

eliminated nutrients found in milk, substitute either fortified soybean milk or green leafy vegetables or a combination of both. A minimum of two cups of soybean milk is recommended for adults and three cups for children, adolescents, and pregnant women. Fortified soybean milk is not a complete substitute for cow's milk, since it provides only ¼ as much (72 milligrams) calcium, ⅓ as much (10 milligrams) riboflavin, and ½ as much (0.5 milligrams) vitamin B_{12}. One cup of cooked greens provides on an average 200 milligrams of calcium. The NRC Recommended Dietary Allowance of calcium for children and adults is 800 milligrams per day. During adolescence, pregnancy, and lactation, the calcium RDA is 1200 milligrams per day. The total vegetarian must include a source of vitamin B_{12} either as fortified soybean milk or as a dietary supplement.

Since the quality of plant protein is generally lower than the quality of animal protein, the total vegetarian must carefully plan a diet that ensures that the essential amino acids of vegetable proteins complement each other's amino acid pattern. The following foods are complementary protein combinations and when eaten at the same meal will provide all the essential amino acids:

— Grains with dried beans or wheat germ;
— Dried beans with grains, nuts and seeds or wheat germ;
— Nuts and seeds with dried beans or wheat germ.

Large populations of the world have lived for centuries on diets considered near vegetarian because of economic necessity and availability of little or no animal products. Today, however, in an affluent society where food supplies are abundant, an interesting trend has been developing in that more and more Americans, particularly young adults, are becoming vegetarians. . . .

Protein in the Vegetarian Diet

Quantitative Aspects

German physiologists recommended high protein intakes based on their opinion that protein need was proportionate to muscular activity. Voit based his recommendation for an intake of 120 grams protein on his survey among German workers who were eating a high-protein diet. However, controlled experiments using the nitrogen-balance method showed that normal subjects can maintain nitrogen equilibrium on protein intakes of from 30 to 35 grams per day.[1]

In 1946, Hegsted et al. studied adults on an all-plant diet in which cereals provided 62 percent of the protein. They concluded that on this type of diet, 30 to 40 grams of protein per day would meet minimal requirements of a man weighing 70 kilograms.[2]

A comprehensive nutritional study by Hardinge and Stare in 1954 compared nutritive intake and nutritional, physical, and laboratory findings of 200 subjects on three types of diets: twenty-six pure vegetarians, who used *no* animal products; eighty-six lacto ovo vegetarians, who used milk and eggs; and eighty-eight nonvegetarians.[3] No evidence of deficiency was found, and each group met or surpassed the Recommended Dietary Allowances. These results showed that the average protein intake of the adult men on the pure vegetarian diet was 83 grams; on the lacto ovo vegetarian diet, 98 grams; and on the nonvegetarian, 125 grams. Results for women were 61, 82, and 94 grams, respectively. Dietitians accustomed to computing meatless menus find it difficult not to exceed the protein allowances when caloric needs are met.

Hegsted and the Harvard group have commented that for adults "it is difficult to obtain a mixed vegetable diet which will produce an appreciable loss of body protein without resorting to high levels of sugar, jams, and jellies, and other essentially protein-free foods." Similar experiences have been found in our laboratories.

Total serum protein, albumin, and globulin values and the hematologic findings for the vegetarian and nonvegetarian groups in Hardinge and Stare's study were not statistically different. The pure vegetarians averaged 20 pounds less in weight than the others who averaged 12 to 15 pounds above their ideal weight.

Although protein has been singled out for attention in populations where malnutrition is prevalent, the problem is often compounded by a total caloric deficit. Even when an adequate amount of protein is provided, symptoms of protein deficiency may still appear if the diet does not also provide sufficient calories since, under these circumstances, some of the protein is utilized for energy.

In a review of cereal diets in which 10 percent or less of the protein calories were derived from animal sources, Ohlson reported that the adult protein requirements, as analyzed by FAO, probably could be met if sufficient calories were available.[4] She found that 2,500 kilocalories from such a food mixture would, on the average, supply 67 grams protein—almost 50 percent more protein than estimated to be adequate for 98 percent of the adult population.

In India, the average caloric intake is about 2,050 kilocalories per day, supplying a total of 57 grams protein, of which 51 grams come from plant sources. By contrast, in the United States, the average intake is approximately 3,200 kilocalories with a total of 97 grams protein, of which 31 grams is from plant sources. By increasing the Indian diet 1,000 kilocalories (comparable to the caloric level in American diets), there would be an increase of 25 grams plant protein. With this caloric increase, the total protein level in the Indian diet would be 82 grams, considerably exceeding recommendations.

In a review of current concepts of protein nutrition, Scrimshaw of Massachusetts Institute of Technology asks: "How do we allow adequately for individual variation without recommending a wasteful margin of safety?"[5] To answer this question, at least for young adults, he studied 100 young men, all university students, who were given a diet adequate in calories but lacking in protein. His studies indicated that generally an amount less than 30 grams protein daily is adequate for normal activities. Nitrogen balance at these low levels of intake was possible only because a protein of excellent quality, that of freeze-dried whole egg, was used. A correction for the lesser protein quality of ordinary mixed diets must be made. Scrimshaw makes the point that absolute requirements for protein in healthy adults are much lower than commonly suggested, provided the quality is good.

Scientific studies continue to confirm Sherman's findings that 1 gram protein per kilogram body weight provides a liberal margin of safety for adult maintenance.[6] This is reflected in the 1980 revision of the Recommended Dietary Allowances, which are practical and desirable levels. The importance of planning adequate diets to meet these allowances has been amply substantiated, not only by research but by clinical studies and human experience. Table 47.2 shows how easily protein needs can be met on a lacto ovo vegetarian diet. It will be noted that the protein total for two meals is about 60 grams, approximately twice the minimum requirement for adult man.

Qualitative Aspects

The extensive fund of knowledge supplying information in regard to the amino acid composition of foods has been achieved through a number of methods of experimentation. Among these are animal growth studies, biologic-value methods, nitrogen-balance studies, and dietary surveys, as well as chemical and chromatographic determinations.

A number of the very early studies used the rat-growth method for evaluating the quality of single proteins. By this method, the quality of plant proteins was generally undervalued. However, the concept of mutual supplementation evolved. As pointed out in *The Lancet*: "Formerly vegetable proteins were classified as second class and regarded as inferior to first-class proteins of animal origin; but this distinction has now been generally discarded. Certainly some vegetable proteins, if fed as the *sole* source of protein, are of relatively low value for promoting growth; but many field trials have shown that the proteins provided by suitable mixtures of vegetable origin enable children to grow as well as children provided with milk and other animal proteins."

Table 47.2 Two Menus to Meet Protein Needs from Typical Lacto Ovo Vegetarian Meal Patterns

Food	Protein (grams)	Food	Protein (grams)
Menu I		**Menu II**	
Oatmeal and raisins	4.0	Lettuce and tomato salad	2.0
Milk, 1 glass	8.5	(with cottage cheese)	15.0
Bread, 2 slices whole		Entrée	12.0
wheat toast	5.0	Peas	5.0
Fruit, 1 serving	1.0	Potato	3.0
Egg or meat analog		Bread, whole wheat	2.5
(1–2 ounces) *or*		Milk, 1 glass	8.5
nuts (½ ounce), *or*		Dessert	3.0
peanut butter (1 tablespoon)	5–6.0		
Total	24.0	Total	36.0

Note: Total for two meals equals approximately 60 grams protein; values for the third meal are not included.

Bressani and Behar have stated: "From a nutritional point of view, animal or vegetable proteins should not be differentiated.[7] It is known today that the relative concentration of the amino acids, particularly of the essential ones, is the most important factor determining the biological value* of a protein. . . . By combining different proteins in appropriate ways, vegetable proteins cannot be distinguished nutritionally from those of animal origin. The amino acids and not the proteins should be considered as the nutritional units."

Since wheat is so widely used, early studies of the supplementary value of wheat protein with other proteins were carried out in this laboratory.[8] Because wheat is low in lysine, foods that are relatively high in this amino acid were tested. We found that when 70 percent of the protein in the diet was from wheat protein and the remaining 30 percent from milk, yeast, nuts, soybeans, and other legumes, excellent supplementary action occurred as judged by rat growth.

In a study by Sanchez, Porter, and Register, a week's hospital vegetarian diet containing milk and eggs was fed to a group of animals, and their growth was compared with that of a group of animals receiving the same diet in which meat replaced the plant protein entrées.[9] The results showed no significant difference. The average growth of the animals on the meat and meatless diets was 39 and 37 grams per week, respectively.

Sanchez et al. designed a study to evaluate by the biologic-value method the protein content of complete meals.[10] All basal meal patterns consisted of portions from plant foods and were tested together with supplements of lysine, soybean milk, cow's milk, or a combination of these supplements. When diets were formulated to contain grain-legume mixtures as eaten in most countries, biologic values were above 70 and compared favorably with diets containing meat, milk, and lysine. These results suggest the possible supplementary value of proteins in diets of peoples of many countries which include large quantities of cereals, some legumes, and possibly some other vegetables, fruits, and nuts, and little or no animal foods.

Using the nitrogen-balance method, Register et al. evaluated in human subjects the protein quality of diets containing vegetable protein mixtures prepared to simulate meat products.[11] The results were compared with similar diets containing milk and beef. Six university students served as subjects in each of four tests. At an approximately 60-gram

---

*Editors' note: Biological value (BV) is a measurement usually made in growing animals. BV is the ratio of protein or nitrogen retained within the tissues and body fluids to the protein or nitrogen absorbed from the gastrointestinal tract. The ratio is used as a measure of protein quality since more protein is assumed to be retained when all the essential amino acids are present in adequate amounts to meet the needs of growth.

protein level, selected diets containing prepared vegetable protein mixtures with soybean milk or cow's milk maintained nitrogen balance. Such diets also compared favorably with the nonvegetarian diet in maintaining nitrogen balance.

The metabolic response of eighteen-year-old adolescent girls to a lacto ovo vegetarian diet was studied by Marsh and co-workers.[12] The calculated essential amino acid intake was far in excess of the minimal requirement for women for every amino acid.

Edwards et al. did nitrogen balance studies on twelve men at the beginning and end of four fifteen-day intervals following the ingestion of wheat diets containing 46 grams protein per day. They found that nitrogen balance was maintained over a period of sixty days.[13]

In studying vegetarians, Hardinge, Crooks, and Stare analyzed the essential amino acids of the dietary proteins of the subjects.[14] Their figures showed that the intake of all groups ranged from more than twice to many times the minimum essential amino acid requirements. . . .

Evaluating protein quality by various methods has resulted in a large body of information that provides scientific basis for planning vegetarian diets that are quantitatively and qualitatively adequate. Understanding of protein nutrition has progressed to the point where an all-vegetable combination, such as Incaparina, is completely adequate in feeding very young children, even those suffering from malnutrition.

In the developing countries, this concept of mutual amino acid supplementation has sparked investigations into many single plant sources to determine combinations of available supplies which supplement each other. Rao and Swaminathan summarized a number of these studies: peanut proteins supplement wheat, oat, corn, rice, and coconut proteins to a significant extent; being rich in lysine and valine, soybean proteins supplement those of wheat, corn, and rye; a mixture of soy and sesame proteins has a high nutritive value comparable to milk proteins; and the proteins of legumes and leafy vegetables remarkably supplement those of cereals.[15]

In a paper on current concepts of protein nutrition, Scrimshaw declares: "Vegetable mixtures supplying the amino acids in appropriate proportions are as efficient in meeting protein needs at minimum levels of intake as proteins of animal origin."[16] Recent advances in our understanding of protein requirements, he says, free us "from dependence on the concept of the need for animal protein or amino acids from conventional food alone and allows us to concentrate on ways of most efficiently and economically meeting man's need." He further states that the "bulk of present and future needs will be met by conventional plant proteins."

Information from studies on the supplementary relationship of plant proteins has resulted in the development and marketing of a number of formulated plant protein foods referred to as "meat analogs."

A number of these products combine various proportions of legumes, nuts, and cereals. One advantage of all of these foods is that, since they are made of plant sources, they do not contain cholesterol or saturated animal fats.

Soy Products

Vegetable proteins that are finding special consumer interest are the spun soy and textured soy protein products. They offer great potential and versatility because they can be formulated to any protein, fat, or carbohydrate level desired, and proteins may be blended to accomplish a very favorable amino acid composition.

Since spun soy isolates are the purified protein fraction of soybeans, it is important that they be fortified or used in combination with foods which contain the essential nutrients, such as iron and a number of the B vitamins which meat proteins provide in the diet. The U.S. Department of Agriculture's Agricultural Research Service has set up compositional requirements for textured vegetable protein products for use in the school lunch program.

Based on casein as a standard with a protein efficiency ratio (PER)* of 2.50, ham analog has a PER of 3.10; smoked turkey analog, 2.81; plant protein wieners, 2.50; textured protein sausage, 2.40; and chicken analog, 2.34. Meat analogs also usually contain less fat than their meat counterparts. Ham analog has only 12 percent fat compared with about 30 to 35 percent for ham; plant protein wieners, 12 percent compared with up to 30 percent for meat wieners; and beef analog, 12 percent compared with 18 to 23 percent for beef.

In a study by Koury and Hodges, prison volunteers were hospitalized and placed on a diet for twenty-four weeks with soy protein foods as the only source of protein.[17] The diet was well accepted, weight was maintained, and all subjects remained in good health. Laboratory results showed normal findings for hemoglobin, hematocrit, and urea nitrogen, indicating that the protein was well utilized. Serum cholesterol and triglyceride values were markedly influenced by the diets. The average decrease in serum cholesterol was approximately 100 milligrams per milliliter.

Bressani et al. compared the protein quality of textured soy protein with meat and milk in experimental animals and children.[18] Growth was

---

Editors' note: Protein efficiency ratio (PER) is a method of evaluating the quality or nutritive value of a protein by calculating the weight gain of a growing animal per gram of protein eaten. The ratio is determined under experimental conditions in which the intake of calories or other nutrients are adequate and the protein intake is 10 percent by weight of the diet.

the same for dogs fed soy protein as for those fed meat. Even when large amounts of soy protein were given, no adverse physiologic effects were observed.

Nitrogen absorption and retention were essentially the same for both the milk and soy protein diets of children. It was concluded that the protein quality of soy protein was high, about 80 percent of the protein quality of milk, with adequate digestibility.

As the world protein supply dwindles in relation to the population growth, textured protein products will be used to supplement and extend existing protein sources. A recent Cornell University study forecasts that meat analogs and extenders may reach 10 percent of all domestic meat consumption by 1985, certainly by year 2000.[19] This would represent an increase from the present level of 145 million pounds per year to approximately 2.45 billion pounds in fifteen years.

Adequate and Inadequate Vegetarian Diets

Worldwide studies of properly selected vegetarian diets support the adequacy of such a dietary pattern. True, many reports have been published of nutritional diseases prevalent in underprivileged areas of the world. These generally show that the diseases are due, not to a vegetarian diet as such, but to a gross shortage of food, or to a diet consisting largely of such foods as refined cornmeal, cassava root, tapioca, or white rice, with practically no milk, eggs, leafy vegetables, legumes, or fruits. Lack of suitable postweaning foods affects young children, particularly. Parasitic infestations frequently accentuate the symptoms of nutritional diseases in these areas.

Hardinge and Crooks reviewed the scientific literature on vegetarian and near-vegetarian diets.[20] They conclude that "widely differing dietary practices appear among vegetarians and near vegetarians. A reasonably chosen plant diet, supplemented with a fair amount of dairy products, with or without eggs, is apparently adequate for every nutritional requirement of all age groups.

"Pure vegetarian diets, the use of which produced no detectable deficiency signs, contained adequate calories obtained mainly from unrefined grains; legumes; nuts and nut-like seeds; a variety of vegetables, including the leafy kinds; and usually an abundance of fruits.

"Vegetarian and near vegetarian diets that have proved inadequate include: (1) vegan diets which have been reported to produce vitamin B_{12} deficiency in some individuals; (2) grossly unbalanced near vegetarian diets in which as much as 95 percent of the calories were provided by starchy foods extremely low in protein, such as cassava root; (3) diets dependent too largely on refined cereals, such as cornmeal or white rice, even though small amounts of animal foods were included;

and (4) intake of total calories insufficient for maintenance requirements.''

Plant Dietaries and Serum Lipids

Experimental studies and epidemiologic findings on the lipid-lowering effect of plant dietaries may have great significance for current problems in nutrition and public health. The pure vegetarians in a study by Hardinge and Stare had significantly lower serum cholesterol than either the lacto ovo vegetarians or nonvegetarians.[21]

Serum cholesterol and the dietary habits of a voluntary group of 466 Seventh-Day Adventists (SDA) were studied to determine the influence of diet on serum cholesterol in an adult population whose main environmental differences related to their adherence to a vegetarian diet. West and Hayes matched vegetarians with nonvegetarians from the same base population and examined the effects of various levels of meat, fish, and fowl consumption (degrees of nonvegetarianism) on serum cholesterol levels.[22] The difference between serum cholesterol of the vegetarians and nonvegetarians was statistically significant. Several degrees of nonvegetarianism were noted, and the evidence was clear that as the degree of nonvegetarianism increased, the serum cholesterol increased.

Lemon and Walden, in their study of California Adventists, showed that male SDAs suffered their first heart attack a full decade later than most Americans, and the incidence of heart disease was only 60 percent of the average California male population.[23] Hodges et al. fed a diet to men in which the source of protein was meat analogs; they reported a significant decrease in serum cholesterol.[24]

Although the type and amount of fat, as well as the cholesterol content of the diet, have usually been singled out in relation to elevated serum lipid levels, within recent years a number of studies have suggested that people with diets rich in fiber have lower blood cholesterol levels.

Leguminous seeds, twice as rich as cereals in fiber content, have been considered in animal experiments and in human subjects. In India, male volunteers ate 247 grams Bengal gram (chick peas), consuming 16.0 grams fiber daily. Even while eating a high-fat diet (156 grams butter fat per day), they had a decrease in mean serum cholesterol from 206 milligrams to 160 milligrams per 100 milliliters. It was necessary to eat the diet for twenty weeks to produce the maximal hypocholesteremic effect. Excretion of all bile salts was significantly increased on the high-fiber diet.

In 1963, a Japanese dietary survey reported an average daily per capita consumption of 5.7 grams ordinary beans—similar to the United

States figure of 7.5 grams—but a total of 69.4 grams leguminous seeds, used largely as *miso, tofu,* and other processed forms. Since leguminous seeds appear to have a cholesterol-depressing effect, this feature of the Japanese diet may contribute to the maintenance of the low serum cholesterol level characteristic of that population.

Practical Considerations for Dietary Change

It is fortunate that the planning of a vegetarian diet is not difficult. In essence, it is the application of the basic concepts of good nutrition with a relatively few but important modifications. If one were to state the fundamental consideration, it would be to choose a wide variety of foods with a minimum number of refined products. (This basic principle is appropriate to the planning of any type of diet.)

The Lacto Ovo Vegetarian Diet

The Basic 4 food pattern provides a reliable guide for planning vegetarian diets with the major change in the meat or protein-rich group. In applying the Basic 4 pattern to a lacto ovo vegetarian diet, the following recommendations are important:

1. Since in a vegetarian diet fewer concentrated sources of protein, such as meat, are used frequently, it is necessary to decrease significantly the "empty" calories. It has been estimated that approximately 35 percent of calories in the typical American diet are from sugars and visible fats. Unrefined foods, on a caloric basis, with few exceptions, supply their quota of protein to the diet. In evaluating the diet of anyone changing from a nonvegetarian to a vegetarian diet, the dilution of nutrients by empty calories should be checked and corrected.

2. Meat in the protein group will be replaced by a generous intake of a variety of legumes, nuts, meat analogs made from wheat and/or soy proteins, and other formulated plant proteins. Although commercially prepared plant proteins are not essential to a well-balanced vegetarian diet, these products do facilitate menu planning and preparation. Their use in the meal replaces the meat entrée with little further change in the menu needed. A number of canned, dehydrated, and frozen meat analogs are available in an expanding number of markets. Many combinations, consisting of legumes, cereals, and nuts, with or without milk and eggs, can be made in the home. Vegetarian recipe books are available, and a homemaker can make many tasty vegetarian entrées.

3. In the milk group, greater use of nonfat or low-fat milk products, such as cottage cheese, contribute to protein intake and provide

vitamin B$_{12}$. The recommendation of the milk group will supply vitamin B$_{12}$ sufficient to meet the average adult need.

4. Since the cereal and bread group also supplies some protein, as well as iron and B vitamins, intake of this group, preferably in the whole grain form, should be somewhat increased. However, care must be observed that this increase does not take place at the expense of the other food groups.

5. The fruit and vegetable group is usually well represented in the vegetarian diet. Perhaps because of this, a vegetarian diet is often associated in the minds of the general public as consisting largely of vegetables. This class of foods is an important part of the diet, but other food groups are an integral part of a balanced vegetarian diet.

Actually, the lacto ovo vegetarian diet does not differ markedly from the average Western diet. The main difference is that it replaces meat with a variety of legumes, meat analogs, cereals, and nuts and more generous intake of milk and milk products and some eggs. In practice, the nutritional composition of this type of diet is strengthened by the variety of foods which replace meat. Ohlson has pointed out that "many Americans, particularly adult men, eat diets which are poorly balanced because of the large intakes of muscle meat, sweets, and fats and almost complete omission of cereals, except as refined flour entering into the preparation of sweet rolls or desserts. The vegetables and fruits are limited in both amount and variety."[25]

The Pure Vegetarian Diet

Several difficulties may be encountered when diets completely devoid of animal foods are eaten. In the first place, many plant foods are low in calories; consequently, the sheer bulk of food to meet caloric needs can become a problem if the selection is not well planned. Second, although a lacto ovo vegetarian diet provides adequate amounts of vitamin B$_{12}$, no presently known practical source of vitamin B$_{12}$ is present in plant foods. Some individuals appear to maintain good health for many years on a pure vegetarian diet without developing symptoms of deficiency, while others develop symptoms in a shorter time. The reason for this variation is not clear. Until more information is available, a pure vegetarian should include a source of vitamin B$_{12}$ in his diet.

The following recommendations are important in changing from a lacto ovo vegetarian diet to a pure vegetarian diet.

The same consideration for the protein and cereal-bread groups which has already been made applies to a pure vegetarian diet. There will be, of course, increased use of the foods of these two groups, as well as from the fruit-vegetable group, to meet caloric needs. An adequate intake of calories is important. When caloric intake is inadequate, the body will preferentially use protein to meet its energy needs.

The milk group requires special attention. In the lacto ovo vegetarian diet, the milk group supplies 75 percent of the calcium, 43 percent of the riboflavin, 22 percent of the protein, and practically 100 percent of vitamin B_{12}. One way to obtain an adequate intake of these nutrients is to use sufficient quantities of fortified soybean milk. For an adult, this would be a minimum of two glasses a day. The label must be checked to make certain that the soybean milk is *fortified*.

Green leafy vegetables, on a weight basis, supply as much calcium and riboflavin as milk. . . . A large serving (about 1 cup, 200 grams) of such greens as collards, kale, turnip, and mustard, provides as much calcium as 1 cup milk. It is interesting that the Chinese Medical Association recommended an intake of 500 grams green leafy vegetables per day.[26] In addition to greater consumption of dark green leafy vegetables, the use of cabbage, broccoli, and cauliflower will contribute lesser amounts of calcium but more than most other vegetables. Other plant sources which are fair to good sources of calcium include: legumes, particularly soybeans; some nuts, particularly almonds; and dried fruits. An evaluation of a pure vegetarian diet must be made to determine how often and in what quantity these plant sources are used. Occasional use cannot be counted on to replace the calcium and riboflavin of milk.

Hardinge and Stare found that diets of the pure vegetarians they studied usually consisted of cooked cereals and bread, legumes, nuts, large quantities of fruits and vegetables, especially large salads,[27] vegetable oils, and olives. Minimal quantities of refined and commercially prepared foods were used. Few desserts were eaten. . . .

One-Day Vegetarian Menu

Breakfast

- orange juice—4 ounces
- cooked oatmeal—1 cup
- milk (LV)*—4 ounces
- soymilk (PV)**—4 ounces
- whole wheat toast—1 slice
- peanut butter—tablespoon
- clear, hot cereal beverage, if desired

Noon Meal

- soy patties with tomato sauce—2
- baked potato—1
- margarine—1 pat

- cooked fresh or frozen peas — ⅔ cup
- shredded carrot salad — ½ cup scant
- dressing — ½ tablespoon
- wheat roll
- margarine — 1 pat
- strawberries, fresh or frozen without sugar — ¾ cup
- milk (LV) — 8 ounces
- soymilk (PV) — 8 ounces

Evening Meal

- vegetable soup — 1 cup (200 grams)
- sandwich: whole wheat bread — 2 slices; garbanzo-egg filling (LV)
- savory garbanzos (PV)
- sliced peaches — ½ cup
- walnut-stuffed dates — 4
- milk (LV)8 ounces
- soymilk (PV)8 ounces

*LV = lacto ovo vegetarian.
**PV = pure vegetarian

Properly selected lacto ovo vegetarian diets are tasty and attractive and require no supplementation. A pure vegetarian diet can be planned that is adequate in quantity and quality of protein, as well as all other known nutrients, if supplemented with vitamin B_{12}. The approximate values of certain essential nutrients and amino acids for a one-day vegetarian diet are given in tables 47.3 and 47.4

Table 47.3 Approximate Nutrient Composition of One-Day Vegetarian Diet

Nutrient	Lacto Ovo Vegetarian	Pure Vegetarian	Recommended Allowance*
Kilocalories	2,030.0	2,040.0	2,000.0
Protein (grams)	78.0	75.0	55.0
Fat (grams)	76.0	77.0	—
Carbohydrate (grams	260.0	265.0	—
Calcium (milligrams)	1,110.0	740.0	800.0
Iron (milligrams)	18.0	24.8	18.0
Vitamin A (IU)	12,600.0	14,600.0	5,000.0
Thiamine (milligrams)	2.5	2.9	1.0
Riboflavin (milligrams)	2.2	2.3	1.5
Niacin (milligrams)	18.6	22.9	13.0
Ascorbic acid (milligrams)	185.0	185.0	55.0

* For women, 22 to 35 years of age.

Table 47.4 Amino Acid Content of One-Day Lacto Ovo Vegetarian and Pure Vegetarian Diets

Amino Acid (grams)	Lacto Ovo Vegetarian	Pure Vegetarian	Minimum	Recommen-dation*
Isoleucine	3.74	3.40	0.7	1.4
Leucine	6.59	5.66	1.1	2.2
Lysine	3.39	4.09	0.8	1.6
Methionine	1.36	1.08	—	—
Cystine	1.15	1.27	—	—
Total sulphur	2.51	2.34	1.1	2.2
Phenylalanine	4.13	3.76	—	—
Tyrosine	3.10	2.56	—	—
Total aromatic	7.23	6.32	1.1	2.2
Threonine	2.93	2.75	0.5	1.0
Tryptophan	0.92	0.89	0.25	0.5
Valine	4.34	3.74	0.8	1.6

* For average man.

The dimensions of change in food patterns and products, in attitudes and habits during the 1960s have been extensive. The seventies and eighties will continue to present challenges to the dietetic practitioner to become concerned and involved in meeting the nutritional needs of the changing life-style of our contemporary world.

Notes:

1. L.E. Boeher, "Economic Aspects of Food Protein," in M. Sahyun, ed., *Protein and Amino Acids in Nutrition,* (New York: Reinhold, 1948), p. 158.

2. D.M. Hegsted et al., "Protein Requirements of Adults," *Journal of Laboratory and Clinical Medicine* 31 (1969):261.

3. M.G. Hardinge and F.J. Stare, "Nutritional Studies of Vegetarians" 1. "Nutritional, Physical, and Laboratory Findings," *American Journal of Clinical Nutrition* 2 (1954):73.

4. M.A. Ohlson, "Dietary Patterns and Effect on Nutrition Intake," *World Review of Nutrition and Dietetics* 10 (1969):13.

5. N.S. Scrimshaw, "Nature of Protein Requirements," *Journal of American Dietetic Association* 54 (1969):94.

6. H.C. Sherman, "Protein Requirement of Maintenance in Man and the Nutritive Efficiency of Bread Protein," *Journal of Biological Chemistry* 41 (1920):97.

7. R. Bressani and M. Behar, "The Use of Plant Protein Foods in Preventing Malnutrition," in E.S. Livingston, ed., Proceedings of the Sixth International Congress of Nutrition, 1964, p. 182.

8. G.G. Porter, "Some Supplementary Studies with Wheat Proteins," Master's thesis, Loma Linda University, 1957.

9. A. Sanchez, G.G. Porter, and U.D. Register, "Effect of Entrée on Fat and Protein Quality of Diets," *Journal of American Dietetic Association* 49 (1966):492.

10. A. Sanchez, J.A. Scharffenberg, and U.D. Register, "Nutritive Value of Selected Proteins and Protein Combinations," 1. "Biological Value of Proteins Singly and in Meal

Patterns with Varying Fat Composition," *American Journal of Clinical Nutrition* 13 (1963:243.

11. U.D. Register et al., "Nitrogen-Balance Studies in Human Subjects on Various Diets," *American Journal of Clinical Nutrition* 20 (1967):753.

12. A.G. Marsh, D.L. Ford, and D.K. Christensen, "Metabolic Response of Adolescent Girls to Lacto-Ovo-Vegetarian Diet," *Journal of the American Dietetic Association* 51 (1967):441.

13. C.H. Edwards et al., "Utilization of Wheat by Adult Man: Nitrogen Metabolism, Plasma Amino Acids and Lipids," *American Journal of Clinical Nutrition* 24 (1971):181.

14. M.G. Hardinge, H. Crooks, and F.J. Stare, "Nutritional Studies of Vegetarians," 5, "Proteins and Essential Amino Acids," *Journal of the American Dietetic Association* 48 (1966):25.

15. M.N. Rao, and M. Swaminathan, "Plant Proteins in the Amelioration of Protein Deficiency States," *World Review of Nutrition and Dietetics* 11 (1969):116.

16 N.S. Scrimshaw et al., "Nature and Protein Requirements."

17. S. Koury and R.E. Hodges, "Soybean Protein for Human Diets? Wholesomeness and Acceptability," *Journal of the American Dietetic Association* 52 (1968):480.

18. R. Bressani et al., "Protein Quality of a Soybean Textured Food in Animals and Children," *Journal of Nutrition* 93 (1967):349.

19. T.M. Hammonds and D.L. Call, "Utilization of Protein Ingredients in the U.S. Food Industry," Department of Agriculture, Economics Research 320 and 321. Ithaca, N.Y.: Cornell University, 1970.

20. M.G. Hardinge and H. Crooks, "Nonflesh Dietaries," 3. "Adequate and Inadequate," *Journal of the American Dietetic Association* 45 (1964):537.

21. M.G. Hardinge and F.J. Stare, "Nutritional Studies of Vegetarians," 2. "Dietary and Serum Levels of Cholesterol," *American Journal of Clinical Nutrition* 2 (1954):83.

22. R.O. West and O.B. Hayes, "Diet and Serum Cholesterol Levels. A Comparison between Vegetarians and Nonvegetarians in a Seventh-Day Adventist Group," *American Journal of Clinical Nutrition* 21 (1968):853.

23. F.R. Lemon and R.T. Walden, "Death from Respiratory System Disease among Seventh-Day Adventist Men," *Journal of the American Medical Association* 198 (1966):117.

24. R.E. Hodges et al., "Dietary Carbohydrates and Low Cholesterol Diets: Effects on Serum Lipids of Man," *American Journal of Clinical Nutrition* 20 (1967):198.

25. G.G. Porter, "Supplementary Studies on Wheat."

26. Commission on Nutrition, Council of Public Health, Chinese Medical Association, "Minimum Nutritional Requirement for China," *Chinese Medical Journal* 55 (1939):301.

27. A. Sanchez, J.A. Scharffenberg, and U.D. Register, "Nutritive Value of Proteins."

Selection 48   A Guide to Good Eating the Vegetarian Way

Elizabeth B. Smith

Editors' Introduction

The following selection presents another alternative for an eco-logically oriented diet that will also lower cholesterol and satur-ated-fat levels of the diet and thus reduce these risk factors that are associated with the development of heart disease. The follow-ing suggestions differ from those presented in previous selections. They were developed in Canada in response to an expressed need for assistance in the selection of nutritionally adequate meals by those who had recently turned to vegetarianism. Work on the project began with trial menus for a seventy-kilogram man for one week. All the menus provided twelve ounces of milk and one and one-half eggs daily.

Since this project was initiated in Canada, computer checks of energy and nutrient levels indicated that adjustments were needed for adequacy according to Canadian Dietary Standard (CDS) which differ from the RDA. Serving sizes were altered for other age and sex categories of the CDS and their adequacy was checked. Foods of similar composition were classified in four groups, standard servings described, and numbers of servings for each family member tabulated. These guidelines together with instructional materials were designed to assist novice vegetarians in selecting nutritionally adequate, varied, and appetizing meals.

Those races and ethnic groups who, for religious or ethical rea-sons, have traditionally practiced vegetarianism without benefit of the science of nutrition have acquired—by a sort of evolutionary process—certain rules of thumb for selection of prudent and healthful diets. More recently the ranks of the so-called vegetarians have been greatly swollen by those who, for economic or a variety of other reasons (all valid to the practitioners), have given up meat eating.

When the "new vegetarian" goes to the market place, his/her approach will almost certainly be found to fall into one of three classes if

Source: Adapted from Elizabeth B. Smith, "A Guide to Good Eating the Vegetarian Way," *Journal of Nutrition Education* 7, no. 3 (July–September 1975):109–11. © Society for Nutrition Education. Reprinted by permission. Complete notes and references and selected tables appearing in this article have been omitted here; for further information consult the original version.

at least some rudimentary forethought before selection of grocery items may be assumed. The first will simply choose foods as usual but rigorously omit any meats, fish, and poultry and possibly such animal products as milk and eggs. This vegetarian will end up eating larger quantities of a random assortment of plant foods to satisfy appetite. Nutritional adequacy of the daily meals will also be random.

A second group, perhaps with more education and less resistance to Canada's or other food guides than is frequently found, will try to apply the principles of these plans. Although lip service is given to "meat alternates" in these guides, such cavalier treatment of a rather complex matter cannot be expected to automatically ensure inclusion of sufficient protein in the daily meals. The third class of meal planner will rationally choose substitutes of roughly equivalent value to the missing animal foods. The degree to which energy and nutrient needs are met is a function of his/her knowledge and skill in performing this task.

Hazards of Vegan Diet

The hazards of adhering to a strictly based dietary, as practiced by the vegan or by the Zen Macrobiotic, have been pointed out by a number of workers and groups. On the basis of these studies the most serious shortcomings of such diets are the quality and quantity of protein. Other nutrients likely to be marginal are calcium, iron, zinc, riboflavin, niacin, and vitamin D with vitamin B_{12} entirely absent. As stated above, many individuals and population groups have practiced vegetarianism on a long-term basis and have demonstrated excellent health. Study of the diets of such people will invariably show some dependence on such foods as soya beans, nuts, milk and milk products, and eggs, alone or in combination.

That plant-based diets supplemented with milk, or with milk and eggs, can be entirely nutritional has been demonstrated under a variety of conditions including long-term usage of the diets. Firm support that vegetarians can be well nourished *if* they meet certain stipulated conditions was lent by the National Academy of Sciences' Food and Nutrition Board when it issued a statement on vegetarian diets in 1974. The conditions to be met are: a variety of plant foods; inclusion of foods rich in calcium, riboflavin, iron, and vitamin A; sources of vitamin D and vitamin B_{12}.

In our community, the frequency of inquiries for help in adapting to the vegetarian way of life and the many expressions of concern as to the nutritional quality of the meals eaten by the "amateur" vegetarian alerted us to the need for a more structured set of guidelines for food usage than is presently available.

Objective of Project

The project objective was to meet this need by providing an easily understood guide for selection of nutritionally sound vegetarian meals for individuals of all ages and families of all sizes. The project had a secondary aim of explaining the assignment of foods into groups, namely their nutrient contribution in the quantities specified, in order to meet the needs of the body in accordance with the Canadian Dietary Standard (CDS). That is, the vegetarian food guide should become a tool for some basic nutrition education to show the linkup between foods, nutrition, and health. Additional information designed to assist the vegetarian in serving varied, attractive, and tasty meals was to be placed in the text of a small booklet.

Other desirable characteristics of a food guide are that it should offer a pattern of food usage adaptable to people of varying cultural, ethnic, or economic backgrounds; descriptive of conventional or newly developed protein foods available at market sites; flexible enough to permit a three-meal-a-day or a more casual eating pattern; obtainable at various cost levels adaptable to income; permit opportunity for creativity and, while not demanding it, should permit the exercise of culinary skill.

For reasons already described, the guide was designed for lacto ovo vegetarian meals. The nutrient levels of the CDS represented the standard for nutrient adequacy of the meals but not necessarily the energy allowances. Energy levels were met by the meals, plus snacks where required, of moderate- or high-calorie foods. This plan facilitates planning calorie-reduced meals.

Development of the guide involved the following stages:

1. Planning menus for seven days for an adult man, including twelve ounces milk or its equivalent and 1 and a half eggs daily. (For the first set of menus, amounts of food selected were in accordance with our best estimates of what might be needed for nutritional adequacy. The twelve ounces milk was in agreement with *Canada's Food Guide*. The daily egg intake was selected to permit the use of one whole egg in a meal, plus an additional fraction that might be needed for a baked item or a mixed dish. Thus, practical considerations had an overriding influence on the milk and egg allowances. At the same time, protein quality and the levels of several nutrients stood to be enhanced by these quantities of egg and milk.)

2. Calculation of nutrient and energy content in accordance with Handbook No. 8 food composition tables programmed for computer analysis.

3. Adjustment, where necessary, of foods or sizes of servings to meet the CDS.

4. Classification of foods used into groups on the basis of the nutrient content of the amounts set forth.
5. Determination of the minimum number of servings of each food group needed daily to meet the CDS for nutrients. Energy shortages were to be made up by means of snack items.
6. Checking protein quality by calculation of the essential amino acid content of daily menus for comparison with the FAO provisional reference pattern.
7. Testing the validity of the guide at this stage by using it as the only resource for compiling an additional seven days of menus, followed by calculation of the nutrient value of the meals and the total energy value of meals plus snacks.
8. Extension of the guide for all the other age and sex categories of the CDS with adjustments of numbers and sizes of servings to meet their needs (as in stages 2 through 6).
9. Preparation of descriptive and instructional material to assist in interpretation of the guide.
10. Testing and evaluation of the effectiveness of the guide as a tool for the would-be vegetarian.

A more detailed description of these procedures has been published. Food groupings, size of servings (see table 48.1), [and] numbers of servings for each family member (see table 48.2) [were determined]. . . .

Results and Evaluation

As judged by results of preliminary testing by high school and university students who were asked to prepare a one day's menu in accordance with a skeleton form of the guide, clarification of the actual procedure was needed, even for these groups with better-than-average

Table 48.1 Food Groups and Serving Sizes

Group I: Bread, cereal, pasta, and rice
  1 slice of whole grain or enriched white bread with butter or margarine
  ⅓–½ cup granola-type cereal
  ¾ cup cooked whole grain or enriched cereal
  1 cup cold whole grain or enriched cereal
  2–6 tablespoons uncooked farina, cracked wheat, oatmeal, etc.
  ¾ cup cooked, enriched, whole grain or soy macaroni, noodles, etc.
  1 of biscuit, muffin, pancake, slice of nut loaf, fruit bread, with butter or margarine
  1 tablespoon wheat germ
  ¾ cup cooked brown, converted or enriched rice
  1 large cookie
  3–4 crackers

Table 48.1 (continued)

Group II: Vegetable protein foods

TVP: This is a textured vegetable protein usually made from soy beans. It is available in a dried form and needs reconstitution with water during preparation. TVP is used mainly in casserole-type entrées in combination with foods from other groups. One 3-ounce package will be sufficient in a casserole to serve five. Check the label for serving information.

Legumes: 1 cup of cooked soybeans, chic-peas, brown or orange lentils, pinto, kidney or navy beans, etc.
¼ cup of peanuts or peanut butter
6 ounces soybean curd

Meat analogs: These are usually canned or frozen meat-like foods derived from vegetable protein (often soy, gluten, or nut protein). Three ounces of these imitation foods are usually sufficient. These are available as chicken, beef, pork, sausage, or bacon types. They vary in many ways so check the label for information.

Nuts and seeds: 1½ ounces or 3 tablespoons provides one serving. These are usually to be used as snack foods or in combination with Group I or IV foods several times a week. To replace legumes occasionally the quantity should be doubled or tripled. Nuts include cashews, cashew butter, pignolias, pistachios, walnuts, Brazils, pecans, among others. Sunflower, sesame, pumpkin, and squash seeds are the most readily obtained seeds in this country.

Group III: Milk and eggs

Milk: The standard serving of milk is one cup of whole, 2 percent, skim (added vitamins A and D), or other milk drinks. To substitute for one cup of milk you may use:
1¼ ounces cheddar cheese or processed cheese, etc.
1 ounce Swiss cheese
4 ounces cream cheese
4 tablespoons (¼ cup) cottage cheese
1 cup yogurt
1½ cups ice cream

Milk should be supplemented with vitamin D for all growing children and pregnant women.

Eggs: One and a half eggs on the average are recommended by the guide. This includes those used in baked items, scrambled, fried, in omelettes, souffles, custards, and casseroles, etc.

Group IV: Fruits and vegetables

	Serving
Whole, raw, baked, e.g., corn on cob, apple	1 medium
Leafy raw bulky vegetable, e.g., lettuce, bean sprouts	1 cup
Cooked, e.g., canned peas, cherries	½ cup
Large, e.g., grapefruit, melon (5″)	½
Small, e.g., grapes	15
plums	3–4
Juice, e.g., tomato, apple	½ cup (4 ounces)
Dried, e.g., raisins, figs	2 tablespoons

Fruits are numerous: apples, apricots, bananas, berries, melons, citrus (orange, grapefruit), grapes, pears, peaches, plums, rhubarb, pumpkin, and many more. Vegetables include: asparagus, beans, bean sprouts, beets, cauliflower, carrots, celery, greens (lettuce, endive, etc.), onions, parsnips, peas, potatoes, squash, tomatoes.

Table 48.2 Guide to Numbers of Standard Servings

Food Group		Number of Standard Servings Needed Every Day									
	Adult Male	Adult Female	Pregnant Adult Female	Age 18-19 Male	Age 18-19 Female	Age 13-15 Male	Age 13-15 Female	Age 10-12 Both	Age 7-9 Both	Age 4-6 Both	Age 2-3 Both
I. Breads, cereals, pasta, and rice	8	6	6	9	5	7	5	5	4	3	3
II. Vegetable protein foods											
Legumes, meat analogs, TVP	1	¾	¾	1½	¾	¾	½	½	½	¼	⅛
Nuts and seeds	1	1	1	2	1	1	¾	¾	½	¼	⅛
III. Milk and eggs											
Milk	1½	1½	4	2-3	2-3	4	4	4	2	2-3	2-3
Eggs	1½	1½	1½	1½	1½	1½	1½	1½	1	1	1
IV. Fruits and vegetables	6	5	5-6	6	5	5	5	4	4	3	2
Extra foods*	No requirements										

Note: Amounts were determined by computer analysis of nutrients of test menus.

* These foods may provide calories, but few nutrients. They include sugar, jams, seasonings, beverages including alcohol, cream, pickles, foods used in garnishing, etc., and are useful mainly in providing flavor and color interest.

education. In consultation with professional colleagues, the explanatory material was revised, the glossary of terms expanded, and the reading level lowered to meet that of an individual with about grade 8 education. Finally, the food guide was submitted to the staff of the Home Economics Directorate of the Manitoba Department of Health and Social Development to arrange for printing in booklet form for consumers in our province.

The actual process of menu planning, preferably done on a weekly basis, is set forth as a series of eight steps, initially, which should be reducible to a minimum following a little practice. A series of cross-checks requires pen-and-paper work at the outset but should soon become a mental process, except for the weekly shopping list which requires careful calculation. Examples of entrée dishes and a sample menu for a family of four carried through these planning stages plus the cross-checks are added to ease the entry of the novice into the new life-style.

As a further evaluative procedure, the material has been presented at a workshop attended by about 100 home economists, dietitians, and nutritionists. They are the professionals who will assist the consumer by interpreting and supplementing the printed material where required. A consensus of the evaluations was that it was rather complex and initially time-consuming compared to other plans now in use. However, it was felt that with practice and interpretation where required, both of these objections could be overcome and that the vegetarian food guide could truly point the way toward a nutritional and rewarding eating style.

Selection 49 Unconventional Food: Menu for Tomorrow

Nevin S. Scrimshaw

Editors' Introduction

Novel food resources and unconventional technologies for food production, assuming they can be applied on a mass scale, may well avert the world famine that appeared inevitable only a few

Source: Adapted from Nevin S. Scrimshaw, "Unconventional Food: Menu for Tomorrow," *Technology Review* (October/November 1977):53–57. Reprinted by permission. Photos appearing in this article have been omitted here; for further information consult the original version.

years ago. These new nutritional technologies involve the production of vitamins, minerals, amino acids, and protein concentrates that can be used for fortification of traditional foods and formulation of new ones. The most promising approaches are enrichment and fortification with synthetic nutrients and fortification with biologically produced protein concentrates.

Enrichment and Fortification with Synthetic Nutrients

Food quality can be upgraded through enrichment and fortification during processing. Missing nutrients can be supplied with synthetically produced vitamins, minerals, and essential amino acids, thereby increasing the nutritive value of traditional foods. Although enrichment and fortification are common practices in affluent nations, mass use of the idea to benefit the Hungry World is relatively new. For example, since World War II, a number of industrial countries have passed regulations requiring the addition of synthetic B-vitamins to refined flour to replace the nutrients lost in processing. In developing nations where polished rice is a staple food, beriberi, the thiamine-deficiency disease characterized by degenerative changes in the nervous system, is still prevalent. In the Philippines, Taiwan, and elsewhere in the Far East the experimental introduction of thiamine-enriched rice has resulted in a decline in the incidence of thiamine deficiency.

The use of iodized salt in some developing countries is a new application of a standard concept of fortification used in Canada and the United States. As pointed out by Alan Berg, author of *The Nutrition Factor,* in the goiter belt of India, the prevalence of goiter among those consuming fortified salt declined from 38 percent of the population to 15 percent in five years and to 3 percent in ten years. Similar results were reported in Guatemala, where endemic goiter dropped from 39 percent of the population in 1952 to 15 percent in 1962 and to 5 percent in 1965. As Berg further points out, in neighboring Central American countries where salt remained unfortified, the goiter rates did not decrease during the same period.

Studies indicate the nutritional status of population groups subsisting on cereal diets may possibly be improved by adding synthetic forms of limiting amino acid(s). For example, the quality of wheat has been improved with addition of lysine; the quality of maize has been improved with addition of lysine and tryptophan; and the amino acid pattern of rice has been improved with addition of lysine and threonine. However, although such measures enrich and fortify cereals and improve the quality of vegetable protein consumed, they do not solve the problem of low-protein and low-calorie intake typical in developing countries. Also, although the cost of vitamin and mineral supplementation of traditional foods is relatively low, the cost of protein fortification is still prohibitive. Furthermore, a great deal of caution is needed to avoid adding too much of the limiting amino acid and perhaps causing an amino acid imbalance. Such programs, feasible where cereals are milled in a central facility, are not feasible in rural areas where the people grow and grind their own cereal products. Thus, only urban populations have access to such fortified foods.

Fortification with Biologically Produced Protein Concentrates

Foods may be fortified with biologically produced concentrates such as oilseeds, fish protein concentrates (FPC), single-cell protein (SCP), and leaf protein.

Oilseeds. One of the most promising means of increasing the quantity and quality of protein in the diets of people in developing countries is the use of oilseeds. Oilseed meal is manufactured as a by-product of vegetable oil production from cottonseed, soybean, sesame, and sunflower. The residue, cake or meal, from the production of oil (when properly refined and processed) is fit for human consumption and is probably the world's least expensive source of protein, containing 40 to 50 percent good-quality protein. The quality of protein in oilseeds, although considerably higher than protein in any individual cereal, is not as high as animal protein. Oilseed protein is low in the essential amino acid methionine. A combination of cereal with oilseeds yields a better combination than when either are eaten alone, since most oilseeds are low in methionine found in cereals but high in lysine and the other essential amino acids that cereals lack.

Oilseed meal is used to fortify such foods as dry milk solids and flour. In schools oilseed meal is often added to soups, stews, and mixed dishes. It also serves as a protein base for such formulated foods as Incaparina, a mixture of vegetable proteins designed as a milk substitute to prevent malnutrition among children in Central America. Incaparina contains 25 percent or more of high-quality protein as well as vitamins and minerals to prevent nutrient deficiencies that usually accompany kwashiorkor. Similar products have been used in Africa and India, where they have been engineered to meet the specific nutrient needs of target groups in these countries and provide calories. According to some experts, if oilseed meals were used fully for human consumption, 10 grams of additional protein per capita daily could be added to the diets of people in developing countries. Unfortunately, many of these protein-deficient countries export much of their domestically produced oilseed meals to affluent countries where they are used as fertilizer or animal feed.

Recently soybean meal has been developed for human consumption in the form of soy flour, soy concentrate, and soy isolate; each of which vary in their protein content and contain from 50 to 90 percent protein. They are used in infant foods, beverages, cereals, breads, cakes, and cookies and to produce simulated milk products (soybean milk), textured meat analogs, and meat extenders. Soybeans provide the base for a high-protein soft drink, Vitasoy, popular in Hong Kong. Similar beverages are being marketed on a trial basis in Brazil, Guyana, and other countries.

Meat analogs, or textured protein product (TPP), are made by spinning soy isolate into fibers that are then formed into bundles and fashioned into various textured forms. With the addition of flavorings and colorings, they become facsimile foods. They may taste and look like chicken, ham, hot dogs, bacon, or hamburgers, but they contain less saturated fat, particularly cholesterol, than meat. When textured soy protein meat extenders are added to ground meat, for example, the amino acid pattern of the vegetable protein is supplemented by the methionine in meat, resulting in a product with an excellent amino acid pattern at a much lower cost. In the coming years meat analogs and meat extenders may make up from 10 to 20 percent of the U.S. meat supply. The popularity of such soy products may price developing countries out of the soy food market just as they have been priced out of the high-quality animal protein market.

Fish protein concentrate (FPC). A tasteless, colorless powder, called fish protein concentrate that contains 80 to 90 percent protein of high quality can be made from trash fish, otherwise unacceptable to humans, by removing all the oil and water. Small amounts of FPC are added to flour, infant foods, soups, and other traditional foods as well as to livestock feed and pet foods. Adding 5 to 10 percent FPC to cereal boosts the nutritional composition to a level comparable to the composition of animal protein. Large amounts of imperfectly processed FPC prove objectionable in taste, odor, or color. FPC is a rather expensive fortifying additive. The UN Protein Advisory Group's working committee on FPC has, therefore, concluded that FPC could not be recommended to developing countries because its cost would not generally be competitive with the cost of other supplements. In the future less expensive, but more sophisticated, techniques will probably be developed to eliminate the fish taste and odor and to facilitate the production of less expensive, bland forms of FPC.

Single-cell protein (SCP). Certain strains of microorganisms, including the bacteria and yeast, may be cultivated to increase the supply of protein. Single-cell protein, labeled SCP, has been identified by the UN Protein Advisory Group as a potentially new protein source. One common method of production involves the cultivation of these microorganisms on oil, natural gas, sewage, and paper to provide a source of preformed energy to support growth. In addition, inorganic nitrogen such as ammonia or ammonium salts is also introduced into the medium. The bacteria and yeast utilize the inorganic nitrogen that is not utilizable by higher animals to synthesize protein. The dried extracted product or powder contains about 40 percent protein and is colorless and flavorless. Since SCP is unpalatable as a food in itself, it is now used as an ingredient in animal feed. Technological procedures are being developed to extract the high content of nucleic acid in SCP, since it may cause kidney disease and gout in humans. However, technological breakthroughs are developing to eliminate this substance and other possible toxic materials and thus render a purer product fit for human consumption. The economics of such processes are still questionable and will determine whether SCP will be a feasible protein fortifier for widespread use.

Leaf protein. The green leaves and stalks of grasses, shrubs, and trees contain some protein. However, these food sources cannot be consumed directly by humans because of their high-fiber content and their bitter taste. Although still in the experimental stage, efficient protein-extraction equipment has been developed in recent years. In the tropical and subtropical areas, where there is a great protein gap, a continuous supply of green leaves that are available all year round exists. The quality of leaf protein is second only to soy protein and may be further improved by adding methionine.

In the following selection Dr. Nevin S. Scrimshaw, Head of the Department of Nutrition and Food Science at MIT, reviews some of the above-mentioned technologies and discusses other novel materials and approaches. He also stresses the need for a great deal of toxicological research to determine reasonable regulatory standards that can be applied in the development of new foods. With the development of novel foods we must also educate people to use foods that are around them but that for cultural reasons they often overlook. We must bear in mind, however, that when energy intake is deficient, the provision of protein without significant improvement in energy intake is unlikely to improve nutritional status.

Since 1950, the world has had to find food for an additional billion people, and the time in which to increase food production for the next billion will be even shorter.

Before World War II only Europe was a net importer of food, but since then, virtually all other regions of the world have become increasingly dependent on food imports from North America and, to a lesser extent, from Australia and Argentina. In most countries food production has failed to keep up with population increases and the food demands occasioned by rising affluence and living standards.

A National Research Council report, "Population and Food: Crucial Issues," emphasizes that the scale, severity, and duration of the world food problem are so great that a massive, long-range innovative effort unprecedented in history will be required to master it. More recently, the NRC's "World Food and Nutrition Study: The Potential Contributions of Research" has confirmed this prognosis. In fact, the study finds that malnutrition will not be alleviated unless developing countries can double their own food production by the end of this century. Although these countries were able to increase production by 38 percent between 1965 and 1975, the additional 100 percent increase" ... will not be easy to achieve and sustain," according to the NRC's report. Furthermore, if developing countries continue to import increasing amounts of food from the United States, our own productivity must increase at an appreciable rate.

There is little doubt that the production of traditional food sources can be tremendously increased by the application of currently available technology. Future research gives promise of continuing gains, but we must also look to development of unconventional technologies for food production and of novel food sources as potential resources. Indeed, such development is among the priorities of both NRC reports.

Drawing upon a recent study conducted by MIT for the National Science Foundation under its Research Applied to National Needs (RANN) Program, I will review the contributions experts foresee from novel food sources and unconventional technologies of food production in the decades ahead.

The Fixation of Nitrogen

An example of unconventional research to improve traditional agricultural crops is the work on biological nitrogen fixation. It is necessary to pay particular attention to protein foods in view of their critical importance in human nutrition. Proteins are key components of the enzymes controlling all body processes, as well as the fundamental component of muscle, brain, and nerve tissue, and all body cells.

Nitrogen is vital to increased food production, but the cost of nitrogen fertilizer has increased sharply with rising energy costs. We know that some plants—notably the legumes—host microorganisms that have the ability to convert atmospheric nitrogen into chemical forms that are useful as plant nutrients. The protein nature of the nitrogenase complex that catalyzes nitrogen fixation in such microorganisms in soybean and lupine nodules is fairly well understood. But enhancement of such biological fixation—whether by symbiotic microorganisms attached to the plant roots, or nonsymbiotic, through introduction of the enzyme complex into the plant itself, requires greater understanding of the processes themselves and of the organisms that have this capacity. For example, research is needed to determine the enzyme mechanisms and the forces that power the overall reaction. The genes coding for nitrogenase in bacteria have been successfully transferred from one species to another. Thus, a potential exists to improve the nitrogen-fixing capacity of organisms by means of genetic manipulation. Useful application of biological nitrogen fixation to grasses might even be achieved once we understand more fully the genetic and biochemical compatibility of hosts and endophytes.

Milk from Whey

Casein, caseinates, certain milk protein and whey proteins from modified and fermented whey are secondary dairy products, connected with cheese technology and casein manufacture. All are highly nutritious. Unfortunately, these proteins are now largely wasted; they deserve attention because they can improve the protein yield of cheese and casein production. Whey could be formulated with full-fat soya flour, vegetable fats, carbohydrates and vitamin-mineral supplements to provide a low-cost, highly nutritious milk for infants and children.

Amber Waves of Grain

Low-cost cereal grains and their underutilized milling by-products such as brewers' spent grains, corn gluten meal, shorts, bran, and mill feed grains are abundant in this country. Scientific and technological effort could upgrade their food use and nutritional value. The potential benefits of producing protein concentrates from cereals seem particularly promising for both domestic and foreign markets. For example, wheat protein concentrates prepared from dry milling or wet milling of wheat or wheat by-products are becoming available. Nutritious and low-cost oat protein products have been prepared experimentally from the wet milling of oats.

Corn germ flour is now commercially prepared by dry millers for the food industry by refining the germ separated from the corn after oil is extracted. Formerly used for animal feed, it is now expected to contribute nutrient value to many processed foods. Additional food-technology research is needed on corn germ protein isolate, and on corn proteins isolated from corn endosperm by the wet milling industry — another by-product normally consigned to animal feed.

Blood, Bones, and Broken Eggs

The potential for expanded development, production, and use of unconventional products from the meat and poultry industries is also great. Centralized packaging of meat prior to distribution in retail outlets has already increased the use of bones and fat because they can be used for pet food rather than discarded as household waste.

Blood, a by-product of slaughter, contains 17 percent protein and is usually processed into animal feed. The total recovery of this material as food could result in the production of over 400 million pounds of protein per year in the United States alone.

Approximately 5 percent of the eggs used for hatching prove to be infertile; these eggs, identified by shining a light through them, could be removed from incubators at an early stage and processed for human food. A similar proportion of U.S. egg production intended for human consumption is designated unfit when received at processing plants because the eggs have embryos, cracked shells, blood spots, and other minor defects. This represents a substantial loss of safe, edible protein.

At present, federal regulations limit the addition of plant proteins to meat products. For example, sausage must be labeled "imitation" if it contains more than 2 percent of isolated soy protein. The requirement makes no nutritional sense, and as long as no deception is involved, it is not in the consumer's interest.

The Sea's Untapped Harvest

Most of the fish species from U.S. waters that are traditionally eaten by the American consumer are either fully exploited or depleted.

But species exist that remain largely unexploited or underexploited. For example, bottom fish, unpalatable in their original form, could be harvested to yield between 100,000 and 500,000 tons per year and could be offered in the form of engineered, fabricated foods simulating fish products more familiar to the general public.

"Trash fish" (species not desired for human consumption) are caught during shrimping operations and discarded. They could be used as raw material for the manufacture of fish meal. Between 250,000 and 500,000 tons are available per year and are now wasted.

Squid populations are so generous that the U.S. catch on the East and West Coasts could be increased from 13,000 to 500,000 tons per year, once technologies for locating, harvesting, preserving, and processing squid are developed and a market is created for domestic consumption or for export. Squid is now eaten directly as food, but it could also be used in textured and engineered food products.

A further source of aquatic protein stands in a class by itself: Antarctic krill, the single largest natural source of animal protein in the world. A conservative estimate of the krill resource puts the standing crop at 100 million tons, and possibly 50 million tons per year could be harvested without diminishing the resource. If the United States were able to take even one-tenth of this annual potential harvest, we could in theory equal our yields from all conventional aquatic sources. Krill also represents a source for chitin, an important natural polymer capable of replacing certain petroleum-derived products. . . . Management of this resource, however, raises a series of very difficult problems, among them the difficulties of catching and processing the fish in hostile Antarctic waters and finding acceptable ways to use them.

Many of these increased aquatic food resources will consist of raw material derived from species largely unfamiliar to the average U.S. customer. For psychological and economic reasons, such new food products will probably have to be presented to the U.S. consumer in a processed form so that the original raw material is no longer recognizable.

Food Grown on Oil and Gas

Nonphotosynthetic single-cell protein (SCP) is a generic term for protein produced by single-cell organisms such as yeasts or bacteria that ferment petroleum derivatives or organic wastes. Some forms of SCP have been used in human food for millennia; any fermented food product—yogurt, wine, and many cheeses, for example—contains significant quantities of cellular organisms as diverse as bacteria, yeast, and fungi. Thus there should be nothing fundamentally objectionable in the food use of these species.

The raw material chosen for SCP production depends, to a very large extent, on local availability. Natural gas or methane would be reasonable choices in areas where they are available in abundance and where they are now even discarded as flare gas. Less desirable petroleum fractions could be used, and local economics will determine whether any of these—crude, semipurified gas and oil, or refined fractions—are the most feasible substrates. A number of research groups have concentrated on processes that use a relatively pure paraffin distillate for production of either food or feed.

Methane is frequently available at low cost. Its direct fermentation appears limited to bacteria, however, and no large-scale, continuous process has yet been developed that provides sufficiently high cell growth rates and cell concentrations to be economically attractive.

Alcohols, particularly methanol and ethanol, can be derived from gaseous hydrocarbons via catalytic hydration, and both of these can be utilized by a wide variety of microorganisms. They can be prepared with purity adequate for use in food, they are totally water soluble, and leave no residues to contaminate the cell mass. Because these lower alcohols exhibit advantages of both hydrocarbon and carbohydrate fermentations, they currently have the best potential for SCP processing, and they are particularly attractive as a source of food protein.

There are also a variety of fermentable carbohydrate sources. Sulfite waste liquor and whey are good candidates in some geographic areas. Cellulose is the most abundant carbohydrate raw material, available from waste paper, bagasse, wood pulp, sawdust, etc. In the USSR, hydrolyzed wood pulp supports a feed yeast industry estimated at approximately 1 million tons per year. Solid cannery waste and citrus waste are possible sources of carbohydrate, but seasonal processing schedules and the fact that the material is sometimes dilute present problems. Even animal waste and manure can be recovered and refed to livestock after microbiological processing.

Starch is much more readily hydrolyzed than cellulose, and the potential exists for direct fermentation of starch by fungi in a continuous process. Starch may be of particular interest in tropical areas that produce high yields of starch root crops such as cassava. Sugars such as molasses are similarly useful substrates for fermentation. Both are sometimes available in excess in tropical regions. Bacteria, yeast, and fungi are all being considered for use in pilot or commerical scale food processes.

The high content of ribonucleic acid (RNA) relative to protein in SCP is the major limitation to using SCP in food at higher than food additive levels of 3 to 5 percent. Methods have been devised for RNA removal, although they add to the cost of processing. Selective isolation of proteins might be a method to avoid the RNA problem. Chemical, mechanical, and enzymatic means of cell disruption have been tried, but their expense is discouraging. Possible genetic solutions involve isolating "fragile" mutants (mutants with cell walls that break more readily) and temperature-sensitive hyperlytic mutants. Research has yet to be done on how SCP can be applied in the manufacture of food; studies are needed of engineering properties, interactions of SCP with food constituents, and the use of SCP in the production of textured protein.

The protein nutritional quality of SCP is high, but because SCP is deficient in sulfur amino acids, it does not compare well with the nutritional quality of animal proteins. Studies at MIT indicate problems of human tolerance to some SCPs that were not revealed in extensive toxicological studies in experimental animals. We believe that this problem can be overcome by relatively simple processing procedures.

Nutrition from Ponds, Protein from Leaves

Photosynthetic single-cell protein: a long label for a simple organism, algae. It is found suspended in shallow, illuminated ponds in whose waters are dissolved simple salts such as carbonates, nitrates, and phosphates. Depending on growth conditions and genera, algae may contain between 8 and 75 percent protein, and the biological value of algae varies from about 50 to 70 percent of that of egg. Nutritionists have concentrated primarily on three genera—*Chlorella, Scenedesmus,* and *Spirulina*—which, when separated, form a dark green slurry or paste containing 5 to 15 percent solids that may be consumed directly by animals or preserved by freezing or dehydration. For poultry and livestock, algae have been mixed with cereals and manufactured into pellets. For feeding hogs the nutritional value of waste-grown algae appears equivalent to that of meat and bone meal and superior to an equal weight of soybean meal. Waste-grown algae could also be a good supplement to the range feed of such stock as cattle, sheep, and goats. Heat-dried algae flakes or chips can be ground into a very fine, green flour, but only a fanatic would call it palatable.

Green leaves provide the primary and largest supply of protein in the world, but leafy plants are also rich in structural materials—cellulose, lignin—that are largely indigestible by man and other single-stomached animals. Animals such as cattle and sheep that have a rumen (a gastric compartment that breaks down cellulose) or animals such as horses and sheep that have a functional caecum (a blind pouch where the large intestine begins) can digest cellulose through the action of symbiotic microorganisms. Leaves from forage crops such as alfalfa and from wastes in the production of vegetable crops are a prodigious protein resource. For example, in 1973 and 1974, the protein in U.S. alfalfa amounted to almost twice the protein in the 13.8 million tons of soybean meal marketed in this country.

Typically, such forage has been used for animal feed as fresh, whole forage, by field-curing prior to storage, or as silage. We now know that leafy crops dehydrated by pressing yield a product superior to conventionally preserved forage for many reasons, not the least significant of which is the higher retention of nutrients. The juice that is pressed out contains 25 to 50 percent of the leaves' protein and may be used as a protein source. The juice needs no further treatment and can be mixed in pig rations just prior to feeding. It may also be heated or acid treated to coagulate the protein as a curd that may be used as a poultry or swine feed, or as a human food. Further, the juice may be treated to separate a chlorophyll-containing fraction for animal feed plus a colorless fraction suitable for human consumption; both the feasibility and economics of this process remain uncertain. The nutritional value of whole-leaf protein products is in the range of that of soybean meal and may be further improved if supplemented with methionine.

Better Nourishment through Chemistry

Satisfying some human food needs by chemical synthesis is a remote possibility. For example, "formose" (heated glucose and formaldehyde) can be combined as a polymer with hydrogen cyanide (HCN) to produce amino acid mixtures, but yields are very low and many problems remain to be solved, including toxicity of other compounds in the mixture, poor taste and texture, and high cost. Stimulated largely by the demand for food during World War II, German scientists developed several processes by which fatty acids can be synthesized from petroleum hydrocarbons at current costs of about 10 to 20 cents per pound. Much more extensive studies of the products will be necessary, including tests for toxicity.

The synthesis of glycerol for human food has also been investigated, most energetically by NASA, as a potential energy source for a space colony. Commercial synthesis began with propane and resulted in a product costing about 40 cents per pound. However, another approach through formose sugars is potentially much cheaper, largely because it promises greater yield. However, the nature of the other reaction products, including their safety and potential uses, will need investigation.

Novel Food from Shelf to Kitchen

Novel food products will be slow to penetrate the market because many will be expensive and because the food industry and the consumer may be reluctant to accept them. The more innovative a food product, the more the consumer is asked to learn about its benefits and uses. The harder the consumer is to persuade, the higher are the risks for a commercial producer to develop and market the product. Such risks, the long period required to develop and test the product, and the large amounts of capital required all work to make the food industry extremely cautious in evaluating radically new food products.

Safety is an essential consideration when novel proteins or proteins processed in novel ways are to be used for human consumption. Extensive tests using experimental animals are essential, but in many cases symptoms that may appear in human trials do not appear in experimental animal tests. So studies on experimental animals are not sufficient to eliminate all possibilities of adverse reactions in man, and animal tests must be followed by cautious and systematic tolerance studies using human subjects. The need for thorough studies is particularly evident for such proposed new sources as single-cell protein, forage and leaf protein concentrate, and new legume and oilseed plants. Even soy protein should be carefully tested when it is processed in wholly new ways.

Bureaucrats in the Supermarket

Food laws will constrain the introduction of new protein foods from both unconventional sources and unconventional processes in a variety of ways. Present standards were developed or amended by the Food and Drug Administration only after long research and protracted public hearings. Depending on their novelty, protein concentrates produced by fermentation on chemical substrates are sure to be considered food additives.

The Food Additives Amendment of 1958 has now been applied through FDA regulations to any component or even ingredient of food; thus the legislation is a fundamental constraint on the development of novel foods. Food yeast grown on an unconventional substrate, or a new genetic variety of a grain cultivated for high lysine content, could be subject to FDA review. Given the FDA's historical opposition to filled milk (made by adding vegetable oil rather than higher priced butterfat to reconstituted dried skim milk), vitamin-mineral fortified sugar, and whole fish protein concentrate, we cannot expect that future FDA policy will facilitate the introduction of radically new protein resources.

Present and prospective world food needs demand careful vision and judgment. We must not only remove unnecessary legal constraints, but we must go still further to encourage the technological development of new food resources. A great deal more toxicological research on food than is conducted at present will be necessary both to identify reasonable regulatory standards and to produce new food products that will meet those standards.

Real innovation almost always threatens someone, at least in the short run. It is for this reason that many of the disagreements that result from attempts to introduce new protein foods are resolved in the political arena, or even come to litigation. When the many opportunities available to any one group for blocking an innovation are multiplied by the many groups that may oppose the innovation, the effect on a new proposal is often debilitating and occasionally fatal. Consumer pressure for traditional or "natural" foods may also obstruct the marketing of new proteins.

We may be sure that incorporating new foods into human diets will continue at a pace that must increase as pressures on traditional food supplies grow more severe and as costs rise. But economic, nutritional, safety, legal, political, and marketing obstacles will delay the process so that a calendar for these new developments is difficult to predict.

Before novel food resources and processing techniques can be tested in the legislature and the marketplace, problems of supply and nutritional value must be resolved. Even then, basic food science and technology problems of processing protein resources will remain. To solve them, protein fractions and protein molecular species must first be isolated and analyzed. Next, the interaction of these protein materials as food must be examined. And finally, the properties, quality, and acceptability of the final food products must be evaluated. Unconventional protein resources can be tapped most effectively by breaking down the raw materials and combining selected components into edible products. This approach will be more costly than processing protein concentrate by-products from oil recovery operations, but promises to yield more sophisticated and palatable food—food that people will be willing to purchase and eat. The incorporation of novel materials and technologies in food and feed is even now an evident trend in the United States and Europe. Given fairer and more objective regulatory standards and procedures, innovative marketing and promotion of novel foods, and favorable prices, the trend is likely to accelerate and spread to other parts of the world.

Selection 50 The Greening
of the Future

Noel Vietmeyer

Editors' Introduction

Although botanists have identified 50,000 known plant species, humans cultivate only some 300 of them for food. Human ingenuity is now turning to the overlooked potential of some little-known plants. Our present knowledge about potential food sources is woefully deficient. Little-known plants may, one day, contribute to the solution of the world's food deficits. In the following selection an organic chemist suggests some plants with potential as food and as a means to control population.

The 1940s were the decade of wonder chemicals—DDT, sulfa drugs, herbicides, plastics—many of them derivatives of petroleum. Man-made was modern. The laboratory seemed like a limitless cornucopia spewing forth synthesized chemical miracles.

Petroleum itself is a fossil residue of planetary vegetation, but in our euphoric dependence on it, we have forgotten the thousands of plant species that are themselves solar-powered refineries of important chemicals—and this in disregard of the fact that within a generation or two, the petrochemical explosion that began in the forties will have exhausted itself.

Now, with a growing sense of urgency, botanists around the world are reassessing the plant kingdom's genetic and chemical potential, scrutinizing species that can make commercial crops significant to global nutritional needs, and to industry and medicine as well.

Developing new crops is a complex and time-consuming task. There are plant varieties to collect and compare, tests to run on adaptability to soil types, temperatures, day lengths, and rainfall. Crop products must be analyzed and retested in every different application, and often years of research must be repeated should a minor toxin or impurity be spotted.

With today's vast technical capabilities and speedy communications networks, these scientific problems can be surmounted more easily than at any time in human history. It took thousands of years to domes-

Source: Adapted from Noel Vietmeyer, "The Greening of the Future," Quest/79. Reprinted from the September issue of Quest/79 by special permission. Copyright © 1979, Ambassador International Cultural Foundation. All rights reserved.

ticate wheat, but barely a generation to develop cranberries, the rubber tree, the kiwi fruit, and the cinchona tree (the source of quinine). . . . [Here] we sample an array of the sometimes startling new plants that promise to figure more prominently in world agriculture over the next ten to fifteen years.

People and Plants

Human survival has always depended on plants. Early man relied on them for food, medicine, clothing, and shelter, and his botanical skills should not be underestimated. All of the world's major crops were brought in from the wild and domesticated in prehistoric times.

Agriculture is easiest in the temperate and subtropical semihumid climatic zones—not the tropics. Ideally, seasons of adequate rainfall alternate with dry seasons, making soils rich and deep. Starting with a few wild grasses, tubers, beans, and fruits, early man began assisting nature in the selection of crop strains best suited to different human uses and different microenvironments. Some of these crop species now exhibit as much variety as the domestic dog and are equally unsuited to living outside of symbiosis with human beings. And yet, of the hundreds of thousands of known plant species, only about 150 have been commercially cultivated for food. Of these, a mere 30 species provide almost 85 percent of human food by weight, 95 percent of our calories and protein. It has been estimated that three-fourths of all human food energy comes from just eight species of cereal: wheat, rice, maize, barley, oats, sorghum, millet, and rye, of which the first three alone account for three-quarters of the total.

Although humans have not domesticated a single major food crop since prehistoric times, all 30 of the species on which world civilization depends today have been brought to 10 or 20 times their productive capacity of a few centuries ago. Should modern botany succeed in domesticating even one major new crop, the effect on the human future would, to say the least, be revolutionary.

Supermarket on a Stalk

For more than a century after Benjamin Franklin brought the first soybeans to the United States from France, American farmers snubbed the plant. The few soybeans harvested in this country were considered a second-rate crop fit only for export to the teeming masses of the Far East.

A meteoric rise in the soybean's cultural status began in the 1920s when scientists at the University of Illinois subjected it to serious botanical research. Today soybeans are the premier protein crop throughout the world. Soybean products are found in many American processed foods, and huge amounts of protein-rich derivatives are shipped to needy countries

As a global food source, however, the soybean suffers a fundamental limitation. A native of northern China's highland plateaus, it grows well only in temperate climates — Iowa and Argentina for example. But the world's most protein-deficient regions are hot and humid, and though millions of dollars have been spent to adapt the soybean to tropical conditions, the yields have been disappointing.

Three years ago a powerful alternative weapon in the fight against malnutrition gained attention. A new crop, the *winged bean*, was "discovered" growing in peasant gardens in remote areas of Papua New Guinea and Southeast Asia. Descriptions of the winged bean's remarkable properties were scattered through botanical literature and folklore, but few scientists had grasped the crop's global potential — in part because the winged bean, like the soybean before it, had long been ostracized as a "poor man's crop."

Today many normally cautious scientists are downright exuberant about the winged bean's future. Agronomists in at least seventy countries are testing what just may be the long sought "soybean of the tropics."

The plant looks like a pole bean, climbing with almost incredible vigor to a height of fifteen feet or more if the support pole is tall enough. A leafy mass of twining tendrils, the plant is decked from top to bottom with flowers of white or blue that quickly develop into pods.

The pods themselves, which may be green or purple or red, are as long as a man's forearm in some varieties. They are four-sided with a square or oblong cross section. A distinctive flange, or "wing," projects from each corner. Picked young, these pods are a succulent green vegetable that can be eaten raw, steamed, boiled, or stir fried to make a crisp, chewy delicacy.

But pods are just one of six different foods provided by this "supermarket on a stalk." There's no part of the winged bean plant that can't go into the pot. The leaves, cooked and eaten like spinach, could easily correct the vitamin A deficiency that blinds thousands of children annually throughout the tropics. The winged bean also sprouts succulent tendrils that look like lacy-thin asparagus. The flowers themselves can be made into a sweet-tasting garnish with the black appearance and texture of steamed mushrooms.

Perhaps the winged bean's most astounding feature is the tuberous root that swells to the size of a small potato in the soil beneath the plant. Its firm, ivory-white flesh has a delicate nutty flavor esteemed so highly by the highland tribesmen of Papua New Guinea that they hold winged bean *sing-sings* (festivals) at harvesttime. Like potatoes, these tubers can be boiled, baked, fried, or roasted, but they are four times richer in protein than potatoes and ten times richer than the more common tropical protein source, the cassava.

This is especially significant in terms of infant care, for in the tropics mothers customarily wean their babies from the breast to starchy root crops like cassava. The immediate plunge in the level of protein intake regularly induces malnutrition, marasmus, and kwashiorkor, damaging both brain development and the infant's general health.

Weaning infants to the winged bean promises to avoid this precipitous loss of protein.

For all the food value and savoriness of the pods, leaves, tendrils, flowers, and tubers, it is actually the winged bean seed that has created the greatest excitement.

If pods are left hanging on the vine, they dry out and harden, but the soybean-like seeds inside continue to swell and mature. Rich in protein (up to about 40 percent) and edible oil (about 17 percent), the seeds have a nutritional value equivalent to that of soybeans. Amino acids that make up the seed protein of both beans are present in similar proportions, as are vitamins and other nutrients. Once cooked, both beans are highly digestible and both are rich in iron and vitamin E.

In Ghana and the Ivory Coast, teams of Czech, Ghanaian, and Swiss scientists have demonstrated that winged bean seeds can be made into soups and purees suitable for very young children. Flour made from the seeds can also be used as a milk substitue to treat victims of extreme protein deficiency.

The protein that pervades the winged bean comes from a rather unexpected source—air. Air is four-fifths nitrogen, and it is a paradox that this abundant element is the key ingredient in both protein and nitrogenous fertilizer—each in short supply in the world today. Nitrogen as a gas is inert, requiring a complex chemical reaction to convert it into protein and fertilizer. The winged bean and other leguminous plants do it themselves.

The winged bean's greatest promise is as a small-scale crop in market gardens and village and backyard plots throughout the tropics, and the plant is catching on in scores of countries where it was previously unknown while undergoing more intense cultivation where it is indigenous.

In January 1978 a First International Winged Bean Conference was held in the Philippines. Some 200 participants from 29 nations on 6 continents attended. The crop even has its own newsletter, a University of Papua New Guinea publication called the *Winged Bean Flyer*. The San Francisco–based Asia Foundation has set up an office to coordinate research on the winged bean as well as seed and information exchanges.

Man-Made Grain

Triticale is a remarkable new cereal grain that is entirely a product of imaginative curiosity and scientific skill. The highest yielding of all grains, triticale is on its way to becoming the first viable crop achieved through the hybridization of two different plant species.

Since 1876 it has been known that pollen from rye could be used to fertilize wheat flowers, but the resulting hybrid remained a curiosity until the 1950s when botanists learned how to induce it to produce fertile seeds. Neither a wheat nor a rye, the hybrid has been dubbed *triticale*—from *Triticum* and *Secale,* the Latin names for the two parent grasses.

Today, the breeding of this artificial genus is spearheaded jointly by Canada's University of Manitoba (where the fertile seeds were first produced) and in Mexico by Dr. Norman E. Borlaug, whose development of high-yielding wheats earned him the Nobel Peace Prize in 1970.

In Mexican tests, an acre of triticale has yielded 3,380 pounds of grain, compared with 2,934 for wheat—results so astonishing that the hybrid is under trial cultivation on about one million acres in over 50 countries. Triticale promises to suppplement the world supply of bread, cereals, and animal feeds in addition to brewed and distilled drinks.

The new grain is seen not as competition for wheat, but as a supplement to it, for triticale inherits the vigor and hardiness of rye and can be grown in climates and soils insufficiently arable for use as wheatland.

Research shows that triticale is also equal or possibly superior to wheat in palatability and nutritive value as well. It is especially rich in lysine, an amino acid essential for human and animal health but rarely present in sufficient quantity in other cereal proteins.

Triticale is a model of what can be achieved by modern plant breeding. Its great promise to hungry developing nations has already been corroborated in trials in both Ethiopia and India.

Poor People's Rich Protein

Because the major centers of scientific research are located in the temperate zone, botanists long focused mainly on plants found in these climates. But now the needs of tropical populations have dramatically widened botany's horizons. Researchers are discovering all sorts of exotic plants that turn out to be useful in very different ways. One good example is *tarwi.*

Practically unknown outside South America's Andean region, tarwi is a common crop of the Indians of Peru, Bolivia, and Ecuador. Indeed, along with corn (maize), potatoes, and quinoa (another promising but little-known crop), tarwi is a staple of the highland diet. Pre-Inca peoples domesticated this lupine at least 1,500 years ago, and today tourists visiting Cuzco, the ancient Inca capital, will find baskets of tarwi seeds a common sight in the marketplace.

To the Indians in their poverty, meat is a luxury. But tarwi is extremely rich in protein, richer in fact than peas, beans, soybeans, or peanuts, and, for this reason, about a dozen researchers scattered around the globe have begun intensive study of the Andean plant.

Like other poor man's crops, tarwi is hardy and adaptable. It is easily planted and can tolerate frost, drought, a range of soils, and many pests. It grows vigorously, sometimes reaching a height of two meters, with masses of foliage and showy purplish flowers. Held high about the leaves are many tiers of pods, each containing bean-like seeds of white or black or a mottled combination of the two.

Tarwi seeds are exceptionally nutritious. Protein and oil make up more than half their weight, the protein content alone averaging 46 percent. With oil content ranging from 5 to more than 20 percent, the tarwi seed is roughly comparable to the soybean in composition and nutritional value.

Before tarwi becomes a widespread crop, researchers will have to solve one major problem. Unprocessed, the seeds taste quite bitter due to the presence of toxic alkaloids. The Indians soak the seeds in running water for a day or two to wash out the alkaloids. But this inconvenience may eventually be unnecessary: preliminary research indicates that botanists will succeed in developing tarwi strains entirely lacking in these bitter chemicals.

New Fruits for the Table

In the last few years, a fuzzy, brown, egg-shaped fruit known as the *kiwi* has begun appearing at stands and supermarkets throughout the United States. A decade ago, kiwis didn't exist—at least not by that name. Instead they were called Chinese gooseberries after the fruit's country of origin. Because New Zealand has become the center of Chinese gooseberry cultivation, and because exporters glimpsed a huge international market in the fruit's hardy shelf life and sweet mild flavor, a contest was held to come up with a more patriotic name—kiwi, after New Zealand's mascot bird. Today the sprawling kiwi vine is cultivated on huge plantations in California as well as New Zealand.

Indeed, a wealth of other exotic fruits could as easily debut in the U.S. market in the next few years. Among them:

— *Tree tomato (Cyphomandra betacea)*—a South American native that looks like an elongated tomato but is much sweeter;
— *Cape gooseberry (Physalis peruviana)*—a South American relative of

the ground cherry popular among the *Mayflower* pilgrims, it would do spendidly in the United States;

— *Feijoa (Feijoa sellowiana)*—a South American relative of the guava with pineapplelike flavor;
— *Naranjilla (Solanum quitoense)*—the "golden fruit of the Andes" is related to the tomato but tastes more like a cross between pineapple and strawberry;
— *Rambutan (Nephelium lappaceum)*—bright red and bewhiskered, this table fruit is the pride of tropical Southeast Asia;
— *Jaboticaba (Myrciaria cauliflora)*—common in Rio de Janeiro, this grape-like fruit springs directly from the bark of the vine and has a flavor comparable to the finest Concord grapes.

Sugar Substitutes

Worried about the safety of cyclamates and saccharin, and even the high levels of natural sucrose in the American diet, food chemists have launched a feverish search for substitute sweeteners. Some of the best are derived from plants:

— *Licorice*—Licorice roots were known to the ancient Assyrians and were included among the funerary treasures entombed with King Tut. Only recently determined is that the sweetness of licorice comes not from a sugar but from glycyrrhizin, a molecule distantly related to vitamin D. Licorice has no calories and, gram for gram, it is fifty times sweeter than cane sugar.
— *Miracle fruit*—West African children delight in impressing visitors by munching on bitterly sour fruits without wincing. What they don't tell is that beforehand they suck the berries of a native shrub called miracle fruit (*Synsepalum dulcificum*). The active ingredient is a protein, not a sugar, and it appears to work by blocking the sourness receptor sites on the children's taste buds. The protein itself is tasteless and contains no calories. Horticulturists in the Caribbean have begun growing the miracle fruit commercially.
— *Serendipity berry*—In 1965 George Inglett, a researcher now with the U.S. Department of Agriculture, was scouring the West African rain forests for sweet fruits when he chanced to try the red, grape-like berries of *Dioscoreo phyllum cumminsii*. Scientific literature gave no hint of their sweetness and so Inglett coined the name serendipity berry. The berry's sweetness is caused by a protein that is 3,000 times sweeter than sugar. (Saccharin, the familiar synthetic, is 300 times sweeter than sugar.)
— *Katemfe*—Another intensely sweet West African fruit discovered by Inglett, katemfe is already sold worldwide in extract form by

the world's largest sugar company, Tate and Lyle of London, under the trade name Talin. The Food and Drug Administration has not yet approved the substance for sale in the United States.

Population Control

Folktales about plants useful in birth control are told all over the world. But for decades, the pharmaceutical industry has shunned these leads and pursued synthetic contraceptive drugs.

Now, however, a research team at the College of Pharmacy of the University of Illinois has explored the anthropological and botanical literature and confirmed claims of fertility control for over 4,000 plant species of which computer analysis has identified a core of 370 as especially promising sources of contraceptive substances.

Under the sponsorship of the World Health Organization, a network of laboratories around the globe has joined in the research. Thirty-six plants have been selected as initial targets for exhaustive scrutiny. Among these is the *motherwort*, an herb reportedly taken as a contraceptive by Chinese women for over 2,000 years. Others come from Paraguay, Bangladesh, and India.

But the leading candidate currently is *zoapatle* (*Montanoa tomentosa*), a small Mexican shrub that is a member of the sunflower family. Preliminary tests on animals and humans confirm folklore's claims for the plant. A Swedish research institute is about to inaugurate a formal clinical trial and Ortho Pharmaceuticals, a leading U.S. contraceptives company, has taken out patents on molecules isolated from zoapatle. With a molecular structure rather like that of prostaglandins, hormone-like material found in humans, compounds of the humble zoapatle may finally result in a successful "morning-after pill," one of the longest sought and most desperately needed pharmaceuticals in an age of runaway population growth.

Selection 51 Unconventional Foods: The Virtues of Variety

Frank Meissner

Editors' Introduction

Generally, technology includes all the ways of doing things that extend human potential. Rising energy costs place a premium on crops that can be harvested without excessive reliance on mechanized agriculture. Human ingenuity is increasingly challenged to cultivate little-known food crops or to improve our ability to extract foods from the world's waterways. For example, fish farming, the cultivation and harvesting of fish and shellfish in coastal areas (mariculture) and in land-based ponds (aquaculture), has the potential for becoming a major means of providing low-cost protein. Mariculture is already being successfully practiced in the Orient and Southeast Asia, where production relies heavily on extensive methods involving little or no control over the environment. Estuaries, coastal ecosystems where freshwater systems (rivers) and the ocean meet, are being used for this type of fish farming. They provide an excellent environment for the growth of certain marine species because they are natural sinks for the flow of valuable nutrients from the land to the sea. Modern techniques to control fertilization and the nutrient content of the water as well as mortalities due to predation have greatly enhanced the productivity of these areas.

In ponds intensive, factory-like methods are used. Full environmental control is achieved by setting up a complete ecosystem. Drained and dried ponds are fertilized with synthetic fertilizer, animal wastes, or fish wastes. The ponds are then gradually filled and phytoplankton (microscopic plants) such as algae are allowed to develop. The phytoplankton are consumed by zooplankton (microscopic animals) and tiny animals that are in turn consumed by fish. Under ideal conditions, remarkable yields for trout, carp, milkfish, and salmon have been demonstrated in Japan, the USSR, and the Philippines. Experimental projects are now underway in the Orient to determine the feasibility of cultivating fish and shellfish in irrigated rice fields in order to obtain dual crops of rice and fish.

Source: Adapted from Frank Meissner, "Unconventional Foods: The Virtues of Variety," *The Futurist*, February 1980, pp. 58–66. Reprinted by permission of the World Future Society, 4916 St. Elmo Avenue, Washington, D.C. 20014.

Although aquaculture will probably be a significant source of fish in some poorer countries, ecologist G. Tyler Miller has pointed out that since aquaculture frequently competes directly with land that could be used for animal production, aquaculture offers no particular advantage over animal husbandry, except where fish is the preferred protein food. In the past, the tomato was regarded as poison. Some countries still consider corn as food only for farm animals, and the peanut was once so regarded.

Today we know that there are many underutilized foods that are safe to eat and that can make a significant nutritional contribution in the diets of both livestock and humankind. The task is to educate people regarding the use of these foods. Food sources are needed that are ecologically responsible, technologically feasible, and acceptable to consumers. In the following selection, Frank Meissner sets forth some promising avenues for consideration. Is it possible that with proper promotion and advertising, some little-known foods may become the commonplace acceptable foods of the future?

There is no use beating around the bush: massive rural poverty— sustained and spurred on by rapidly increasing populations—is the most difficult problem faced by developing Third World countries around the globe. And it is a problem that no nation, rich or poor, can afford to ignore. The 1978 Annual Report of the World Bank estimates that in 1980, food deficits in the Third World will reach nearly the equivalent of 145 million tons of grain, with most of this shortage occurring in the impoverished nations of Africa and Asia. These nations are too poor to import food and their citizens too numerous to simply be fed and supported by the wealthier countries of the world. The suffering that this poverty and malnutrition engenders, and the political, social, and economic problems that result, can only be alleviated by improving the conditions in which the world's impoverished millions live—most importantly, their diets.

The culprits that conspire to depress nutritional levels and rural income in developing nations are many: slow and erratic increases in food production; ecological variations such as adverse weather; the depletion of necessary resources such as water or fertile land; population growth that tends to gobble up whatever little production gains have been made; economic fluctuations that make tradition-bound farmers reluctant to innovate; inequitable distribution of everything from land and credit to taxes and income; and many others. All this adds up to the chronic inability of many developing nations to feed themselves.

There are suggestions galore about how to improve our efforts aimed at the challenging task of feeding this world. Most of them focus on increasing the production and improving the marketing of traditional crops such as rice, wheat, barley, corn, sorghum, millet, legumes, and root crops, or on finding new ways to get more out of domesticated animals. But many agriculturists overlook another possibility: using nontraditional species of plants and animals to supplement the current system of food production, especially in the world's poorer nations.

Although large-scale mechanized agriculture, as it is currently practiced in the United States and other Western countries, has dramatically, and some would say miraculously, increased food production in the last twenty years, it is only one option among many; and it, too, has limitations. Modern agriculture, for example, requires not only skilled labor and expensive machines but also parts, mechanics, relatively good terrain, and most crucially, energy to fuel farm machines and make fertilizers. As energy prices go up and supplies dwindle, some of the drawbacks of modern agricultural methods, and the tremendous difficulty of importing them wholesale into developing countries, become apparent.

Exploring new possibilities for agriculture is one way to increase the chances that the world's population can at least improve its diet a little bit, even though no new plants or other sources of food should be seen as panaceas. New possibilities for producing food are numerous. They include everything from domesticating wild animals to breeding new strains of traditional crops. But two avenues seem particularly promising: (1) bringing some existing but little-known species of plants under systematic cultivation, and (2) improving man's ability to feed himself from the world's rivers, lakes, and oceans.

The Wealth of Species

There are some 350,000 species of plants in the world. About 20,000 are found in the United States, 30,000 in China, 45,000 in Africa, and 100,000 in South America. Perhaps 80,000 plants are edible. Yet over the course of history, people have used only 3,000 or so species for food, or less than 4 percent of the incredible array of available species. Indeed, some 95 percent of all our calories and protein are supplied by just thirty species. More than half of all human food energy and protein comes from only three species: wheat, rice, and corn. Similarly, for all the enormous productivity of American agriculture, a typical U.S. supermarket seldom offers more than a few dozen different fruits and vegetables.

Considering the vast number of plants available for consumption, it is risky to rely so heavily upon a mere handful. Biologically speaking, there is safety in diversity: bad weather, disease, and long-term climatic change can play havoc with a few widespread crops. This in itself is a worthy reason for exploring the potential of little-known species, especially in developing countries, where overwhelming reliance on a single crop can exacerbate the consequences of natural and political disasters, which so often take such a horrible toll of human life. The current famine in Cambodia is only the most recent case in point.

Furthermore, squeezing out native plant varieties in favor of a few widespread crops reduces the genetic materials that plant breeders have to work with, and thus limits their ability to breed new strains adapted to changing environments. In fact, in "Seeds of Trouble," a recent *Washington Post* editorial, a United Nations official says: "When farmers clear a field of primitive grain varieties, they throw away the key to our future." In addition, the [*Washington*] *Post* notes, private corporations now hold a growing concentration of the world's seed resources, and plant geneticists of the future may have to contend with patents on certain varieties of plants in their efforts to develop new strains. And there is still another fringe benefit in relying on a broad variety of crops rather than a few: Variety can help improve nutrition.

Of course, despite the world's overwhelming reliance on crops such as wheat, corn, and rice, some important new crops gradually do gain acceptance. In the 1920s, for example, scientists at the University of Illinois began intensive research aimed at helping the growing U.S. agroindustry find a source of oil and protein that could be grown and processed on a large scale in the Midwest and shipped throughout the world. The crop they struck upon was the soybean, and the almost 60 million acres of land planted with soybeans in the United States in 1977 (compared with 75 million for wheat and 83 million for corn) prove that a valuable new crop can rapidly make a place for itself in modern agriculture.

Looking toward the future, it seems that agronomists and planners, especially in developing nations, might do well to take a lesson from the soybean and explore the potential of other little-known crops. Plenty of candidates exist. As of this writing, for example, a plant called the winged bean may be on the verge of a takeoff similar to that of the soybean. Virtually unknown in the early 1970s, the winged bean came to the attention of Noel Vietmeyer of the U.S. National Academy of Sciences. In 1973, Vietmeyer stumbled across an article about the winged bean entitled "A Crop with a Future," contacted the author, and in 1975 persuaded the National Academy of Sciences to study the plant. The resulting booklet, *The Winged Bean: A High-Protein Crop for the Tropics,* became an agricultural bestseller of sorts. Requests for the booklet and for more information poured in from all over the globe.

By the end of 1979, the winged bean had been introduced into more than seventy countries. Indonesia and the Philippines have designated the plant a "priority research crop," and agricultural scientists throughout the world are now experimenting with the winged bean. Today, it is at the point that soybeans were in the United States in the 1920s—the winged bean could become an important new crop in the last two decades of this century. [See pages 434–35.]

Barriers to Broader Selection

But despite the success of the soybean, and the apparent potential of the winged bean, very few new crops gain acceptance without a struggle. And there is no lack of reasons why humankind depends heavily on so few crops. In Third World countries, for example, today's consumption patterns were formed during the colonial period of the nineteenth century. Rulers then encouraged development of a few native crops that could be grown on a large scale, such as oil palm, coffee, cocoa nut, bananas, and others. At the same time, European colonial administrators introduced food crops that they were accustomed to: potatoes, cabbages, barley, etc. To a great extent, native crops that had been sustaining local populations for centuries were pushed into the background as people in Third World countries grew to depend on food imported by colonial administrations, and as these administrations focused their efforts at agricultural research on valuable export crops. To some degree, this pattern still persists today. In recent years, however, native crops that were long in the background have started to get some of the attention they deserve.

Similarly, in the highly mechanized and energy-intensive agriculture of the United States, high-yield crops that can be planted and harvested by machine, mass-processed, and mass-marketed have been the main beneficiaries of the financial, technical, and scientific support given to agriculture. Unfamiliar species simply have few backers. Furthermore, the perils of the marketplace, both in the United States and in other countries, make developing a new crop a risky business. Often consumers are slow to accept new foods.

But perhaps the most important reason that little-known foods are slow to gain popularity is simply a lack of communications. Peanuts, for example, were a relatively unimportant crop until George Washington Carver's work at the Tuskegee Institute in Alabama got them on the road to worldwide acceptance. Soybeans, which are native to Northern China, were first brought to the United States by Benjamin Franklin, who stumbled upon them at the Botanical Gardens of Paris while he served as U.S. envoy to France. Their central place in American agriculture today illustrates how easily valuable crops can become victims of centuries of "benign neglect," only to be "discovered" and exploited much later.

Promising New Crops

Agricultural scientists around the world are now beginning to see the importance of finding productive new crops. As a result, new species from many countries are now coming under scientific scrutiny. Sam Iker explores the possibilities of several little-known species, some of which are included below, in his article "Are You Ready for the New Foods?" in the July/August 1979 issue of *International Wildlife* magazine. And both the U.S. National Academy of Sciences and the U.S. National Science Foundation have recently released studies on unfamiliar plants. Some particularly promising species for the future include:

Winged bean. Winged bean seeds have as much oil and protein as soybeans, and the firm, white flesh of their starchy roots contains many times the protein of potatoes. The flowers, pods, and shoots are all edible, and the leaves, when cooked, make a leafy green vegetable that tastes like spinach. Viny varieties of the winged bean are already being grown in Southeast Asia and New Guinea, and scientists are trying to develop shorter, bushy varieties that could be grown throughout the tropics.

Lablab bean. Already widespread throughout the tropics, the lablab bean is extremely versatile and adaptable. The pods, when young, make a tasty table vegetable; the leaves and flowers can be eaten like spinach, the seeds can be made into high-protein concentrate; and the plant itself is good forage and ground cover. One or another of the many varieties of the lablab bean thrives in arid or semiarid regions, subtropics, and rain forests, lowlands and highlands, and in a variety of soils. The dried seeds contain 20–28 percent protein and are rich in amino acids, so they are a good addition to cereal diets.

Cocoyam. A native of Central and South America and West Africa, the cocoyam is just as nutritious as the potato, does well in various soils, and can be cultivated at various altitudes. Cocoyams can be prepared in as many different ways as potatoes, and could one day be an important tropical crop.

Ye-eb. A small bush native to East Africa, the ye-eb yields seeds that are almost a nutritionally balanced diet in themselves. The seeds contain fat, protein, starch, minerals, and sugar, and are high in energy. The ye-eb grows well in extremely arid regions, and could perhaps become an important export crop for nations with low or irregular rainfall.

Marama bean. High in protein and energy, the marama bean could one day be an important crop for semiarid regions. Roasted, both the beans and the roots are edible and tasty. The marama bean contains about as much protein as the soybean and almost as much oil as the peanut.

Amaranths. Amaranth grains are exceptionally high in protein and were a mainstay of the Aztec diet before the invasion of the Spaniards in the sixteenth century. Amaranth leaves can be boiled and eaten as a green vegetable. The hardy amaranth still grows in Latin America, experiments with it are underway in the United States, and it is becoming increasingly popular in certain areas of Africa and Asia.

Buffalo gourd. The protein-rich seeds of the buffalo gourd have long been a part of the diets of western American Indian tribes. The edible root of the buffalo gourd can weigh as much as sixty pounds. Buffalo gourds are rugged perennials that thrive in dry regions and do well on even marginal cropland. Today, the plants are under cultivation in parts of Mexico and Lebanon, and in the future they could become an important food in many arid and semiarid regions of the world.

Quinua. A grain-like crop of the High Andes, quinua yields seeds that are high in protein. Soaking quinua seeds in water removes their hard, bitter coating. Scientists are already attempting to breed nonbitter strains, which could become significant sources of protein on other continents.

Tarwi. Tarwi seeds contain up to 50 percent protein and between 14 and 24 percent oil, making tarwi, a native of South America, a good candidate for high-protein meal and cooking oil. Tarwi seeds, like quinua, must be soaked to remove bitterness, but nonbitter strains could make tarwi a major crop for temperate regions and tropical highlands around the world.

These brief vignettes far from exhaust the list of little-known crops that could help allleviate world hunger. And although these plants should not be seen as a new generation of "supercrops" destined to supplant corn, wheat, and rice in the world's diet, they could add variety and vegetable protein to diets, and even help people save money to boot. More importantly, as inexpensive sources of protein, starch, and minerals in developing countries, new crops can fill agricultural niches—and hungry bellies—that might otherwise be left empty.

Food from the Waters

Like unfamiliar species of plants, the world's oceans represent sources of valuable protein that haven't been fully exploited as yet.

Oceans, lakes, and rivers cover over 70 percent of the world's surface. Yet, today, marine foods make up only a fraction of 1 percent of total food production. Some 20,000 species of fish are known to exist in salt and freshwater environments. As is the case with plants, only a few dozen of this array of species are being used commercially.

Current annual fish production is hovering around 70 million tons per year, having reached a peak of 73.5 million tons in 1978. More than 85 percent of the world's fish catch comes from the sea, with almost two-thirds consisting of pelagic (surface-dwelling) fish such as anchovies, herring, mackerel, and tuna. Demersal (bottom-dwelling) fish such as cod, snapper, and flounder make up the rest, together with a few invertebrates such as mollusks and squids, and some larger crustaceans such as prawns, lobsters, and crabs. Since the early 1970s, production from inland waters, rivers, and lakes has remained steady at about 10 million tons annually.

There seems to be a consensus that current fishing methods and technologies limit the conventional marine harvest to somewhere between 70 and 100 million tons per year. But the recurring failure of certain fisheries—the anchovy fishery in Peru, for example—make a target of even 80 to 90 million tons difficult to achieve. Because catches are declining, many coastal nations have now extended their jurisdiction to a 200-mile exclusive economic zone.

The mix of species caught in the oceans is also changing over time because victims of overfishing tend to be replaced by newly developed fish stocks. The previously noted anchovy fishery in Peru is an example of an extremely productive fishing ground already in decline. On the other hand, the recent discovery of blue whiting in waters off the coast of the United Kingdom offers prospects of a fishery yielding about 1 million tons per year in an area where in the mid-1970s the catch exceeded 0.1 million tons for the first time.

Although the mix of species that makes up the world fish catch may be changing, a rapid increase in world fish production is not at hand. The rise and fall of various species of fish is usually a response to changing currents in the ocean, or overfishing: as certain species are depleted, others have more room to expand. Many of the most valuable and most sought after species are already either fully exploited or actually overfished. In the Pacific, fish stocks of anchovies, haig, halibut, salmon, sardines, and large tuna are now either fully exploited or already on the decline. In the Atlantic, herring and cod stocks are being fished to their limits. And the shrimp and large tuna of the Indian Ocean are almost fully exploited.

Furthermore, the amount of fish available for human consumption also depends in part on the proportion that is converted to fishmeal for animal feed. Today, about 30 percent of the catch goes to make fishmeal. More importantly, every year millions of tons of fish are discarded at sea because keeping them would contravene fishing regulations or reduce boat space for more profitable species. Five million tons of fish are also lost to spoilage every year.

Together, all these considerations suggest that, in the 1980s, any increase in the contribution of fish to human nutrition will depend not so much on catching more fish but on better distribution of the fish already caught, reducing waste, and changing current patterns of consumption and use.

Trends in Distribution

On a global scale, the 1980s may see a larger share of the world fish catch going to developing countries than in previous decades. By extending their jurisdiction over marine resources, Third World nations have to some degree curtailed the roving fleets of other countries, especially the Soviet Union and Japan. Developing nations may also be able to feed their populations with some of the fish that the fleets of advanced nations would have taken home to be turned into fishmeal for animal feed.

Within developing nations, the 1980s may see more emphasis on catching fish for consumption at home rather than the continued development of modern fishing fleets that catch tuna and shrimp, for example, for export. Indeed, in the race to develop commercial fishing fleets based on Western models, small, artisanal fishermen who catch most of the fish for local consumption in Third World nations have been exposed to benign neglect.

Since the mid-1970s, however, the situation has begun to change. The concern of many developing nations over protecting their marine resources has focused attention closer to home. It is now evident that many coastal stocks, as well as fish in lakes and rivers, can be harvested with simple fishing gear operated from small boats or from shore. Labor-intensive fisheries can successfully exploit fish stocks too small to support capital-intensive commercial fishing fleets. In short, with more support and the use of appropriate technologies, small-scale fisheries can provide more food for millions of hungry people and give an economic boost to small fishermen as well.

Improved Use of By-Catch

Making commercial fishing in developing countries more productive, and bringing the price of fish within the reach of poorer populations, might also be accomplished by improving the use of the less profitable species of fish that are unintentionally hauled in by commercial fishing fleets. Commercial shrimping boats, for example, may catch four to twenty times as much fish as shrimp, and much of this "by-catch," amounting to five million tons annually, is simply thrown overboard because the fish bring only 10-20 percent of the price of shrimp, or are not commercially viable for some other reason.

Unfortunately, making use of by-catch is easier said than done. The main purpose of the shrimping industry in developing nations is to supply exports, which today amount to about $1 billion annually. The shrimpers are in business to catch shrimp, not fish, and their business is most profitable when the hold is full of shrimp and nothing else. Furthermore, in contrast to northern temperate waters, catches in tropical waters often contain unpalatable species, and some that are outright poisonous.

But the reason that making better use of by-catch from commercial fishing boats is so attractive is simply that the by-catch consists of fish already caught—throwing them back in the ocean wastes the effort it took to catch them and deprives poorer consumers of a valuable source of protein. The challenge of the future for developing countries is to combine commercial fishing with a method of handling and processing the by-catch.

Reducing Postharvest Losses

Finding a way to use by-catch and relying more on small fishermen raises another problem that must be addressed if poor nations are to increase their take from the sea: reducing postharvest losses.

In small landing places with low daily catches, preserving fish with even the simplest of chilling or freezing techniques is far too expensive for small fishermen. Some of the catch is sold immediately in the neighborhood, and some processed by traditional methods such as smoking, sun drying, pickling, and fermentation. All of these methods can reduce the nutritive value of the fish, and generally make it less appealing. The rest of the catch is simply wasted.

The possibilities for preserving more fish include everything from simple techniques like shading the catch from the sun and gutting the larger fish immediately to processing the fish into fish protein concentrate (FPC), a high-protein powder that can be used to fortify a whole range of other foods. But aside from improving traditional preservation techniques such as smoking and drying, the best hope for reducing postharvest losses depends on adapting a few modern processing technologies to the conditions of Third World countries. Technologies such as the meat-bone separator—which can quickly clean the flesh of all kinds of different fish—might enable developing countries to feed their populations with some of the species that are now being made into animal feed, take better advantage of small pelagic species that can readily be converted into minced fish by these technologies, and perhaps preserve species such as anchovies and menhaden, which are as nutritious as more common food fish but, because of their higher oil and fat content, more perishable.

Broadening Resources with Unconventional Fisheries

In addition to making better use of by-catch and wasting fewer fish, a few unconventional species and techniques could also help augment the harvest from the waters. Krill (a tiny shrimp-like crustacean), oceanic squid, and a few other types of fish may be more fully exploited in the coming decades, and many experts are now looking to aquaculture to make a significant contribution to world food production in the years ahead.

Squid. Edible squid are rich in protein, can be caught by a variety of methods that are suitable for small fishermen, need no preparation on board, and freeze well without loss of quality. The main source of squid is the Northwest Pacific, where Japan, South Korea, and China currently catch nearly a million tons a year. The oceans may hold as much as 500 million tons of various kinds of squid, but in many countries, particularly the United States, the prejudices of consumers make them unmarketable today.

Krill. The harvesting and processing of Antarctic krill has enjoyed rapid development in recent years. Krill are the natural food of many species of whales, and as the whale population has declined, the possibilities of harvesting krill have improved. As recently as 1975, experts were predicting that many years of research would be needed to find out how to catch and process krill. But in 1976, experimental fishing by West Germany, the Soviet Union, and Japan was well on the way to success. Similar progress has been made in freezing the harvested krill and processing it into an edible paste.

Another possibility is to introduce salmon into southern oceans where they could feed on krill. It is conceivable that a salmon fishery producing several million tons per year could thus be established. And if natural migration patterns can be preserved, the salmon would return to the vicinity of their release every year.

Aquaculture

Experiments with releasing artificially hatched larvae, aimed at increasing production of stocks of wild fish, go back to the nineteenth century. In the past, it was difficult to rear larvae large enough to survive. Furthermore, countries were not willing to invest in expanding fish populations that other countries could exploit. Recent advances in aquaculture, however, coupled with the extension of national jurisdiction in coastal areas, have removed these barriers. In 1950, Norway therefore resumed experimental work, which had been abandoned at the beginning of the twentieth century, and released large numbers of cod larvae in the Oslo fjord. Japan revitalized a failing scallop fishery along the coast of the Okhotsk Sea, with production increasing from about 100 tons in 1970 to 4,200 tons by 1975.

Aquaculture offers particularly good prospects from both marine and fresh water. At present about 600 species of plants and animals are being cultivated experimentally or commercially. World production in 1976 was over 6 million tons. If the necessary scientific, organizational, and financial help were to be forthcoming, increases of up to 30 million tons are feasible by the end of the century.

Yet, so far, aquaculture has not been the pathway to cheap protein. This is because there has been a tendency to look for species that command high prices in the marketplace of affluent countries. People with the greatest purchasing power — rather than those in greatest need — have been the main beneficiaries of intensive aquaculture. The chances are excellent, however, that with redirected research priorities, simple, labor-intensive, and energy-saving technologies can help us put to use the vast underdeveloped and underutilized waters of the world — natural and man-made lakes and ponds, rivers, irrigation canals, estuaries, and coastal waters — that are potentially suitable for aquaculture.

The advantages of aquaculture compared to conventional fishing, are many:

— Fish are cold-blooded animals; they adapt to the temperature of the surrounding water rather than wasting energy keeping warm. Fish are therefore about 50 percent more efficient feed converters than hogs, and perhaps thirty times more efficient than cattle.
— Fish grow faster in warm waters. For every 10° C rise in water temperature, the speed at which they grow doubles, as demonstrated by experiments with halibut off the coast of Scotland. Consequently, the potential for fish production in warm tropical waters in Third World countries is enormous. In cooler climates, some tropical fish that thrive in warm waters, such as the tilapia, can be raised in water that has been warmed by waste heat from power plants or even atomic reactors. Pilot experiments are already underway at power plants run by the Tennessee Valley Authority, Oak Ridge National Laboratories, and Texas Power and Light Company.

— Fish occupy a three-dimensional space. Thus they can be grown in a "polyculture," a system in which different species of fish that habitually feed at different depths live together in the same body of water. A pond with a surface area of one hectare stocked with compatible species of fish can have a tremendous productive capacity because it produces fish at different depths.

— With adequate recycling of water, fish require little space. Trout can grow to their maximum size in a body of water no greater than their own volume. In the coastal water of Singapore, mussel cultures have produced forty-five times as much protein per acre as protein-rich soybeans.

— Aquaculture is closer to husbandry than to hunting. It is therefore more compatible with farming than with conventional fishing. Farmers can relate to aquaculture. Even the terminology—stocking and breeding, feed and fertilizer—is familiar.

Betting on the Waters

In addition to the 50 million tons of fish now available for human consumption, diverting more of the catch to production of food for humans and away from animal feeds, making better use of by-catch, reducing postharvest losses, and improving processing and distribution in developing countries could yield another 25 to 30 million tons of fish per year by the end of the century. Catches far in excess of 100 million tons per year can be achieved if we are willing to invest in aquaculture and increase the exploitation of unconventional resources such as krill.

Some futurists suggest that the protein now obtained from the seas could be increased six or sevenfold. As overly optimistic as such a forecast might seem, it could be translated into reality if nations around the world learn to control pollution, which threatens valuable nursery grounds, in coastal and inland waters, and systematically manage the living resources of oceans, lakes, and rivers by suitable variations of aquaculture.

Filling in the Future

Focusing on alternative means of increasing food production, such as cultivating little-known species of plants and developing aquaculture, does not mean that conventional modern agriculture should be either ignored or abandoned. Rather, exploring the potential of new plant species and foods from the sea gives developed and developing nations alike a chance to fill in the unexploited niches in their food production systems. The gravity of the world food problem demands that every promising avenue for increasing food production be explored.

Even if none of the "new" fish or plant species ever becomes a predominant contributor to world food production, they could still spell the difference between adequate nutrition and malnutrition in many regions of the world.

Selection 52 Summary of World Food Conference Resolutions

UNICEF

Editors' Introduction

World hunger is a pressing problem confronting international organizations. They have spurred such consciousness-raising events as World Hunger Day and Food Day, during which persons are asked to fast and contribute the cost of missed meals to hunger relief agencies. The following selection consists of excerpts and summaries from resolutions made as a result of the World Food Conference in 1974 in which international experts considered the world food situation and prospects to 1985.

Summary of World Food Conference Resolutions

1. *Objectives and strategies of food production.* This resolution resolves that all governments should accept the removal of the scourge of hunger and malnutrition. It calls upon the developing countries to give high priority to formulating plans, both short and long term, for food production through agricultural and fisheries development; to promote changes in rural socioeconomic structures; and to develop adequate supporting services. Governments are called upon to increase their development assistance, facilitate greater access to inputs by developing countries, support the UN Special Program and the Agricultural Development Fund, and reduce the waste of food and agricultural resources.

2. *Priorities for agricultural and rural development.* This resolution calls for appropriate agrarian reforms and institutional improvements aimed at generating employment, income, and integrated development

Source: From "Annex: Summary of World Food Conference Resolutions," *The World Food Situation and Prospects to 1985*, pp. 87–90. UNICEF.

in rural areas; eliminating any exploitative patterns of land tenure, lending, and marketing; improving credit, marketing and input distribution systems, and promoting cooperative organizations for farmers and rural workers.

3. *Fertilizers.* This resolution asks developed countries and various international agencies to help meet developing countries' fertilizer needs by providing material and financial support for the International Fertilizer Supply Scheme; extending grants and concessional loans for fertilizer and raw material imports; organizing a joint program to improve fertilizer plant efficiency; assisting in building new fertilizer production capacity in appropriate developing countries; and by assisting all developing countries to establish storage facilities, distribution services, and related infrastructures.

4. *Food and agricultural research, extension, and training.* [This resolution] recommends increased support for programs related to the survey, conservation, and effective utilization of all agricultural resources, particularly soil, water, and plant and animal resources. A global network of plant genetic resource centers is urged, to be followed by work on animal genetic resources.

5. *Policies and programs to improve nutrition.* [This resolution] recommends that each country formulate integrated food and nutrition plans and policies based on careful assessments of malnutrition in all socioeconomic groups and preconditions for improving their nutritional status. The objective is "to eliminate within a decade hunger and malnutrition." FAO, in cooperation with the World Health Organization, the UN Children's Fund, the World Food Program, the World Bank, the UN Development Program, and the UN Educational, Scientific and Cultural Organization and assisted by the Protein Advisory Group is to prepare a project proposal by mid-1975 for assisting governments in developing broad food and nutrition plans. The resolution calls for a worldwide control program to reduce deficiency of vitamins A and D, iodine, iron/folate, riboflavin, and thiamine; an inventory of noncereal vegetable food resources and a study of possibilities of increasing their food production and consumption; a food-contamination monitoring program to provide early warning to national authorities, FAO, WHO, and UNICEF; a global nutrition surveillance system to monitor food and nutrition conditions; and an internationally coordinated program in applied nutritional research.

6. *World soil charter and land capability assessment.* [This resolution] recommends that governments apply soil protection and conservation measures to all attempts to increase agricultural production. It also recommends that FAO, UN Educational, Scientific and Cultural Organization, UN Development Program, the World Meteorological Organization, and other international organizations prepare an assessment of

remaining cultivatable land, taking account of forestry for protection of catchment areas required for alternative uses. FAO is urged to establish a World Soil Charter as a basis of international cooperation for most rational use of the world's land resources.

7. *Scientific water management: irrigation, drainage, and flood control.* [This resolution] calls for corrected action by governments, FAO, World Meteorological Organization, and other international agencies to undertake extensive surveys of climate, water, irrigation potential, hydropower potential, energy requirements for irrigation, and expand irrigation as rapidly as possible; develop safe uses of brackish water; reclaim areas affected by waterlogging, salinity, and alkalinity; identify and exploit groundwater resources and develop better ways of improving crop production in arid areas; complement flood protection and flood control measures; establish drainage systems to control salinity in swampy areas; develop controls for desert crops; and develop better water technology and delivery systems. Extensive aid to developing countries and extensive research into the use of solar, geothermal and wind energy in agricultural production are urged.

8. *Food and women.* [This resolution] calls on governments to involve women fully in the decision making for food-production and nutrition policies; promote equal rights and responsibilities for men and women and include in national-development plans provision for education and training of women in food-production and agricultural technology, marketing and distribution techniques, as well as credit and nutrition consumer information; and provide women with full effective access to all medical and social services, food for pregnant women and lactating mothers, means to space their children, and child health and development education.

9. *Achievement of a desirable balance between population and food supply.* [This resolution] points to the increasing difficulty in meeting the food needs of a rapidly growing world population and to consensus on a World Population Plan of Action reached at the August 1974 World Population Conference. The resolution calls on governments and peoples everywhere to support rational population policies which ensure couples the right to determine the number and spacing of births, freely and responsibly, in accordance with national needs within the context of an overall development strategy.

10. *Pesticides.* This resolution recommends international coordination of efforts to assure an adequate supply of pesticides, including where possible the local manufacture and establishment of reserve stocks; programs to increase the efficiency of protection measures taking into account the elements of supply, information, training, research, and quality control; and the promotion of a strong continuing program of research into the mechanism of resistance in both plants and pests—

especially as applicable to the development of integrated pest management in tropical and subtropical areas—and on the residual effects of pesticides.*

11. *Program for the control of African animal trypanosomiasis.* [This resolution] asserts that an integrated economic development plan for Africa should begin with trypanosomiasis and tsetse control. It calls for a small coordinating unit at FAO to immediately initiate as the first phase of the program training, pilot field-control projects, and applied research, in preparation for future large-scale operations for the control of African animal trypanosomiasis.

12. *Seed industry development.* [This resolution] urges developing countries to make continuing commitments of manpower, institutional, and financial resources for seed industry development; recommends policies and legislation for the production, processing, quality control, distribution, marketing and promotion of quality seed and education of farmers in their use; and proposes that the FAO Seed Industry Development Program be strengthened to meet demands for seed production, seed export, and training of competent technical and managerial manpower.

13. *International fund for agricultural development.* [This resolution] resolves that an International Fund for Agricultural Development should be established immediately to finance agricultural development projects, primarily for food production in the developing countries.

14. *Reduction of military expenditures for increasing food production.* [This resolution] calls on countries to rapidly implement all UN resolutions pertaining to the reduction of military expenditures on behalf of development, and to allocate a growing proportion of these sums to finance food production in developing countries and establish reserves for emergency cases.

15. *Food aid to victims of colonial wars in Africa.* [This resolution] requests FAO and the World Food Program "to take immediate action to intensify food aid to Guinea-Bissau, Cape Verde, Mozambique, Angola, Sao Tome, and Principe"; and requests the UN secretary-general and other UN organizations "to assist the national liberation movements or the governments of these countries to formulate a comprehensive plan of national reconstruction."

16. *Global information and early warning system on food and agriculture.* [This resolution] cites the urgent need for a worldwide food information system to identify areas with imminent food problems, monitor world food supply-demand conditions, and contribute to the effective functioning of the proposed International Undertaking on World Food Security.

*Includes insecticides, herbicides, fungicides, acaricides, rodenticides, growth regulators, and other pest control measures.

17. *International undertaking on world food security.* [This resolution] endorses the objectives, policies, and guidelines of the proposed IUWFS and urges its adoption and implementation. The resolution affirms common responsibility of the international community for adequate policies on world food, asks all states to participate, and calls for national stocks, particularly of grain, to be maintained with the objective of ensuring a globally sufficient amount.

18. *An improved policy for food aid.* [This resolution] affirms the needs for forward planning of a continuous, augumented amount of food aid. Donor countries are asked to provide commodities or financial assistance for a minimum of 10 million tons of grain for food aid a year, in addition to other food commodities, starting in 1975. Donor countries are also urged to channel more food aid through the World Food Program, increase the grant component of bilateral food aid, consider applying part of food-aid repayments to supplementary nutrition programs and emergency relief, and where possible to purchase such food for aid from developing countries.

19. *International trade and adjustment.* [This resolution] requests that all states cooperate in expanding and liberalizing world trade and improving the trading position of exports from developing countries.

Selection 53 Food Security for the World's Poor

Lance Taylor
Alexander H. Sarris
Philip C. Abbott

Editors' Introduction

Formulating food policy is a sensitive and complex issue. The food crisis stirs our humanitarian impulses. At the same time the economic ramifications of food production, distribution, and consumption affect international relations to a remarkable degree. The nations of the world agree on one point—that an interna-

Source: Adapted from Lance Taylor, Alexander H. Sarris, and Philip C. Abbott, "Food Security for the World's Poor," *Technology Review* (February 1978):44–54. Reprinted by permission. Tabulated matter appearing in this article has been omitted here; for further information consult the original version.

tional reserve of food should be maintained to stabilize food prices and feed the starving when famine strikes. However, deciding how to implement such a policy is not so easy. How much should be saved? What prices should be established? Where should food reserves be stored?

In the following selection Lance Taylor, a professor of both economics and nutrition and food science, sets forth with his colleagues, economists Alexander H. Sarris and Philip C. Abbott, some of the problems and issues inherent in formulating famine-relief policies.

Laying in stores of food for hard times ahead is an ancient and honored public activity—at least as ancient as the biblical Joseph and his predecessors in the riverine civilizations of the Middle East. Most cultures still honor the activity in folk tales. We're all familiar with the story of the thrifty ant who demonstrates civic virtue, saving seeds for itself while leaving the frivolous grasshopper justly to starve.

Those who now make public policy were reared with this cultural background. So their current indecision about setting up grain reserves looks a bit surprising. Why wasn't a coordinated international food-reserve system set up years (or centuries) ago? Outside of fairyland and the bible world in which Pharaoh's vizier *knew* that there would be seven bad years, of course, are many institutional, political, and economic obstacles against any attempt to further the public good by establishing food reserves.

A discussion of political economy cannot be avoided in this context: All governments intervene in grain markets to obtain more freedom in formulating internal agricultural and food-consumption policies. Any negotiated agreement about an international food security scheme must accede to the fact that national rulers will continue to play a major role in assuring food supplies to their people.

The 1972 Food Crisis:
Causes and Response

From before the Great Depression until 1972, food security was not a major issue on the world scale (though repeatedly at the level of famine-stricken regions and countries, it was of paramount importance). World grain markets were a haven of stability, with prices fluctuating a few percentage points per month, at most. But from late 1972 to early 1974 the situation changed drastically, as prices of major traded grains almost tripled. For example, the New Orleans export price of U.S. wheat went from $63.80 per metric ton in August, 1972, to $103.60 in December, 1972, and rose to an astonishing $221.60 the following February.

A number of factors led to these developments:

— A decline in world grain production in 1972–73 was caused by unfavorable weather and acreage restrictions in major producing countries.
— The reduced Peruvian anchovy catch in 1972 led to increases in demand for soybean meal and ultimately to an increased demand for feed grains.
— The USSR purchased over 15 million tons of grain to make up in an unexpectedly vigorous way for production shortfalls in that country.
— The U.S. dollar was devalued.

Econometric analyses suggest that 60 to 80 percent of the observed food price increases can be attributed to these factors. The remaining inflation is best explained by a desire for "liquidity" in staples on the part of many governments that control their nations' grain trade. The Soviet purchases in 1972 exhausted U.S. and Canadian stocks. The knowledge that North America could no longer fulfill its historical role as a reliable residual grain supplier spread fast, causing panic buying among importers. Fears of food shortage persisted for some time, even though 1973–74 was a record world crop year. And widespread dissatisfaction with the structure and functioning of the worldwide supply system led to the Rome World Food Conference in November 1974.

The current discussion of grain reserves really began with the preparatory papers for that conference. During the formal discussions, reserve schemes and food aid were viewed almost as panaceas. According to Resolution XVII, a reserve/aid combination should ". . . assure the availability at all times of adequate world supplies of basic foodstuffs, primarily cereals, so as to avoid acute food shortages in the event of widespread crop failures or natural disasters; sustain a steady expansion of production; and reduce fluctuations in production and prices."

Clearly, the Rome conferees envisaged a world food security agency that at the very least could transfer supplies so that everyone would "have enough," assure that unanticipated local supply shortfalls would be made good, and stabilize prices and production. We shall refer to these goals as "food aid," "emergency relief," and "stabilization," respectively. We deal with all three issues here, trying to understand their significance in terms of both political economy and magnitude.

Market Stabilization through Buffer Stocks

How can stabilization be attained, and how can we measure its benefits once achieved? When we address these questions, a number of conceptual problems arise:

Should quantities or prices be stabilized? Price stabilization seems the more logical answer. Although the Rome conferees preferred to think in terms of quantity, this goal is unattainable in our uncertain world. A completely unprecedented crop shortfall could always occur in the next growing season, in such magnitude as not to be offset by any conceivable amount of food in storage.

The usual approach to such essential uncertainty is to set up the problem in probability terms—to design a reserve large enough to be sure that if historical crop fluctuation patterns persist, then world supply will not be more than (say) 30 million metric tons (mmt) short in (say) 99 years out of 100.

In the wake of the Rome conference, a number of calculations of this sort were carried out. Typically, these indicated that 25 or 30 million metric tons each of wheat and feed grains "ought to be" stored. The rationale is simple: the standard deviation of world production of either major class of grains has been about 12 to 15 million metric tons over the past 20 years. Having two standard deviations' worth of both crops in storage would allow the world to make up for bad harvests in all but the worst year or two in a century. Q.E.D.

The economist's problems with this approach are readily apparent. Unless those who manage the stores in a probability-based reserve scheme approach both omniscience and omnipotence in their responses (recall Joseph once again), the market will compensate for their mistakes via changing prices. Why not then *plan* to let price increases absorb moderate supply shortfalls, and store only enough grain to preclude extreme reactions such as those occurring during the food crisis of 1972–1974?

A buffer stock that is accumulated when grain is cheap and is sold when it is dear would stabilize both quantities and prices. This would offset most of the ill effects of bad crop years and maintain market incentives. Unlike a simple probability scheme, the costs of a buffer stock integrated with the market are easily calculated, and its benefits are assessable. Also, a price-stabilizing buffer stock is the only scheme that could possibly function under twentieth century socioeconomic arrangements for disposing of the world's food.

How should the reserve's benefits be measured? Once we agree that prices are to be stabilized, the next task is to ascertain who gains and who loses from the operation. Consider, for example, the 1972–1974 period, characterized by unprecedented increases in grain prices. As a direct consequence, the food import bill of cereal-deficit countries increased dramatically, while exporters reaped the profits. Within all countries, grain producers and processors prospered, and real incomes of consumers (especially the poor) went down because of the food price inflation. As a result, a series of compensating macroeconomic adjustments took place.

From this catalog of effects of grain price inflation, we gather that one way to evaluate a price-stabilizing buffer stock is through foreign exchange gains and losses from stabilization. Had prices been stabilized in 1972–1974, exporting countries would have lost foreign exchange, and importing countries would have gained. Within countries, producers would have sold a stock—with a level fixed by the harvest—at a lower price, and lost from stabilization. Consumers would have purchased this same stock more cheaply, and also would have gained by consuming the grain put on the market from its stores by the buffer stock agency. The agency itself would have built up cash reserves from its sales, though these would presumably have been earmarked for future purchases when grain prices fell again. In an oversupply situation, the losers and gainers would be reversed, but the analysis is similar.

Adding up probable losses and gains over the years for relevant economic groups would allow us to foresee who might favor or oppose price stabilization: A wheat buffer stock would probably help consumers and importers, and harm producers and exporters. The inference is much less clear for feed grains because demand curves are more nearly linear, producer response is greater, and trade is more open.

So far, we have been somewhat ambiguous about how a price-stabilizing buffer would operate. We have implied that it might buy either when worldwide crops are large, or when the relevant international grain price is low. These two response patterns are said to be induced by quantity and price triggers, respectively.

Any functioning buffer would, of course, utilize all information available, whether in the form of prices, quantities, or forecasts of either. Also, it would not announce its decision rules explicitly, since at best market participants could then offset any interventions it might make and at worst it could be ruined by speculation. Central bankers, the most influential market stabilizers in the world, are dour characters for just these reasons.

In practice, however, a functioning buffer stock would base most of its decisions on price signals. World grain markets are active and clear quickly, so price movements can indicate trends in supply and demand. For this reason, it is realistic to analyze a stock operating on the basis of price triggers, entering the market to buy (sell) when the world price falls (rises) to some lower (upper) bound. In other words, there is a "price band" that determines the buffer stock's activity. If the price in some market year stays within the band, the buffer stock agency does nothing. If the price reaches a limit, the agency intervenes until either the price returns within the band, or the stock's capacities are exhausted. Two parameters describe the capabilities of the stock: The width of its price band, and the maximum amount of grain it can buy for storage when the price is low. . . .

Besides the annual costs incurred on the grain it has in storage, the other major items in the buffer stock's accounts are the cash inflows and outflows it would realize on sales and purchases. Even an agency that bought cheap and sold dear might well have storage costs large enough to make it run a net loss over time. The larger the average amount of grain stored and the longer it remains there, the more likely is the buffer stock agency *not* to be profitable (even abstracting from the initial costs it will incur in stocking up). The determining factors seem to be:

— A wider price band means a longer waiting time between buying and selling operations, and higher storage costs. On the other hand, the margin between buying and selling prices would be greater, possibly by enough to cover the increased costs. The relationship between price band and buffer stock profits is ambiguous, since it also depends on the stock's capacity.

— As capacity increases for a given price band, so does the average amount stored, and profits decline.

— The magnitude of buy-sell operations will be influenced by demand elasticities in the current year and the exuberance of farmer supply response subsequently.

— As a necessary part of its operations, a buffer stock will increase world trade for other market participants. That is, its purchase and holding of stocks must increase the value of exports or reduce the value of imports for nations already in the market before the reserve commences operations. In effect, the buffer stock "finances" a decrease in net imports (or an increase in net exports) of the rest of the world via its own deficit. Which countries will actually gain foreign exchange because of price stabilization depends on the elasticities, but clearly the likely beneficiaries should help make good the buffer stock's paper losses.

Even after this trade effect is netted out, a buffer stock may be expected to lose money over time, especially for tight price bands. When this likelihood was first discovered, it created some surprise. But a second thought clarifies: a buffer stock would protect consumers against uncommon events—crop failures every five years or so. Even if five- to ten-year grain futures contracts existed, the market would not hedge against major crop failures, because of private risk aversion and the storage costs involved: ". . . there are no profits to be earned by consistently investing in improbable prospects. . . ."

In effect, we are advocating a price-stabilizing buffer stock to stabilize and control the market. Price increases would bear part of the effects of crop shortfalls, but timely sales by the stock agency would keep the inflation within limits, and dampen the kind of panic which swept around the world between 1972 and 1974. The events of those years already demonstrate that the market is incapable of stabilizing itself in extreme situations.

Defining Emergency Relief

International consciousness about food aid in general is usually raised by unpleasant television pictures and news stories of disaster and famine in underdeveloped parts of the world. Timely procurement and distribution of grains in these instances is of incalculable human value. The main questions involve triggering and delivering that kind of relief.

Droughts and natural disasters are impossible to predict, and occur quite randomly across the world. Even so, a given region has a high probability of experiencing serious drought (or other catastrophe) over a long period of time, say thirty years. Therefore, emergency relief is better viewed in *flow* than in *stock* terms. Any commitment by the community of nations to assist one another in the case of food emergencies should be a continuing one, since catastrophes will continue to occur. In the case of food, flexibility of response is the main issue. It could be provided easily by cash instead of cereal commitments, since the actual tonnages of cereals required in emergencies are likely to be miniscule in comparison to world production or even trade.

Two bottlenecks slow most relief efforts. The discovery and announcement of an emergency can be stalled; and organization and delivery of supplies to the stricken area is often disorganized and slow. Famine strikes at random across time and location. So food reserves dispersed idly over the globe would serve only to accumulate storage costs; a speedier response could be guaranteed by centralizing the relief agency.

At the international level, most famine relief can be activated only *after* the government of the afflicted country announces that severe food shortages exist. One assumes that in most cases national authorities would act rapidly on behalf of their people. But this is not always the case. Famine may conveniently decimate groups within the population opposed to the current regime, or the rulers may fear loss of face in requesting help from abroad. Cases of belated requests for help certainly occur — as in Ethiopia, where the government suppressed news of famine conditions in the early 1970s literally for months. If governments behave irresponsibly, international action might be called for, but the matter is inevitably delicate.

Bypassing this touchy issue, let us suppose that a relief fund has been established. Suppose also that severe threat of famine arises in some underdeveloped country. The government of that country would presumably import grain in an attempt to cover the shortfall. After exhausting both its foreign exchange capacity and its international credit, the country might still be in need. In such a case, it would presumably ask for international aid, and a portion of the famine fund could be used to buy the additional needed supplies.

Since both imports and famine-relief supplies paid for by the fund would have to be obtained in international markets, world grain prices would have an evident impact on the financing of relief. In a tight market year the international price would be high. The stricken country, even with the relief fund, could purchase only a quantity limited by its foreign exchange capabilities. The large single purchase would raise the price of grain still further. Adverse international market conditions can frustrate famine-relief operations, even though funds are available.

Under these circumstances, a price-stabilizing grain buffer stock would be selling its supplies to dampen price increases. These sales would incidentally stabilize the purchasing power of the famine-relief fund, and could even be directed to the afflicted countries. We discover another rationale for a grain buffer stock—it would lend order and effectiveness to international efforts for famine relief.

Magnitude of Relief Requirements

The actual magnitude of required relief efforts is probably so small as to have minimal impact on the grain buffer stock or the world market in general. We can calculate this amount, as we did with the buffer stock, either by using a probability-based model or on the basis of economic considerations. Not surprisingly, the probability calculations can be juggled to produce extremely high estimates of "necessary" reserves. Though psychologically reassuring, storing stocks of the size that comes out of the "worst case" assumptions of these studies is of dubious economic value. Holding tens of millions of tons of grain idle for several years awaiting doomsday is a very costly proposition. Even when the stocks are used, they need not bring any great benefits, since even in a crisis consumption can adjust somewhat without overwhelming hardship. Much more useful would be a guaranteed flow of funds to a relief agency, which could bring quick succor by using the world market and shipping facilities (or the stores of a price-stabilizing grain reserve).

We base our conclusion on the following facts. The major economic impact of a severe crop failure in a poor, agricultural country is on purchasing power. The resulting internal loss of aggregate demand will not be remedied unless emergency food supplies are both donated from abroad and directed to those harmed economically by the disaster. Emergency grain reserves must therefore be viewed as supporting food aid, but aid of a special kind: its destinations will vary from region to region and time to time. An estimate of required yearly average flows can be inferred from recent grain-import patterns for underdeveloped countries. The Most Severely Affected (MSA) countries, currently numbering forty-four, obtain most of their imports through commercial channels and another significant portion through food aid. FAO estimates that in 1975–76 there was a shortfall in MSA import capacity of about 2 million metric tons. Emergency relief requirements in 1975–76 would presumably have been less than this figure, since MSA countries are still recovering from their reduced import capacities due to the oil and food price explosions of 1972–1974. Hence, some part of the shortfall must be attributed to simple lack of purchasing power and not disaster per se.

Another estimate of the required flow is embodied in a Swedish proposal to the World Food Conference that enough grain be on hand to feed 2 million famine victims for a year. At 250 kilograms of grain per person, this works out to 500,000 metric tons. If these two estimates are taken as spanning the range of potential MSA grain needs that would not otherwise be covered, then a yearly *flow* of about 1 million metric ton seems a reasonable guess of the amount of required emergency supplies. The crudeness of this estimate is apparent—it should be supplemented with analyses both of magnitudes of recent relief efforts and likely future production shortfall-induced import requirements in MSA countries under realistic assumptions about world food prices and foreign exchange positions.

Translated into dollars, 1 million metric ton of grain amounts to a flow of only about $100 to $150 million, including transport costs to the afflicted regions. This is of course only a very small fraction of the total aid currently directed to the MSA countries.

The machinery for delivering emergency supplies is currently supplied through the World Food Program, the UN Disaster Relief program, the Red Cross, and various other charitable organizations. Their problem in past disasters has not been lack of organization but lack of timely available funds and supplies. But their status prevents them from delivering resources for relief efforts until after the disaster reaches headline proportions. They must wait until the overworked parliaments of the donor countries go through their established procedures for appropriating funds for unilateral or multilateral action. The essentials lacking for timely delivery of aid are a mechanism for rapid certification that a disaster has occurred, and assurance that in a given year stocks of food or funds will be at hand for emergency use. If stocks were to be guaranteed, then of course any unused portions could carry over to subsequent years.

India is particularly concerned about famines, and has in effect established its own emergency reserve. Given the difficulties of storage in the tropics, this is likely to prove an expensive exercise. If, for instance, 1 million metric ton of wheat is bought (or not sold) internationally by India, stored domestically for five years before it is needed, and then distributed to famine-stricken areas, the total cost to the government, including purchasing costs, storage cost, and opportunity cost of the funds is about $250 million. If instead this sum were saved as foreign exchange reserves, the government might be more flexible in the time of the crisis.

Apparently, the outcry of underdeveloped countries during the recent food crisis was due not only to high international prices but also to the unavailability of supplies—a much more dangerous situation from a subsistence country's point of view. The existence of an international stabilization grain reserve would provide the needed assurances for the third world. Poor countries might choose to supplement it with their own physical or monetary reserves, but their perceptions about the magnitudes required might be considerably reduced.

Food Aid: A Policy Dilemma

Food aid and grain reserves are inextricably intertwined in politician's pronouncements about food problems, although to a large extent they are economically separate entities. In the following paragraphs, we will outline briefly the major issues arising in past debate about food aid, and summarize the evidence regarding how it is utilized by recipient countries.

If we ignore public condemnation of blatantly political uses of food aid, then we are left with three main questions which have figured in past debate. Who should pay for food aid? Who should receive food aid? How can food-distribution systems be set up within the recipient country to minimize interference with agricultural production incentives?

The question of payment came to the fore recently as excess grain and other food stocks in exporting countries declined. Around 1971 or 1972, aid ceased to be useful as a vent for surpluses generated by the United States, for example, to support high producer-price agricultural policies. Subsequent Atlantic Community pressure on oil producers to help bear the cost of food aid shipments is an obvious corollary of the new world trade situation.

On the other side of the ethical ledger, the feeling exists in some policy-making circles that poor countries have an absolute "need" for aid, which should be satisfied by the rich. The U.S. Congress has been said to be a bastion of this doctrine. If this is so, then a strong political case can be made for food donations. Moreover, if the chronic oversupply situation of the 1960s reappears (a not improbable development), then the United States and Canada would again be tempted to act as discriminating oligopolists, selling their own grain surpluses to poor countries at reduced prices in the form of "source-tied" foreign aid. These arguments suggest that the problem of who should pay for aid in the future may not be pressing. If the present trend of good crop years continues, the exporters will be hastening to shoulder the burden.

Politics entered into the selection of food aid recipients when in the early 1970s Congress sought to curtail the use of food aid as a means for supporting the war in Vietnam. Legislators now are more conscious of the politically coercive uses of food, and a few are pushing to direct food flows to more humanitarian ends.

This internal U.S. discussion overlapped with new international awareness of the plight of the MSA countries and the wide publicity given the Bangladesh and Sahel famine-relief efforts. The notion of need implies that countries with unclosable food supply or foreign exchange gaps are, and ought to be, the first in line for continuing international help. Ethically appealing as this is, it provides no guidance as to the magnitude of aid required, nor does it imply any criteria which may be used to judge the effectiveness of food donations. So the question arises: What do recipient countries do themselves to absorb food aid inflows?

Food donations may have the effect of reducing a country's incentive to increase its agricultural production. Guaranteed aid could diminish government enthusiasm for research and financing extension services, and so on. This alleged impact on policy is of somewhat mystical nature and would be extremely hard to quantify, but no doubt has been important in some cases.

A more mundane market effect can also be identified. The possibility exists that in a domestic market where the government does not intervene to separate consumer and producer prices, food aid inflows will add to short-run supply, depress the price level, and so influence farmers to curtail output in the next few harvests.

If aid is really added to marketed supply, the reduction of price—and subsequently output—depends on demand and supply elasticities. If on the other hand the food is distributed *gratis* to those who could not otherwise afford to enter the market, domestic price and production would not be affected. If the government sells the donated food through the country's usual commercial channels, the revenue can be categorized as a domestic counterpart of general economic aid. Similarly, reexport of the donations can be a convenient source of foreign exchange.

As in any balance of payments problem, this internal market elasticity approach can be supplemented by asking how the economy adjusts macroeconomically to absorb the extra foreign exchange inflow that the donations represent. This amounts to asking whether the donations increase the supply level that commercial imports would otherwise have provided. If the aid is *not* additional, and merely replaces imports, then on the domestic front it would not depress internal producer prices. In balance of payments terms it would be equivalent to general economic aid. An important question arises—how much does aid add to the quantity imported, and how much does it replace imports that the government would have been making in any case?

The empirical evidence on this "additionality" question is suggestive, but not clear-cut. A plausible model has the government of a representative underdeveloped country setting a target for the amount of food it will make available in urban areas to satisfy the demands of the politically potent middle- and low-income groups there. The necessary supplies of grain can be acquired either from the rural interior of the country or from abroad. Internally, the power of the state can be mobilized to obtain a fixed amount of grain from the countryside, which implies that harvest shortfalls are borne by the rural poor. In the exterior, it is rational to buy grain from the cheapest supplier; hence available food aid at concessional terms will first be acquired by the government. But the fact that food aid can be obtained does not mean that the government will import much more than it otherwise had planned. If imports don't increase, then food aid is not additional; it is better treated as general economic aid, *not* as a device for channeling food to "the hungry people who need it most."

In light of this model, special steps within the poor country are required to make donated food additional to otherwise targeted imports, and really useful to the poor. Econometric analysis of import data for a number of countries for the last twenty-five years suggests that few have taken the requisite internal distributional steps. India with its Fair Price Shops seems to be an exception. This system of distributing food has probably been able to utilize imports to increase the total supply, in particular the quantity rationed out to the undernourished poor.

How Much Food to Supply?

Food available for aid seems likely to increase in the near future, as stocks build up in the grain exporting countries. If the recipient poor countries continue to use the concessionally available grain as general purpose foreign aid, then it is reasonable to ask whether food aid is economically efficient. Both product tying of aid (forcing the aid to be food) and source tying (forcing the food to be purchased from the donor) can exact a high price from the recipient. If the donated food is converted to foreign exchange, then its value is diminished by the constraints placed on the recipient by the donor. If it is used as food, then source tying—forcing it to come from a specific place—may increase transport costs, reduce perceived quality, and so on.

A second issue to be addressed is whether reserves should be set aside specifically for food aid. Remember that by its very nature, food aid has to be a flow—a constant diversion of some fraction of world supplies to poor countries, year after year. The flow can be characterized in several ways:

— It should be separate from and additional to grain allocations for emergency relief.
— Recipient governments ought to be assured of the amount of aid they can expect over the next few years, for their own planning purposes. Of course, they should also be able to count on emergency relief aid when necessary.
— Since the evidence indicates that most importing governments set cereal-inflow targets that they will satisfy, the magnitude of food aid flows becomes almost a question of foreign exchange budgeting: How much of the $X hundred million per year of food that country A will almost surely be importing should be covered by donors? If most countries use the flows as general aid, then the type of calculations used to determine the volume of the latter become relevant.
— Insofar as some countries make special efforts to transform the food inflows into extra supplies directed toward poor people, they should receive favorable consideration for larger allocations.

Programming all these flows would presumably be simplified if world grain price stability could be guaranteed. A buffer stock thus enters as an important component of future food aid deliberations. The buffer could also conceivably be used as a working stock to help keep aid flows moving, although this would be mostly a matter of convenience. As with emergency relief, the buffer stock is important because it would stabilize prices and make planning for disbursement and use of aid much easier.

Finally, if food aid flows have little direct impact on poor country import demand functions, then they will not have much feedback on an international grain buffer stock either. The buffer would basically operate as an $N + $ 1st country in international trade, and our results indicate that there would be minimal impact from aid through cereal trade on its operations. If aid flows begin to shift poor country import demands in the future, then they might make the task of price stabilization easier by smoothing trade flows.

Proposals for a Reserve Policy

Wheat reserves would have to be the pivot of any viable price stabilization scheme. Wheat is by far the most extensively traded grain, and its price is the most volatile. Since wheat is a major component of most advanced country diets, control of its price could stave off inflation-ary pressures in the rich countries as well as helping ease foreign exchange constraints on growth in the underdeveloped part of the world. Finally, substitution relationships among wheat and feed grains are such that stabilization of the world wheat price would help stabilize other grain markets as well.

Our econometric analysis . . . suggests that the size of an interna-tional wheat reserve could be quite modest, preferably smaller than 15 million metric tons, and most likely in the range of 10–15 million metric tons. These sizes are far smaller than those appearing in many proposals for grain reserves that appeared in wake of the World Food Conference. The reserve should be built under easy market conditions . . . when the world wheat price is around \$110–130/million metric tons. Reserves should be held *firmly* until a time such that world (real) price is in the vicinity of \$170–190/million metric tons at which point they would be released at these prices, with priority given to countries that are par-ticipating in a reserve scheme, especially less developed countries.

If a policy of this type is followed, our results indicate that price fluctuations can be substantially reduced—the number of times the wheat price rises above \$200 per ton (from a normal price of \$140) might be expected to fall from three years out of 20 down to one. The costs of stock operations required to achieve this degree of stabilization would be relatively small: an expenditure of between \$1 billion and \$1.5 billion over a period of years to build up the reserve, and operating costs of about \$100 million per year thereafter.

The reserves should preferably be held internationally, but if this proves a political impossibility, then certainly they should be held publicly rather than privately (since private storage efforts are likely to be quite inadequate). With a wide price band and small magnitude, international reserves need not interfere with the normal workings of the market, but instead would prevent abnormal behavior during times of crises. Nationally held reserves would be a good substitute for an inter-national program only if the holding government(s) acted in a stabilizing fashion, purchasing when prices were low and selling when prices were high. United States behavior during 1972–73 is not reassuring on this point, since it sold its stocks early to the USSR at very low price levels and then let speculators take advantage of the ensuing panic. Insulation of the management of a reserve scheme from the kind of foreign policy pressures which gave rise to the United States-USSR grain deal would be an unavoidable prior condition for its successful functioning. How then to prevent this "management" from degenerating into yet another proliferated UN agency becomes a question which must be faced and *answered* before the scheme can be set up. The fact that the reserve will have to participate in an active, competitive market is perhaps a hopeful omen on this front.

Within the United States, farm groups oppose grain reserve sales in periods of high prices because they want to reap the excess profits. However, when prices are low they are very vocal in advocating reserve purchases and support of falling prices. Since consumers pay taxes to finance reserve stocks in periods of glut, it is only reasonable that they recoup some of their investment via lower prices and less inflation in periods of shortage. The reserve stock we advocate incorporates a wide price band, so that farm groups might be less vocally opposed than they would be to more stringent stabilization.

In the case of internationally held reserves the burden of financing should fall on the large developed trading countries, such as the United States, Canada, Australia, Japan, the European community, and especially the USSR as the major likely beneficiary. Since there appears to be some offset between gainers and losers in wheat and feed grain reserves, it is possible that joint establishment of two buffer stocks would make economic sense.

In any case, participation in the reserve scheme should be the criterion for eligibility to purchase in periods of high prices, and as many countries as possible should be encouraged to join.

Turning to the issue of emergency relief, our rough analysis suggests that required annual flow of grain is likely to be quite small on the average, on the order of 1 million metric ton per year. Establishment of famine-relief stockpiles in remote parts of vulnerable countries might be worthwhile, but it is likely that their cost and flexibility would limit their usefulness. Rather, readily available emergency relief funds earmarked specially for disaster could prove to be a better solution. Disbursement of these funds for purchase of grain in world markets would be requested by afflicted countries, and decided upon in light of their foreign exchange positions and internal relief efforts. The annual flow of funds toward relief might be expected to amount to $100–$200 million, a small share of total foreign aid given to MSA countries.

The fact that disasters are of random location and magnitude—but almost invariably highly localized—points to the necessity of timely organization and assurance of relief funds or supplies. Given the relatively small magnitude of the probable costs, a scheme designed specifically for famine relief (but perhaps with the right of rapid withdrawal from internationally held stocks) would be both feasible and potentially of incalculable value in alleviating human suffering.

With the notable exception of India, food aid seems to have been used in the past by recipient countries as a source of general economic assistance, and not as a means for improving the nutritional status of vulnerable groups within the population. In strictly economic terms, food aid as a device for transferring foreign exchange from rich countries to poor ones is not efficient. In fact, it probably served as a vehicle for discriminatory oligopoly pricing by North American grain exporters during the surplus years of the 1960s.

The strictly *economic* conclusion we draw is that in principle food aid should be phased out and replaced by general economic assistance in the future, except for countries such as India which undertake the domestic policies necessary to make donated food flows add to normal levels of imports.

To this general recommendation, a number of qualifications must be added. First, it is distinctly possible that political decisionmakers in many advanced countries, and especially the United States, look with more favor on donations of food than donations of money (especially if a condition of generalized excess supply of cereals occurs again). A large amount of food aid used inefficiently as a form of general economic assistance is clearly preferable to a small amount of the real thing. Second, some countries are simply chronically unable to satisfy domestic food demand with their own resources (Egypt being a case in point). Since such countries will be importing anyway, there is much to be said for giving them favorable terms (instead of seeing them forced to borrow short-term money at 20 percent interest to pay for irreducible imports, as occurred during the food crisis). Again, interactions between price stabilization and needs for other forms of aid become apparent, but efforts to direct all possible aid flows toward MSA countries remain paramount.

Finally, it is worth recalling that general food aid, like emergency relief, is essentially a flow, with new commitments required year after year. An international buffer stock might in normal times be used as a pipeline reserve to support such flows, but for practical purposes new resources will have to go into aid programs with each advanced country budget exercise. Stabilization and guarantee of the amounts of aid flows over time would be of inestimable use to recipient countries in planning their own internal food policy and agricultural development efforts.

Snags in the World Forum

Many proposals for "food reserves" have appeared since the Rome World Food Conference in 1974. Even in some of the more recent ones, the three food security objectives—price stabilization, food aid, and emergency relief—are confused. We simply reiterate here that both food aid and emergency relief are *flows* of grain that must be maintained indefinitely, while price stabilization can be abetted by adroit manipulation of a *stock*. Holding very large stocks in some corner of the world as insurance against an emergency that might occur just there is likely to be expensive, and the total shortfall will not be large in comparison to world trade. Hence, it makes economic sense to divert flows of grain to the region at the appropriate time. Contrariwise, flows of food (manna excepted) will not be forthcoming when the world as a whole has a bad harvest year; stocks in the control of some sort of Buffer Stock Agency would be desirable to moderate food price inflation and soothe market disruption and panic.

So serious food security proposals boil down to discussion of price-stabilizing stocks, with provision for emergency relief operations and food aid to countries that under one sort of allocation rule or another deserve it.

There are three probable points of divergence in the negotiations about grain reserves that are now progressing in various international fora (the London-based International Wheat Council, the "Tokyo Round" of tariff-reduction talks in Geneva, the discussions in UN-related agencies such as the Food and Agriculture Organization and the World Food Council in Rome): size of reserves; triggering mechanisms; and burden-sharing. On at least a few of these broad issues, there seems to have been some progress.

As discussed . . . the reserve proposals that were offered . . . [a few] years ago tended to cluster around stocks of 25 to 30 million metric tons, a horrendously expensive quantity of grain to maintain. Press reports suggest that recent proposals run to from 10 to 20 million metric tons for wheat, a much more reasonable quantity in view of our econometric results.

. . . there was substantial disagreement between the major negotiators on triggers. The United States, tacitly backed by other exporting countries, favored quantity triggers for a grain reserve, to its own benefit in times of shortage because statistically reliable information about crop shortfalls at a global level usually arrives late, long after prices have skyrocketed.

As grain stocks have increased and prices softened, the exporting countries have come to look more benignly on market regulations. The Common Market, the other major trader, in any case inclines toward this point of view because of its Common Agricultural Policy (whereby farmer subsidy payments are tied to world prices) and more basically because of its *dirigiste* ideological approach to economic problems.

The current discussions focus around a U.S. proposal of September 1977 to the International Wheat Council for a price-triggered reserve of (according to the press leaks, but not the proposal) 15 million metric tons. Who is to pay for the relatively modest losses that such a reserve would run remains unclear. Both the econometric analysis of the type discussed here and the broader political issues in terms of worldwide attempts to exit from the present conjuncture will have some role in fixing what share of the burdens of grain reserves the nations will shoulder, if they shoulder them at all.

Selection 54   The Roots of Power

Ed Cowan

Editors' Introduction

The conversion of organic matter (biomass) into fuel is seen by some as an energy alternative for the future. The process of replacing fossil fuels with fuels produced by converting various grains into alcohol and adding a small amount of gasoline to produce "gasohol" has been discussed as a possible solution to the shortage and rising costs of fossil fuels. The utilization of manioc—known as tapioca by the American consumer—has been discussed for the production of alcohol instead of foodstuffs. Scientists desiring to utilize the entire plant may find ecologically responsible ways to provide both food and fuel.

The following selection details some of the problems associated with the introduction of such an innovative technology and prompts us to ask how far we are willing to go to convert foodstuffs into alcohol and eventually gasohol.

If you were a farmer and were offered a crop that would power your car and tractor, provide more starch than a potato, readily convert to any one of several sugars for the processed-food industry, yield more protein for human consumption from its leaves than a good soybean crop, subsist on the poorest of soils, use little fertilizer, and resist drought and insects—would you give it a try? And particularly so if you found that in replacing some of the crops you are now growing you would raise their price on the world market and thus generally raise the income of farmers worldwide?

Sounds like the idle musings of farmer-President Jimmy Carter? In fact, such a plant not only has long been a staple in the diet of the

Source: From Ed Cowan, "The Roots of Power," *The Humanist* 40, no. 2 (March/ April 1980):26–30, 54. This article first appeared in *The Humanist*, March/April 1980, and is reprinted by permission.

Third World peoples, but also since 1977 has been converted into automobile fuel. Biomass the latter is called—the conversion of organic matter into fuel. Of late it's received a lot of attention in American energy circles. There are numerous studies for producing alcohols, methane, and oils from wood, grasses, corn and other grains, sugar cane and sugar beet, coffee pulp, manure, crop residues, municipal wastes, pond algae, kelp, and even newsprint. In the Midwest and the South there are already pilot projects for converting various grains into alcohol, and "gasohol," a blend of a small percentage of alcohol with gasoline, can be bought at select service stations in Nebraska, Indiana, Illinois, and Iowa.

However, the world leader in alcohol fuels at the moment is Brazil. Its goal is to have alcohol comprise 20 percent of its motor fuel by the early eighties. The byproduct syrup of Brazil's sugar-cane production has been the major feedstock of the alcohol program, but increasingly the feedstock will be the plant in question: cassava (*Manihot esculenta crantz*).

Manoic it is also called. We know it only as tapioca, but its yard-long tuberous root of nearly pure starch is the potato of the tropical world. Although the Brazilians have a headstart on cassava-alcohol production, their methods are crude and unimaginative compared to the scheme of Dr. Dick McCann, formerly a research chemist at Sydney University in Australia. His comprehensive studies reveal why this versatile, productive shrub of the spurge family may eventually rival rice and wheat as the world's most important plant.

McCann has been studying cassava for several years, and his scheme calls for an agro-industrial system that would use the entire plant. The leaves, for example, contain up to 30 percent protein on a dry-weight basis, and they would yield slightly more crude protein than even a very good (forty bushels per acre) soybean crop. The protein would first be extracted from the leaves at $210 a tonne (a metric ton, 2204 pounds) of concentrate containing from 50 to 60 percent crude protein, which is protein produced at a slightly cheaper cost than that of soybeans. (All figures are in U.S. dollars converted from Australian dollars at a 1.13 exchange. McCann's study was made in 1975 Australian dollars.)

The remains of the leaf, the rest of the aboveground portion of the plant, and the peels and fibrous residue of the tubers would be converted into methane through anaerobic fermentation. The methane would be burned to power the entire processing operation, from the peeling of the tubers to the final distillation of the alcohol, and some methane would even be available as tractor fuel. Any organic material can be rendered into fuel, but with most, the process would consume more energy than it produced. McCann's figures reveal a net energy yield for the entire operation at a ratio of 1.5 to 1.

By converting the tops and peels (the bagasse) into methane instead of burning it directly as in the sugar-cane industry, potassium, phosphorus, and other soil nutrients remain in the waste liquids and would be returned to the soil. Theoretically, none of the nutrients would be lost except nitrogen, so that once the soils were fertilized to adequate levels, only nitrogen fertilizer would need be reapplied. In the McCann scheme that would come mainly every fourth year with a nitrogen-fixing legume such as alfalfa or soybeans. However, McCann surmises that some other soil nutrients would be lost in the process and would need to be periodically reapplied.

The tubers, once peeled, would be pulped and hydrolyzed into glucose (sugar), which would then be fermented into ethanol, the same ethyl alcohol that brings relief to Americans at happy hour. But this two-step process is costly. Thus, McCann's first priority has been to develop a yeast that will ferment the starch directly into alcohol. He is experimenting with various fermentation techniques, and he has been most successful with a continuous tower fermenter, similar to those used in some breweries. It speeds up the process to just a few hours, which helps keep costs low.

McCann showed in 1975 that alcohol could be produced at a cost of $285 a tonne, but that was using World War II technology. Cassava yields have reached 20 tonnes of tubers per acre on unirrigated land in Australia, but tests there under ideal conditions suggest an optimum yield of from 32 to 36 tonnes per acre can be achieved. At a yield of 32 to 36 tonnes of tubers per acre and with the full development of a one-step fermentation process, alcohol could be produced at $170 a tonne. However, McCann reports that the current cost is about $215 a tonne. That is the total cost, from sowing the seed to pouring off the alcohol. It is a conservative figure. It includes a 25 percent return on capital and three times the current cost of irrigation, even though irrigation is not mandatory.

McCann's calculations are based on a complex producing 230,000 tonnes of alcohol and 63,000 tonnes of leaf protein a year. The complex would service a farming community of 116,000 acres of cropped land; each year 86,400 acres would be sown in cassava and 29,000 sown in a nitrogen-inputting legume. And best of all, the capital cost of a single complex that would farm 116,000 acres of land and produce 230,000 tonnes of alcohol per year is $72.8 million, small potatoes indeed when compared with a nuclear-power plant, a coal-liquefaction plant, or even a new refinery.

As a result of the new militancy and long-standing unrest in the oil-producing nations, refined gasoline is ranging from $150 to $250 a tonne on the world market, and the December 1979 round of OPEC talks threatens to send crude oil to $60 a barrel. With President Carter's decontrol of domestic oil, all refined gasoline in the United States will be selling in that range within several years. McCann's current price of $215 a tonne is now slightly high.

However, a two-tier tax policy can make cassava alcohol competitive right now for any country that imports a sizable percentage of oil and that is capable of growing cassava. Once again, Brazil is doing just that. Initially it assured the sale of all of its ethanol and encouraged the switch to alcohol-burning engines by selling gasoline taxed at $1.50 a gallon and ethanol untaxed at $1.00 a gallon, but now there are only a few cents difference in price. In the United States, at the beginning of 1979, alcohol added to gasoline as a fuel supplement is exempt from federal excise tax, and the states that have a gasohol program have exempted it from a state tax as well.

A nontax or low-tax policy for a new energy source would bring only economic benefit. The excise-tax base would be lowered slightly, but that would be recovered by the payroll and corporate taxes on the increase in the domestic production of energy. Most important, the currency flow abroad to pay for imported oil—which for us now runs $40 billion a year—would be eliminated. Brazil is already well on the way to eliminating it altogether. And generally the domestic economy would be stimulated with an increase in the gross national product and a decrease in imports.

Manoic's greatest feature is its inexhaustible productivity. Twenty tonnes of tubers per acre per year would produce 912 gallons of alcohol per acre per year. The energy potential of this plant can be realized when one considers that at that yield, and even with one-quarter of the land in a "green manure," Brazil alone has enough uncultivated, tillable land to produce ethanol in excess of the entire world production of oil, most of which is refined into some form of liquid fuel.

This is not to suggest that we raze the Brazilian rain forest, which has been described as the lungs of the world, and replant it all with cassava. Brazil will never get the opportunity to satisfy the world's fuel thirst even if the country were so foolish as to try. As another example, Australia, which receives less than half the rainfall of South America, could produce—depending on just how much of its arid land would actually support cassava—between 2.5 and 5.7 times its current consumption of petroleum fuels and do so with no appreciable reduction in its current crops. These two examples give some indication of the potential of cassava as biomass; it should be remembered that there are more than a hundred countries in the world that have a suitable climate for growing cassava somewhere within their borders.

Although the prospect in the United States is not quite so sanguine, it is nevertheless good. Figures supplied by Paul Boden, agronomist with the U.S. Department of Agriculture in Albuquerque, New Mexico, indicate that the irrigated and unirrigated acres that could likely support cassava in Hawaii, California, New Mexico, Texas, Louisiana, Florida, and Puerto Rico—even allowing for a third lower yield on the unirrigated land—would produce 27 billion gallons of alcohol annually, 24 percent of the gasoline consumed in the United States in 1976.

Climate is the big question mark, for most South American varieties will not tolerate frost. But some species of cassava reach maturity within six months, and Boden points out that glass or plexiglass caps could be placed over the young plants to extend the growing season and possibly even allow for a slightly staggered harvesting season. Furthermore, one of the 130 known species of cassava, *Manihot carthaginensis* (more commonly called Ygilla, Yuca de Monte, and Xcache), is indigenous to the South and Southwest. Since we still have an agricultural policy of paying farmers not to produce and still have large agricultural surpluses, we have room for the introduction of another large crop that would more than pay its own way with both energy and protein. Cassava would simply move in and send the crops it replaces further north or onto soil-banked land.

However, some of that southern acreage now supports crops, such as citrus fruits, that cannot be grown anywhere else. And since our consumption of gasoline continues to increase, it would seem that if a cassava agronomy could replace 10 percent of America's gasoline consumption within fifteen years, it would be very successful. If, however, agronomists can use our domestic *carthaginensis* to develop frost-tolerant hybrids suitable to the North American climate, Texas alone, with one hundred million acres of pasture and range land, could probably double that figure to 20 percent by the turn of the century.

Brazil's successful alcohol program has already aroused interest here. Calvin Sherman, a consultant to the Florida Solar Energy Center, has submitted a grant request to the Department of Energy to study cassava as an energy source. He has aligned subcontractors from Hawaii to Brazil that will help study everything from cassava cultivators to distillery equipment, and his effort already has been sufficiently impressive to garner him promises from more than one large food producer should the government fail to find the requested $1.3 million, three-year grant.

Cassava is so right for large-scale agricultural development that it almost seems bred for it. The plant has no mandatory harvest period. It just keeps growing until the farmer gets around to it, although after ten months of growth there would be some leaf drop, which would lower protein production. Unlike sugar cane, which must be processed eight hours after chopping, there is a forty-eight-hour period after harvesting before the tubers develop serious deterioration. Furthermore, the tops can be harvested and processed and the tubers left in the ground indefinitely without spoiling. Or they can be dried and stored. All of which means that McCann's processing complex would operate routinely twelve months a year in areas where the climate would permit staggered planting for continuous harvesting.

Not the least of cassava's several favorable characteristics is its hardiness. The plant produces hydrocyanic (prussic) acid, and even in the so-called sweet varieties, it must be squeezed or boiled out before human consumption. The presence of this poison throughout the plant makes it naturally resistant to insect and disease attack, and there is some evidence that the bitter varieties, because of their greater inherent protection from predators, develop larger, starchier tubers. Cassava is such an efficient scavenger of nutrients that it can grow in soils so poor that they would support almost no other plant life. Some species are swamp-type plants, capable of growing in standing water. Others not only can flourish on about half the water and fertilizer of sugar cane, but also are drought resistant. During long periods without rain, the leaves drop off and the plant slips into dormancy until new rains come, at which point it draws on the reserves in the roots and spouts new leaves.

Alcohol makes an excellent automotive fuel and can also replace most of the liquid fuels derived from petroleum. The one major drawback is that it has a lower calorific value (energy content) than petroleum fuels; the heating of your home or factory would require a greater volume of alcohol than fuel oil. In spite of this, Brazil is experimenting with alcohol as a fuel for power stations.

However, when added in small quantities to gasoline, alcohol actually increases the octane and lowers the noxious emissions, and it can be added to gasoline in portions as high as 20 percent without entailing alterations to the car engines on the road today. With the use of dual carburetors it can be burned with diesel fuel on a 50:50 ratio in diesel trucks and buses. But most important, a Brazilian engineer, who for years has studied alcohol as a fuel, has shown that a properly designed engine, because it can use a higher compression ratio and can burn a cleaner mixture, can burn 100 percent alcohol and cause up to 50 percent less pollution with slightly better mileage—all this despite the lower calorific value of alcohol.

Fuel need not be the exclusive end product of a cassava economy. The alcohol can be the feedstock of the chemical industry just as petroleum is today, and Brazil has already laid plans to make this possible. In countries woefully short of protein or in a period of fuel glut, the cassava starch can be hydrolyzed into single-cell protein. Or it can be hydrolyzed into the various sugars used in the processed-food industry. In an area where the energy source is supercheap (perhaps geothermal), the tops could be processed into a protein-rich animal feed instead of fermented into methane to fuel the process.

It is for the Third World—most of whose countries lie in the tropical belt in which cassava is now grown in family plots as a table vegetable—that cassava alcohol production holds the greatest promise. These underdeveloped countries grow sugar cane, coffee, bananas, rubber, and other produce that are sold in the developed countries to the north, often at fluctuating prices that wreak havoc with the local economy. Sugar, for instance, has dropped from over 50 cents a pound years ago to a few cents a pound today. By cutting back on its production of sugar, cotton, coffee, fruit, rubber, and other products, the Third World would decrease the supply of these commodities. That would raise the commodities' world prices and thereby increase the export income of the Third World countries that produce them. They would make much more by producing less. And by converting the available acreage to cassava, they would cut their oil-import bill and generally stimulate their economy as they satisfy their own energy needs.

Because of cassava alcohol's importance to the underdeveloped world, McCann and an associate made a study and preliminary design for a village-scale project in 1978. In the village context sophistication and fermentation speed are not important factors; the equipment is simple, the process slower. Labor is cheap and distribution costs nil. His study predicts that alcohol at the village level could be produced at 22 cents a gallon—alcohol that would power electrical generators, outboard canoes, motorcycles, minitrucks, and other forms of local transportation that now run on petroleum products at five to eight times that price.

Brazil's leadership in severing the OPEC lifeline and the obvious economic gain of biomass will undoubtedly induce much of the tropical world to follow suit. An inevitable rise in world food prices will follow — good news for the farmer of the tropical world but bad news for the consumers of North America and Europe. Yet a successful cassava agronomy will be more effective in raising the living standard of the underdeveloped world than all of the aid programs of the past. We can at least look forward to a reduction in those foreign-aid programs as well as to a larger, healthier world market for all goods and services.

In particular, a rise in world food prices will enable American agricultural products to become more competitive on the world market. If the price of rice rises sufficiently, Americans are going to sell more wheat to China and India, and in time we will be able to greatly enlarge our export of protein-rich crops such as beans, which we can grow in enormous quantities. A higher price is the essence of the recent farmers' protest in Washington. A cassava economy will bring higher prices *and* expanded markets. And Washington should be happy with the cuts in agricultural subsidies and surpluses—and the slight anti-inflationary impact of reduced budget deficits that result.

However, the one detriment to a cassava economy abroad and here at home would be the inflationary impact of rising food prices. But inflation is inevitable whichever way we turn. If the world does not develop alternate energy sources, the cost of oil and gas will continue to soar as it becomes ever more scarce. Coal and nuclear power, Washington's star substitutes at the moment, entails enormous capital costs, high operating costs (most estimates peg oil-from-coal at twice the current world price of oil), and environmental costs, which are only now being perceived and may prove intolerable.

The one solid criticism of biomass is that it grows energy on land needed to grow food for an overpopulated, undernourished world. But today political barriers, market barriers, joblessness, poverty, ignorance, and poor distribution are the causes of malnutrition and undernourishment—not insufficient land. Cassava itself offers an example of malnutrition caused by ignorance. *Kwashiorkor*, the protein-deficiency disease, is a common ailment of the 300-million people who eat cassava because they consume only the root, not the protein-rich leaves. And what finer example could there be of the way political barriers and poverty keep half the world in a state of hunger than our agricultural policy of paying farmers not to sow and storing the supluses produced from the land they do sow. Yet unless there is a drastic change in the population growth rate, at some point in the next decade or two mass hunger and starvation will dictate that energy production give way to food production. Even then an energy crop that delivers 63,000 tonnes of protein for every 230,000 tonnes of fuel and that gives way every fourth year to another protein crop will be hard to stop.

Selection 55 Goals for Mankind

Ervin Laszlo et al.

Editors' Introduction

Public opinion polls are a measure of popular attitudes toward current issues. In 1975 pollster Louis Harris found that people were willing to make changes in their consumption habits and move toward a more ecological life-style. Political leaders, nutritionists, home economists, educators, behavioral psychologists, and sociologists must work together to develop strategies to help people move in this direction.

Goals in Canada and in the United States

Americans comprise 6 percent of the world's population (now 5 percent), but consume 40 percent of the world's production of energy and raw materials. The following responses were made to a number of questions asked in connection with this level of consumption:

— 74 percent said this uses up our own natural resources and those of others abroad;
— 74 percent said this makes products and raw materials scarce, thereby driving prices up;
— by 50 percent to 31 percent, most thought that, sooner or later, this will turn the rest of the world's people against us;
— by 55 percent to 30 percent, most believed that this hurts the well-being of the rest of the world;
— by 61 percent to 23 percent, almost a three-to-one majority, most felt that this is "morally wrong."

In this same survey, more than two out of three people admitted that they themselves are "highly wasteful." Ninety percent thought that "we are going to have to find ways to cut back on the amount of things we consume and waste." Some 64 percent agreed that such a cutback will mean lowering the U.S. standard of living. When the alternative was posed between "changing our life-style" in order to consume fewer physical goods, and "enduring the risks of continuing inflation and unemployment due to raw material shortages," a 77 to 78 percent

Source: Adapted from Ervin Laszlo et al., "A World Atlas of National and Regional Goals," *Goals for Mankind*, pp. 39–40. Copyright © 1977 by The Research Foundation of the State University of New York. Used by permission of E.P. Dutton.

majority of the American people opted for a change in life-style (see table 55.1 for the specific changes people were willing to make).

A number of additional viewpoints are being advocated in the United States as alternatives to the established view. Many of them embody the overall intent of . . . global goals. . . . Some half-dozen groups in the United States have enunciated some type of "declaration of interdependence," hoping to create a new ethical standard for the nation. Which of these viewpoints—if any—will rise to predominance in the future is not clear. What is certain is that the decade-long series of poll data indicates a continuing erosion of confidence in the policies that govern the nation, especially when these policies are compared with other more stable social indicators.

Table 55.1 Responses to a Louis Harris and Associates Survey Taken between August 30 and September 6, 1975

The following questions were put to a stratified sample of 1,497 persons, with this preamble: "Now let me ask you about certain specific areas which have been suggested for people to cut down on the amounts they consume. Would you personally be willing, or not, to . . ."

	Willing (%)	Not Willing (%)	Not Sure (%)
Have one meatless day a week?	91	7	2
Stop feeding all-beef products to pet animals?	78	15	7
Do away with changing clothing fashions every year?	90	7	3
Wear old clothes, even if they shine, until they wear out?	73	22	5
Prohibit the building of large houses with extra rooms that are seldom used?	73	19	8
Make it much cheaper to live in multiple-unit apartments than in single homes?	57	34	9
Eliminate annual model changes in automobiles?	92	5	3
Sharply reduce the amount of advertising urging people to buy more products?	82	11	7

Source: Louis Harris & Associates, Inc. (personal communication).

Appendix

Appendix A: RDA Charts

Table A–1 Recommended Dietary Allowances, Revised 1980

Age and Sex	Weight		Height		Protein	Fat-Soluble Vitamins				
						Vit. A	Vit. D	Vit. E	Vit. C	Thiami
	kg.	lb.	cm.	in	gm.	μg. R.E.[1]	μg.[2]	mg. αT.E.[3]		mg.
Infants										
0.0–0.5 yr.	6	13	60	24	kg. × 2.2	420	10.0	3	35	0.3
0.5–1.0 yr.	9	20	71	28	kg. × 2.0	400	10.0	4	35	0.5
Children										
1–3 yr.	13	29	90	35	23	400	10.0	5	45	0.7
4–6 yr.	20	44	112	44	30	500	10.0	6	45	0.9
7–10 yr.	28	62	132	52	34	700	10.0	7	45	1.2
Males										
11–14 yr.	45	99	157	62	45	1,000	10.0	8	50	1.4
15–18 yr.	66	145	176	69	56	1,000	10.0	10	60	1.4
19–22 yr.	70	154	177	70	56	1,000	7.5	10	60	1.5
23–50 yr.	70	154	178	70	56	1,000	5.0	10	60	1.4
51 + yr.	70	154	178	70	56	1,000	5.0	10	60	1.2
Females										
11–14 yr.	46	101	157	62	46	800	10.0	8	50	1.1
15–18 yr.	55	120	163	64	46	800	10.0	8	60	1.1
19–22 yr.	55	120	163	64	44	800	7.5	8	60	1.1
23–50 yr.	55	120	163	64	44	800	5.0	8	60	1.0
51 + yr.	55	120	163	64	44	800	5.0	8	60	1.0
pregnancy					+30	+200	+5.0	+2	+20	+0.4
lactation					+20	+400	+5.0	+3	+40	+0.5

Note: The allowances are intended to provide for individual variations among most normal persons as they live in the United States under usual environmental stresses. Diets should be based on a variety of common foods in order to provide other nutrients for which human requirements have been less well defined. The allowances are designed for the maintenance of good nutrition of practically all healthy people in the United States.

[1] Retinol equivalents; 1 retinol equivalent = 1 μg. retinol or 6 μg. β-carotene. See text for calculation of vitamin activity of diets as retinol equivalents.

[2] As cholecalciferol: 10 μg. cholecalciferol = 400 I.U. vitamin D.

[3] αtocopherol equivalents: 1 mg. d-α-tocopherol = 1 αT.E.

[4] 1 N.E. (niacin equivalent) = 1 mg. niacin or 60 milligrams dietary tryptophan.

[5] The folacin allowances refer to dietary sources as determined by *Lactobacillus casei* assay after treatment with enzymes ("conjugases") to make polyglutamyl forms of the vitamin available to the test organism.

Ribo-flavin	Niacin	Vit. B	Folacin[5]	Vit. B12	Calcium	Phosphorus	Magnesium	Iron	Zinc	Iodine
	mg.N.E.[4]	mg.	μg.		mg.					μg.
0.4	6	0.3	30	0.5[6]	360	240	50	10	3	40
0.6	8	0.6	45	1.5	540	360	70	15	5	50
0.8	9	0.9	100	2.0	800	800	150	15	10	70
1.0	11	1.3	200	2.5	800	800	200	10	10	90
1.4	16	1.6	300	3.0	800	800	250	10	10	120
1.6	18	1.8	400	3.0	1,200	1,200	350	18	15	150
1.7	18	2.0	400	3.0	1,200	1,200	400	18	15	150
1.7	19	2.2	400	3.0	800	800	350	10	15	150
1.6	18	2.2	400	3.0	800	800	350	10	15	150
1.4	16	2.2	400	3.0	800	800	350	10	15	150
1.3	15	1.8	400	3.0	1,200	1,200	300	18	15	150
1.3	14	2.0	400	3.0	1,200	1,200	300	18	15	150
1.3	14	2.0	400	3.0	800	800	300	18	15	150
1.2	13	2.0	400	3.0	800	800	300	18	15	150
1.2	13	2.0	400	3.0	800	800	300	10	15	150
0.3	+2	+0.6	+400	+1.0	+400	+400	+150	[7]	+ 5	+25
0.5	+5	+0.5	+100	+1.0	+400	+400	+150	[7]	+10	+50

e RDA for vitamin B12 in infants is based on average concentration of the vitamin in human milk. The wances after weaning are based on energy intake (as recommended by the American Academy of Pediatrics) consideration of other factors, such as intestinal absorption.

e increased requirement during pregnancy cannot be met by the iron content of habitual American diets or by existing iron stores of many women; therefore, the use of 30 to 60 milligrams supplemental iron is mmended. Iron needs during lactation are not substantially different from those of nonpregnant women, but tinued supplementation of the mother for two to three months after parturition is advisable in order to enish stores depleted by pregnancy.

rce: Reproduced from *Recommended Dietary Allowances*, 1980, with permission of the National Academy of nces, Washington, D.C.

Table A–2 Estimated Safe and Adequate Daily Dietary Intakes of Additional Selected Vitamins and Minerals

Age Group	Vitamins			Trace Elements*		
	Vitamin K	Biotin	Panto-thenic Acid	Copper	Man-ganese	Fluoride
	μg.			mg.		
Infants						
0.0–0.5 yr.	12	35	2	0.5–0.7	0.5–0.7	0.1–0.5
0.5–1.0 yr.	10–20	50	3	0.7–1.0	0.7–1.0	0.2–1.0
Children and Adolescents						
1–3 yr.	15–30	65	3	1.0–1.5	1.0–1.5	0.5–1.5
4–6 yr.	20–40	85	3–4	1.5–2.0	1.5–2.0	1.0–2.5
7–10 yr.	30–60	120	4–5	2.0–2.5	2.0–3.0	1.5–2.5
11 + yr.	50–100	100–200	4–7	2.0–3.0	2.5–5.0	1.5–2.5
Adults	70–140	100–200	4–7	2.0–3.0	2.5–5.0	1.5–4.0

Note: Because there is less information on which to base allowances, these figures are not given in the main table of the RDAs and are provided here in the form of ranges of recommended intakes.

Table A–3 Mean Heights and Weights and Recommended Energy Intake

Category	Age (years)	Weight		Height		Energy Needs (with range)	
		(kg)	(lb)	(cm)	(in)	(kcal)	(MJ)
Infants	0.0–0.5	6	13	60	24	kg × 115 (95–145)	kg × .48
	0.5–1.0	9	20	71	28	kg × 105 (80–135)	kg × .44
Children	1–3	13	29	90	35	1300 (900–1800)	5.5
	4–6	20	44	112	44	1700 (1300–2300)	7.1
	7–10	28	62	132	52	2400 (1650–3300)	10.1
Males	11–14	45	99	157	62	2700 (2000–3700)	11.3
	15–18	66	145	176	69	2800 (2100–3900)	11.8
	19–22	70	154	177	70	2900 (2500–3300)	12.2
	23–50	70	154	178	70	2700 (2300–3100)	11.3
	51–75	70	154	178	70	2400 (2000–2800)	10.1
	76+	70	154	178	70	2050 (1650–2450)	8.6

Trace Elements*			Electrolytes		
Chromium	Selenium	Molybdenum	Sodium	Potassium	Chloride
		mg.			
0.10–0.04	0.01–0.04	0.03–0.06	115–350	350–925	275–700
0.02–0.06	0.02–0.06	0.04–0.08	250–750	425–1,275	400–1,200
0.02–0.08	0.02–0.08	0.05–0.1	325–975	550–1,650	500–1,500
0.03–0.12	0.03–0.12	0.06–0.15	450–1,350	775–2,325	700–2,100
0.05–0.2	0.05–0.2	0.1–0.3	600–1,800	1,000–3,000	925–2,775
0.05–0.2	0.05–0.2	0.15–0.5	900–2,700	1,525–4,575	1,400–4,200
0.05–0.2	0.05–0.2	0.15–0.5	1,100–3,300	1,875–5,625	1,700–5,100

* Since the toxic levels for many trace elements may be only several times usual intakes, the upper levels for the trace elements given in this table should not be habitually exceeded.

Source: Reproduced from *Recommended Dietary Allowances*, 1980, with permission of the National Academy of Sciences, Washington, D.C.

Category	Age (years)	Weight (kg)	Weight (lb)	Height (cm)	Height (in)	Energy Needs (with range) (kcal)	Energy Needs (with range) (MJ)
Females	11–14	46	101	157	62	2200 (1500–3000)	9.2
	15–18	55	120	163	64	2100 (1200–3000)	8.8
	19–22	55	120	163	64	2100 (1700–2500)	8.8
	23–50	55	120	163	64	2000 (1600–2400)	8.4
	51–75	55	120	163	64	1800 (1400–2200)	7.6
	76+	55	120	163	64	1600 (1200–2000)	6.7
Pregnancy						+300	
Lactation						+500	

Note: Recommended Dietary Allowances Revised 1980. The data in this table have been assembled from the observed median heights and weights of children shown in table A–1 together with desirable weights for adults given in table A–2 for the mean heights of men (70 inches) and women (64 inches) between the ages of 18 and 34 years as surveyed in the U.S. population (HEW/NCHS data).

The energy allowances for the young adults are for men and women doing light work. The allowances for the two older groups represent mean energy needs over these age spans, allowing for a 2% decrease in basal (resting) metabolic rate per decade and a reduction in activity of 200 kcal/day for men and women between 51 and 75 years, 500 kcal for men over 75 years and 400 kcal for women over 75. . . . The customary range of daily energy output is shown for adults in parentheses, and is based on a variation in energy needs of ± 400 kcal at any one age. . . . emphasizing the wide range of energy intakes appropriate for any group of people.

Energy allowances for children through age 18 are based on median energy intakes of children of these ages followed in longitudinal growth studies. The values in parentheses are 10th and 90th percentiles of energy intake, to indicate the range of energy consumption among children of these ages. . . .

Appendix B: The Requirements of Human Nutrition

Table B-1 Essential Amino Acids and Fatty Acids

	RDA for Healthy Adult Male (milligrams)	Dietary Sources	Major Body Functions	Deficiency	Excess
Essential Amino Acids					
Aromatic		From proteins:	Precursors of structural protein, enzymes, antibodies, hormones, metabolically active compounds	Deficient protein intake leads to development of kwashiorkor and, coupled with low energy intake, to marasmus.	Excess protein intake possibly aggravates or potentiates chronic disease states.
Phenylalanine	1,100	*Good sources:*			
Tyrosine	1,100	Legume grains			
Basic		Dairy products	Certain amino acids have specific functions:		
Lysine	800	Meat			
Histidine	Not known	Fish	(a) Tyrosine is a precursor of epinephrine and thyroxine		
Branched Chain		*Adequate sources:*			
Isoleucine	700	Rice	(b) Arginine is a precursor of		
Leucine	1,000	Corn			
Valine	800	Wheat			
Sulfur Containing		*Poor sources:*			
Methionine	1,100	Cassava			
Cystine	1,100	Sweet potato			

Other Tryptophan Threonine	250 500		(c) Methionine is required for methyl group metabolism (d) Tryptophan is a precursor of serotonin	
Essential Fatty Acids Arachidonic Linoleic Linolenic	6,000 6,000	Vegetable fats (corn, cotton-seed, soy oils) Wheat germ Vegetable shortenings	Involved in cell membrane structure and function Precursors of prostaglandins (regulation of gastric function, release of hormones, smooth-muscle activity)	Poor growth Skin lesions Not known

Note: Essential amino acids and fatty acids cannot be synthesized in the body and must be present in food. Amino acids are the building blocks of body proteins; essential fatty acids are involved in the maintenance of cell membrane structure and function and serve as precursors of the prostaglandins, a family of hormone-like compounds that have diverse physiological actions in the body.

Table B-2 Vitamins

Vitamin	RDA for Healthy Adult Male (milligrams)	Dietary Sources	Major Body Functions	Deficiency	Excess
Water Soluble					
Vitamin B₁ (Thiamine)	1.5	Pork, organ meats, whole grains, legumes	Coenzyme (thiamine pyrophosphate) in reactions involving the removal of carbon dioxide	Beriberi (peripheral nerve changes, edema, heart failure)	None reported
Vitamin B₂ (Riboflavin)	1.8	Widely distributed in foods	Constituent of two flavin nucleotide coenzymes involved in energy metabolism (FAD and FMN)	Reddened lips, cracks at corner of mouth (cheilosis), lesions of eye	None reported
Niacin	20.0	Liver, lean meats, grains, legumes (can be formed from tryptophan)	Constituent of two coenzymes involved in oxidation-reduction reactions (NAD and NADP)	Pellagra (skin and gastrointestinal lesions, nervous, mental disorders)	Flushing, burning and tingling around neck, face and hands
Vitamin B₆ (Pyridoxine)	2.0	Meats, vegetables, whole grain cereals	Coenzyme (pyridoxal phosphate) involved in amino acid metabolism	Irritability, convulsions, muscular twitching, dermatitis near eyes, kidney stones	None reported
Pantothenic Acid	5–10.0	Widely distributed in foods	Constituent of coenzyme A, which plays a central role in energy metabolism	Fatigue, sleep disturbances, impaired coordination, nausea (rare in man)	None reported
Folacin	0.4	Legumes, green vegetables, whole wheat products	Coenzyme (reduced form) involved in transfer of single-carbon units in nucleic acid and amino acid metabolism	Anemia, gastrointestinal disturbances, diarrhea, red tongue	None reported

Vitamin B$_{12}$	0.003	Muscle meats, eggs, dairy products, (not present in plant foods)	Coenzyme involved in transfer of single-carbon units in nucleic acid metabolism	Pernicious anemia, neurological disorders	None reported
Biotin	Not established. Usual diet provides .15–.3	Legumes, vegetables, meats	Coenzyme required for fat synthesis, amino acid metabolism and glycogen (animal-starch) formation	Fatigue, depression, nausea, dermatitis, muscular pains	Not reported
Choline	Not established. Usual diet provides 500–900	All foods containing phospholipids (egg yolk, liver, grains, legumes)	Constituent of phospholipids. Precursor of putative neurotransmitter acetylcholine	Not reported in man	None reported
Vitamin C (Ascorbic Acid)	45.0	Citrus fruits, tomatoes, green peppers, salad greens	Maintains intercellular matrix of cartilage, bone and dentine. Important in collagen synthesis	Scurvy (degeneration of skin, teeth, blood vessels, epithelial hemorrhages)	Relatively non-toxic. Possibility of kidney stones
Fat Soluble Vitamin A (Retinol)	1.0	Provitamin A (beta-carotene) widely distributed in green vegetables; retinol present in milk, butter, cheese, fortified margarine	Constituent of rhodopsin (visual pigment); maintenance of epithelial tissues; role in mucopolysaccharide synthesis	Xerophthalmia (keratinization of ocular tissue), night blindness, permanent blindness	Headache, vomiting, peeling of skin, anorexia, swelling of long bones
Vitamin D	0.01	Cod liver oil, eggs, dairy products, fortified milk, and margarine	Promotes growth and mineralization of bones. Increases absorption of calcium	Rickets (bone deformities) in children; osteomalacia in adults	Vomiting, diarrhea, loss of weight, kidney damage

Table B-2 (continued)

Vitamin	RDA for Healthy Adult Male (milligrams)	Dietary Sources	Major Body Functions	Deficiency	Excess
Vitamin E (Tocopherol)	15.0	Seeds, green leafy vegetables, margarines, shortenings	Functions as an antioxidant to prevent cell-membrane damage	Possibly anemia	Relatively non-toxic
Vitamin K (Phylloquinone)	0.03	Green leafy vegetables Small amount in cereals, fruits, and meats	Important in blood clotting (involved in formation of active prothrombin)	Conditioned deficiencies associated with severe bleeding, internal hemorrhages	Relatively non-toxic Synthetic forms at high doses may cause jaundice.

Note: Vitamins are organic molecules needed in very small amounts in the diet of higher animals. Most of the water-soluble (B complex) vitamins act as coenzymes, or organic catalysts; the four fat-soluble vitamins (A, D, E, and K) have more diverse functions. Although low vitamin intake can result in deficiency disease, the misguided use of high-potency vitamin pills can also have undesirable effects.

Editors' Note: The figures given in table B-2 are based on the 1974 edition of the Recommended Dietary Allowances. Some changes have been made in the 1980 edition. (see Tables A-1, and A-2, pp. 486-87). For example, the recommended allowance for vitamin C has been increased substantially. For the first time, ranges of estimated safe and adequate intakes of biotin, pantothenic acid, and vitamin K are given in the 1980 edition of the Recommended Dietary Allowances.

Source: From Nevin S. Scrimshaw and Vernon R. Young, "The Requirements of Human Nutrition," *Scientific American* (September 1976):63. Copyright © 1976 by Scientific American, Inc. All rights reserved. Reprinted with permission.

Table B–3 Essential Mineral Elements

Mineral	Amount in Adult Body (grams)	RDA for Healthy Adult Male (milligrams)	Dietary Sources	Major Body Functions	Deficiency	Excess
Calcium	1,500.0	800	Milk, cheese, dark green vegetables, dried legumes	Bone and tooth formation Blood clotting Nerve transmission	Stunted growth Rickets, osteoporosis Convulsions	Not reported in man
Phosphorus	860.0	800	Milk, cheese, meat, poultry, grains	Bone and tooth formation Acid-base balance	Weakness, demineralization of bone Loss of calcium	Erosion of jaw (fossy jaw)
Sulfur	300.0	(Provided by sulfur amino acids)	Sulfur amino acids (methionine and cystine) in dietary proteins	Constituent of active tissue compounds, cartilage and tendon	Related to intake and deficiency of sulfur amino acids	Excess sulfur amino acid intake leads to poor growth
Potassium	180.0	2,500	Meats, milk, many fruits	Acid-base balance Body water balance Nerve function	Muscular weakness Paralysis	Muscular weakness Death
Chlorine	74.0	2,000	Common salt	Formation of gastric juice Acid-base balance	Muscle cramps Mental apathy Reduced appetite	Vomiting
Sodium	64.0	2,500	Common salt	Acid-base balance Body water balance Nerve function	Muscle cramps Mental apathy Reduced appetite	High blood pressure

Table B-3 (continued)

Mineral	Amount in Adult Body (grams)	RDA for Healthy Adult Male (milligrams)	Dietary Sources	Major Body Functions	Deficiency	Excess
Magnesium	25.0	350	Whole grains, green leafy vegetables	Activates enzymes Involved in protein synthesis	Growth failure Behavioral disturbances Weakness, spasms	Diarrhea
Iron	4.5	10	Eggs, lean meats, legumes, whole grains, green leafy vegetables	Constituent of hemoglobin and enzymes involved in energy metabolism	Iron-deficiency anemia (weakness, reduced resistance to infection)	Siderosis Cirrhosis of liver
Fluorine	2.6	2	Drinking water, tea, seafood	May be important in maintenance of bone structure	Higher frequency of tooth decay	Mottling of teeth Increased bone density Neurological disturbances
Zinc	2.0	15	Widely distributed in foods	Constituent of enzymes involved in digestion	Growth failure Small sex glands	Fever, nausea, vomiting, diarrhea
Copper	0.1	2	Meats, drinking water	Constituent of enzymes associated with iron metabolism	Anemia, bone changes (rare in man)	Rare metabolic condition (Wilson's disease)
Silicon	0.024	Not established	Widely distributed in foods	Function unknown (essential for animals)	Not reported in man	Industrial exposures: Silicon—silicosis

Vanadium	0.018	*	*	*	*	Vanadium—lung irritation Tin—vomiting Nickel—acute pneumonitis
Tin	0.017	*	*	*	*	
Nickel	0.010	*	*	*	*	
Selenium	0.013	Not established (Diet provides .05–1 per day)	Seafood, meat, grains	Functions in close association with Vitamin E	Anemia (rare)	Gastrointestinal disorders, lung irritation
Manganese	0.012	Not established (Diet provides 6–8 per day)	Widely distributed in foods	Constituent of enzymes involved in fat synthesis	In animals: poor growth, disturbances of nervous system, reproductive abnormalities	Poisoning in manganese mines: generalized disease of nervous system
Iodine	0.011	.14	Marine fish and shellfish, dairy products, many vegetables	Constituent of thyroid hormones	Goiter (enlarged thyroid)	Very high intakes depress thyroid activity
Molybdenum	0.009	Not established (Diet provides .4 per day)	Legumes, cereals, organ meats	Constituent of some enzymes	Not reported in man	Inhibition of enzymes
Chromium	0.006	Not established (Diet provides .05–.12 per day)	Fats, vegetable oils, meats	Involved in glucose and energy metabolism	Impaired ability to metabolize glucose	Occupational exposures: skin and kidney damage
Cobalt	0.0015	(Required as vitamin B$_{12}$)	Organ and muscle meats, milk	Constituent of vitamin B$_{12}$	Not reported in man	Industrial exposure: dermatitis and diseases of red blood cells

Table B-3 (continued)

Mineral	Amount in Adult Body (grams)	RDA for Healthy Adult Male (milligrams)	Dietary Sources	Major Body Functions	Deficiency	Excess
Water	40,000 (60 percent of body weight)	1.5 liters per day	Solid foods, liquids, drinking water	Transport of nutrients Temperature regulation Participates in metabolic reactions	Thirst, dehydration	Headaches, nausea Edema High blood pressure

Note: Essential mineral elements are involved in the electrochemical functions of nerve and muscle, the formation of bones and teeth, the activation of enzymes and, in the case of iron, the transport of oxygen. The trace minerals nickel, tin, vanadium and silicon, previously considered to be health hazards, are now known to be essential for animals. Although they are so widely distributed in nature that primary dietary deficiencies are unlikely, changes in the balance among them may have important consequences for health.

Editors' Note: The figures given in table B-3 are based on the 1974 edition of the Recommended Dietary Allowances. Some changes have been made in the 1980 edition (see tables A-1 and A-2, pp. 486–87). The most significant change is the addition of ranges of safe and adequate intakes for copper, manganese, fluoride, chromium, selenium, and molybdenum.

* Same as silicon.

Source: From Nevin S. Scrimshaw and Vernon R. Young, "The Requirements of Human Nutrition," *Scientific American* (September 1976):64. Copyright © 1976 by Scientific American, Inc. All rights reserved. Reprinted with permission.

A Food/Ecology Glossary

Abiotic. The nonliving components in an ecosystem which include the sun, various physical forces such as wind, and all the chemical factors that influence the living organisms.

Adenosine Triphosphate (ATP). This special molecule is found in the cells of all living organisms. It is the common energy currency used in the organism in biochemical reactions. ATP is formed when a phosphate group is hooked on to adenosine diphosphate (ADP). When there is a demand for energy, ATP is broken down to ADP releasing large amounts of chemical energy. The ADP can be converted back to ATP when an energy-rich phosphate becomes available as the chemical bonds in glucose, fatty acids, and amino acids are broken down and energy is released.

Agribusiness. A corporate combine that includes: (1) agricultural input firms, (2) agricultural output firms, (3) corporations directly involved in farming, and (4) corporations indirectly involved in farming.

Amino Acid. An organic compound composed of carbon, hydrogen, and nitrogen. Each amino acid molecule contains one or more amino group ($-NH_2$) and at least one carboxyl group ($-COOH$). In addition, some amino acids (methionine and cystine) contain sulfur. Amino acids form the building blocks of protein. They link together in a definite sequence to form a particular protein. The structure of an amino acid is

$$\underset{H}{\overset{H}{\diagdown}}N - \underset{\underset{H}{|}}{\overset{\overset{R}{|}}{C}} - C\underset{OH}{\overset{O}{\diagup}}$$

R represents one of a number of groups that may be attached to the central atom of an amino acid.

Anemia. A reduction of the amount of hemoglobin in red blood cells and/or a reduction in the number of red blood cells themselves that reduces the amount of oxygen available to all body cells. The symptoms of anemia include general weakness, fatigue, paleness, brittle nails, loss of appetite, abdominal pain, and dizziness. Iron, protein, copper, folic acid, and vitamins B_6, B_{12}, and C are all necessary for the normal formation of red blood cells. Nutritional anemia may be caused by the lack or poor absorption of one or more of the above nutrients. Iron-deficiency anemia is the most common form of the condition. Infants, adolescents, and women (particularly during pregnancy) are vulnerable to iron deficiency and may require iron supplements. *See* Iron-Deficiency Anemia, Pernicious Anemia, and Megablastic Anemia.

Antibiotic. A chemical substance produced by a microorganism that has the capacity to inhibit the growth of and even to destroy bacteria and other microorganisms. Penicillin, streptomycin, and other antibiotics are used in the treatment and prevention of infectious diseases of humans, animals, and plants.

Arable Land. Farmland, land that can be used to cultivate crops without extensive modifications to compensate for such limitations as the nutrient content of the soil and/or lack of water or other climatic factors, is considered potentially arable land.

Arteriosclerosis. A disease characterized by the hardening, thickening, and inelasticity of the walls of the arteries.

Ascorbic Acid (Vitamin C). A water-soluble vitamin essential for formation of collagen in the body. Collagen, a protein, is the connective tissue that holds the cells and tissues together. Collagen is necessary for the structural integrity of bones, teeth, connective tissue, skin, cartilage, and small blood vessels. The synthesis of this protein requires the presence of hydroxyproline, an amino acid formed by the addition of the hydroxyl group, —OH group, to the amino acid proline. Hydroxyproline can only be formed from proline in the presence of vitamin C. Vitamin C also has a significant relationship with other nutrients. For example, it enhances the absorption of iron. It also plays an important role in converting folinic acid to folacin the active form of the vitamin.

Atherosclerosis. A form of arteriosclerosis in which mushy deposits of fatty substances (cholesterol) partially obstruct blood flow. Evidence indicates that an elevated serum cholesterol level is one, but not the only, risk factor in the development of atherosclerosis. Other risk factors include smoking, high blood pressure, diabetes mellitus, and advancing age. Men are more susceptible to atherosclerosis than women in their childbearing years. More than half the deaths in the United States are due to heart disease. The underlying condition that contributes to a large proportion of these deaths is atherosclerosis.

Basal Metabolism. The amount of energy required to carry on vital bodily processes during physical, emotional, and digestive rest. These vital processes include rspiration, glandular activity, cellular metabolism, and the maintenance of body temperature.

B-Complex Vitamins. The water-soluble vitamins function as coenzymes, or enzyme helpers. They include thiamine, riboflavin, niacin, pantothenic acid, pyridoxine, biotin, folacin, and vitamin B_{12} (also known as cobalamin). The B-complex vitamins are vital to the release of energy as a result of the metabolism of carbohydrates, fats, and proteins. They also help maintain the normal functioning of the nervous system and the muscle tone of the gastrointestinal tract.

Beriberi. The final form of thiamine deficiency. The gastrointestinal tract, nervous system, and muscles are affected by this deficiency disease.

Biogeochemical Cycles. The mechanisms by which nutrient elements such as carbon, oxygen, phosphorus, nitrogen, and water circulate between biological organisms and their environment. A biogeochemical cycle has the following characteristics: movement of the nutrient element from the environment to the organism and back to the environment; involvement of biological organisms (plants and/or animals, especially microorganisms); a geological reservoir, the atmosphere (air), the hydrosphere (water), and the lithosphere (soil); chemical change.

Biological or Ecological Succession. The orderly process whereby an ecosystem changes from a simple community into a complex and relatively stable one. The final stage or community in a succession (called the climax community or mature ecosystem) is one in which a diverse set of species is interacting through complex food-web patterns.

Biological Value (BV). A term used to describe protein quality or the efficiency of a protein in meeting the body's need for protein. It is defined as the percentage of absorbed nitrogen retained by the body and depends primarily upon the amino acid composition of a dietary protein. The biological value (BV) of protein may be calculated by determining the nitrogen (N) of the food intake minus the urinary and fecal excretion by using the formula

$$BV = \frac{\text{dietary N} - (\text{urinary N} + \text{fecal N})}{\text{dietary N} - \text{fecal N}} \times 100$$

BV measurements do not take into account food N that is not absorbed (urinary N comes from absorbed N). The following formula can also be used:

$$BV = \frac{\text{retained N}}{\text{absorbed N}} \times 100$$

The biological value of some proteins fed to humans is shown in the accompanying table. When 70 percent of the intake of nitrogen is retained, a biological value of 70, the protein will support growth and maintenance provided that the caloric content of the diet is adequate. With biological values of less than 70, questionable growth occurs.

Food	BV for Adults
Egg	100
Milk	93
Fish	75
Beef muscle	75
Rice	86
Corn	72
White flour	60
Soy flour	72
Navy bean	46

Biotic. The living components in an ecosystem that interact in a consistent way.

Biotin. A vitamin of the B-complex group. Biotin functions as a coenzyme that can accept carbon dioxide removed from one molecule and can add it to another. This capability makes biotin necessary for a number of reactions that are essential for the utilization of carbohydrates, fats, and proteins as sources of energy.

Calcification. *See* Mineralization.

Calcium. This nutrient is essential for the mineralization of bones. The term *mineralization* refers to the process by which calcium, phosphorus, and other minerals crystallize on the protein (collogen) matrix of the bone, and thus harden and strenghthen the bone. Adequate amounts of the dietary calcium are needed during periods of growth to ensure the normal development of bones and also during the adult life to maintain normal bone structure. Actually, bone is a dynamic, metabolic active tissue with mineralization and dissolution constantly occurring. Because of this dynamic state adults still have a dietary requirement for calcium. Calcium is also necessary for the normal formation and maintenance of teeth. The calcium that circulates in the body fluids represents about 1 percent of the calcium in the body, but it performs a number of vital functions. The mineral is essential for normal blood clotting. The transmission of impulses between nerves and muscles is also dependent on normal levels of blood calcium. Calcium is believed to promote the release of a substance (acetylcholine) that bridges the gap between nerve and muscle fibers and allows nerve impulses to pass to the muscles.

Calorie. (1) The heat required to raise the temperature of 1 kilogram of water 1 centigrade degree, from 14.5° to 15.5° C. The calories given for food values are actually kilocalories, which are sometimes represented by using a capital C.

$$1 \text{ kilocalorie (kcal)} = 1 \text{ Calorie} = 1,000$$

(2) calorie. The standard unit for heat that is equivalent to the amount of heat required to raise the temperature of 1 gram of water 1 centigrade, from 14.5° to 15.5° C.

Carbohydrate. All carbohydrates are composed of glucose and other simple sugars that contain carbon, hydrogen, and oxygen. There are three types of carbohydrates: mono-, di-, and polysaccharides. Monosaccharides consist of a single sugar molecule like glucose, fructose, and galactose. Disaccharides are composed of two sugars linked together. Polysaccharides are long chains built up by the linkage of many sugar molecules, usually glucose. Mono- and disaccharides are commonly referred to as sugars. Polysaccharides are commonly described as starches. The body derives energy from carbohydrates, fats, and proteins in the food we eat. Carbohydrates provide four calories per gram when oxidized.

Cardiovascular Disease. A disease that affects the heart and/or the circulatory system.

Carnivores. Animals that eat other animals, thereby obtaining their energy and nutrients indirectly from primary producers.

Carrying Capacity. The maximum population that a given habitat can support indefinitely is known as its carrying capacity.

Cassava. A tropical fruit of the spurge family with edible starchy roots.

Chlorine. This nutrient is found in the body primarily as chloride and helps regulate acid-base balance to control the pH of the blood at 7.4 (7.38 to 7.42). Chloride also stimulates the production of hydrochloric acid, which is necessary for digestion. Chloride activates the starch-splitting digestive enzyme of saliva — salivary amylase.

Cholesterol. The most common member of the group of sterols; cholesterol is present in many foods and can also be made in the body. Cholesterol, like other sterols, is composed of carbon, hydrogen, and oxygen arranged in rings. Many nutritionists believe that there is a link between high levels of blood cholesterol and the development of atherosclerosis. The typical American diet is high in cholesterol and also contains large amounts of animal fats that are high-saturated fatty acids (such as the fat in meat, eggs, butter, hard cheeses, and whole milk). These dietary factors cause elevations in blood cholesterol.

Chromium. There is evidence that this mineral element increases the effectiveness of insulin. It seems to facilitate the binding of insulin to the cell membrane, which in turn facilitates the transfer of glucose from the blood into the cells of the body.

Cobalt. This trace mineral is an essential part of vitamin B_{12} or cobalamin. There is evidence that cobalt activates a number of enzymes necessary for the absorption of iron.

Coenzyme. A small nonprotein molecule that is in class association with an enzyme (often termed the body's protein catalyst). Without coenzymes, enzymes cannot function. Each of the B-complex vitamins — thiamine, riboflavin, niacin, pantothenic acid, pyridoxine biotin, folacin, and vitamin B_{12} (also known as cobalamin) — functions as a coenzyme.

Collagen. This protein forms the chief constituent of connective tissue, cartilage, tendon, bone, and skin.

Complete protein. Protein-yielding foods differ in their amino acid composition. A complete protein contains all the eight or nine amino acids essential for humans; it may or may not contain all the nonessential amino acids. Complete proteins are far more commonly found in animal sources (fish, poultry, meat, egg, cheese, and milk) than in vegetable sources.

Consumers. Organisms that depend for life on other organisms; they are generally divided into primary consumers (herbivores), secondary consumers (carnivores), and microconsumers (decomposers that cause the chemical disintegration of dead plants and animals).

Copper. There is evidence to suggest that copper enhances the utilization of iron: It seems to be necessary for the normal absorption of iron from the gastrointestinal tract to be incorporated into certain iron-containing enzymes; it also acts as a catalyst in reactions involving the incorporation of iron into the hemoglobin molecule.

Coronary Heart Disease. The impairment of the heart's functioning due to a reduction in the flow of blood to the heart muscle. The reduction of the flow of blood is caused by atherosclerosis.

Cretinism. A severe iodine deficiency during fetal development and early infancy may cause cretinism, a disease characterized by retarded growth and mental retardation. The condition is frequently encountered among children born to mothers who had very low iodine intake during adolescence and pregnancy. Cretinism is endemic—that is, it occurs in areas where the soil and water are low in iodine and where fish is not commonly eaten. If treatment is started soon after birth most of the symptoms are reversible. However, if the iodine deficiency is allowed to continue beyond early childhood, permanent mental retardation and dwarfing cannot be prevented. Some experts believe that genetic factors may also contribute to development of cretinism.

DDT. Chlorinated hydrocarbons such as DDT and its derivatives are insecticides used to kill insects that destroy crops or that transmit such human diseases as malaria. These synthetic chemical poisons attack the central nervous system of insects causing convulsions, paralysis, and death. DDT is usually sprayed from airplanes over the target crops and marsh but much of the chemical drifts for many miles in the air, water, and on land. DDT and its derivatives are highly stable and resist disintegration for fifteen or twenty years. These poisons are fat soluble, therefore, they tend to be recycled through the food chains and affect nontarget organisms. Any substance that is not degraded as it moves through the food will become more concentrated. Derivatives of DDT have been found in all animals on earth that have been examined. Although chlorinated hydrocarbons are relatively nontoxic for humans, concern is growing about the possible long-term genetic and health effects on humankind because of the increasing levels of DDT in our food and water.

Delaney Clause. When the 1958 Food Additives Amendment to the Pure Food and Drug Act of 1938 was passed a rider to the amendment, the Delaney Clause, was added to prohibit the use of an additive in any quantity if it is found to induce cancer when ingested by humans or animals.

Demography. The study concerned with the analysis of populations including such items as births, deaths, and age is known as demography.

Denitrification. One of the processes involved in the nitrogen cycle is denitrification, the conversion of nitrates into atmospheric nitrogen accomplished by certain soil bacteria. When plants and animals die, nitrogen is converted by decomposers to ammonia gas (NH_3) and certain ammonium (NH_4) salts. These are in turn converted by other groups of bacteria into atmospheric nitrogen N_2.

Diabetes Mellitus. This chronic, hereditary disease is characterized by an absolute or relative lack of insulin that leads to abnormalities in carbohydrate (glucose) metabolism and abnormalities in the metabolism of protein and fat. The individual with diabetes mellitus is unable to regulate the blood glucose level normally because the hormone insulin, secreted by the beta cells of the pancreas, controls glucose metabolism by facilitating the transfer of glucose from the spaces around the cell into the cell interior. Adult onset diabetes is frequently associated with obesity. Many physicians and nutritionists believe that susceptibility to diabetes mellitus is increased by obesity combined with inactivity. In fact, studies indicate that weight reduction alone often results in improvement in the obese diabetic patient.

Cardiovascular disease occurs much more often in diabetic patients than in the general population.

Doubling Time. The number of years it takes for a population to double in size is referred to as the doubling time of the population. The human population has continued to increase from the Stone Age to modern times at an ever-increasing rate; each doubling has taken place in less time.

Ecology. Ecology is the science that studies the interrelationships between living organisms and their habitat; the study of the structure and function of an ecosystem.

Ecosphere, Biosphere, or Global Ecosystem. These terms are used to refer to the sum total of all the various systems on the earth necessary to support life. This total concept includes every relationship that binds living things together. It includes the sphere of air, water, and land in which life exists.

Ecosystem. A self-sustaining complex network and self-regulating community of organisms considered in relation to each other and with their nonliving environment (including the media through which they exchange matter and energy as they interact).

Emulsifier. A chemical food additive used to prevent the separation of oil and water. Processed foods such as salad dressing contain emulsifiers.

Endemic. A condition (such as goiter) that occurs infrequently in the general population but more or less constantly in the population of a particular area.

Endosperm. The starchy portion within the kernel of wheat, corn, or other cereal. When the germ and fibrous outer layer are removed from the endosperm, refined flour is produced.

Energy. The capacity to do work. It derives from radiant energy, chemical energy, electrical energy, heat energy, or mechanical energy.

Enrichment. The addition of nutrients to specific foods to replace those that have been lost during processing. Legal standards are set for the enrichment of foods. For example, refined flour, bread, and certain cereals have standards of identity that require the addition of thiamine, riboflavin, niacin, and iron. When the Pure Food Drug and Cosmetic Act of 1938 was enacted, bread and flour were given "Standards of Identity"—that is, published standards stating what ingredients must be in the product and in what amounts.

Entropy. The degree of disorder or randomness—that portion of energy that is not available for useful work.

Enzyme. An enzyme is a chemical compound produced by the body from protein and other molecules that helps initiate or speed up specific chemical reactions. Enzymes are often called biological catalysts.

Essential Amino Acids. Amino acids that are needed by the body but cannot be synthesized in the body from other substances are termed *essential amino acids*. Eight amino acids are known to be essential for human adults: methionine, threonine, tryptophan, isoleucine, leucine, lysine, valine, and phenylalanine. Children and possibly adults also require histidine.

Essential Fatty Acid. Linoleic acid, a polyunsaturated fatty acid, has been demonstrated to be necessary for growth and the prevention of certain types of dermatitis (infection or inflammation of the skin) in infants. The body cannot synthesize linoleic acid, which is therefore considered an essential fatty acid. (The word *essential* refers to the fact that it must be supplied by eating food that contains it; it cannot be manufactured in the body from other foodstuffs.) Corn, cottonseed, soybean, and wheatgerm oil are excellent sources, and margarine, vegetable shortenings, and peanut oil are good sources of linoleic acid.

Exponential Growth. A quantity exhibits exponential growth when it increases by a constant percentage of the whole in a constant time period. Doubling time (or the time it takes a growing quantity to double in size) occurs at shorter and shorter intervals.

Fabricated or Synthetic Foods. These foods are prepared principally from ingredients specifically designed to achieve a particular function not possible with common food ingredients.

Fats or Lipids. Almost 95 percent of the lipids in the diet are triglycerides, a compound composed of carbon, hydrogen, and oxygen arranged as a molecule of glycerol linked with three fatty acids. Glycerol is an alcohol with the formula $C_3H_5(OH)_3$. A fatty acid consists of a long chain of carbon atoms with attached hydrogen atoms and an acid group, a carboxyl group (−COOH) at one end. The properties of the different fats depend on their fatty acids. Fats serve many important functions. They are an important source of concentrated energy. When metabolized by the body, they yield more than twice the energy per gram than either carbohydrates or proteins. One gram of fat can yield nine calories whereas one gram of carbohydrate or protein can provide only four calories. Fats are the sole source of the essential fatty acid, linoleic acid. This essential fatty acid cannot be manufactured in the body from other foodstuffs. Linoleic acid has been demonstrated to be necessary for growth and also for the health of skin in infants. Fats serve as carriers of vitamins A, D, E, and K, the fat-soluble vitamins. The recommended intake of fat is 30 to 35 percent of the total intake of calories, but typical diets in the United States contain approximately 45 percent of the calories from fat. Dr. Fredrick Stare states that the recommended intake of linoleic acid should be at least 1 percent of the day's kilocalories. Vegetable oils are good sources of linoleic acid.

Fatty Acid. An organic compound composed of a carbon chain with hydrogens attached and an acid group (the carboxyl group) at one end.

Stearic acid

Feedback. All systems maintain themselves through feedback — that is, the unique capacity to receive input that helps in regulating and maintaining the system. Positive feedback occurs when input sent back to the system causes the system to change continuously in the same direction. As a result of this accentuation of a tendency, the system can go out of control.

Fertilizer. A substance that makes land or soil capable of producing more vegetation or crops. The two types of fertilizers are inorganic and organic. Synthetic plant nutrients that have been produced by man are known as inorganic fertilizers. Among the most common inorganic fertilizers are ammonium sulfate and calcium nitrate. Animal manure and other naturally derived organic material are used as plant nutrients and considered organic fertilizers.

Fluorine. Recent evidence indicates that this mineral may reduce tooth decay by discouraging the growth of acid-forming bacteria. This nutrient is found in the body in compounds known as fluorides.

Folacin or Folic Acid. A member of the B-complex vitamin group. Folacin is a coenzyme with a chemical structure that enables it to receive single carbon units from one molecule and transfer them to another. This transfer mechanism is vital in the formation of nucleic acids such as DNA and RNA. DNA is a substance found in the nucleus of living cells that functions in the transfer of genetic characteristics. RNA is found in the cytoplasm of cells. RNA is replicated from DNA and functions as the code determining the amino acid sequence of a protein. The folic acid coenzyme is needed in many other single transfer reactions occurring in the body such as the formation of porphyrin (the constituent of hemoglobin) and in the inter-conversion of various amino acids (phenylalanine to tyrosine).

Food Additive. Any substance or mixture of substances intentionally or unin-tentionally added to food and consumed with the food. Intentional, or direct, additives are those that (1) preserve and prevent spoilage, (2) add or enhance flavor, (3) maintain or improve nutritional value, (4) produce an acceptable consistency. The legal definition set forth by the Food and Drug Administration includes only intentional additives. It does not include incidental or indirect additives that are not deliberately used. These sub-stances have become part of the food as a result of some phase of the production, processing, storage, or packaging of food.

Food and Agriculture Organization of the United Nations (FAO). This branch of the United Nations was established in 1945 for the purposes of raising levels of nutrition and standards of living and securing improvements in the efficacy of the production and distribution of food. Most of the FAO's activities are directed toward improving the production of and trade in food and other commodities within the context of the national and international policies established by UN member countries.

Food Chain. With the passage of energy as food from one trophic level to another only about 10 percent of the energy from one level can be captured by organisms on the next highest trophic level. The loss of usable energy at each step in the food chain is frequently depicted in a food pyramid.

Food Web. Many animals feed on a variety of species at different trophic levels resulting in the crosslinking and interconnection of different food chains to form a relatively complex system known as a food web.

Foodstuff. A substance or material suitable for food. Proteins, carbohydrates, and fats are sometimes referred to as the three foodstuffs, or the basic organic chemicals in our diet.

Formulated Foods. Mixtures of two or more foodstuffs (or ingredients other than seasonings) processed or blended together.

Fortification. The addition of one or more nutrients to a food in amounts in excess of those normally found in the food. Milk, for example, is often fortified with vitamin D.

Fossil Fuel. Coal, oil, and natural gas are fossil fuels. They are the remains of once-living plants and animals that can be burned to release energy.

Glycerol. An alcohol that is composed of a 3-carbon chain, each with an alcohol (−OH) group attached. Glycerol serves as the framework of the fat molecule.

$$
\begin{array}{c}
\text{H} \\
| \\
\text{H}-\text{C}-\text{OH} \\
| \\
\text{H}-\text{C}-\text{OH} \\
| \\
\text{H}-\text{C}-\text{OH} \\
| \\
\text{H}
\end{array}
$$

Goiter. A lack of iodine results in a simple goiter—a swelling of the neck reflecting the enlargement of the thyroid gland. The gland enlarges in an attempt to compensate for the lack of iodine that is essential to the manufacture of thyroxine. The primary function of the hormone thyroxine is the regulation of basal metabolism or the use of energy for vital internal processes. The simple goiter is endemic—that is, a condition that is particular to those areas where the soil and water are low in iodine and where saltwater fish is not eaten. Many nations have adopted laws requiring the iodization of salt. Other countries require the iodization of oil. These practices have proved beneficial in reducing the incidence of endemic goiters.

GRAS (Generally Recognized as Safe). A list of food additives maintained by the Food and Drug Administration that are considered nontoxic when used in the food supply under normal manufacturing processes.

Green Revolution. A general term referring to a variety of methods and technologies used to increase agricultural yield per acre. These methods include the introduction of new crops in an area, the use of fertilizers, increased irrigation, better protection against pests that destroy crops, and the introduction of specially bred seeds that are more productive and more resistant to disease. The term *Green Revolution* is also used when referring to the introduction into an area of new, scientifically bred or selected varieties of food crops.

Greenhouse Effect. The warming of the lower atmosphere and the surface of the earth because of the trapping of heat in the atmosphere. Ecologist G. Tyler Miller explains that as solar radiation, mostly visible light, reaches the earth, it is absorbed by the land, sea, and clouds and is reradiated back into the atmosphere as heat thus cooling the earth. Because of the process termed the *greenhouse effect,* carbon dioxide and water vapor absorb much of this heat. Carbon dioxide and water vapor then reradiate a portion of the absorbed heat (that would normally be lost fairly rapidly into space) back to the earth thus warming the atmosphere. As the carbon dioxide content of the atmosphere increases, more heat is retained, the atmosphere becomes warmer, and the earth's climate could possibly change. The carbon dioxide content in the atmosphere is primarily increasing from the burning of fossil fuels.

Habitat. The place or area in which a group of organisms naturally lives and grows. Eugene Odum refers to the habitat as the species "profession."

Hemoglobin. Performs the basic function of carrying oxygen from the lungs and transporting it to all the tissues of the body where it is released for use. On return to the lungs, hemoglobin carries a portion of the carbon dioxide formed in the cells for release in the lungs.

Herbivores. Animals that eat plants to obtain their energy and nutrients.

High-Quality Protein. A protein of high quality supplies all the essential amino acids in the relative amounts and proportions needed by the human body for protein synthesis. High-quality proteins include those of eggs, milk, cheese, fish, poultry, and meat.

Homeostasis. As long as a system remains in a state of dynamic equilibrium or homeostasis (where inputs and outputs are balanced below the maximum limits of the system and its surroundings), the system remains functional. All systems maintain themselves through feedback—that is, the unique capacity to receive output from the system back as input that helps in regulating and maintaining the system. The open system has the capacity to maintain its integrity despite inputs from and outputs to one or more systems outside itself. All living organisms, including humans, are open systems. They must receive inputs in the form of air, food, and water and eliminate wastes. Deprivation of air, even for a few minutes, is fatal. Deprivation of the ability to obtain any input or to dispose of any output is fatal in a relatively short time. Furthermore, the human being is in a state of homeostasis because of the body's regulatory mechanisms that act to maintain the constancy of the body's internal environment. Many of these regulatory mechanisms operate on the principle of negative feedback—that is, deviations from a given normal set are detected by a sensor. Signals from the sensor trigger compensatory changes that continue until the set point or ideal state (homeostasis) is again reached.

Horizontal Integration. The expansion of a business establishment by absorbing or constructing additional facilities to meet an increased volume of an aspect of food production and thus have exclusive control over a farm commodity in a market or control that makes possible the manipulation of the food product.

Hormone. A secretion produced in the body (by endocrine glands) and carried in the bloodstream to other parts of the body. Each hormone has a specific influence on the functioning of a tissue, organ, and the body as a whole. For example, thyroxine is a hormone secreted by the thyroid gland; insulin is a hormone secreted by the pancreas.

Human Ecology. The study of the relationships and interactions of humans with other humans, their habitat, environment, and the rest of the nonliving (abiotic) and living (biotic) world. How ecosystems affect and are affected by human beings is also studied.

Hypervitaminosis. Undesirable symptoms produced by taking an excess of a vitamin concentrate or pure vitamin. Huge doses of vitamins A, D, and K may cause serious injury to health.

Incaparina. This special high-protein, low-cost infant food was developed for use in Central America. It consists of a combination of corn, high-protein cottonseed meal, vitamin A, and tortula yeast (a source of the B-complex vitamins).

Insecticide. A substance or preparation used to kill insects.

Iodine. This mineral is an essential part of thyroxine, a hormone produced by the thyroid gland. The primary function of thyroxine is the regulation of the rate of cellular oxidation (the "burning" of the nutrients with the release of energy).

Iron. The mineral necessary for the formation of hemoglobin, the oxygen-carrying protein in red blood cells. Iron is found in the muscle cells in two forms: myoglobin and a constituent of certain enzymes. Myoglobin, like hemoglobin, is made up of an iron-containing pigment and a protein. Myoglobin may be considered the heart and muscle version of hemoglobin and is the recipient of oxygen carried by hemoglobin to the cells. The cytochromes, iron-containing enzymes, are needed to catalyze the final steps of biological oxidation where water is formed and useful energy is trapped in the form of ATP.

Iron-Deficiency Anemia. This condition can be caused by either a lack of dietary iron (a form of nutritional anemia) or by excessive blood loss (hemorrhagic anemia). Infants, adolescents, and women (particularly during pregnancy), are vulnerable to nutritional anemia due to iron deficiency and may require iron supplements. Iron-deficiency anemia, due to a lack of iron over a prolonged period of time, is characterized by smaller than normal sized red blood cells (microcytic anemia) and by a reduced hemoglobin level in the red blood cells (hypochromic anemia). Because of the limited ability to transport oxygen to tissue and remove carbon when hemoglobin levels are reduced, people with iron-deficiency anemia often suffer from general weakness, dizziness, loss of appetite, abdominal pain, and increased susceptibility to infection.

J-Curve. A curve with the shape of the letter J depicts exponential or geometric growth 1, 2, 4, 8, 16, . . .).

Joule. The unit of energy in the metric system. One calorie is equivalent to 4.184 joules (J).

Kwashiorkor. The form of protein-calorie malnutrition that results from a diet that is high in calories but deficient in protein. This condition is prevalent among children aged two to five in developing countries. In Africa, Central

America, South America, the Near East, and the Far East, mother's milk is the only reliable and readily available source of protein for the infant. However, when infants are weaned, they are typically given enough food to meet their caloric needs but in the form of starchy gruel that is low in protein. The main symptoms of kwashiorkor are failure to grow in weight and height, wasting of muscles, irritability, edema (the accumulation of fluid in the tissues), especially in the lower half of the body, drying and peeling of the skin resulting in the formation of ulcers, changes in the hair pigmentation that result in a characteristic reddish color, loss of appetite, vomiting and diarrhea, enlargement of the liver, and anemia. Dr. Stare, a world-famous nutritionist, points out the usual pattern is that a protein-deficient child will have mild degrees of kwashiorkor until he or she contracts some illness. At the time of illness, the protein deficiency becomes more intense, and advanced kwashiorkor is likely to develop often with fatal results.

Leaching. The downward movement of dissolved nutrients and solids through the soil to groundwater (water beneath the surface of the ground that is in a saturated zone).

Legume. The botanical family Leguminosae is referred to as a legume. Peas, beans, lentils, alfalfa, and peanuts are all legumes, and their seeds are high in protein content. The fruit of nearly all the members of the pea family are legumes. Legumes have a higher protein content than any other plant product. The protein value of legumes is not as high as animal protein because legumes are low in the essential amino acid methionine. However, legumes are rich in lysine. Many cereals are deficient in the essential amino acid lysine. A combination of legumes and cereals may have a nutritive value equal to animal protein. Legumes are a good source of B-complex vitamins (except for riboflavin). Legumes are also important in maintaining soil fertility. Most legumes have nodules on their roots that contain bacteria capable of fixing atmospheric nitrogen. Later, when the nodules disintegrate, nitrogen is returned to the soil. All plants other than legumes must use nitrogen in the soil.

Magnesium. This mineral acts as a catalyst in reactions involving the utilization of carbohydrates, fats, and proteins as sources of energy. It is necessary for the normal transmission of nerve impulses and for muscular contraction.

Malnutrition. A state of impaired health resulting from a deficit (too little), an excess (too much), or an imbalance in nutrients. Malnutrition includes undernutrition as well as overnutrition. The term *undernutrition* refers to a caloric deficit (a lack of calories) and the across-the-board deficiency of nutrients that accompanies calorie deficiency or "hunger." Overnutrition can result from excessive intakes (particularly of calories, saturated fats, and sugar). It includes conditions such as obesity, diabetes mellitus, and atherosclerosis that are directly or indirectly related to the overconsumption of these dietary factors. It also includes the excessive intake of the fat-soluble vitamins A and D.

Manganese. This trace mineral is necessary for normal skeletal development. It activates a number of enzyme systems that occur in man, although a human deficiency has never been demonstrated.

Marasmus. This disease causing wasting away and emaciation occurs when children are almost completely deprived of food. The severe calorie deficit is usually accompanied by a protein deficiency. The disease occurs most commonly in children from six to eighteen months of age in the overpopulated slums in Asia, Africa, and South America. Usually the marasmic child is weaned early and abruptly and then given inadequate amounts of very dilute milk or commercial milk formulas prepared under unsanitary conditions. Repeated infections develop, especially of the gastrointestinal tract. The mother often treats the infection by starvation therapy—feeding only water, rice water, or other nonnutritious fluids for long periods of time. Marasmus is associated with early weaning in contrast to the late weaning, often extending over two years, associated with kwashiorkor. The marasmic child has many, although not all, of the same symptoms that the child with kwashiorkor has. The symptoms of the marasmic child include failure to grow in weight and height, wasting of muscles, irritability, apathy, diarrhea, and increased susceptibility to infection. A wizened and shrunken appearance makes these children look like little, old people. Most of the infants are ravenously hungry, but a few exhibit anorexia.

Maslow's Hierarchy of Human Needs. Psychologist Abraham Maslow postulates that humankind's needs arrange themselves in a hierarchy—one need must be reasonably satisfied before the need at the next higher level emerges. Gifft, Washbon and Harrison, experts on nutrition and behavior, point out that Maslow's theoretical framework for analyzing human motivation provides useful guidance for the nutrition educator. The hierarchical pattern Maslow proposes includes five, possibly six, steps. In order of precedence they are: (1) *physiological needs* (e.g., hunger and thirst), (2) *safety needs* (e.g., security and order), (3) *love and belonging* (e.g., affection and a place in the group), (4) *esteem needs* (e.g., self-respect and recognition by others), (5) *self-actualizing needs* (e.g., self-fulfillment), (6) *desire to know and understand* (e.g., curiosity, exploration, and the desire for knowledge). Maslow suggests that the sixth need may not be experienced by everyone. Physiological needs take precedence over all other considerations because they are the survival needs. As Maslow said, "For the man who is extremely and dangerously hungry, no other interest exists but food." Maslow also said that, "He dreams food, he remembers food, he thinks about food, he emotes only about food, and he wants only food."

Matter. Anything that has mass, or has weight when subjected to gravitational forces, and occupies space is known as matter.

Meat Analogs. Foods made from various proportions of legumes, nuts, and cereals flavored to resemble beef, ham, chicken, and fish. Many of the meat analogs provide nutrients comparable to those of the animal products they are intended to replace.

Megaloblastic Anemia. A deficiency of folacin and/or vitamin B_{12} may result in megaloblastic anemia characterized by large, immature red blood cells with nuclei called megaloblasts. As with a severe deficiency, the bone marrow becomes megaloblastic—that is, the normal red blood cells in the marrow are replaced by megaloblasts. Many of these cells fail to mature and are destroyed within the marrow itself; those that do enter the bloodstream are short-lived.

Metabolism. The term refers to all the chemical and energy transformations involved in the utilization of nutrients in the body. Body metabolism has two parts: *catabolism,* which includes those reactions in which large molecules are broken down into smaller ones releasing energy; and *anabolism,* which includes constructive reactions in which small molecules are put together to form large ones thereby synthesizing new compounds that are used to build, maintain, and repair tissue. Anabolic reactions require energy.

Methemoglobin. Nitrites are derived from nitrates used as food additives and from certain vegetables that are naturally high in nitrates. When absorbed into an infant's blood, nitrites combine with hemoglobin in the red blood cell to form abnormal methemoglobin, a compound incapable of carrying oxygen. Nutritionist Helen Guthrie notes that the low acidity of the stomach of young infants is conducive to the microorganisms that facilitate the conversion of nitrates to nitrites. Since infants also lack the enzymes necessary to reform hemoglobin from methemoglobin, Guthrie believes the ingestion of nitrates in the first few months of life should be minimized. For this reason she recommends that nitrates be used in infant food only to control the growth of *Clostridium botulinium* and not as a color enhancer. For the same reason the use of vegetables such as spinach, broccoli, and beets that are high in nitrates should also be avoided early in life.

Mineralization. The process by which calcium, phosphorus, and other minerals crystallize on the protein (collagen) matrix of the bone and thus harden and strengthen the bone. Calcification is a type of mineralization. Adequate amounts of dietary calcium are needed during periods of growth to ensure the normal development of bones and during adult life to maintain normal bone structure. Actually, bone is a dynamic, metabolically active tissue with mineralization and dissolution constantly occurring. Approximately one-fourth of the calcium in the blood is exchanged with calcium in the bones.

Minerals. These nutrients have no caloric value but are important constituents of bones, teeth, soft tissue, muscle, blood, and nerve cells. They also function as body regulators in coenzymes and hormones. Minerals help maintain the body's water balance and acid-base balance and thereby keep tissue from becoming too acid or too alkaline. Minerals also help to draw chemical substances in and out of the cells of the body.

Monoculture. The growth of some single crop such as corn or wheat to the exclusion of other crops on a piece of land.

Monounsaturated Fatty Acid. A fatty acid that lacks two hydrogen atoms and has one double bond between carbons.

Oleic acid

Fats of animal origin are high in saturated fatty acids and in monounsaturated fatty acids.

Natural Restraints. Two major factors have influenced population growth. One is the availability of food, water, and other necessary resources; the other is what clergyman and economist Thomas Malthus called natural restraints. By this phrase he meant disease, famine, war, crime, and natural disasters. With overpopulation (more people than the environment can support), disease, starvation, warfare, and crime set in to limit and reduce population density to within the environment's capacity to support it.

Negative Feedback. All systems maintain themselves through feedback—that is, the unique capacity to receive output from the system back as input that helps in regulating and maintaining the system. Negative feedback is corrective feedback occurring when the input sent back to the system slows down and eventually halts or reverses a tendency or movement away from homeostasis—that is, the state or point at which the system can maintain itself. Thus negative feedback helps to preserve the stability of the system.

Net Protein Utilization (NPU). Protein quality can be measured by an index known as net protein utilization that is defined as the proportion of nitrogen intake retained. NPU is a single measurement for both the digestibility of the protein and the biological value of the amino acid mixture absorbed from the intestines. NPU can be expressed as follows:

$$NPU = \frac{N \text{ retained}}{N \text{ intake}}$$

or

$$NPU = BV \times \text{coefficient of digestibility}$$

Values for single foodstuffs and mixed tests using humans as test animals are difficult to obtain, but values for tests using rats are relatively easy to obtain. The following table gives the results of a series of NPU tests conducted by the FAO/WHO:

The Net Protein Utilization of Some Common Food, FAO/WHO, 1972

Protein	NPU Determined on Children	NPU Determined on Rats
Maize	36	51
Millet	43	44
Wheat	49	48
Soya flour	67	65
Whole egg	87	94
Human milk	94	87
Cow's milk	81	82

Most good mixed diets have an NPU value of approximately 70. As the noted nutritionist Sir Stanley Davidson points out, this figure is hardly affected by the amount of protein of animal origin in the diet. However, when 70 percent or more of the dietary proteins come from a single staple food such as maize, cassava, or wheat, Davidson underscores the fact that the NPU value of the food becomes of great importance and may determine whether or not protein requirements are met.

Niacin. This vitamin is a member of the B-complex group. It is a component of two coenzymes—nicotinamide-adenine dinucleotide (NAD) and nicotinamide-adenine dinucleotide phosphate (NADP)—that are essential for a series of reactions vital to the use of carbohydrates, fats, and proteins as sources of energy.

Niche. The role played by an organism or a population in relationship to the living and nonliving environment is known as its niche (or ecological niche). Ecologist Eugene Odum refers to a species niche as its "address."

Nitrification. The conversion of ammonia and ammonium salts to nitrates by certain groups of bacteria in the soil. The nitrates are dissolved in soil and water, taken up by roots of plants, and used to synthesize protein.

Nitrogen Balance. The relationship between the nitrogen content of all food eaten and the amount of nitrogen excreted in the urine and feces. The rationale for using the nitrogen-balance technique as a means of determining protein requirement is based on the fact that, on the average, protein contains 16 percent nitrogen, therefore, every gram of nitrogen going in or out of the body is equivalent to 6.25 grams of protein. If the nitrogen or protein in the diet is equal to the amount necessary to replace losses, *nitrogen balance* or equilibrium exists. This state is normal for adults and indicates a status quo exists between concurrently occurring processes in which tissues are constantly being broken down (catabolism) and tissues are constantly being synthesized (anabolism). If the intake is greater than the output, *positive nitrogen balance* exists, which means that new tissues are being synthesized in a normal process during growth in childhood, pregnancy, and lactation. If the intake is less than the output, the subject is said to be in *negative nitrogen balance* and a net decrease in body protein exists. This undesirable state occurs in an otherwise healthy individual when the quantity or quality of protein in the diet is inadequate for tissue replacement or when the diet does not contain adequate amounts of carbohydrates and fats, and protein is used as a source of energy.

Nitrogen Fixation. The conversion of gaseous nitrogen to nitrates by certain groups of bacteria and algae in soil, in water, and on the roots of leguminous plants. The nitrates dissolved in soil or water are taken up by the roots of plants and used to synthesize protein.

Nutrient. A chemical substance necessary for the growth of an organism. Plants get their nutrients from the soil. Animals obtain nutrients, carbohydrates, fats, proteins, vitamins, minerals, and water from the food they eat. The nutrients in food function in one or more of the following ways: as sources of energy (calories), as building materials, and as body regulators.

Nutrient Density. The concentration of nutrients in a serving of a food in relationship to its caloric value. Nutrient density is expressed by the Index of Nutritive Quality (INQ)

$$\text{INQ} = \frac{\text{\% of daily requiement (i.e., U.S. RDA) for a specific nutrient supplied by a quantity of food}}{\text{\% of total energy requirement supplied by same quantity of food}}$$

If the INQ for a nutrient is one or more, the food is making at least as great a contribution to the needs for the specific nutrient as the needs for energy. A good or excellent food source for a nutrient has an INQ of 1.5. Nutritionist Helen Guthrie noted that it has been proposed that if food has an INQ of 1 or more for four nutrients or an INQ of 2 for two nutrients, it makes a significant contribution to the nutrient content of the diet and may be identified as nutritious.

Nutrient Profile. The relative amounts of various nutrients in a given food expressed in a bar graph that provides a comparative measure for the nutritive quality.

Obesity. A major health problem in the United States and Canada, obesity is present when the body is loaded with excess fat. Often obesity is defined as weight 15 or 20 percent or more above the average weight for age, height, sex, and body frame. The relationship between moderate degrees of over-weight (weight in excess of the average) and obesity (excessive fatness) is not always clear.

Omnivores. Animals that eat a mixed diet of plant and animal food.

Osteomalacia. Adult rickets, osteomalacia, is a disease in which the bone becomes soft because of loss of calcium. This disease is prevalent among women in the Orient and parts of the Near East. Typically these afflicted women have gone through a series of repeated pregnancies and periods of lactation, have little exposure to sun, and have a low dietary intake of vitamin D. During pregnancy and lactation, the requirement for calcium is greatly increased above the usual adult need in order to satisfy the demands of the infant's developing skeleton and the mother's manufacture of milk, respectively. Adequate amounts of vitamin D are essential to stimulate the absorption of calcium and regulate the utilization of calcium.

Pantothenic Acid. This vitamin is a member of the B-complex group. It is essential in the body because it is a component of coenzyme A (CoA) that is vital to metabolic reactions involved in the release of energy from car-bohydrates, fats, and proteins. Coenzyme A is involved in the synthesis of fatty acids and cholesterol.

Pasteurization. This process involves heating a fluid at a moderate temperature for a definite period of time in order to destroy undesirable bacteria without changing to any extent the chemical composition of the fluid except for a loss of about 20 percent of the vitamin C content. In the pasteurization of milk, pathogenic bacteria (disease-producing bacteria) are destroyed by heating the milk to 140° F for twenty minutes. If higher temperatures are used, the time of exposure to heat is reduced.

Pellagra. A disease due to niacin deficiency. The skin, gastrointestinal tract, and nervous system are affected by the deficiency. The symptoms progress through dermatitis (the inflammation of the skin), diarrhea, and depression preceding death in the four D's of pellagra.

Pernicious Anemia. A megaloblastic anemia caused by the inability to absorb vitamin B_{12} due to a lack of intrinsic factor. Normally intrinsic factor is secreted by the parietal cells of the gastric mucosa. Intrinsic factor forms a complex with vitamin B_{12} to be actively transported across the intestinal membrane. To prevent pernicious anemia in people lacking intrinsic factor, vitamin B_{12} is injected directly into the blood stream on a regular basis throughout life.

Pesticide. A chemical used to kill or control weeds, insects, algae, rodents, or other pests. Pesticide is a general term that includes insecticides.

Phenylketonuria (PKU). An inborn error of metabolism in which the enzyme responsible for the breakdown of the amino acid phenylalanine is not produced in the body. In its absence, phenylalanine accumulates in the blood to toxic levels, eventually causing irreversible brain damage characterized by mental retardation. Early diagnosis is essential for successful treatment and prevention of mental retardation. A diet that is very low in phenylalanine is prescribed.

Phosphorus. This nutrient is essential for the mineralization of bones. Phosphorus compounds play a role in the storage and release of energy. As Corrinne Robinson, Professor Emeritus of Nutrition at Drexel University, explains, certain phosphate compounds trap large amounts of energy and are known as high-energy phosphate compounds. Adenosine triphosphate (ATP) is one such compound. It contains three phosphate groupings, two of which are held to the rest of the molecule by high-energy bonds. On demand ATP gives up one of its phosphate groups releasing energy that can be used by the cell for its work. The energy required to reconvert adenosine diphosphate (ADP) to ATP is supplied by the oxidation of carbohydrates, fats, or proteins. Phosphorus is a constituent of the nucleic acids deoxyribonucleic acid (DNA) and ribonucleic acid (RNA), the substances that control heredity and protein synthesis.

Photosynthesis. The process by which plants containing chlorophyll are able to synthesize carbohydrates (chemical energy) by utilizing sunlight (radiant energy) and combining carbon dioxide from the air and water from the soil.

Plasma. Unclotted blood with the cells removed.

Pollutant. Any material or set of conditions that create a stress or unfavorable alteration of an individual organism, population, community, or ecosystem beyond that found in normal environmental conditions.

Polyunsaturated Fat. A triglyceride composed of glycerol and three polyunsaturated fatty acids is known as polyunsaturated fat. Polyunsaturated fats have a low melting point and are liquid at room temperature.

Polyunsaturated Fatty Acid (PUFA). A fatty acid that lacks four or more hydrogen atoms and has two more unsaturated bonds between carbons is known as a polyunsaturated fatty acid.

```
  H  H  H  H  H        H        H  H  H  H  H  H  H
  |  |  |  |  |        |        |  |  |  |  |  |  |        O
H-C--C--C--C--C--C=C--C--C =C--C--C--C--C--C--C--C--C
  |  |  |  |  |  |  |  |  |    |  |  |  |  |  |  |  |        OH
  H  H  H  H  H  H  H  H  H    H  H  H  H  H  H  H  H
```

Linoleic acid

Vegetable fats have a relatively high content of polyunsaturated fatty acids and a lower content of salty-acid fatty acids. Corn, cottonseed, soybean, and wheat germ oil are excellent sources, and margarine and peanut oil are good sources of polyunsaturated fatty acids.

Producers. An organism, such as a photosynthetic plant, capable of converting radiant energy from the sun into chemical energy, glucose. Such an organism can synthesize its own organic substances from inorganic substances.

Protein. A protein is a large molecule made up of many smaller units called amino acids that contain carbon, hydrogen, oxygen, and nitrogen, and sometimes other elements. Adequate dietary protein is required to supply the essential amino acids that cannot be manufactured in the body in sufficient amounts and to supply the nitrogen needed by the body for the synthesis of nonessential amino acids. All the different kinds of amino acids, essential and nonessential, in a particular protein must be available simultaneously and in the correct amounts for protein synthesis, the process by which proteins are built up from amino acids, to take place. Protein synthesis is necessary for making and repairing body tissue. Approximately 15 to 20 percent of the human body is protein, and that protein exists in many forms. Protein is present in every cell and is an essential component of enzymes, such as the digestive enzymes and hormones, including insulin and thyroxine.

Protein-Calorie Malnutrition (PCM). The broad spectrum of protein-calorie malnutrition varies from a diet that is relatively high in calories and deficient in protein (as seen in the condition known as kwashiorkor) to one that is low in both calories and protein (as seen in the condition known as marasmus). Those most apt to show severe symptoms of protein-calorie malnutrition are young children in the years immediately following weaning. Their symptoms include stunted growth, mental retardation, and lack of muscle development. They also have a lowered resistance to infection and recover from illness more slowly and with greater difficulty than adequately nourished children.

Protein-Efficiency Ration (PER). This method of evaluating the quality or nutritive value of a protein is determined by calculating the weight gain of a growing animal per gram of protein consumed.

$$PER = \frac{\text{weight gain (grams)}}{\text{protein intake (grams)}}$$

PER is based on the assumption, which may be questioned, that the extent of growth is an indicator of how well the protein meets requirements for essential amino acids. In modern PER experiments the following standard procedures have been established in studying rats: The intake of calories and other nutrients must be adequate, the intake of protein must be 10 percent by weight of the diet, and the study must be carried out for at least twenty-eight days. The PER of the protein studied is compared to the PER of casein, the major protein in milk. The PER of casein is 2.5. High-quality proteins have a PER equal to or better than casein. Currently, in nutritional labeling in the United States, proteins are divided into three quality classes based on the PER of 2.5—that of casein. The U.S. RDA for high-quality proteins (those that have a PER equal to or better than casein) is set at 45 grams. For those proteins with a PER between casein and 20 percent of casein, the U.S. RDA is set at 65 grams. The FDA in 1973 stated that very poor quality protein with a PER less than 20 percent of casein "shall not be stated on the label" and are designated "not a significant source of protein."

Protein Quality. Protein-yielding foods differ in their amino acid composition. The term *protein quality* refers to whether or not the protein supplies all the eight or nine essential amino acids in the relative amounts and proportions needed by the body for protein synthesis.

Pulse. The edible seeds of the pea (Leguminosae) family including peas, beans, and lentils are known as pulses. According to Sir Stanley Davidson, noted physician and nutritionist, the English word *pulse* is taken from the Latin *puls*, meaning pottage or thick pup.

Pyridoxine. This vitamin is a member of the B-complex group and is sometimes referred to as vitamin B_6. Pyridoxal phosphate and pyridoxine phosphate are the active coenzyme forms of vitamin B_6. These coenzymes are necessary for normal carbohydrate and protein metabolism. The coenzyme pyridoxal phosphate is essential for transamination, the transferring of an amino group of an amino acid to certain compounds to manufacture new nonessential amino acids in the body.

Recommended Dietary Allowances (RDA). The Food and Nutrition Board of the National Research Council sets recommended daily intakes for certain nutrients known as the Recommended Dietary Allowances. They are meant to be standards to serve as a goal for good nutrition for practically all healthy individuals in the United States. Except for calories, the allowances are designated to afford a safety margin that exceeds the requirements of most individuals and thereby ensures that the needs of nearly all healthy people in the population are met.

Riboflavin. A member of the B-complex group, riboflavin is a component of two coenzymes: flavin mononucleotide (FMN) and flavin adenine dinucleotide (FAD). These coenzymes are attached to enzymes known as flavoprotein. The flavoprotein enzymes are necessary for normal cellular respiration. They act closely with other enzymes containing niacin and thiamine in a number of reactions that are essential for the release of energy from glucose and fatty acids derived from the breakdown of carbohydrates, fats, and proteins.

Rickets. In the absence of adequate vitamin D, infants and children develop rickets, a disease characterized by poor mineralization of bones resulting in weak, soft bones rather than strong, rigid ones. Rickets is a major public health problem in developing areas of the world where there is little sunlight or cultural factors prohibit the exposure of babies to sunlight until they are a year old and little or no vitamin D or calcium is provided in the diet. The disease has virtually been eradicated in most developed countries primarily as a result of the fortification of milk with vitamin D and because pediatricians routinely prescribe cod liver oil for infants.

Saturated Fat. A triglyceride composed of glycerol and three saturated fatty acids. Saturated fats such as butter or lard have a high melting point and are solid at room temperature. A diet high in saturated fats tends to significantly raise serum cholesterol levels.

Saturated Fatty Acid. A fatty acid carrying the maximum number of hydrogen atoms is referred to as a saturated fatty acid.

$$H-\overset{\displaystyle H}{\underset{\displaystyle H}{C}}-\overset{\displaystyle H}{\underset{\displaystyle H}{C}}-\overset{\displaystyle H}{\underset{\displaystyle H}{C}}-\overset{\displaystyle H}{\underset{\displaystyle H}{C}}-\overset{\displaystyle H}{\underset{\displaystyle H}{C}}-\overset{\displaystyle H}{\underset{\displaystyle H}{C}}-\overset{\displaystyle H}{\underset{\displaystyle H}{C}}-\overset{\displaystyle H}{\underset{\displaystyle H}{C}}-\overset{\displaystyle H}{\underset{\displaystyle H}{C}}-\overset{\displaystyle H}{\underset{\displaystyle H}{C}}-\overset{\displaystyle H}{\underset{\displaystyle H}{C}}-\overset{\displaystyle H}{\underset{\displaystyle H}{C}}-\overset{\displaystyle H}{\underset{\displaystyle H}{C}}-\overset{\displaystyle H}{\underset{\displaystyle H}{C}}-\overset{\displaystyle H}{\underset{\displaystyle H}{C}}-\overset{\displaystyle H}{\underset{\displaystyle H}{C}}-\overset{\displaystyle H}{\underset{\displaystyle H}{C}}-\underset{\displaystyle OH}{\overset{\displaystyle O}{C}}$$

Stearic acid

Most of the fats of animal origin are relatively high in saturated fatty acids.

Schistosomiasis. Disease caused by a parasite worm, a fluke, that is transmitted by snails. It afflicts humans who wade or bathe in water contaminated by the fluke in its free-swimming stage or are bitten by snails. When the parasite enters the body, the victim develops a wasting anemia-type disease because the parasite feeds on the blood cells and destroys them. Life expectancy after infection is about two to three years unless the patient is treated. The disease is widespread throughout Asia, Africa, and tropical America.

Scurvy. Disease caused by a severe lack of ascorbic acid (vitamin C). Early symptoms include listlessness, fatigue, muscle cramps, aching of the bones, joints, and muscles and hemorrhaging of the eyes and gums. Later, as full-blown scurvy develops, degeneration of many tissues, particularly skin, teeth, gums, blood vessel walls, bone cartilage, and muscle tissue is present. Subacute or latent scurvy occurs among infants fed a diet that almost exclusively consists of heat-treated milk and/or cereal gruels, when sources of vitamin C are not given. The children develop the following symptoms characteristic of latent scurvy: failure to grow properly, weakness, irritability, swollen joints, and tenderness of the lower extremities.

Selenium. This micromineral works with vitamin E as an antioxidant, a substance that inhibits the oxidation of other compounds. Both vitamin E and selenium protect the fat-soluble vitamins and polyunsaturated fatty acids from oxidation. Selenium may reduce the requirement for vitamin E.

Serum. The watery portion of the blood that remains after the cells and clot-forming material have been removed is known as serum.

Serum Lipid Levels. Elevation in the level of cholesterol and/or triglycerides are factors known to increase the risk of developing atherosclerosis and coronary heart disease. Normal serum cholesterol levels range from 180–240 milligrams/100 milliliters. Normal serum triglyceride levels range from 50 to 150 milligrams/100 milliliters.

Sodium. This nutrient helps maintain normal fluid balance in cells.

Stabilizer. A substance put into a food to keep the texture of the product smooth and stable is known as a stabilizer. Stabilizers are classified as intentional food additives.

Starvation. The level of caloric deprivation that, if permitted to continue without suitable amounts of food, will eventually lead to death. Loss of weight and wasting of vital tissue occur in the effort to meet the energy requirements needed for survival.

Sulfur. The mineral sulfur is found in every cell of the body. Sulfur-containing amino acids are methionine, cystine, and cysteine. Sulfur is a component of thiamine and biotin. Recent evidence indicates that sulfur is necessary for the synthesis of collagen, the protein that is found in skin, tendons, bones, and cartilage.

System. A collection of interdependent parts called components, elements, or subsystems that can be seen as a single whole. No part of the system can be affected without other parts being less, equally, or more affected.

Thermodynamics. The type of physics mainly concerned with the transformations of heat into mechanical work and the opposite transformations of mechanical work into heat. *The First Law of Thermodynamics* is the principle of the conservation of energy and states that energy is neither created nor destroyed during physical and chemical processes but can be transformed from one form to another form such as heat, light, and electrical, mechanical, and chemical energy. *The Second Law of Thermodynamics* (the law of entropy) states that each time energy is transferred in physical or chemical processes, it tends to go from a more organized and concentrated form to a less organized and more dispersed form. Thus as energy is transferred from one usable form to another, some energy is always wasted or lost to the system.

Thiamine. A member of the B-complex group, thiamine, is a component of the coenzyme thiamine pyrophosphate (TPP), which is required for the utilization of carbohydrates. Glucose is broken down (oxidized) in the body's cells to supply energy. The oxidization of glucose occurs through a series of reactions. TPP (also known as cocarboxylase) is involved in a number of these reactions, those that involve the removal of carbon dioxide from carbohydrate derivatives formed in the breakdown of glucose.

Toxicity. The quantity of a substance that makes it poisonous is referred to as its level of toxicity.

Toxicity Test. The Food Additives Amendment of 1958 places additives into two groups: (1) regulated food additives that are toxic at some levels, and (2) GRAS-list chemicals and ingredients that are not toxic under normal use. The regulated food additives are limited in the amount that can be used in foods because they are toxic to humans if too high a level is consumed. Before a food company can introduce a chemical into the food supply the FDA requires that the chemical be tested for safety. Among other tests, three kinds of toxicity tests are generally required: acute, subacute, and chronic. Theodore P. Labuzza, professor of Food Science at the University of Minnesota, describes these tests as: (1) The *acute toxicity test* is the initial toxicity test—a procedure for determining the lethal dose of the chemical for 50 percent of the experimental animals; (2) The *chronic toxicity test* is a three-year test procedure for determining the long-range and cancer-causing effects of a chemical; (3) The *subacute toxicity test* is done after the chronic toxicity test is completed. This test is a method of determining whether or not there are biologically adverse effects derived from using a specific amount of a chemical. Based on these toxicity tests and other tests, the FDA determines if the chemical or additive can be used in food and specifies the amount that may be used in foods.

Trophic Level. The link in the food chain to which an organism belongs. An organism's trophic level is determined by the number of steps from the primary production of food energy. Thus, producers transfer food energy to consumers, herbivores, and carnivores, which exist at different trophic levels.

U.S. Recommended Daily Allowance (U.S. RDA). The Food and Drug Administration's (FDA's) standards for daily quantities of specified vitamins, minerals, and proteins that are used for nutritional labels are known as the U.S. RDA. The values are derived from the 1968 Recommended Dietary Allowances developed by the Food and Nutrition Board of the National Research Council. They usually represent the highest recommended levels of intake for any age group (except for pregnant and lactating women) proposed in the 1968 Recommended Dietary Allowances. Nutrient information on nutritional labels is expressed as a percentage of the U.S. RDA.

Vanadium. There is some evidence that this trace mineral may inhibit the formation of cholesterol.

Vegetarian Diets. This eating pattern excludes meat, poultry, and fish. Although vegetarian diets differ in the kinds of food they contain, they usually include vegetables, fruits, whole grain and enriched breads and cereals, dry beans and peas, lentils, nuts, peanut butter, and seeds. A *lacto ovo vegetarian diet*, the most popular type, includes eggs and dairy products as a supplement to vegetable foods. The *lacto vegetarian diet* includes only dairy products and not eggs as a supplement to plant foods. *Vegans, strict* or *total vegetarians,* avoid all foods of animal origin including eggs and dairy products.

Vertical Integration. The movement of agricultural input and output firms into the production stage of the food system. According to Richard Merrill, an expert on agribusiness, this movement may be direct or indirect. Direct movement occurs when a processing plant buys or leases land to produce commodities for its operation. Indirect movement occurs when an agribusiness firm contracts with a farmer to produce a certain quantity and quality of a certain commodity at a certain time and for a certain price. In both cases Merrill emphasizes a degree of control over production passes from the farmer to the agribusiness corporation.

Vitamins. These nutrients have no caloric value but are important body regulators. Vitamins are constituents of enzymes that function to initiate or speed up metabolic reactions. They may be classified as either fat- or water-soluble.

Vitamin A. This fat-soluble vitamin is essential for the formation of cells (particularly in the skin) and for normal vision. It also aids in maintaining resistance to infections.

Vitamin B_{12} (Cobalamin). This water-soluble vitamin is a member of the B-complex group. Although vitamin B_{12} is necessary for the adequate functioning of all the cells of the body, it is particularly essential for those of the nervous system, gastrointestinal tract, and bone marrow. The B_{12}-coenzymes catalyze reactions necessary for the release of energy from carbohydrates, fats, and proteins and are essential for the formation of nucleic acids in DNA. A deficiency of vitamin B_{12} results in megaloblastic anemia. Intrinsic factor, a constituent of gastric juice, forms with vitamin B_{12} allowing vitamin B_{12} to be actively transported across the intestinal membrane. A deficiency of vitamin B_{12} due to the absence of intrinsic factor results in a condition known as pernicious anemia. The symptoms of pernicious anemia include fatigue, weakness, megaloblastic anemia, smoothness of the tongue, sore cracked lips, degeneration of the nervous system, and a decrease in the amount of hydrochloric acid in the stomach. To treat this condition, vitamin B_{12} is injected directly into the blood stream on a regular basis throughout life.

Vitamin D. This fat-soluble vitamin promotes the absorption of calcium from small intestines and is necessary for the normal mineralization of bones.

Vitamin E. This fat-soluble vitamin functions as an antioxidant in the body. In other words, it opposes chemical processes by which substances combine with oxygen (oxidized). When substances such as vitamins A and C and polyunsaturated fatty acids are oxidized, they cannot react in the unique ways that are essential to the body. For example, vitamin E prevents the oxidation of vitamin A and polyunsaturated fatty acids in the red cell membrane thus preventing the rupture (hemolysis) of the erythrocytes.

Vitamin K. This fat-soluble vitamin is often called the antihemorrhagic vitamin because it promotes blood clotting (the process of blood coagulation).

Water. Approximately 55 to 60 percent of the body weight of an adult man and 45 to 50 percent of an adult woman is water. Water is used as a building material in every cell. Cells and tissues differ in their water content. Some specific functions of water include acting as a solvent in facilitating digestion. Water helps to regulate body temperature. Heat is eliminated by means of evaporation of water from the lungs and surface of the skin. In addition, water is essential for the transport of nutrients to the cells and waste from the cells as part of the circulatory system.

Zero Population Growth (ZPG). When the birth rate equals the death rate, the population no longer grows. Zero population growth is achieved. ZPG is the name of an organization dedicated to achieving this goal.

Zinc. This mineral is a component of insulin, the hormone that regulates carbohydrate metabolism. Zinc is also a constituent of a protein-splitting enzyme (cocarboxypeptidase) of pancreatic juice and thus plays a role in the digestion of proteins. The enzyme carbonic anhydrase of red blood cells contains zinc. Carbonic anhydrase facilitates the transport of carbon dioxide within the body and its elimination from the body. In addition to a number of other important roles zinc aids in wound healing. Recent evidence indicates that zinc concentrates in wound tissues and plays a role in incorporating the amino acid glycine into the protein of the skin and the amino acids glycine and proline in skin collagen.

Bibliography

Part I

Baker, J.J., and Allen, G.E. *Matter, Energy, and Life.* Reading, Mass.: Addison-Wesley, 1970.

Burton, Benjamin T. *Human Nutrition.* 3d ed. New York: McGraw-Hill, 1976.

Calloway, Doris H. "Recommended Dietary Allowances for Protein and Energy, 1973." *Journal of the American Dietetic Association* 64 (1974):157–62.

Campbell, J.A. "Canadian, U.S., and International Standards Compared— Approaches in Revising Dietary Standards." *Journal of the American Dietetic Association* 64 (1974):175–78.

Deevey, E.S. "Mineral Cycles." *Scientific American* 223 (1970):148–59.

Delwiche, C.D. "The Nitrogen Cycle." *Scientific American* 223 (1970):136–47.

Dubos, Rene. "The Crisis of Man in His Environment." *Ekistics* 27 (1969):151–54.

Food and Agricultural Organization. *Calorie Requirements, FAO Nutrition Study.* No. 15. Rome, Italy: Food and Agriculture Organization, 1957.

——. *Protein Requirements.* Report of a Joint PAO/WHO Expert Group. Rome, Italy: Food and Agriculture Organization, 1965.

Food and Nutrition Board. *Recommended Dietary Allowances.* 9th ed. Washington, D.C.: National Academy of Sciences–National Research Council, 1980.

Greenwood, Ned, and Edwards, J.M.B. "The Ecological Basis." In *Human Environments and Natural Systems,* pp. 40–68. No. Scituate, Mass.: Duxbury Press, 1973.

Hardin, Garrett. "The Tragedy of the Commons." *Science* 164 (1968):1243–48.

Harper, A.E. "Recommended Dietary Allowances: Are They What We Think They Are?" *Journal of the American Dietetic Association* 64 (1974):151–56.

Hertzler, Ann A., and Anderson, Helen L. "Food Guides in the United States." *Journal of the American Dietetic Association* 64 (1974):19–28.

Jacobson, Michael F., and Wilson, Wendy. *Food Scorecard.* Washington, D.C.: Center for Science in the Public Interest, 1974.

Klippstein, Ruth and Washbon, Majorie. *Food Makes a Difference.* Cornell Miscellaneous Bulletin 92. Ithaca, N.Y.: An Extension Publication of New York State College of Home Economics, Cornell University, July 1968.

Kormondy, Edward J. *Concepts in Ecology.* Englewood Cliffs, N.J.: Prentice-Hall, 1969.

Lamb, Mina W., and Harden, Margarette L. *The Meaning of Human Nutrition.* Elmsford, N.Y.: Pergamon Bio-Medical Science Series, 1973.

Levine, Norman D. "The Physico-Chemical Habitat." In *Human Ecology* by Norman D. Levine et al., pp. 8–38. No. Scituate, Mass.: Duxbury Press, 1975.

Livingston, Sally K. "What Influences Malnutrition?" *Journal of Nutrition Education* 3 (1971):16–26.

Martin, Ethel A. *Nutrition in Action.* 3d ed. New York: Holt, Rinehart and Winston, 1971.

McGill, Marion, and Pye, Orrea. *The No-Nonsense Guide to Food and Nutrition.* New York: Butterick, 1978.

Odum, Eugene P. "The Strategy of Ecosystem Development." *Science* 164 (1970):262–70.

——. *Fundamentals of Ecology.* 3d ed. Philadelphia: Saunders, 1971.

Penman, H.L. "The Water Cycle." *Scientific American* 223 (1970):98–109.

Russwurm, Lorne H. "A Systems Approach to the Natural Environment." In *Man's Natural Environment: A Systems Approach* edited by Lorne H. Russman and Edward Sommerville, pp. 1–16. No. Scituate, Mass.: Duxbury Press, 1974.

Sears, Paul B. "Ecology, The Intricate Web of Life." In *As We Live and Breathe: The Challenge of Our Environment.* Washington, D.C.: National Geographic Society, 1971.

Stare, Fredrick J., and McWilliams, Margaret. "Nutrition from the Physiological Viewpoint." In *Living Nutrition,* pp. 244-403. New York: Wiley, 1973.

Sutton, David B., and Harmon, Paul N. *Ecology: Selected Concepts.* New York: Wiley, 1973.

Woodwell, George M. "Toxic Substances and Ecological Cycles," March 1967. In *Food* readings from *Scientific American.* San Francisco: Freeman, 1973, pp. 72–79.

Part II

Asimov, Isaac. *Earth Our Crowded Spaceship.* Greenwich, Conn.: Fawcett, 1974.

Bengoa, J.M. "Hunger and Malnutrition in the World Today." *World Health Magazine* (1974):4.

Bird, David. "A Hungry World Struggles for More Food." *New York Times,* January 26, 1975, pp. 85–86.

Borgstrom, Georg. *The Hungry Planet.* New York: Collier Books, 1967.

Brown, Lester R. *In the Interest: A Strategy to Stabilize World Population.* New York: Norton, 1974.

——, and Eckholm, Erik P. *By Bread Alone.* New York: Praeger, 1974.

Brown, R.E. "Some Nutritional Considerations in Times of Major Catastrophe." *Clinical Pediatrics* 11 (1972):334.

——. "Breast Feeding in Modern Times." *The American Journal of Clinical Nutrition* 26 (1973):556–62.

Cravioto, J. "Complexity of Factors Involved in Protein-Calorie Malnutrition." *Bibliograph of Nutrition and Dietetics* 14 (1970):7–22.

Davis, Kingsley. "Zero Population Growth: The Analysis and Meaning." *Daedalus* 104 (1973):15–30.

Economic Research Service, U.S. Department of Agriculture. "The World Situation and Prospects to 1985." Foreign Agricultural Economic Report No. 98, Washington, D.C., 1974.

Ehrlich, Paul R. *The Population Bomb.* rev. ed. New York: Ballantine, 1971.

——, and Ehrlich, Anne H. *Population, Resources, and Environment.* 2d ed. San Francisco: Freeman, 1972.

——, and Holdren, John P. "Impact of Population Growth." *Science* 171(1971):1212–17.

Frejka, Tomas. "The Prospects for a Stationary World Population." *Scientific American* 228 (1973):15–23.

Gause, G.F. *The Struggle for Existence.* New York: Hafner, 1969.

Gebre-Medhin, Mehari, and Vahlquist, Bo. "Famine in Ethiopia—The Period 1973–1975." *Nutrition Reviews* 35 (1977):194–201.

Gillie, Bruce R. "Endemic Goiter," June 1971. In Food Readings from *Scientific American*, San Francisco: Freeman, 1973, pp. 63–71.

Harrar, J.G. "Nutrition and Numbers in the Third World." *Nutrition Reviews,* 32 (1974):97–104.

Jacobson, Michael. "Our Diets Have Changed, but Not for the Best." *Smithsonian* (1975):96–102.

Jelliffe, D.B. "Commerciogenic Malnutrition? Time for a Dialogue." *Food Technology* 25 (1971):55.

——**, and Jelliffe, E.F.P.,** guest eds. "The Uniqueness of Human Milk." *American Journal of Clinical Nutrition* 24 (1971):968–1024.

Keys, A. et al. *The Biology of Human Starvation,* vols. I and II. Minneapolis: University of Minnesota Press, 1950.

Malthus, T.R. *Population: The First Essay.* Ann Arbor, Mich.: University Press, 1959.

Nutrition Canada Summary Report. Information Canada, 171 Slater Street, Ottawa K.I.A. 059.

Peccei, Aurelio. "Controlling the Population." *Development Forum.* (September–October 1974):4.

Poleman, Thomas T. "World Food: A Perspective." In *Food: Politics, Economics, Nutrition and Research,* pp. 8–16. Washington, D.C.: American Association for the Advancement of Science, 1975.

Population Bulletin. Published six times yearly by the Population Reference Bureau, Inc., 1755 Massachusetts Ave., N.W., Washington, D.C. 20036.

Population Information Program. Department of Medical and Public Affairs, The George Washington University Center. "The 29th Day," *Population Reports,* series E, No. 5, Washington, D.C. (January 1978).

Population Reference Bureau. Washington, D.C., *Population Data Sheet,* published annually.

Preliminary Findings of the First Health and Nutrition Examination Survey. "United States, 1971–1972: Dietary Intake and Biochemical Findings." National Center for Health Statistics, U.S. DHEW/PHS Publication No. (HRA) 74–1219–1, January 1974.

"The Prevention of Xerophthalmia." *WHO Chronicle* 28 (1974):220–28.

Salomon, Joao B.; Boianovsky, David L.; and Pereira, Mauricio G. "The Epidemiological Triad." In Proceedings Western Hemisphere Nutrition Conference III (1971):248–52.

Ten State Nutrition Survey, 1968–1970. Center for Disease Control, HSMHA. DHEW Publications No. (HSM) 72–8130 through 72–8134.

Trowell, Hugh C. "Kwashiorkor," December 1974. In *Food* readings from *Scientific American.* San Francisco: Freeman, 1973, pp. 52–56.

United Nations, Department of Economics and Social Affairs. "Methods of Appraisal of Quality of Basic Data for Population Estimates," Population Studies No. 23. New York: United Nations, 1955.

U.S. Committee for UNICEF. "Teaching about World Hunger." U.S. Committee for UNICEF, 331 East 38th St., New York, N.Y. 10016.

Winick, M., and Rossee, P. "The Effects of Severe Early Malnutrition on Cellular Growth and the Human Brain." *Pediatric Research* 3 (1969):181.

Young, Vernon R., and Scrimshaw, Nevin S. "The Physiology of Starvation," October 1971. In *Food* readings from *Scientific American.* San Francisco: Freeman, 1973. pp. 44–51.

Zero Population Growth. "Benefits of Zero Population Growth." Zero Population Growth, Inc., 1348 Connecticut Ave., N.W., Washington, D.C. 20036.

Part III

Baker, George L. "The Invisible Workers: Labor Organization on American Farms." In *Radical Agriculture,* edited by Richard Merrill, pp. 143–67. New York: Harper & Row, 1976.

Bender, R.J. "Why Water Desalting Will Expand." *Power* 113 (1971):171.

Billard, Jules B., ed. "The Revolution in American Agriculture." *National Geographic* (February 1970):117.

Bloom, Gordon F., and Curhan, Ronald C. "Technological Change in the Food Industry." *Technology Review* (December 1974):20–29.

Borlaug, Norman E. "The Green Revolution: For Bread and Peace." *Science and Public Affairs* (June 1971):6–9, 42–48.

Brown, Lester R. "Human Food Production as a Process in the Biosphere," September 1970. In *Food* readings from *Scientific American.* San Francisco: Freeman, 1973, pp. 205–14.

——, **and Finsterbusch, G.W.** *Man and His Environment: Food.* New York: Harper & Row, 1972.

Chapman, Duane. "An End to Chemical Farming?" *Environment* 15 (1973): 12–17.

Ehrlich, Paul R.; Ehrlich, Ann H.; and Holdren, John P. "Food and Fuel." *Scientific American* 230 (1974):48.

——. *Human Ecology.* San Francisco: Freeman, 1973.

Enloe, Cortez F. "A Tale of Two Farms." *Nutrition Today* 10 (1975):42–50.

Food and Agricultural Organization. *Things to Come: The World Food Crisis—The Way Out.* Rome, Italy: Food and Agricultural Organization, 1974.

Hall, Ross H. "A Concept of Fertility." "Global Greening." and "Agribusiness." In *Food for Nought,* pp. 129–42, 143–62, 163–71. San Francisco: Harper & Row, 1974.

Harlan, Jack R. "Our Vanishing Genetic Resources." In *Food: Politics, Economics, Nutrition, and Research,* edited by Philip H. Abelson, pp. 157–60. Washington, D.C.: American Association for the Advancement of Science, 1975.

Heady, Earl O. "The Agriculture of the U.S." *Scientific American* 235 (1976):106–28.

Hightower, Jim. *Eat Your Heart Out.* New York: Crown, 1975.

——. "Hard Tomatoes, Hard Times: The Failure of the Land Grant College Complex." Schnenkman Publishing Company, Inc. and the Land Grant

College Task Force, part of the Agribusiness Accountability Project, an
independent nonprofit research organization, 1000 Washington Avenue,
Washington, D.C., 1972.

Holt, S.J. "The Food Resources of the Ocean," September 1969. In *Food* readings
from *Scientific American*. San Francisco: Freeman, 1973, pp. 139–51.

Jennings, Peter R. "The Amplification of Agricultural Production." *Scientific
American* 235 (1976):180–94.

Kotz, Nick. "Agribusiness." In *Radical Agriculture*, edited by Richard Merrill,
pp. 41–51. New York: Harper & Row, 1976.

LaBuza, Theodore P. *Food and Your Well Being*. St. Paul, Minn.: West, 1977.

Loomis, Robert S. "Agricultural Systems." *Scientific American* 235 (1976):
98–105.

McLeod, Daryl. "Urban-Rural Food Alliances, a Perspective on Recent
Community Food Organizing." In *Radical Agriculture*, edited by Richard
Merrill, pp. 188–223. New York: Harper & Row, 1976.

Mellor, John W. "The Agriculture of India." *Scientific American* 235 (1976):
154–63.

Miller, Robert R., ed. *Agricultural Outlook*. Washington, D.C.: Superintendent of
Documents, Government Printing Office January–February, 1978/AO–29.

The National Dairy Council. "The Role of Processing in Extending the Food
Supply." *Diary Council Digest* 48 (1977):19–23.

Nickerson, J.T.R., and Ronsivivalli, L.J. *Elementary Food Science*. Westport,
Conn.: Avi, 1976.

Olson, Christine M., and Bisogni, Carole A. "The Impact of Technology," *Forum*
(Fall/Winter 1977):10–13.

Paddock, William. "How Green Is the Green Revolution?" *Bio-Science* 20
(1970):890–902.

Perelman, Michael. "The Green Revolution: American Agriculture in the Third
World." In *Radical Agriculture*, edited by Richard Merrill, pp. 111–26. New
York: Harper & Row, 1976.

Pyke, Magnus. "The Evolution of Technology." "Freezing, Drying, Canning,
and Irradiation." In *Man and Food*, pp. 168–85, 186–207. New York: World
University Library, 1972.

———. *Food and Society*. London: John Murray, 1968.

Rappaport, Roy A. "The Flow of Energy in an Agricultural Society." *Scientific
American* 224 (1971):116–33.

Revelle, Rodger. "The Resources Available for Agriculture." *Scientific American*
235 (1976):164–78.

Richard, William R., and Stubbs, Thomas. *Plants Agriculture and Human Society*.
Menlo Park, Calif.: Benjamin, 1978.

Robin, Meyers. "The National Share Croppers Fund and the Farm Co-op
Movement in the South." In *Radical Agriculture*, edited by Richard Merrill,
pp. 129–42. New York: Harper & Row, 1976.

Schmitt, W.R. "The Planetary Food Potential." Ann. N.Y.: Academy of Sciences.
118 (1965):645.

Scrimshaw, Nevin S. "Food," September 1963. In *Food* readings from *Scientific
American*. San Francisco: Freeman, 1973, pp. 197–204.

Steinhart, John S., and Steinhart, Carol E. "Energy Use in the U.S. Food System." *Science* 184 (1974):307–16.

U.S. Department of Agriculture. *From the Earth to Your Table.* Washington, D.C.: Office of Communication, U.S. Department of Agriculture, 1977.

Wade, Nicholas. "World Food Situation: Pessimism Comes Back into Vogue." *Science* 181 (1973):634–38.

Walsh, John. "U.S. Agribusiness and Agricultural Trends." In *Food: Politics, Economics, Nutrition, and Research,* edited by Philip H. Abelson, pp. 29–42. Washington, D.C.: American Association for the Advancement of Science, 1975.

Wellhausen, Edwin J. "The Agriculture of Mexico." *Scientific American* 235 (1976):128–50.

Whitter, S.H. "Food Production: Technology and the Resource Base." In *Food: Politics, Economics, Nutrition, and Research,* edited by Philip H. Abelson, pp. 85–90. Washington, D.C.: American Association for the Advancement of Science, 1975.

Wortman, Sterling, and Cummings, Jr., Ralph W. *To Feed This World.* Baltimore: Johns Hopkins, 1978.

Part IV

"Adapting Ethnic Foods to Nutrition Need." *Forecast for Home Economics.* (May/June, 1971), F86–87.

Austin, James E. "Can Nutrition Sell?" *The Professional Nutritionist* 33 (1976):12–15.

Benarde, Melvin A. *The Chemicals We Eat.* New York: McGraw-Hill, 1971.

"Complexities of Food Standards." *The Professional Nutritionist* (Summer 1976):8–11.

Consolidated Edison Company of New York. *How to Use Electricity and Gas Wisely and Safely and Save Money, Too.* January 1976.

Darby, William J., and Hambraeus, Leif. "Proposed Nutritional Guidelines for Utilization of Industrially Produced Nutrients." *Nutrition Reviews* 36 (1978):65–71.

Fleck, Henrietta. "Buying Food for Good Nutrition." In *Introduction to Nutrition.* 3d ed., pp. 430–53. New York: Macmillan, 1976.

Gifft, Helen H.; Washbon, Majorie B.; and Harrison, Gail G. *Nutrition, Behavior, and Change.* Englewood Cliffs, N.J.: Prentice-Hall, 1972.

Hall, Ross H. *Food for Nought.* San Francisco: Harper & Row, 1974.

Jacobson, Michael F. *Eater's Digest.* Garden City, N.Y.: Doubleday, 1972.

Johnson, Paul E. "Misuse in Foods of Useful Chemicals." *Nutrition Reviews* 35 (1977):225–29.

Jukes, Thomas H. "Fact and Fancy in Nutrition and Food Science." *Journal of the American Dietetic Association* 59 (1971):203–11.

Kottak, Conrad P. "Ritual at McDonald's." *Natural History* 87 (1978):74–82.

LaBuza, Theodore P. *Food and Your Well-Being.* St. Paul, Minn.: West, 1977.

LaChance, Paul A. "A Commentary on the New FDA Nutrition Labeling

Regulations." *Nutrition Today* (January–February 1973):16–23.

Lerza, Catherine, and Jacobson, Michael. eds. *Food for People, Not for Profit.* New York: Ballantine, 1975.

Lowenberg, Miriam, et al. *Food and Man.* 2d ed. New York: Wiley, 1974.

Malik, R.K. "Food Quality and Control." *Food and Nutrition* 2 (1976):12–15.

Martin, Ethel A. "Puerto Rican Diets." "Mexican Diets." "Negro Diets." American Indian Diets." In *Nutrition in Action.* 3d ed., pp. 356–60, 361–64, 365–67, 368–75. New York: Holt, Rinehart and Winston, 1971.

National Dairy Council. "Food Labeling." *Dairy Council Digest* 45 (1974).

National Nutrition Consortium, Inc. with Ronald M. Deutsh. "Nutritional Labeling—How Can It Work for You." Bethesda, Md.: The National Nutrition Consortium, Inc., 1975.

National Research Council, National Academy of Sciences. *World Food and Nutrition Study—The Potential Contributions of Research.* Washington, D.C.: National Academy of Sciences, 1977.

Naylor, John; Ganzin, M.; and Kapsiotis, G. "Food Resources of the Sea: Some Economic Problems Relating to Their Utilization." *Food and Nutrition* 3 (1977):12–15.

Richmond, Fredrick W. "The Role of the Federal Government in Nutrition Education." *Journal of Nutrition Education* 9 (1977):150–51.

Schafer, Robert B. "Factors Affecting Food Behavior and the Quality of Husbands' and Wives' Diets." *Journal of the American Dietetic Association* 72 (1978):138–43.

Scrimshaw, Nevin S. "Through a Glass Darkly: Discerning the Practical Implications of Human Protein—Energy Interrelationships." *Nutrition Reviews* 35 (1977):321–37.

Sebrell, William, and Haggerty, James J. *Food and Nutrition.* New York: Time, 1967.

U.S. Department of Agriculture. *Food for Thrifty Families.* C.F.E. (Adm) 326, Hyattsville, Md.: Consumer and Economics Institute, Agricultural Research Service, USDA, September 1976.

Part V

Berg, Alan. *The Nutrition Factor.* Washington, D.C.: Brookings, 1973.

Boerma, Addeke H. "A World Agricultural Plan," August 1970. In *Food* readings from *Scientific American.* San Francisco: Freeman, 1973, pp. 215–28.

Borgstrom, Georg. "Food Shortage—An Education Challenge." *Nutrition News* 37 (1974):9 and 12.

Brown, P.T. and Bergen, J.G. "The Dietary Status of New Vegetarians." *Journal of the American Dietetic Association* 67 (1975):455–59.

Bruch, Hilde. "The Allure of Food Cults and Nutritional Quackery." *Journal of the American Dietetic Association* 57 (1970):316–20.

Center for Science in the Public Interest. *99 Ways to a Simple Life.* Garden City, N.Y.: Anchor Books, 1977.

Chopra, Joginder G.; Forbes, Alan L.; and Habicht, Jean-Pierre. "Protein in the U.S. Diet." *Journal of the American Dietetic Association* 72 (1978):253–58.

Darby, William J. "Nutrition, Food Needs, and Technologic Priorities: The World Food Conference." *Nutrition Reviews* 33 (1975):225–34.

Dwyer, Johanna T., et al. "The 'New' Vegetarian." *Journal of the American Dietetic Association* 64 (1974):276–382.

Ellis, Frey S.; Path, M.R.C.; and Montegriffo, V.M.E. "Veganism, Clinical Findings and Investigations." *The American Journal of Clinical Nutrition* 23 (1970):249–54.

Erhard, Werner. *The Hunger Project—The End of Starvation Within 20 Years.* San Francisco: The Hunger Project, P.O. Box 789, 1977.

Food and Agriculture Organization. *Energy and Protein Requirements.* Rome, Italy: FAO Nutrition Meeting Report Series, no. 52, 1973.

Frankle, Reva T. and Heussenstamm, F.K. "Food Zealotry and Youth." *American Journal of Public Health* 64 (1974):11–18.

Friedman, Glenn M., et al. "Alternate Approach to Low Fat—Low Saturated Fat—Low Cholesterol Diet." *Journal of Nutrition Education* 6 (1974):8–10.

Handler, Bruce. "The Politics of Water." *Saturday Review* 14 (1977):16–19.

Hardy, R.W.F. and Haveka, U.D. "Nitrogen Fixation Research: A Key to World Food?" in *Food: Politics, Economics, Nutrition, and Research,* edited by Philip H. Abelson, pp. 178–88. Washington D.C.: Association for the Advancement of Science, 1975.

Harland, Barbara F. and Peterson, Michael. "Nutritional Status of Lacto Ovo Vegetarian Trappist Monks." *Journal of the American Dietetic Association* 72 (1978):259–64.

Harpstead, Dale D. "High-Lysine Corn," August 1971. In *Food* readings from *Scientific American.* San Francisco: Freeman, 1973, pp. 245–58.

Hegsted, Mark D. "Protein Needs and Possible Modification of the American Diet." *American Dietetic Association* 68 (1976):317–20.

Humphrey, Hubert H. "Helping the World Solve Its Food Problems." *The Futurist* 9 (1975):303–06.

Lappé, Frances M. *Diet for a Small Planet.* rev. ed. New York: Ballantine, 1975.

———, **and Collin, Joseph.** *Food First.* Boston: Houghton Mifflin, 1977.

Love, Sam. "The Overconnected Society." *Futurist* 8 (1974):293–98.

Mayer, Jean, and Dwyer, Johanna. eds. *Food and Nutrition Policy in a Changing World.* New York: Oxford University Press, 1979.

Oace, Susan M. and Ulrich, Helen D., eds. "Perspective—U.S. Dietary Goals." *Journal of Nutrition Education* 9 (1977):152–57.

Orr, Elizabeth. "The Contributions of New Food Mixtures to the Relief of Malnutrition." *Food and Nutrition* 3 (1977):2–10.

Paarlberg, Don. "A World Food Policy That Can Succeed." *The Futurist* 4 (1975):300–02.

Pirie, N.W. "Orthodox and Unorthodox Methods of Meeting World Food Needs," February 1967. In *Food* readings from *Scientific American.* San Francisco: Freeman, 1973, pp. 229–43.

Register, U.D., and Sonnenberg, L.M. "Principles of The Vegetarian Diet." *Nutrition and the M.D.* 1 (1975).

A Report of the Club of Rome. *RIO Reshaping the International Order.* New York: New American Library, 1977.

Robertson, Laurel; Finder, Carol; and Bronwen, Godfrey. *Laurel's Kitchen.* Berkeley, Calif.: Nilgiri Press, 1976.

Schumacher, E.F. *Small Is Beautiful.* New York: Harper & Row, 1973.

Scrimshaw, Nevin S. "Through a Glass Darkly: Discerning the Practical Implications of Human Dietary Protein — Energy Interrelationships." *Nutrition Today* 35 (1977):321–37.

Seelig, R.A. *A Review of Vegetarianism,* Washington, D.C.: United Fresh Fruit and Vegetable Association, 1019 Nineteenth St., N.W., Washington, D.C., 20038.

Taylor, Lance; Sarris, Alexander H.; and Abbott, Philip C. "Food Security for the World's Poor." *Technology Review* 80 (1978):44–54.

U.S. Senate Select Committee on Nutrition and Human Needs. Reprinted with certain abridgements in *Nutrition Today* 12 (1977):20–30.

Wortman, Sterling, and Cummings, Jr., Ralph. *To Feed This World.* Baltimore: Johns Hopkins, 1978.

Index

Additives. *See* Food additives

Adenosine triphosphate (ATP): 32–34

Adipose tissue. *See* Fats

Adolescents, nutritional requirements of: 340, 342–343

Advertising: 120–121, 319–320

African animal trypanosomiasis: 456

Aged. *See* Elderly

Agent: 96

Agribusiness: 148; economic considerations of, 207–209; energy and, 209–212; green revolution and, 199–200. *See also* Agriculture, technology and

Agricultural revolution: 147–148, 197. *See also* Green revolution

Agriculture, technology and: 202–207; acreage expansion, 130–131; changes in, 211–212; consumers and, 208–209; economic considerations of, 207–208; education and, 138–139; energy use and, 206–207, 209–212; fertilizers, 133; food taste and, 311–312; increasing yield per acre, 131–133; irrigation, 134–136; machinery, 139; monoculture, 208; pest control, 136–137; seeds and breeds, 136; soil erosion, 212–213; trained manpower, 137–138. *See also* Food system, of the U.S.; Green revolution; Plants, innovations in

Alcohol, cassava and: 475–476, 477–481

Alfalfa: 132

Algae: as food, 142, 148; nitrogen fixation and, 14, 15

Amino acids: 24–25, 28; deficiency syndromes and, 167; enriching, 419–420; essential, 25, 58–59, 295, 490; iron deficiency and, 169–170;

limiting, 129, 419–420; vegetarian diet and, 410. *See also* Proteins

Analogs, meat. *See* Meat analogs

Anemia: 492, 493. *See also* Iron-deficiency anemia

Antarctic krill: 426, 450

Appetite: 84

Aquaculture: 440–441, 450–452. *See also* Fishing, innovations in

Aquatic protein: 425–426

Arteriosclerosis: 108, 110

Artificial-coloring: 323

Ascorbic acid: 35, 42, 48, 76, 306, 486

Asia, food chain of: 11

Atherosclerosis: 108

Atmosphere: 3, 13

Baby. *See* Infants

Baby foods: additives and, 119–120; formula, 94, 320–321. *See also* Breast-feeding

Bacteria, nitrogen fixation and: 14–15

Barley: 366, 367, 368. *See also* Grains

Basic 4 food plan: 37–38, 344–348; Four-Food Group plan, 396; vegetarian diet and, 406–407, 417. *See also* Dairy products; Fruit; Grains; Meat; Vegetables

Basic 7 food plan: 37

Bean. *See* Legumes

Beef: alternate protein sources, 292–297; cow taboo and, 216–224; food chain contamination and, 176–186; grading, 290; price of in U.S., 154–165; wasted, 239–240. *See also* Meat

Beriberi: 492

Biogeochemical cycles: 10, 12

Biomass: 474–481

Biomes: 7

Biosphere. *See* Ecosphere

Note: Italicized entries are included in the Glossary.

innovations in; Processed foods

Food pyramid diagram: 11

Food science. *See* Processed foods

Food security: 457; emergency relief, 463–464, 471; food aid, 466–469, 472; market stabilization, 459–463, 469; 1972 food crisis, 458–459; relief requirements, 464–466; reserve policy, 469–472, 473–474

Food sources, innovations in: 143–144, 149, 349–350, 430–431; aquatic protein, 425–426; chemistry and, 429; consumer acceptance of, 430; fortification and enrichment, 419–424; grown on oil and gas, 426–428; meat and poultry industry and, 425; milk from whey, 424; need for, 440–442; nitrogen fixation, 424; oilseeds, 420–421; protein concentrate from grain, 424–425; single-cell protein, 422; synthetics, 142–143, 419–420; U.S. nutritional policy and, 430

Food stamps: 265–266, 271, 272–275

Food supply, population and: 63–64, 80–82, 144–146; demographic transition, 81; developing countries, 74–75; Hungry World, 64; Satisfied World, 64; technology, 73, 75; World Food Conference and, 455; world model and, 65, 66, 71–73. *See also* Hunger; Malnutrition; Technology

Food supply of the U.S., technology and: 122–126, 187, 324, 325; fruits, 190–191; grains, 188–189; health food, 193–194; improvement in, 194–195; meat, 191–192; milk products, 189–190; protein alternatives, 192–193; safety of, 325–326; vegetables, 190–191

Food system, of the U.S.: 147–148; beef prices and, 154–165; contamination in, 176–186; definition, 149–150; energy-intensive, 235; monopolies in, 150–152; processed foods and, 153–154; regulation, 152–153; structure, 150–154; tech-

nology, 127–128, 215–216. *See also* Food waste, Garbage Project and; Green revolution

Food, taste of: 307–310; agricultural technology and, 311–312; chemicals and, 312; cooking and, 310–311; fermentation, 310; umami, 309–310

Food technology: convenience foods, 215–216; education and, 216; elderly and, 276–277; fruits, 190–191; grains, 188–189; women lacking in, 226. *See also* Biomass; Food sources, innovations in; Processed foods

Food waste, Garbage Project and: 234–235, 243; costs of, 241–242; household refuse used in, 236–237; methodology, 237–238; results, 238–242

Food webs: 9, 11

Formose: 429

Formula: 94, 320–323

Fortification: 286, 419–424

Four-Food Group plan: 396

Fruits: guide to eating, 346; new, 437–438; nutritional value, 389; Survival Seven plan and, 388; technology and, 190–191; in vegetarian diet, 396, 407, 416, 417

Fuel, cassava and: 474–481

Garbage Project. *See* Food waste, Garbage Project and

Gas, food grown on: 426–428

Gasahol, cassava and: 475

Gatekeeper, food decisions and: 230

Global ecosystem: 2, 19–20. *See also* Ecosphere

Goiter: 74, 77, 167, 419

Government: agricultural research and, 196–198; nutrition and, 118–120, 122. *See also* United States

Grains: enriching, 419–420; guide to eating, 346; nutritional value, 387, 389; oat, barley, and rye, 366–368; protèin concentrate from, 424–425; as protein source, 294,

129, 294–295, 370–371; recipes,
371–378; Survival Seven plan and,
388; vegetarian diet, 416; winged
bean, 434–435. *See also* Soybeans
Leisure, food patterns and: 232
Less developed countries. *See* Third
World
Licorice: 438
Life cycle, nutrition and: 74
Life-support system: 280. *See also*
Ecosphere
Limiting amino acid: 129, 419–420
Lipids. *See* Fats
Lithosphere: 3–4. *See also* Soil
Liver disease: 109, 110

Magnesium: 49, 173–174, 487, 496
Male, diet of: 337–338, 339–340,
342–343; RDA, 486–487, 488–489
Malnutrition: 73, 75, 82–83; agent
and, 96; in Canada, 106–107, 108;
categorization of countries, 79–80;
causes of, 76; in children, 77; deficiency diseases, 59–60, 76–77, 107;
ecology of, 96–99; environment
and, 96–98; estimating degree of,
78–79; food supply and, 80–82;
host and, 96; ignorance and,
97–98, 100; infection and, 96;
poverty and, 74, 97–98; protein-
calorie, 73, 74, 76, 79, 99, 102;
technology and, 99–100. *See also*
Education; Hunger
Malnutrition, early childhood and:
consequences of, 102; in infancy,
77, 99–102; infections, 102–103;
mental performance, 103–104;
mortality, 102; school failure and,
104–106
Malnutrition, U.S. and: 106–108;
advertising and, 112–113; costs of,
108; diseases, 116–117; education,
114; eliminating, 113–114; food
composition, 112; food prices and,
111; nutritional evaluation and,
112; overabundance, 109–111;
restaurants and, 111; undernutrition, 111
Man-food continuum: 2, 12. *See also*

Ecosystem; Nutrient cycles
Manganese: 488, 497, 511–512
Manoic: 474–481
Maple-syrup-urine disease: 53
Marama bean: 445–446
Marasmus: 76, 490. *See also* Protein-
calorie malnutrition
Mariculture: 440. *See also* Fishing,
innovations in
Matter: 2, 10, 18–19
Meal planning: alternatives,
356–376; families and, 336–343;
vegetarian diet, 414–418
Meat: alternatives to, 292–297,
356–376; guide to eating, 347–348;
occasional consumption of, 392;
technology and, 191–192. *See also*
Beef; Cattle farming; Meat
analogs; Soybeans; Vegetarian diet
Meat analogs: 193, 382–383, 384,
393, 402–403, 406, 416, 421
Meatless diet. *See* Vegetarian diet
Mechanization: 208. *See also*
Technology
Metabolic-balance method: 54–55
Metabolism: 31. *See also* Nutrition
Methane, cassava and: 475–476
Methemoglobinemia: 15
Mexican-American food patterns:
259–260
Micronutrients. *See* Trace elements,
food chain and
Milk: from whey, 424; skim, 387,
389. *See also* Dairy products
Minerals: 26, 34–35, 43, 48–49; defi-
ciency diseases, 76–77; essential,
495–498; RDA, 487. *See also*
Specific minerals
Miracle fruit: 438
Molybdenum: 489
Monoculture: 208
Morbidity rate: 69–71; malnutrition
and, 102, 109; U.S., 110

Natural community: 6
"Natural restraints," on population:
63
Need hierarchy: 225
Negative feedback: 69–71

Vegans diet. *See* Vegetarian diet

Vegetables: nutritional value, 389; Survival Seven plan and, 388; technology and, 190–191; vegetarian diet and, 396, 407, 408, 416, 417; wasted, 240. *See also* Plants

Vegetarian diet: 355–356, 393; adequacy of, 404–405; cholesterol and, 405–406; food guide for, 414–418; Four-Food Group plan, 396, 406–407; lacto ovo diet, 393, 394, 399, 400, 402, 408–410, 414–418; lacto vegetarian diet, 393, 394, 406–407; one-day menu, 408–410; planning and, 395–397; protein in, 397–403; recipes for, 356–376; Survival Seven plan, 392; vegan (pure), 393, 394–395, 397, 404, 407–408, 408–410, 413. *See also* Dairy products; Legumes; Meat analogs; Protein complementarity

Vitamin A: 27, 35, 41, 45, 76–77, 306, 486

Vitamin B$_1$ (*thiamine*): 27, 35, 42, 46, 486

Vitamin B$_2$ (*riboflavin*): 36, 42, 46, 487

Vitamin B$_3$ (*niacin*): 36, 42, 46, 487

Vitamin B$_6$ (*pyridoxine*): 36, 47

Vitamin B$_{12}$: 36, 47, 487

Vitamin C (*ascorbic acid*): 35, 42, 48, 76, 306, 486

Vitamin D: 27, 35, 45, 486

Vitamin E: 35, 45, 486

Vitamin K: 35, 46

Vitamins: 24, 26–27, 35–36, 45–48; deficiency diseases, 76–77; RDA, 486–487, 492–494; sources, 306; synthesizing, 143. *See also* specific vitamins

Water: 3–4, 45; desalination, 135; famine and, 91; irrigation, 134–136, 155; need for, 306; nitrates in, 15; nutrition and, 24, 25; RDA, 498; requirements, 339; surface, 20–21

Wavelength: 5

Weight-reduction: 110–111; menu-planning and, 337–343; Survival Seven plan, 386–387

Welfare program, U.S. nutrition policy and: 263–265

Wheat: food reserve policy and, 469–471, 473–474; recipes, 356–363; as source of protein, 356–357. *See also* Grains

Whey, milk from: 424

Winged bean: 434–435, 443–444, 445

Women: diet of, 338–339, 342–343; food and nutrition policies and, 455

World Food Conference: 453–457

Xerophthalmia: 493

Ye-eb: 445

Yogurt: 190

Zinc: 49, 167, 170–171, 174, 487, 496, 521